APPLICATIONS OF EMG IN CLINICAL AND SPORTS MEDICINE

Edited by **Catriona Steele**

Applications of EMG in Clinical and Sports Medicine
Edited by Catriona Steele

Published by InTech
Janeza Trdine 9, 51000 Rijeka, Croatia

Publishing Process Manager Danijela Duric

Technical Editor Teodora Smiljanic

Cover Designer InTech Design Team

Additional hard copies can be obtained from orders@intechopen.com

Applications of EMG in Clinical and Sports Medicine, Edited by Catriona Steele
p. cm.
ISBN 978-953-307-798-7

For EU product safety concerns:
IN TECH d.o.o., Prolaz Marije Krucifikse Kozulić 3, 51000 Rijeka, Croatia,
info@intechopen.com or visit our website at intechopen.com.

Meet the editor

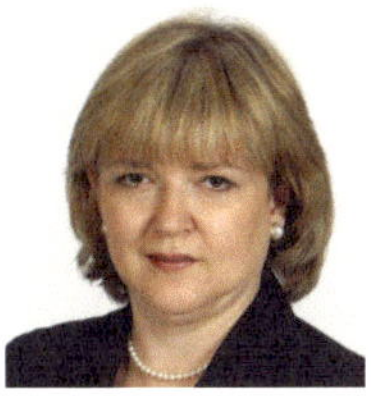

Dr. Catriona M. Steele is the Director of the Swallowing Rehabilitation Research Laboratory at the Toronto Rehabilitation Institute, and an Associate Professor at the University of Toronto. A speech-language pathologist by training, Dr. Steele is particularly known for her use of instrumentation to measure physiological signals in swallowing, including electromyography, electromagnetic articulography and intraoral manometry.She has used surface electromyography as a tool for biofeedback in exercise-based approaches to therapy for people with dysphagia (swallowing disorders) since 1999. Dr. Steele is a frequent speaker at conferences and professional training courses around the world.She is known for her commitment to evidence based practice.

Contents

Preface

This is the second of two books on Electromyography (EMG). In the first book, chapters are focused on the basic principles of using and analyzing EMG signals. This second book addresses the application of EMG in several different clinical contexts, divided into sections on gait, posture and falls prevention, back care, sports medicine, gynecology/urology, and orofacial function, including swallowing.

The first section includes three chapters that deal with surface electromyography and gait and lower limb function. The first chapter is by Fagundes Loss and covers EMG analysis of Pilates Exercise. This chapter unites information from three studies on muscular activation during hip flexion-extension exercise performed in the Cadillac position, including two studies already published about the use of agonist/antagonist muscle groups and trunk stabilizer muscles during the exercise. The second chapter, by Tomelleri, describes EMG analysis methods on robotic gait machines. The purpose of this chapter is to introduce, explain, and compare the methods of different EMG analyses carried out on different robotic gait machines. An understanding of the biomechanical interaction between robotic gait machines and patients during locomotor training on the device is relevant to ensure correct interaction forces applied to the patients' joints and the correct activation of their muscles. The section ends with a chapter by Fratini, who discusses the use and efficacy of surface electromyography to measure muscle response to vibration treatments. A review of the characteristics and analysis of vibration in sEMG recordings is provided, with examples for the *rectus femoris* (RF) and *vastus medialis* (VM) muscles. The authors discuss precautions to be taken in measurements where vibration is present and describe how the two technologies can be used together with recommendations for appropriate procedures to limit artifact. They discuss both locally-applied whole body extended vibration, with consideration of different methods (alternating rotation and vertical oscillation), and resulting parameters of importance (magnitude of vibration and acceleration).

The second section includes five chapters dealing with posture and the prevention of falls, and the extension of the use of EMG with robotics. The section starts with a chapter by Berg on the role of electromyography (EMG) in the study of anticipatory postural adjustments (APAs). These APAs are feed-forward mechanisms initiated by the central nervous system (CNS) in response to expected postural disturbances, and they produce pre-emptive muscle responses to help maintain stability. The second chapter is by Gopura, and it covers the application of surface electromyographic signals to control an upper-limb exoskeleton robot. There is a brief review of signal processing with a useful table to define activated muscles for upper-limb motions. The methods used to apply surface EMG signals for robotic control are also explained. This is followed by a contribution from Kai on trunk muscle activity and its impact on performance level in the context of falls prevention. This chapter examines how excellent body performance levels can be attained by activating trunk muscle activity in seniors at risk for falls. The next chapter by Su and Gu deals with SEMG in people with different heel height conditions. The objective of this chapter was to provide information about surface electromyography (SEMG) activity patterns in lower limb muscles during human locomotion. SEMG signals from the *tibialis anterior, medial* and *lateral gastrocnemius, soleus* and *biceps femoris* muscles were acquired from ten professional female dancers who wore shoes with different heel heights, thereby illustrating the physiological impact of shoes on leg function. Finally, the chapter by Benedetti deals with muscle activation patterns during level walking and stair ambulation. The evaluation of the "on-off" pattern of one or more muscles, particularly when examined together with kinematics (joint angles) and kinetics (joint moments and powers), provides an insight into the performance of muscles and their role in accomplishing a motor task.

The third section includes four chapters that deal with surface electromyography and back care. It starts with a chapter by Chang, discussing the use of EMG for electrophysiological monitoring of fatigue in paralyzed muscles during functional electrical stimulation (FES) treatments in patients with spinal cord injury. Cardozo and colleagues then discuss the assessment of low back muscle function using surface EMG. A global understanding of the parameters that can be used to assess the lower back muscle is presented, with examples showing that EMG can be a reliable tool for evaluating muscle fatigue. The authors review low back muscle fatigue during isometric contractions and look at EMG spectral analysis over time and frequency banding. The possibility of deriving indices to verify muscle fatigue states, such as the electromyographic fatigue threshold (EMGFT), is also explored. The Sorensen test for assessing low back pain and the incorporation of EMG measures during manual load lifting are discussed, with reference to current literature. The third chapter, by Fagundes Loss, explores EMG signals for the posterior-medial trunk musculature in the context of symmetrical load lifting without mechanical restriction. In the final chapter in this section, Bohbot and colleagues discuss methods for analyzing and interpreting electromyography signals in patients with complete and incomplete transections of the spinal cord.

The fourth section of this volume discusses EMG applications in the context of sports and performance medicine. Shan and Visentin open this section by exploring the application of EMG to the performing arts in musicians and dancers. Salamons and colleagues then discuss the use of surface electromyography of *m. ulnaris lateralis* during both standing and walking to understand performance in horses who have undergone different training regimes. Sahu and colleagues then describe the use of

EMG to evaluate shoulder pain and suprascapular nerve neuropathy (SNN). Electromyography of damaged nerves may display a variety of abnormalities, including reduced motor potential amplitudes, increased spontaneous activity, fibrillations, and polyphasic activity, indicating possible denervation of the supraspinatous or infraspinatous muscles. EMG is also useful in confirming traumatic lesions of SSN. Techniques for arthroscopic suprascapular nerve release are described and compared to open surgical techniques with detailed illustrations of the relative success of the arthroscopic intervention.

The fifth section on gynecology/urology starts with a chapter by Vrhovec, who describes uterine EMG activity and its use as a measure of labor progression. The chapter describes the delicate balance to be obtained between the maintenance of tone and the resistance to propagated uterine contractions until the end of gestation and the onset of labor. At the onset of labor, the uterus becomes active and at the labor's end it empties its contents through rhythmic, forceful, organized and synchronous contractions that are crucial for the successful outcome of pregnancy. The second chapter by Martinez-Gomez provides an interesting chapter on pelvic and perineal striated muscles in female mammals, using a rabbit model. The chapter reviews methods for measuring pelvic and perineal muscle EMGs in laboratory rabbits, and describes alterations in this activity associated with dysfunction, particularly urinary incontinence. The third chapter in the section by Lorenzo-Gomes describes EMG in the diagnosis pelvic floor muscle function in women with urinary incontinence.

The final section of this book includes four chapters that deal with surface electromyography in the evaluation of orofacial function and swallowing. In the opening chapter of this section, Steele and colleagues describe electromyography as a biofeedback tool for rehabilitating swallowing muscle function in patients with neurologic swallowing impairment (dysphagia). Several case studies are reviewed, and single-subject methods for monitoring change are illustrated. The second chapter by Kemsley discusses the use of SEMG to monitor facial muscle activity during chewing, and the use of EMG analysis to determine how mastication changes according to the mechanical and sensory properties of food. In this chapter, the authors discuss the hardware and software needed to conduct SEMG of the facial muscles during mastication, and describe the signal that is acquired, as well as options for further data processing of this signal to extract parameters for statistical analysis. The chapter highlights some of the complexities that may be encountered downstream during signal analysis, in particular, teasing out issues of inter-participant and inter-session variability. Sassi and colleagues then describe EMG for the measurement of facial paralysis. EMG data of the *anguli oris* elevator muscles are correlated to the Facial Disability Index in a group of patients with long standing facial paralysis. The fourth and final chapter by Ichiro discusses movement-related cortical potentials in the jaw musculature associated with orofacial functions, such as chewing. The authors provide a useful overview of non-invasive human brain imaging methods, including event-related potentials (ERPs), and other measurement techniques for brain activity, including positron emission tomography (PET), functional magnetic resonance imaging (fMRI), and magnetoencephalography (MEG). They explain how movement-related cortical potentials (MRCPs) and contingent negative variations (CNVs) are classified into ERPs. The authors have investigated MRCPs and CNVs in relation to oral and facial functions in humans to clarify motor preparation processes of the brain and to clarify the neural pathways underlying mastication and swallowing.

Dr. Catriona Steele
Senior Scientist, Toronto Rehabilitation Institute
Associate Professor, Speech-Language Pathology,
University of Toronto,
Canada

Part 1

Gait

1

Evaluating the Electromyographical Signal During Symmetrical Load Lifting

Jefferson Fagundes Loss[1], Débora Cantergi[1], Fábia Milman Krumholz[2], Marcelo La Torre[1,2] and Claudia Tarragô Candotti[1]
[1]*Universidade Federal do Rio Grande do Sul*
[2]*Universidade do Vale do Rio dos Sinos*
Brazil

1. Introduction

Muscular problems account for almost half the cases of work absence, with the back being the region most involved (Kumar, 2011). Bending the trunk forward while performing domestic work or sports related activities is the cause of most back injuries (Fathallah et al., 1998). Small degrees of flexion of the trunk can be considered a medium to high risk factor of injury, mainly when the angle of the forward inclination is greater than 15 degrees and is combined with lifting activities. As the task of lifting objects from the ground exposes spinal structures to muscular-skeletal overload it has been consistently investigated (Simon, 1997). In addition, epidemiological research associates lifting to the risk of developing lumbar back pain (Ferguson & Marras, 1997; Dolan & Adams, 1998; Jäger & Luttmann, 1999; Nachemson, 1999; Wilke et al., 1999; Burdorf, 2000; Kingma et al., 2001; Wilke et al., 2001; Ferguson et al., 2004).

In the early 20th century, the scientific community was already studying back injuries, in particular low back pain (Ghormley, 1933), and its relation with the loads that affect the spine. Due to the invasive nature of measuring these internal loads, models employing indirect means of estimating the loads that act on the lumbar region of the spine during lifting activities began to appear in the 1940s (Wilke et al., 2001). The models found in the literature continue to be primarily concerned with the forces between the muscles, joints and ligaments in only one cross section of the lumbar region (Strait et al., 1947; Cheng, 1998; Gagnon, 2001). While considering the spine as a single rigid structure, these simplified models attempt to provide estimates of what occurs in the spine in situations such as lifting a weight. However, these models are far from representative of the functional anatomical reality of the spine, which consists of several articulated segments and a complex muscle anatomy. The growing interest in producing a more realistic model of the trunk and, consequently, the spine, may have inspired some anthropometric studies (De Leva, 1996; Erdmann, 1997; Zatsiorsky, 2002) to divide the trunk into two or more connected segments. Some models that split the spine into more than one segment are conceived using biomechanical techniques, such as the link segment model (LSM), surface electromyography (EMG) and inverse dynamics (Larivière, 1999; Marras, 1997; La Torre, 2005). The EMG of the trunk muscles has been used as input for biomechanical models that attempt to indirectly estimate the forces acting on the spine (Granata, 1995; Arjmand, 2006).

A review of the literature reveals that, while the segments of the spine are considered in terms of anatomical division, the overwhelming majority of EMG-based research into lifting is concentrated on the analysis of the lumbar region alone (Alexiev, 1994; Mannion et al., 1997a; Gonçalves & Barbosa, 2005), while a few have studied the thoracic region (Basler et al., 1997; Lu et al., 2002) and only one study was found that involved positioning electrodes on the cervical region of the spine (Basler et al., 1997). Another problem is that most of these analyses involved various limitations such as the use of devices intended to impose a mechanical restriction on the subjects' movements, activities with limited amplitude or involved no extra load. Specifically in relation to the lifting of symmetrical loads, some studies use electrodes on only one side of the trunk (Toussaint et al., 1995; Dolan & Adams, 1998). However, though there are those that have collected bilateral signals for different purposes (Nielsen et al., 1998; Granata et al., 1999; Jorgensen & Marras, 2000; Mirka et al., 2000), and some authors have presented results for right and left muscles (Sheikhzadeh et al., 2008), few studies have actually investigated the electromyographical similarity between the right and left sides.
Considering the above-mentioned issues, the aim of the present study was to investigate the electrical activation of the posterior-medial muscles of the trunk when lifting a load from the floor using a symmetrical movement without mechanical restriction and with electrodes positioned at various levels on both sides of the spine.

2. The steps and procedures of the electromyographical evaluation

The study included 16 healthy male individuals. The subjects were right-handers, aged between 20 and 34 years, with mean height of 170.8 ± 10.4 cm and mean weight of 67.0 ± 12.5 kg and no history of spine pathology.
The lifting task started and finished with the individual in a static position without a load and consisted of lifting and lowering an object using both hands, while keeping the knees straight and executing the movement by flexing from the hip. For the purposes of analysis, the gesture was divided into four distinct phases: (1) bending forward without a load (2) lifting the load (3) bending forward with a load (4) returning to the initial position. In the present study, only the data from the load lifting phase were analyzed, because it is the phase which imposes the highest demand on the paraspinal muscles. Together, Figures 1 and 2 illustrate the complete gesture.

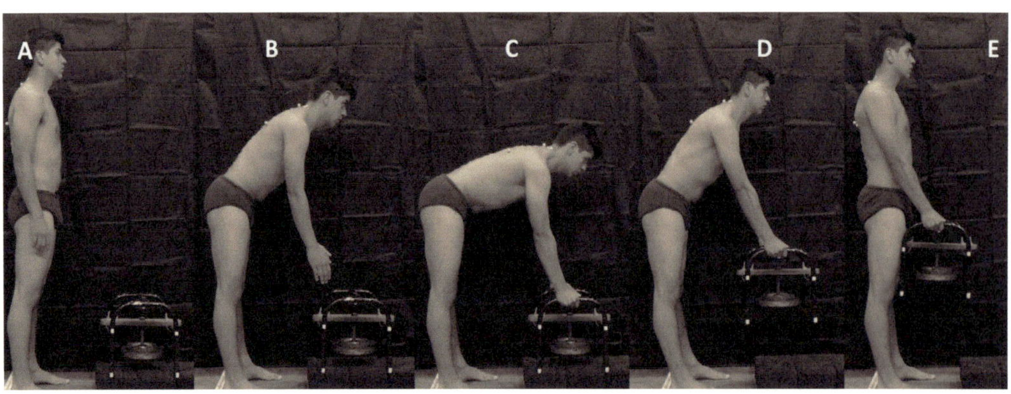

Fig. 1. Phases 1 and 2. The gesture begins with the subject in the standing position (A), the individual bends forward without a load (A to C), lifts the load and returns to an upright position with the load (C to E).

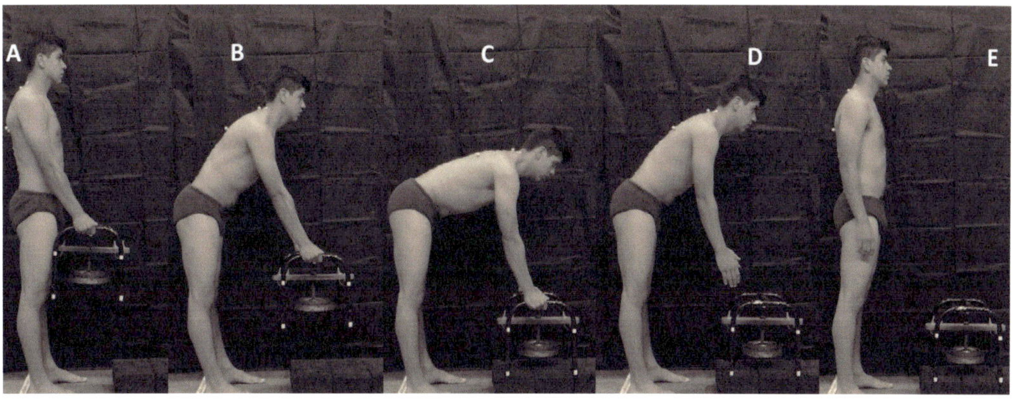

Fig. 2. Phases 3 and 4. The subject bends forward with a load (A to C), and returns to an upright position without the load (C to E).

The object was a fixed size and positioned at a specific height for each subject (Figure 3A). This was done in order to ensure that the curvatures of the spine remained unchanged while executing the task and to avoid unwanted movements of the pelvis due, for example, to muscle shortening. The load of the attached to the object was determined for each individual by calculating the recommended weight limit established in the Guide to Work Practices for the Handling of Loads from the National Institute for Occupational Safety and Health (NIOSH) (Waters et al., 1994). In this study, the load was equivalent to a Lifting Index (LI) of 1.5. The object consisted of a metal structure with a device for supporting weight plates, which allowed the load on the object to be adapted for each participant in the sample (Figure 3B).

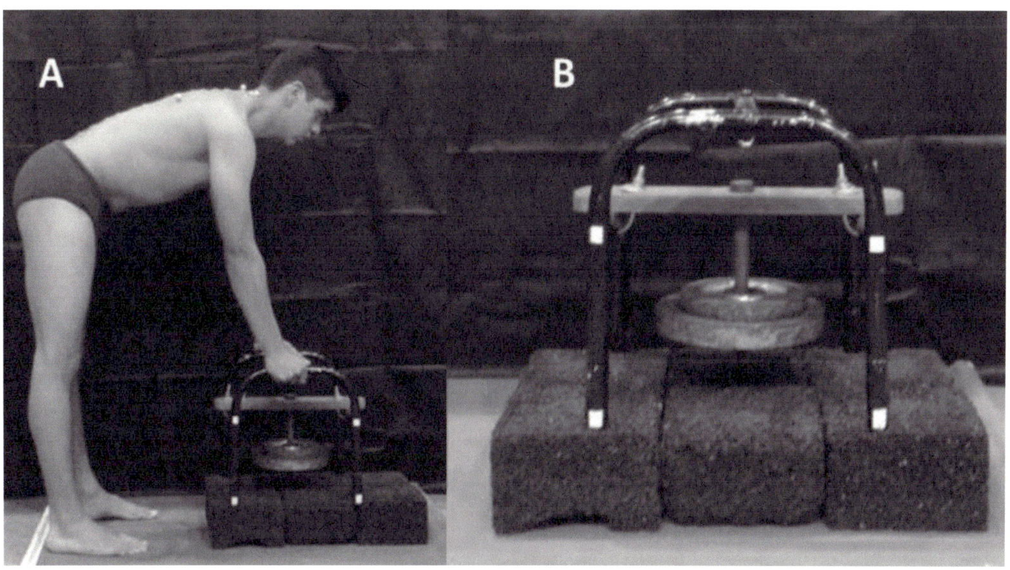

Fig. 3. The lifting task. (A) The object to be lifted is positioned at pre-determined height, according to the individual's anatomical features. (B) The object has a comfortable grip and can be adjusted by including/excluding weight plates like those used in strength training.

Each participant performed two series of ten repetitions of the analyzed gesture. Four devices were used in order to collect electromyographical data, each one with four channels (Miotool 400, Miotec, Porto Alegre, RS, Brazil), totalling 16 analogical input channels. Signals were collected with a sampling rate of 2000 Hz per channel, A/D converter of 14 bits, common rejection mode of 110 db (at 60 Hz), input impedance of the system was 100 Gohms and a band-pass between 0.1 and 1000 Hz. For the kinematic data acquisition, two digital video cameras were used, with a sampling rate of 50 Hz (GR-DVL9800, JVC). The images were captured, stored and reconstructed using Dvideow software - Digital Video for Biomechanics for Windows 32 bits (Figueroa et al., 2003). The data from the two systems (EMG and video cameras) were aligned using a device that simultaneously emitted a light signal, which was visible in one of the cameras, and an electrical pulse signal that was captured by the A/D converter, as described elsewhere (Candotti et al., 2008). Figure 4 shows a schematic representation of the distribution and connections of the equipment used for data collection.

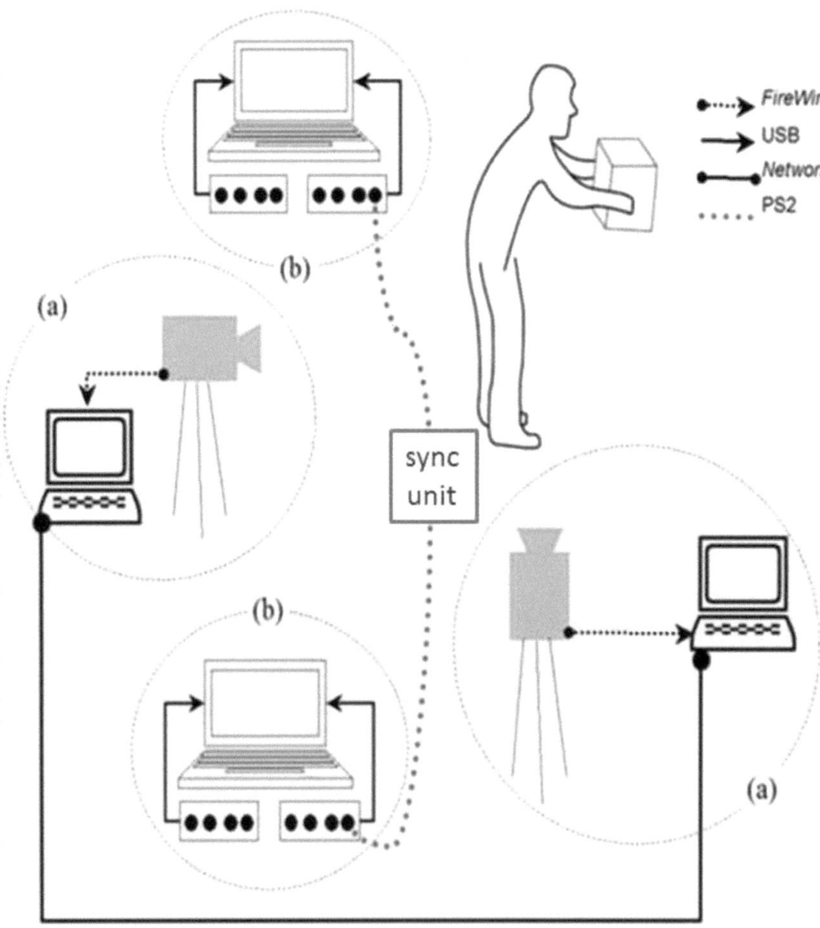

Fig. 4. Schematic representation of the equipment and connections used for the data collection (a) the video cameras connected to the computers, (b) the electromyographical data collection systems.

The subject's skin was prepared according to the guideline from the SENIAM project (Surface Electromyography for the Non-Invasive Assessment of Muscles - www.seniam.org). Fourteen (14) pairs of 10 mm-diameter Ag/AgCl surface electrodes (Tyco Healthcare, Mini MediTrace 100 - Kendall), were used in a bipolar configuration, with 20 mm between the electrodes. They were positioned, according to Basler et al. (1997), bilaterally, with its center 30 mm from the distal region of the spinal processes of C7, T3, T6, T9, L1, L3 and L5 (Figure 5). Reference electrode was positioned on the right anterior-superior iliac spine. Electrode impedance was measured, and considered acceptable when less than 10 kohms.

For later normalization of the EMG data, each subject performed two three-second maximum isometric voluntary contractions (MVC) with a two-minute interval between each one. To execute the MVCs, the individuals lay on a table in the decubitus ventralis position with the trunk suspended beyond the edge of the table and the lower limbs strapped to the table with Velcro straps. Manual resistance applied to the back of the head and verbal encouragements were used to ensure that maximum effort was made during each MVC, while the trunk was aligned to the lower limbs. The resistive force during the MVC data collection was assumed to be maximum and symmetrical.

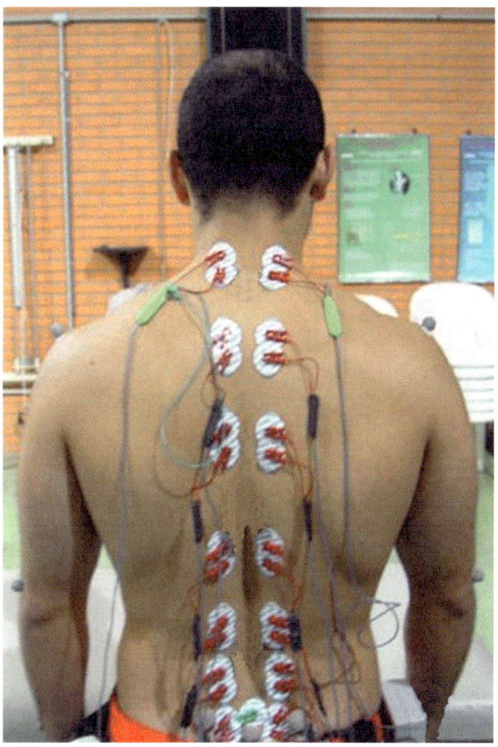

Fig. 5. The positions of the 14 pairs of electrodes placed along the spinal column.

In order to verify the symmetrical execution of the gesture, and divide it into four phases, kinematic data was collected synchronously with the acquisition of the electromyographical data. The phases of the movement were separated using data from digitalized images showing the displacement of the marker placed on T1. Symmetrical execution of the movement was confirmed by analyzing the trajectory of the markers placed on the scapulas. In the case that, based on the kinematic trajectory of the markers, the execution was considered to be asymmetrical it was discarded from electromyographical analysis.

The EMG signals from the task and the MVCs were processed using a 3rd order, Butterworth band-pass digital filter, with cut-off frequencies of 20 Hz and 500 Hz. The EMG signal was then separated according to the movement phases, and the Root Mean Square (RMS) value was calculated. The RMS value of the second phase of the gesture was normalized with the RMS value obtained from the MVC. This normalization generated a percentage of the MVC that was representative of the EMG activity during the execution of phase 2.

To check the symmetry of the electromyographical signal of each vertebral level between the right and left sides, we used the Wilcoxon test. One-way ANOVA was used to compare the activation between adjacent levels, using the average EMG activity obtained between the right side and left side at each level. In order to identify any differences between the levels and also between the anatomical regions, the behaviour of the EMG signal between vertebral regions was analyzed using a Tukey *post-hoc* test, according to the anatomical division of the spine into the cervical, dorsal and lumbar spine. The level of significance for all tests was $p < 0.05$.

3. Symmetry of the electromyographical signal

The electrical activation of the posterior-medial muscles of the trunk was evaluated during the act of lifting the load from the ground. Similarity between the sides of the spine was only found in the lumbar region at levels L1 and L5 (Figure 6).

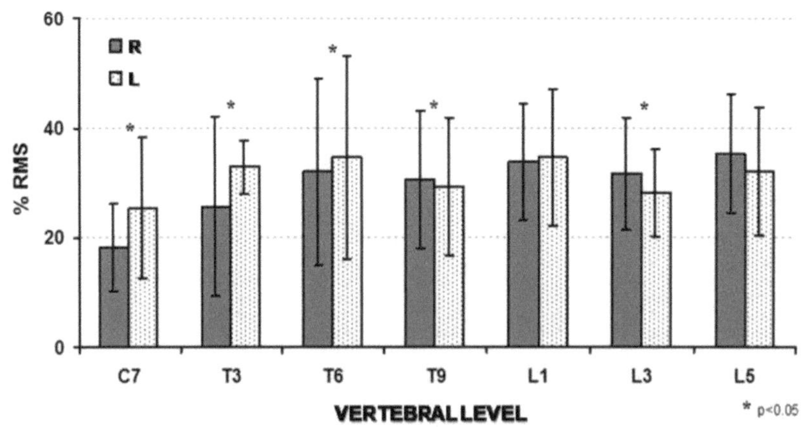

Fig. 6. Means and standard deviations of the electromyographical signal of the symmetrical executions obtained during phase 2 of the act of symmetrical lifting of a load from the ground.

The fact that symmetry was only found to occur at levels L1 and L5 may be related to the anatomy of the spine, particularly the orientation of the facet joints. Facet joints are in the frontal plane in the thoracic spine, permitting rotation, conversely, they are in the sagittal plane in the lumbar spine, providing positive resistance to axial rotations (Qiu et al., 2006).

Thus, symmetrical movement is facilitated in the lumbar region, while rotational and lateral bending movements are facilitated in the cervical and thoracic regions. Considering this structural feature of the posterior pillar of the functional unit, the lumbar spine has less of a propensity to rotate when compared to cervical and dorsal regions. This characteristic implies that the higher the vertebral level, the greater the need for muscle action in order to avoid unwanted movements during the execution of a symmetrical movement (Neumann, 2002).
Figures 7, 8 and 9 illustrate the comparison of the behaviour of electrical activity between right and left sides in each execution of phase 2 of the gesture performed by a single member of the sample. Considering the anatomy of each region, the asymmetry displayed in the upper levels may be related to greater potential to rotate of the thoracic and cervical regions due to the spatial positioning of their facet joint. This factor may explain the similarity between the sides in the lumbar level activation, which may be related to the restricted degree of freedom in this region of the spine in relation to this movement.

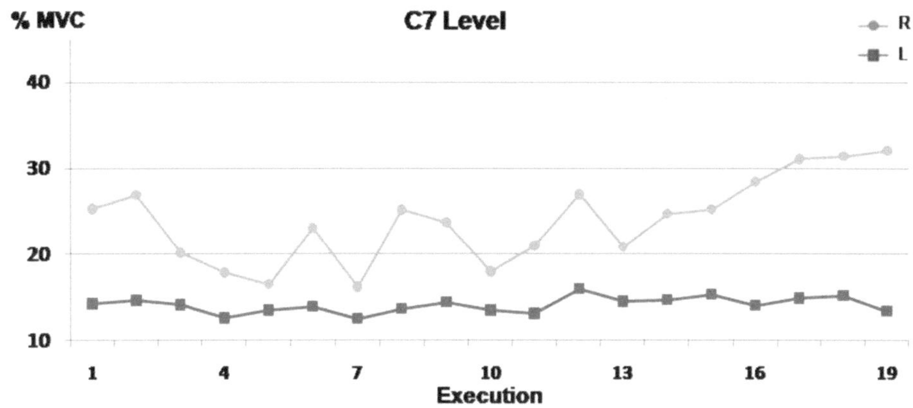

Fig. 7. Comparison of electromyographical activity between right and left sides, at the C7 level in phase 2 of the gesture of symmetrical lifting of a load from the ground, showing all the executions of an individual.

Furthermore, considering the Systems Model of Balance theory, Umphred (1995) explained the necessity for subject/task/ambient interaction in order for dynamic balance to occur. In this model, peripheral and central components act on the motor planning and execution systems at the same time as the sensorial stimulus and the processing system. So sufficient movement is generated in order to maintain balance and perform the task (Thelen, 1989; Umphred, 1995). Muscle actions that help control the symmetry of the movement are automatic postural responses that allow continuous unconscious balance control during the execution of volitional movements. It is speculated that automatic postural responses occur due to the information obtained from the System Model of Balance. These characteristics related to mobility may explain the findings of the present study, in which symmetry was only found at levels L5 and L3.
While the task in the present study was designed to be performed freely, without any apparatus to limit movement, thus mimicking as closely as possible the way in which this task is performed by individuals in their daily activities, some studies, when investigating the occurrence of activation symmetry, have used data obtained from isometric tasks performed with the use of mechanical limitations intended to ensure symmetrical execution

of the movement. Alexiev (1994) found symmetry in 40 individuals and Mannion et al. (1997b) in 34 individuals, and in both studies, the samples consisted of individuals who had no complaint of lumbar pain. Golçalves and Barbosa (2005) also used a healthy, though smaller, sample and found symmetrical activation of the lumbar muscles while researching for data on muscle fatigue. In all the above-mentioned studies data were collected exclusively from the lumbar region.

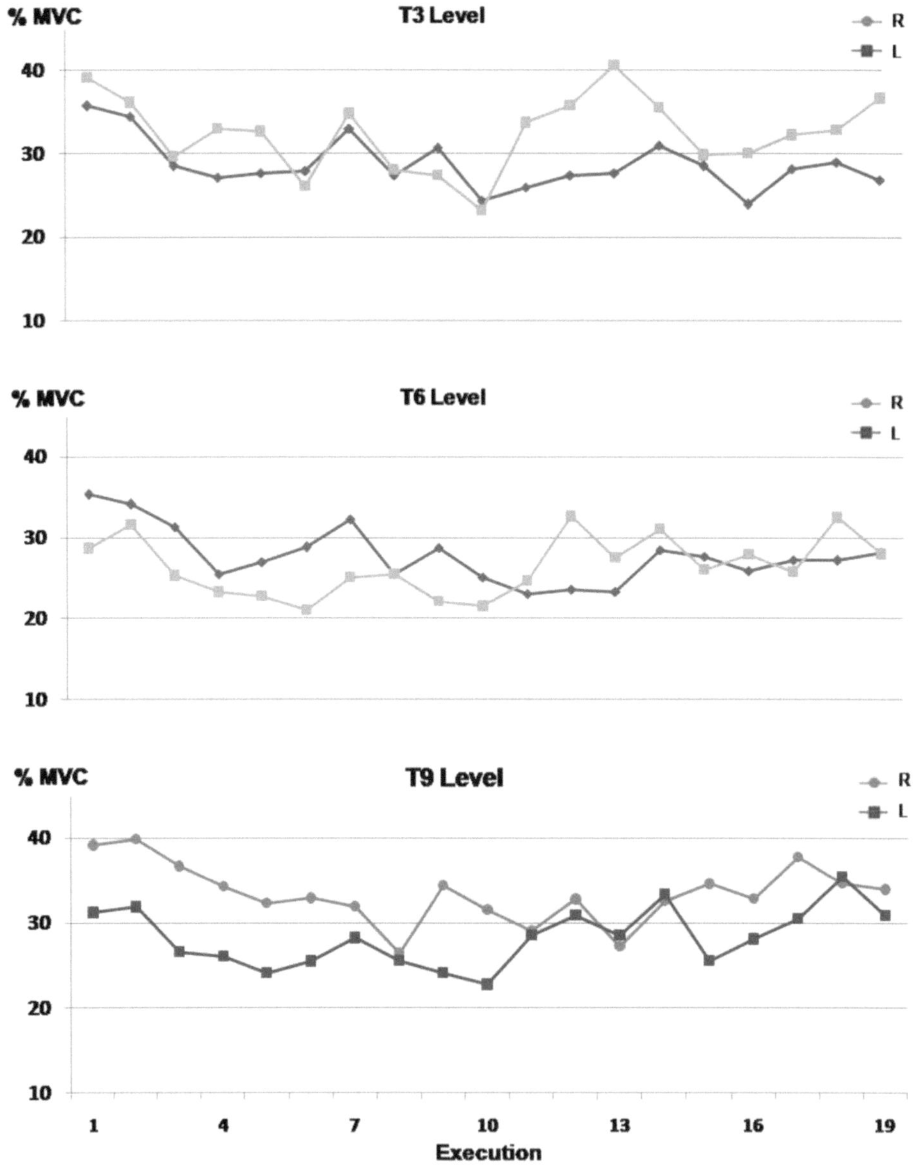

Fig. 8. Comparison of electromyographical activity between right and left sides, at the T3, T6 and T9 levels in phase 2 of the gesture of symmetrical lifting of a load from the ground, showing all the executions of an individual.

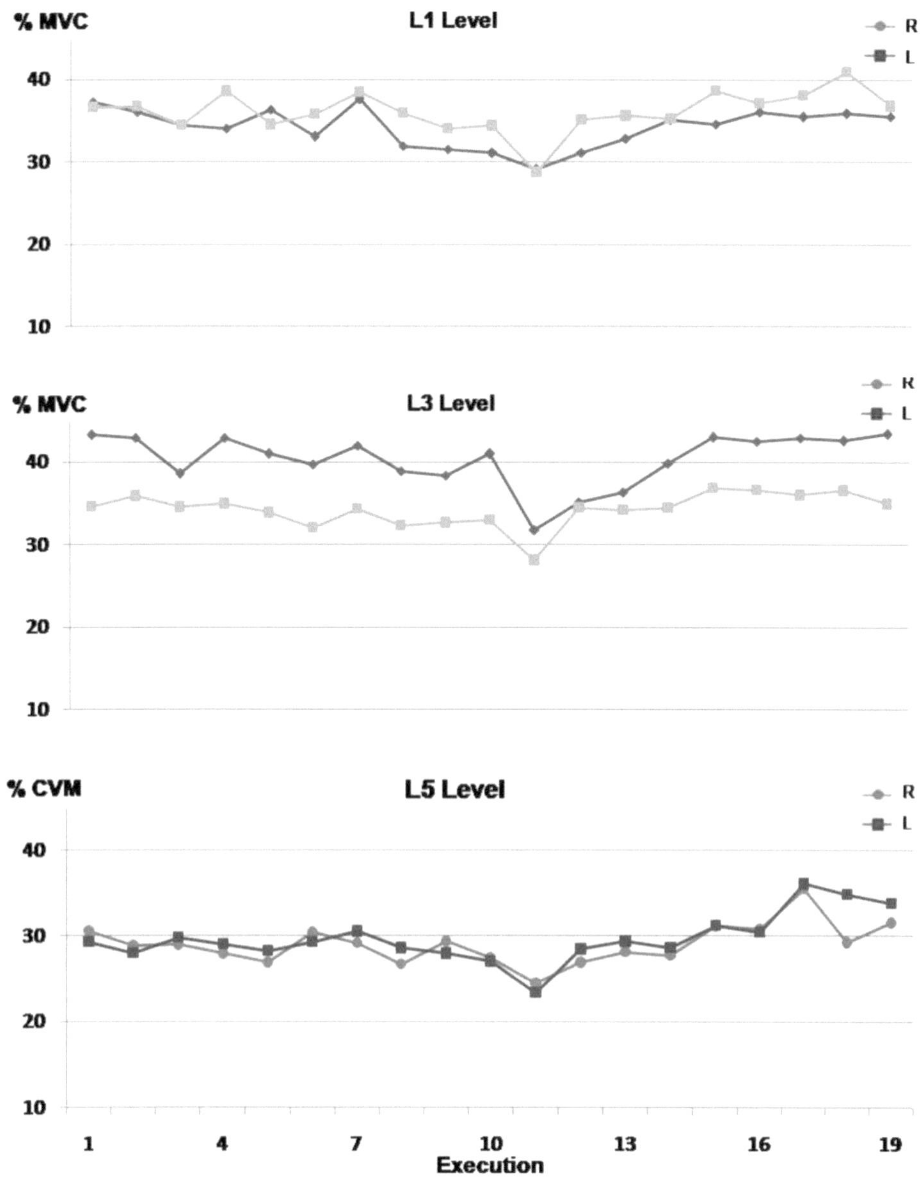

Fig. 9. Comparison of electromyographical activity between right and left sides, at the L1, L3 and L5 levels in phase 2 of the gesture of symmetrical lifting of a load from the ground, showing all the executions of an individual.

Basler et al. (1997) and Lu et al. (2002) investigated the thoracic and cervical regions. The first study analysed the C3-C4, T1, T6 and T9 levels, as well as L3 level, but, in their protocol, the electromyographic signal was captured during isometric contractions without load, with posture correction both in orthostatic and sitting posture. In the second study, electrical activation at the T3-T4, T10-T11 and L2-L3 levels was analyzed during the performance of only two repetitions of the movement without load. Although the latter study did not use any device to ensure execution symmetry, the low number of repetitions made verification easy.

In other studies involving only the lumbar level, the movements were limited to isometric contractions or dynamic activities with mechanical restrictions, which may have influenced the results (Alexiev, 1994; Lu et al., 2002). Only Nouwen et al. (1987) found asymmetry of the activation in the lumbar region in individuals both with and without pain. In that study, the participants performed trunk flexion and extension while having their pelvis held by the examiner.

Thus, when the posterior-medial muscles of the trunk are analyzed during a task involving the symmetrical flexion-extension of the trunk, activation symmetry is only seen in the lumbar region, and this symmetry is more evident the lower the vertebral level being studied. Hence, it may be suggested that studies that analyze the upper levels of the vertebral spine should place electrodes bilaterally, even when the movement is considered symmetrical, while those that study the lumbar level, specially the lower levels, may place them unilaterally.

4. Comparison between the vertebral levels and description of the electrical behavior of different segments of the spine

In order to compare the different vertebral levels, the arithmetic average between the activation of the right and left sides was calculated. Figure 10 shows the average values corresponding to the activation during the load-lifting phase. Similarity in behaviour was only found between the adjacent levels T6-T9 and L3-L5. It should be noted that comparisons were only made between adjacent levels, as there was no justification for comparisons between distant regions. The EMG signal captured in the cervical region showed the lowest level of activation (approximately 22%), probably due to the relative non-involvement of this region in the effect produced by overload imposed by the activity under study.

No data were found in the literature that compared activation between so many vertebral levels. Gonçalves and Barbosa (2005) conducted a study of fatigue-induction using electrodes at levels L2-L3 and L4-L5 and found higher levels of fatigue in the lower region, but they did not relate this finding with a higher degree of electrical activation, but to a predominance of type II muscle fibres, which are less resistant to fatigue. It should also be noted that the greater rhomboid muscle inserts on the spinous process of fifth thoracic vertebra, and thus there may have been a cross-talk effect, due to the need to stabilize the scapulas. However, on the other hand, interestingly, it is in this region that the apex of thoracic kyphosis is found. In contrast, the apex of the lumbar curvature, L3, is precisely the lumbar level with the lowest activation.

These results enable us to identify a non-homogeneous behaviour between adjacent levels. That is, while some comparisons between levels were similar, others presented differentiated muscular demands. Moreover, there was no pattern of increasing or decreasing behaviour along the spine. From this perspective there seems to be no pattern of activation throughout the various levels analyzed during the concentric phase of the symmetrical load lifting task. However, information regarding the intensity of the EMG signal from the posterior-medial muscles of the spine may help in developing models that provide information regarding the load on the spine.

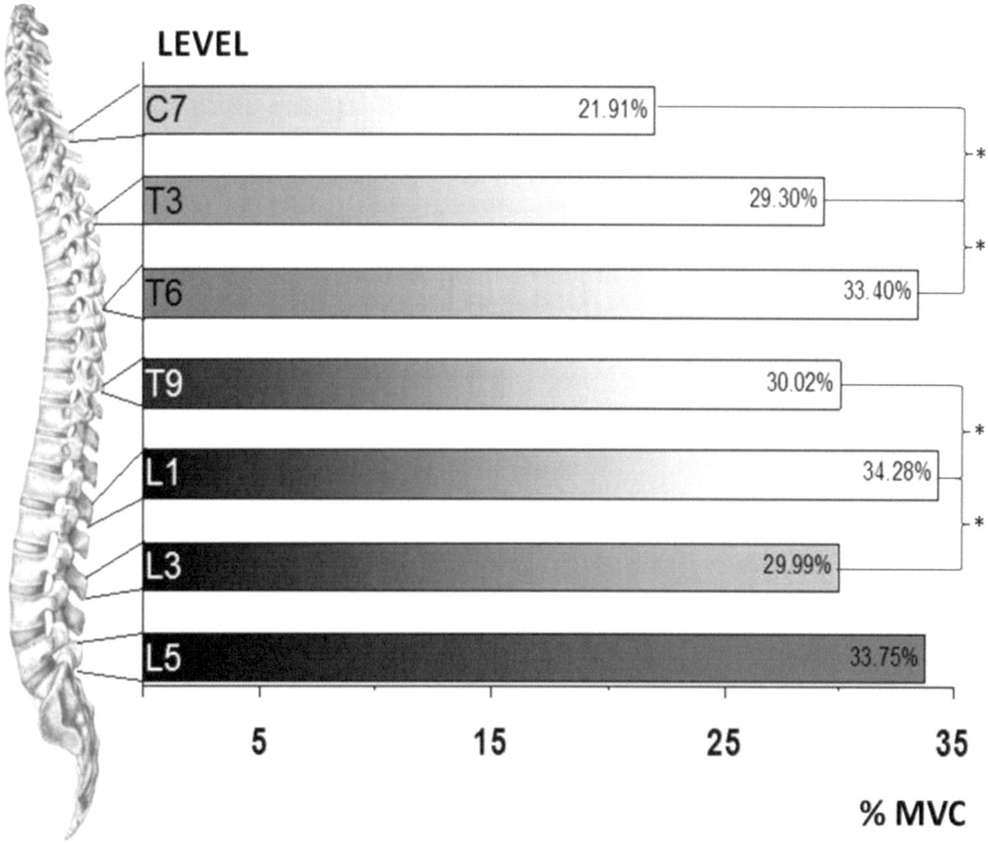

Fig. 10. Mean electrical activation between right and left sides in the seven vertebral levels for all symmetrical executions in phase 2 and their relationship with the sagittal curvatures of the spine. * Significant difference between the marked levels ($p < 0.05$).

It is of great importance to understand the loads imposed on the spine, since these are considered a major risk factor for the acceleration of intervertebral disc degeneration (Wilke et al., 2001). Thus, the scientific community that studies the loads imposed on the spine has developed several methods of measuring or estimating their magnitude. One such method makes use of the EMG technique. Assuming that the muscle force developed by a given muscle contraction depends on the neural excitation applied, the EMG can be considered an indicator of strength. Consequently, different types of biomechanical models of the lumbar spine have used EMG to indirectly estimate the load on the spine during lifting tasks (Granata, 1995; Kingma et al., 1996; Gagnon, 2001; Kingma, 2004; Arjmand, 2006).

According to Dolan et al. (1999), the indirect methods that use biomechanical models to measure loads on the spine can be divided into two basic categories: (1) those that measure the acceleration of body parts and use Link Segment Model (LSM) and (2) those that attempt to directly measure muscle strength by calibrating the electromyographical signal (EMG Models). In addition, there are Hybrids that combine LSM with EMG Models. EMG-assisted models for evaluating dynamic movement have been introduced based on the concept that the EMG signal is a continuous measure of muscle activity, and may be used as a basis for determining the force generating history (Marras et al., 1997).

McGill and Norman (1986) developed a dynamic musculoskeletal model of the lumbar spine that incorporates great three-dimensional detail of the ligaments of musculoskeletal system. The model predicted the resultant moment in the intervertebral articulation between the fourth and fifth lumbar vertebrae (L4-L5) allowing a rough estimate of the compression and shearing forces. The resultant moment obtained using the LSM-3D was divided into separate muscle, ligament and joint components based on information from the literature, radiological archives and the use EMG of techniques. The model was used to analyze the performance of tasks involving the symmetrical lifting of an object from the ground, executed by simultaneous flexion of the hip and knee.

Dolan and Adams (1993) analyzed the compressive forces on the lumbar spine using an EMG-assisted model. The model considered the muscular activity of agonist and antagonist muscles during the movement, as well as aspects related to the speed of contraction, the force-length and force-velocity relationships. The model was evaluated by comparing the results of the trunk extensor moment, obtained from an LSM associated with the inverse solution with the results predicted by the model based on the electromyographic signal.

An auxiliary electromyographic model was developed by Granata and Marras (1995), using information on the muscle activity (EMG), specific tension, physiological cross-sectional area (PCSA) and the force-length and force-velocity relationships to calculate the muscle strength of trunk muscles and the erector joint force at L5-S1. According to Granata and Marras (1995), the main advantage of this model over the LSM, is that it shows the influence of muscle coactivation on the results of compressive strength during the lift.

Dijke et al. (1999) implemented a biomechanical model of load transference from the spine to the pelvis and legs, taking into account the influence of muscles, ligaments and different postures. The geometric data from the model were obtained using Magnetic Resonance Imaging (MRI), which enabled the muscles and ligaments to be modelled in terms of vector forces. The model was characterized as static and three-dimensional. The agonist muscle activity predicted by the model corresponded to the values for electromyographical activity found in the literature.

Considering the possibility of using the results of the present study in models that use electromyography to estimate the forces acting within the spine, and given that there was no activation pattern between the different levels that were analyzed, we attempted to group the various levels into regions to minimize the variability of the signal obtained. For this purpose the established anatomical regions were considered, so that the electrode placed at the C7 level represented the cervical region, the electrodes placed at T3, T6 and T9 represented the thoracic region, and the electrodes placed at L1, L3 and L5 represented the lumbar region. To represent each region, a value was calculated based on the arithmetic mean of the values of each pair of electrodes representing its respective region.

The activation in the cervical region was 21.8% of the MVC, in the thoracic region it was 30.8%, and in the lumbar region it was 32.6% (see Table 1). When analyzing the average EMG levels collected from each region, significant differences were found between all the regions compared ($p < 0.05$). Furthermore, the activation was found to increase from top to bottom; that is, the level of electrical activation is greater when a lower region is compared with that located immediately above it.

If, on the one hand, the results of this study cannot be directly used to implement an EMG-aided model of the spine, on the other the grouping by regions (cervical, thoracic and lumbar) suggests that it is feasible to divide the column in at least three levels. In the same way as there is a classical anatomical division of the spine into these three regions,

Region	Mean Activation	Confidence Interval = 95%	
		Lower Limit	Upper Limit
Cervical	21.85 [a]	20.03	23.67
Thoracic	30.85 [b]	29.80	31.90
Lumbar	32.63 [c]	31.58	33.68

Table 1. Mean values for electrical activation (% of MVC) of the posterior-medial muscles of the spine, grouped into three segments: cervical, thoracic and lumbar. Different letters indicate a difference compared to the other regions.

Zatsiorsky (2002) divided the trunk into three regions and provided anthropometric data for each region. With this in mind, electromyographical monitoring of the posterior-medial trunk muscles seems to provide the means to model the spine in three regions as an alternative to a rigid structure.

5. Conclusions

This study has found that when comparing the electrical activation of the right and left sides of the spine at seven vertebral levels in the cervical, thoracic and lumbar spine while symmetrically lifting a load from the ground, similarity only occurs in part of the lumbar levels. When comparing the mean electrical activation between the different levels during the same gesture it was also found that the electrical activation increases from highest to the lowest studied region, so that the percentage of activation is higher in the lumbar region than in the thoracic region, which in turn, has a higher activation than the cervical level.
Given the highly complex nature of the joint and muscle structures that make up the spine, most of the models found in the literature only provide the results of internal loads on the lumbar spine. The models presented above, despite using detailed views of the muscle and joint structures, are limited by the fact that they consider the spine as a rigid structure, using a single rotating axis, while in reality the column is divided into 7 cervical, 12 thoracic, 5 lumbar and 5 sacral vertebrae, as well as the coccyx and sacrum, and is articulated between each two vertebrae, particularly in three upper areas. Thus, it is understood that the next step in model development will be to split the spine into more segments.
While there are studies that seek to understand the spine as a whole, and include the cervical, thoracic and lumbar spine, studies of the internal loads on the spine are usually limited to the lumbar region. Although most cases of back injury involve the lumbar region, there are also complaints of pain in other regions of the trunk. A model that divides the spine into more segments, while not reflecting the total number of vertebrae in the spine, would bring the study of the internal loads in the spine closer to reality. The results of this study together with those of other anthropometric and anatomical studies provide a contribution towards future studies aimed at creating models of the spine that include more segments, which will in all likelihood provide better estimates of what is happening internally in the spine.

6. Acknowledgements

We thank Miotec Equipamentos Biomédicos Ltda for the loan of the electromyographical equipment and for their technical support during data collection.

7. References

Alexiev, A. R. (1994). Some differences of the electromyographic erector spinae activity between normal subjects and low back pain patients during the generation of isometric trunk torque *Electromyography and clinical neurophysiology* 34(8): 495-499,

Arjmand, N. S.-A., A. (2006). Model and in vivo studies on human trunk load partitioning and stability in isometric forward flexions *Journal of biomechanics* 39(3): 510-521,

Basler, H. D., Keller, S. & Herda, C. (1997). Good postural habits: A pilot investigation using emg scanning of the paraspinals *Applied psychophysiology and biofeedback* 22(3): 171-182,

Burdorf, A. (2000). Work-related musculoskeletal disorders *Annals of Occupational Hygiene* 44(3), 0003-4878

Candotti, C. T., Loss, J. F., Bagatini, D., Soares, D. P., Da Rocha, E. K., De Oliveira, Á. & Guimarães, A. C. S. (2008). Cocontraction and economy of triathletes and cyclists at different cadences during cycling motion *Journal of Electromyography and Kinesiology*,

Cheng, C. K., Chen, H. H., Et Al. (1998). A three-dimensional mathematical model for predicting spinal joint force distribution during manual liftings *Clinical Biomechanics* 13(1): 1223-1230,

De Leva, P. (1996). Adjustments to zatsiorsky-seluyanov's segment inertia parameters *Journal of biomechanics* 13(1): 1223-1230,

Dijke, G. a. H. V., Snijders, C. J., Stoeckart, R. & Stam, H. J. (1999). A biomechanical model on muscle forces in the transfer of spinal load to the pelvis and legs *Journal of biomechanics* 32(9): 927-933, 0021-9290

Dolan, P. & Adams, M. A. (1998). Repetitive lifting tasks fatigue the back muscles and increase the bending moment acting on the lumbar spine *Journal of biomechanics* 31(8): 713-721,

Dolan, P., Kingma, I., Van Dieen, J., De Looze, M. P., Toussaint, H. M., Baten, C. & Adams, M. A. (1999). Dynamic forces acting on the lumbar spine during manual handling: Can they be estimated using electromyographic techniques alone? *Spine* 24(7): 698-703, 0362-2436

Dolan, P. A., M. (1993). The relationship between emg activity and extensor moment generation in the erector spinae muscles during bending and lifting activities *Journal of biomechanics* 26(4-5): 513-522,

Erdmann, W. S. (1997). Geometric and inertial data of the trunk in adult males *Journal of biomechanics* 30(7): 679-688,

Fathallah, F. A., Marras, W. S. & Parnianpour, M. (1998). An assessment of complex spinal loads during dynamic lifting tasks *Spine* 23(6): 706, 0362-2436

Ferguson, S. & Marras, W. (1997). A literature review of low back disorder surveillance measures and risk factors *Clinical Biomechanics* 12(4): 211-226, 0268-0033

Ferguson, S. A., Marras, W. S. & Burr, D. L. (2004). The influence of individual low back health status on workplace trunk kinematics and risk of low back disorder *Ergonomics* 47(11): 1226-1237, 0014-0139

Figueroa, P. J., Leite, N. J. & Barros, R. M. L. (2003). A flexible software for tracking of markers used in human motion analysis *Computer methods and programs in biomedicine* 72(2): 155-165,

Gagnon, D., Larivière, C., Et Al. (2001). Comparative ability of emg, optimization, and hybrid modelling approaches to predict trunk muscle forces and lumbar spine loading during dynamic sagittal plane lifting *Clinical Biomechanics* 16(5): 359-372,

Ghormley, R. K. (1933). Low back pain: With special reference to the articular facets, with presentation of an operative procedure *Journal of the American Medical Association* 101(23): 1773, 0098-7484

Gonçalves, M. & Barbosa, F. S. S. (2005). Análise de parâmetros de força e resistência dos músculos eretores da espinha lombar durante a realização de exercício isométrico em diferentes níveis de esforço *Revista Brasileira de Medicina do Esporte* 11(2): 109-114,

Granata, K., Marras, W. & Davis, K. (1999). Variation in spinal load and trunk dynamics during repeated lifting exertions *Clinical Biomechanics* 14(6): 367-375,

Granata, K. P. M., W. (1995). An emg-assisted model of trunk loading during free-dynamic lifting *Journal of biomechanics* 28(11): 1309-1317,

Jäger, M. & Luttmann, A. (1999). Critical survey on the biomechanical criterion in the niosh method for the design and evaluation of manual lifting tasks *International journal of industrial ergonomics* 23(4): 331-337, 0169-8141

Jorgensen, M. & Marras, W. (2000). The effect of lumbar back support tension on trunk muscle activity *Clinical Biomechanics* 15(4): 292-294,

Kingma, I., Baten, C., Dolan, P., Toussaint, H., Van Dieën, J., De Looze, M. & Adams, M. (2001). Lumbar loading during lifting: A comparative study of three measurement techniques *Journal of Electromyography and Kinesiology* 11(5): 337,

Kingma, I., De Looze, M., Toussaint, H., Klijnsma, H. & Bruijnen, T. (1996). Validation of a full body 3-d dynamic linked segment model *Human Movement Science* 15(6): 833-860,

Kingma, I. V. D., J. H. (2004). Lifting over an obstacle: Effects of one-handed lifting and hand support on trunk kinematics and low back loading *Journal of biomechanics* 37(2): 249-255,

Kumar, S. (2001). Theories of musculoskeletal injury causation *Ergonomics* 44(1): 17-47,

La Torre, M., De Oliveira Melo, M., Et Al. (2005). Cálculo das forças internas na coluna lombar através da técnica da dinâmica inversa *revista brasileira de ciências do esporte* 29(2),

Larivière, C. G., D. (1999). The influence of trunk modelling in 3d biomechanical analysis of simple and complex lifting tasks *Clinical Biomechanics* 14(7): 449-461,

Lu, W. W., Hu, Y., Luk, K. D. K., Cheung, K. & Leong, J. C. Y. (2002). Paraspinal muscle activities of patients with scoliosis after spine fusion: An electromyographic study *Spine* 27(11): 1180,

Mannion, A. F., Connolly, B., Wood, K. & Dolan, P. (1997a). The use of surface enig power spectral analysis in the evaluation of back muscle function *Journal of Rehabilitation Research and Development* 34(4): 427-439,

Mannion, A. F., Dumas, G. A., Cooper, R. G., Espinosa, F. J., Faris, M. W. & Stevenson, J. M. (1997b). Muscle fibre size and type distribution in thoracic and lumbar regions of erector spinae in healthy subjects without low back pain: Normal values and sex differences *Journal of Anatomy* 190(04): 505-513,

Marras, W. S. G., K. P. (1997). The development of an emg-assisted model to assess spine loading during whole-body free-dynamic lifting *Journal of Electromyography and Kinesiology* 7(4): 259-268,

Mcgill, S. & Norman, R. (1986). Partitioning of the l4-l5 dynamic moment into disc, ligamentous, and muscular components during lifting *Spine* 11(7): 666, 0362-2436

Mirka, G., Glasscock, N., Stanfield, P. & Wilson, J. (2000). An empirical approach to characterizing trunk muscle coactivation using simulation input modeling techniques *Journal of biomechanics* 33(12): 1701-1704,

Nachemson, A. (1999). Back pain: Delimiting the problem in the next millennium *International journal of law and psychiatry* 22(5-6): 473, 0160-2527

Neumann, D. A. (2002). *Kinesiology of the musculoskeletal system: Foundations for physical rehabilitation* Mosby, 0815163495, St. Louis

Nielsen, P., Andersen, L. & Jørgensen, K. (1998). The muscular load on the lower back and shoulders due to lifting at different lifting heights and frequencies *Applied Ergonomics* 29(6): 445-450,

Nouwen, A., Van Akkerveeken, P. F. & Versloot, J. M. (1987). Patterns of muscular activity during movement in patients with chronic low-back pain *Spine* 12(8): 777,

Qiu, T. X., Teo, E. C. & Zhang, Q. H. (2006). Comparison of kinematics between thoracolumbar t11-t12 and t12-l1 functional spinal units *Proceedings of the Institution of Mechanical Engineers, Part H: Journal of Engineering in Medicine* 220(4): 493-504, 0954-4119

Sheikhzadeh, A., Parnianpour, M. & Nordin, M. (2008). Capability and recruitment patterns of trunk during isometric uniaxial and biaxial upright exertion *Clinical Biomechanics* 23(5): 527-535,

Simon, M. H., Brogmus, G.E., Courtney, T.K. (1997). Low back pain (lbp) and lifting technique - a review. *International Journal of Industrial Ergonomics* 19(1): 59-74,

Strait, L., Inman, V. & Ralston, H. (1947). Sample illustrations of physical principles selected from physiology and medicine *American Journal of Physics* 15: 375-382, 0002-9505

Thelen, E. (1989). The (re) discovery of motor development: Learning new things from an old field *Developmental Psychology* 25(6): 946–949,

Toussaint, H., De Winter, A., De Haas, Y., De Looze, M., Van Die N, J. & Kingma, I. (1995). Flexion relaxation during lifting: Implications for torque production by muscle activity and tissue strain at the lumbo-sacral joint *Journal of biomechanics* 28(2): 199-210,

Umphred, D. (1995). *Neurological rehabilitation* (Third Edition), Mosby-Year Book Inc, Saint Louis, MO

Waters, T. R., Putz-Anderson, V., Garg, A. & National Institute For, O. (1994). *Applications manual for the revised niosh lifting equation* US Dept. of Health and Human Services, Public Health Service, Centers for Disease Control, National Institute for Occupational Safety and Health, Division of Biomedical and Behavioral Science For sale by NIOSH,

Wilke, H., Neef, P., Hinz, B., Seidel, H. & Claes, L. (2001). Intradiscal pressure together with anthropometric data–a data set for the validation of models *Clinical Biomechanics* 16: 111-126,

Wilke, H. J., Neef, P., Caimi, M., Hoogland, T. & Claes, L. E. (1999). New in vivo measurements of pressures in the intervertebral disc in daily life *Spine* 24(8): 755, 0362-2436

Zatsiorsky, V. (2002). *Kinetics of human motion* Human Kinetics Publishers, Champaign, IL

2

EMG Analysis Methods on Robotic Gait Machines

Christopher Tomelleri[1], Andreas Waldner[1] and Stefan Hesse[2]
[1]Privatklinik Villa Melitta
[2]Medical Park Berlin Humboldtmühle
[1]Italy
[2]Germany

1. Introduction

Gait impairment is one of the consequences of events like stroke, traumatic brain injury, spinal cord injury or neurodegenerative diseases like Multiple Sclerosis or Parkinsons' Disease. The restoration and improvement of walking functions is one of the primary concerns of the rehabilitation of neurological Patients. To achieve this goal, a task specific repetitive training seems the most promising strategy (Jorgensen et al., 1995).

Conventional physiotherapy stresses out the reduction of an elevated muscle tone and the practice of gait preparatory tasks while sitting or standing. Accordingly, the number of steps practised rarely exceeds 50 to 80 steps during one therapy session (Hesse et al., 1995).

To increase the number of steps during therapy, the treadmill training with partial body weight support was a first step. Over the last years, there has been a growing support for the use of manual assisted treadmill training in neurorehabilitation programs. Studies showed that individuals who receive body weight supported treadmill training following stroke, traumatic brain injury and spinal cord injury improve their muscle activity during locomotion and gait symmetry. The main limitation with manual assisted body weight supported treadmill therapy is that a training session relies on several physical therapists to assist the patients' leg and hip movements through the gait cycle by hand. This results in short training sessions because of the physical effort required by the therapists and limits the potential of the treatment for the required training intensity may not be reached (Barbeu & Visintin 2003).

Robotic Gait Machines were developed to bypass these limiting factors. The gait machines move the legs of the patients through specified patterns. This is made either by applying an exoskeleton or an end-effector principle. The exoskeleton devices known so far are the Lokomat (Colombo et al., 2000), the LOPES (Veneman et al. 2007), the AutoAmbulator (Healthsouth Corporation, 2004) and the Sarà (MPD Costruzioni Meccaniche, 2010). Typical end-effector devices are the GangTrainer GT I (Hesse & Uhlenbrock, 2000), the LokoHelp (Freivogel et al., 2008), the Hapic Walker (Schmidt et al., 2005), the 6 Degrees of Freedom Gait Robot (Yoon et al., 2010) and the G-EO Systems (Hesse et al., 2010).

The exoskeleton is equipped with programmable drives or passive elements which flex the knees and hips during the swing phase. With the other principle the feet are placed on foot

plates, whose trajectories simulate the stance and swing phases. The potential risk of Robotic Gait Machines is the introduction of a non physiological gait pattern due the limited degrees of freedom controlled by the machines.
An understanding of the biomechanical interaction between Robotic Gait Machines and patients during locomotor training on the device is relevant to ensure correct interaction forces applied on the patients' joints and the correct activation of their muscles. Typically a gait analysis system is applied on patients or on healthy subjects while walking on the Robotic Gait Machine.
The EMG Analysis on a gait robot aims to prove the correctness of the induced muscle activation while practising on the machines. If the selected muscles are activated in a correct fashion, any concerns about an incorrect training pattern would be inconsistent. The purpose of the present chapter is to introduce, explain and compare the methods of different EMG analyses carried out on different robotic gait machines, i.e. to present the gait robots, the subject pool, the data acquisition and the signal processing strategies. This is made by explaining in detail the choices and techniques represented in the respective Methods section of the studies considered.

2. EMG analysis methods on robotic gait machines

EMG Analyses have been made so far on three different gait robots: the Lokomat (Hidler & Wall), the Haptic Walker (Hussein, 2009) and the G-EO Systems (Hesse et al., 2010). All three studies addressed the essential question of a match between muscle activation patterns of the subjects under test during training on the Robotic Gait Machine and during free walking.
The Lokomat robotic gait orthosis consists of a treadmill, a body weight support system and two light weight robotic actuators to attach to the subjects' legs. The robotic actuators are fully programmable and control the flexion and the extension of the knee and the hip. The actuators are synchronized with the treadmill for setting the correct speed while walking. The movement of the ankle is not controlled; a spring provides for dorsiflexion and avoids the paretic foot to stumble on the treadmill. The Lokomat also controls the speed at which the patient ambulates and the amount of assistance the system provides to the patient.
The HapticWalker is an end-effector robot, designed following the programmable footplate concept. Each of the two foot plates consists of a hybrid serial-parallel robot. The patients' feet are fixed on the foot plates, which move the patients' feet along the natural movement of walking. For the end-effector principle if the last segment of a kinematic chain is moved correctly, all segments and joints in the kinematic chain are moved correctly. It follows that by controlling and moving the foot correctly, the knee and the hip are also moved correctly by the gait robot.
The G-EO Systems follows the end effector principle as well. The patient stands on two foot plates, connected each by a crank arm to two moving units. The G-EO Systems is more compact in the design than the Haptic Walker as it was designed to be a clinically feasible end-effector robot.
The devices differ in their design strategy. The Lokomat follows the exoskeleton principle; the Haptic Walker and the G-EO Systems are end effector based devices. Figure 1 shows the three devices.

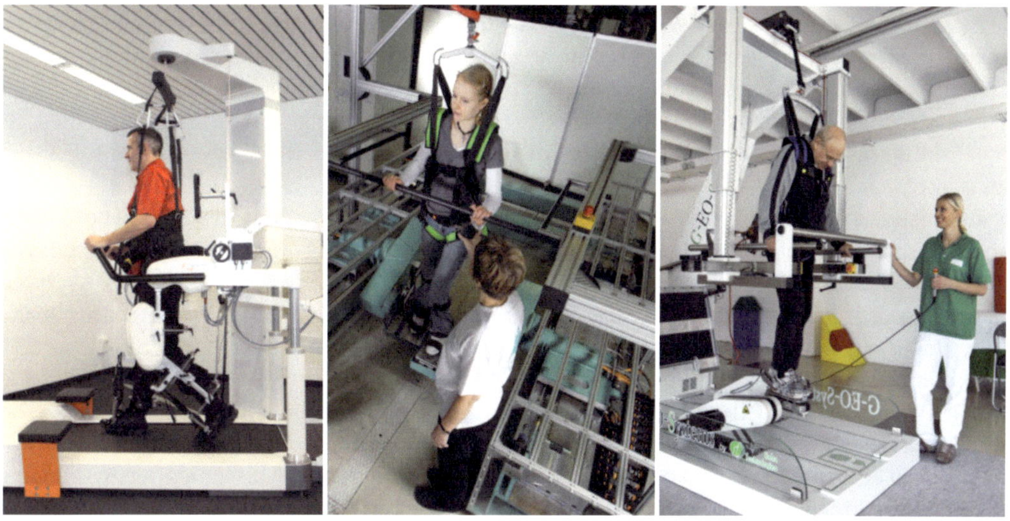

Fig. 1. The Lokomat, the Haptic Walker and the G-EO Systems.

2.1 Test protocol

The Lokomat study enrolled a total of seven healthy subjects with no known neurological injuries or gait disorders, the Haptic Walker study a total of nine healthy subjects. The G-EO Systems Study was conducted on six ambulatory stroke patients.

The Lokomat and the Haptic Walker provided gait velocities suitable to a gait analysis on healthy subjects. It was possible to analyze the gait with no restrictions to gait velocity and cadence of the subjects under test. A restriction of walking speed would have prolonged the duration of muscle activation or altered the timing in the muscle activation patterns. The aim of both studies was to show a match between EMG patterns of real walking and robotic walking.

Having an analysis on the G-EO Systems on healthy subjects would have been senseless, as the trajectories of the Haptic Walker and the G-EO Systems were quite the same. The motion tracking of healthy subjects was made with the same active marker system, but on a different population (Hesse et al., 2010; Schmidt et al. 2005). The aim for the G-EO Systems was not to replicate the results of the Haptic Walker study, which clearly proved a physiological muscle activation on the end-effector robotic gait machine, but to extend these results to another study population.

Furthermore the G-EO Systems was designed for treating gait impaired patients and did not provide gait velocities suitable for an analysis on healthy subjects. A gait analysis on subjects whose own walking speed would have been superior to the one provided by the machine would have altered the EMG patterns. The Authors were looking for subjects able to walk freely on speeds comparable to the maximum speed provided by the G-EO Systems. This was the reason of having the analysis made on ambulatory stroke patients.

2.2 Data acquisition

The Lokomat Subjects walked first on the treadmill without the Lokomat and then with the Lokomat orthoses. The Lokomat linkages were adjusted to the leg lengths of each subject, so that the hip and knee joints of the Lokomat were aligned with those of the subject. During

both Lokomat and treadmill walking, surface EMGs were recorded differentially from the gastrocnemius, tibialis anterior, hamstrings, rectus femoris, adductor longus, vastus lateralis, and gluteus medius and maximus muscles using a 8 channel EMG system.
The gastrocnemius is involved in all standing, walking, running and jumping activities. Its function is the plantar flexion of the foot at the ankle joint and the flexion of the leg at the knee joint.
The tibialis anterior is responsible for dorsiflexing and inverting the foot. The tibialis anterior muscle also allows the ankle to be inverted providing horizontal movement. The muscle stabilizes the ankle as the foot hits the ground during the contact phase of walking through eccentric contraction and acts later to pull the foot clear of the ground during the swing phase by concentric contraction.
The hamstring muscles include three posterior thigh muscles: the semitendinosus, the semimembranosus and the biceps femoris. They act upon the hip and the knee joints. The semitendinosus muscle and the semimembranosus muscle extend the hip when the trunk is fixed. They also flex the knee and provide for medial rotation of the lower leg when the knee is bent. The long head of the biceps femoris extends the hip when starting to walk. Short and long heads of the biceps femoris flex the knee and provide for lateral rotation of the lower leg when the knee is bent.
The rectus femoris muscle is one of the four quadriceps muscles and is situated in the middle of the front of the thigh. The rectus femoris is one of the muscles in the quadriceps involved in the flexion of the hip. By crossing the pelvic femoral joint it can act as a lever to flex the leg at the hip.
The adductor longus is a muscle located in the thigh. The main function is to adduct and laterally rotate the femur. The adductor lies ventrally on the adductor magnus and near the femur.
The vastus lateralis muscle is on the lateral side of the femur and is the largest of the quadriceps muscles. Like all quadriceps muscle its function is to act as an extensor of the knee.
The gluteus medius muscle is one of the three gluteal muscles. With straightened leg the gluteus medius function is to abduct the thigh. During gait the gluteus medius principally supports the body on one leg to prevent the pelvis from dropping to the opposite side. With the hip flexed the gluteus medius rotates the thigh externally. With the hip extended, the gluteus medius rotates the thigh internally.
The gluteus maximus muscle is another gluteal muscle, the largest and most superficial of the three gluteal muscles. Considering the pelvis as fixed the gluteus maximus extends the femur.
Only one leg was instrumented with EMG electrodes since none of the subjects had any gait disorders and walked symmetrically. The EMG data was collected for 60 seconds.
The EMG Signals of the Haptic Walker Subjects EMG were acquired during free walking and during walking on the HapticWalker. For robot assisted walking the same step length as calculated from free walking was used. At least 5 full stride cycles were taken for each trial. The surface EMGs were recorded from the tibialis anterior, gastrocnemius, rectus femoris, biceps femoris, vastus medialis, vastus lateralis, gluteus medius and erector spinae muscles using a 8 channel EMG system.
The biceps femoris belongs to the hamstring muscles and is responsible for knee flexion. The long head is also involved in hip extension. When the knee is semi-flexed, the biceps femoris rotates the leg slightly outward.

The vasus medialis translates the patella medially and provides control of the knee extension together with the vastus lateralis. The vastus medialis is medially located in the quadriceps muscle group.
The Erector spinae is a muscle group. It extends throughout the lumbar, thoracic and cervical regions, and lies in the groove to the side of the vertebral column.
Only one side was instrumented with EMG electrodes since none of the subjects had any gait disorders and walked symmetrically.
The subjects on the G-EO Systems were analysed while walking on the floor at self selected speed and during simulated floor walking on the machine at comparable speed and cadence. The EMG activity was measured on seven lower limb muscles: tibialis anterior, gastrocnemius, vastus medialis, vastus lateralis, rectus femoris, biceps femoris, and gluteus medius of the affected side. The non affected side was not of interest for the purposes of the study. The muscles under analysis were the same as for the Haptic Walker, but did not include the erector spinae. The activation pattern for this muscle group showed to be too weak on hemiparetic patients. The assessment consisted of a 30 seconds long recording of the electromyographic activity during real and simulated floor walking. The subjects were first asked to walk on the floor for at least 30 seconds at a self selected pace. Gait velocity, step length and cadence of free walking were replicated on the gait robot.

2.3 Signal processing

Signal Processing was made for all three studies according to Fourier Analysis (Oppenheim et al., 1996). The bandwidth of the EMG signal was considered as limited, i.e. the Fourier Transform of the EMG Signal is zero outside of a finite band of frequencies. The Fourier transform is a mathematical operation that decomposes a signal into its constituent frequencies. The Fourier Transform for a continuous time signal is given by

$$X(f) = \int_{-\infty}^{+\infty} x(t)\, e^{-j2\pi f t}\, dt \quad (1)$$

Every continuous time signal may be also represented by his frequency content. A signal with infinite bandwidth can be lowpass filtered to a finite bandwidth signal. In the time domain this operation would consist in a convolution operation between the infinite band signal x(t) and the function in the time domain of the lowpass filter h(t), resulting in the finite band signal y(t) given by

$$y(t) = x(t) * h(t) \quad (2)$$

$$y(t) = \int_{-\infty}^{+\infty} x(\tau)\, h(t-\tau)\, d\tau \quad (3)$$

The convolution in the time domain between x(t) and h(t) becomes a multiplication operation in the frequency domain between X(f) and H(f) , due to duality proprieties of the Fourier Transform. The Fourier Transform Y(f) of the limited band signal y(t) is given by

$$Y(f) = X(f)\, H(f) \quad (4)$$

Mind that lowpass filtering a infinite band signal results in a loss of information or a lossy compression. The cut-off frequency of the lowpass filter H(f) should therefore be chosen adequately. Figure 2 shows an infinite band signal, an ideal lowpass filter and a finite band signal as the product in the frequency domain of the infinite band signal and the lowpass filter.

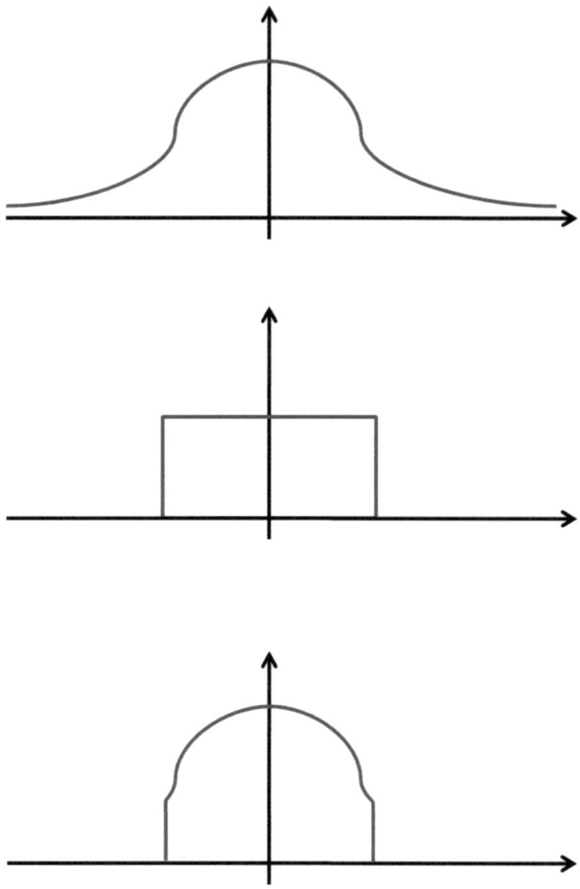

Fig. 2. Infinite band signal, ideal lowpass filter and finite band signal as product in frequency of the infinite band signal and the lowpass filter.

If the samples of the signal are taken sufficiently close together in correspondence to the highest frequency of the signal, then the samples uniquely specify the signal. The correct frequency for sampling a limited band signal is given by the Sampling Theorem which states:

Let x(t) be a band-limited signal with X(f) = 0 for | f | > f_M. If the Sampling Frequency $f_S > f_M$, Then x(t) is uniquely determined by its samples x(nT), n = 0, ±1, ±2,..., where T = 1/f_S. The signal can be reconstructed by an ideal lowpass filter with gain T and cut-off frequency f_C, where $f_M > f_C > f_S - f_M$.

The usual way of representing a finite band signal in regular intervals is the multiplication of the continuous-time signal x(t) and a periodic impulse train p(t). This is known as impulse train sampling. In the time domain the signal $x_p(t)$ results from

$$x_p(t) = x(t)\, p(t) \tag{5}$$

where

$$p(t) = \sum_{n=-\infty}^{+\infty} \delta(t - nT) \tag{6}$$

Multiplying x(t) by a unitary impulse train samples the values of the signal at the points at which the impulses were located. The signal $x_p(t)$ therefore is an impulse train with the amplitudes of the impulses equal to the samples of x(t) at intervals spaced by T; that is

$$x_p(t) = \sum_{n=-\infty}^{+\infty} x(nT)\,\delta(t-nT) \tag{7}$$

Again by duality proprieties between the time domain and the frequency domain, the multiplication in the time domain becomes a convolution in the frequency domain

$$X_p(f) = \frac{1}{2\pi}\int_{-\infty}^{+\infty} X(\varphi)P(f-\varphi)d\varphi \tag{8}$$

with

$$P(f) = \frac{1}{T}\sum_{k=-\infty}^{+\infty} \delta(f-f_s) \tag{9}$$

The convolution with an impulse $\delta(f_0)$ shifts a signal X(f)

$$X(f) * \delta(f-f_0) = X_p(f-f_0) \tag{10}$$

it follows

$$X_p(f) = \frac{1}{2\pi T}\sum_{k=-\infty}^{+\infty} X(f-f_s) \tag{11}$$

It means that $X_P(f)$ is a periodic function of f consisting of a superposition of shifted replicas of X(f) scaled by $1/2\pi T$. If the sampling frequency is chosen according to the Sampling Theorem, there is no overlap between $X_P(f)$ and its replicas. The signal x(t) can be reconstructed correctly using the lowpass filter suggested by the Sampling Theorem.

If the signal is not sampled according to the Sampling Theorem, there would be an overlap between X(f) and its replicas. The overlap results in the higher frequency components in the band of the signal summing and introducing distortion in $X_P(f)$. The signal x(t) could not be reconstructed correctly any more, this phenomenon is referred to as Aliasing. For finite band signals the Sampling Frequency has to be chosen correctly, for infinite band signals there has to be a lowpass filtering prior to sampling. As the aim of this filtering is to avoid the Aliasing Phenomenon, it is also called Anti-Aliasing or Anti-Alias Filtering.

Figure 3 shows the replicas of an infinite band signal overlapping, the result of overlapping and the same signal filtered by an ideal lowpass filter to prevent overlapping.

It is important to notice that the pre-filtering has to be an analogical lowpass filtering and has to happen before sampling. It is good practice to pre-filter finite bandwidth signals as well. Although the band of this kind of signals is finite, there could be spurious components outside the signal band, i.e. disturbances at higher frequencies which superimpose to the signal to sample. Sampling without pre-filtering would sample the disturbances too. If the Sampling Frequency is chosen correctly for the signal to sample, but does not match the Sampling Theorem for the high frequency disturbances, the replicas of the disturbances would overlap on the signal introducing distortion. Pre-filtering with a cut-off frequency equal or below the Sampling Frequency would eliminate disturbances to the signal from the beginning.

Figure 4 shows a finite band signal and a disturbance, the sampled signal with the disturbance overlapping on the signal and the signal filtered prior to sampling by an ideal lowpass filter to prevent disturbances.

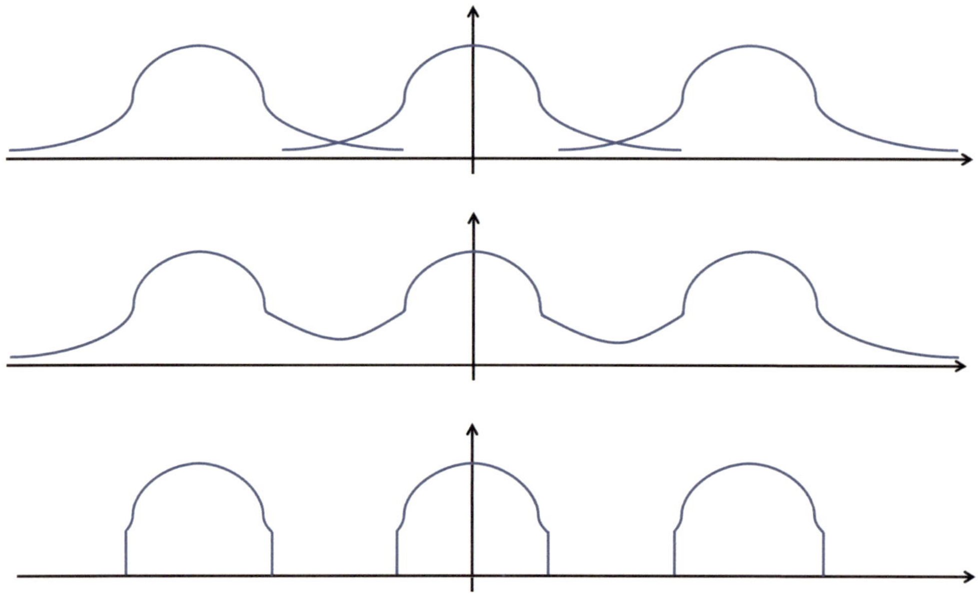

Fig. 3. Aliasing phenomenon resulting in overlapping replicas summing up and result of an Anti-Alias Filtering.

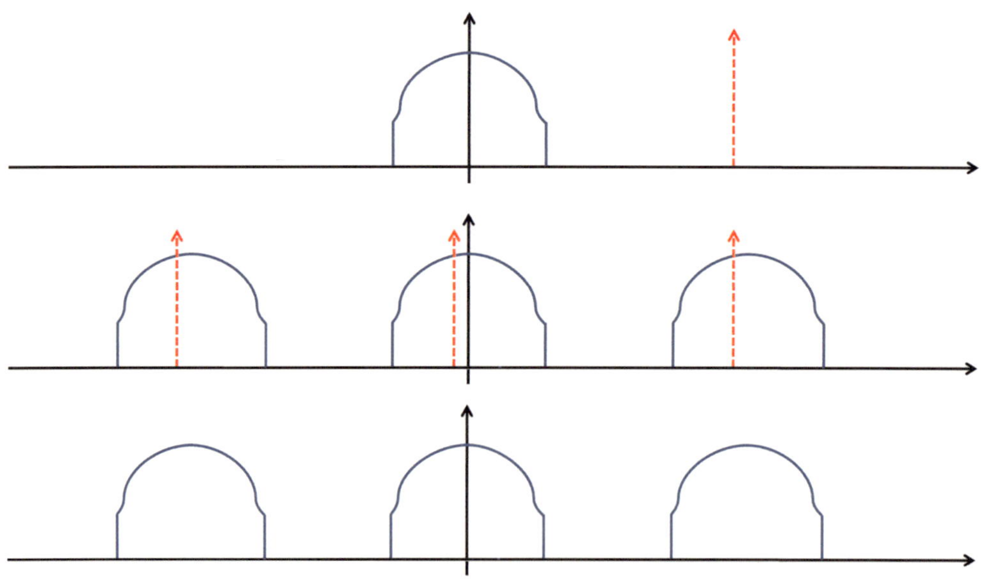

Fig. 4. High frequency disturbances on a finite band signal and result of ideal lowpass filtering prior to sampling.

After sampling all signal processing strategies would be digital. Digital lowpass filtering after sampling would not be a Anti-Alias Filtering. Mind that the signal would be already aliased and that lowpass filtering with a cut-off frequency equal to the Sampling Frequency would be useless. Digital filtering can improve proprieties of the correctly sampled signal as it can provide for smoothing or compression of the signal itself, but it can never provide for Anti-Aliasing.

The EMG signal is not a finite band signal, although the information content above 500 Hz is negligible. A good choice of the cut-off frequency of an ideal lowpass filter for pre-filtering purposes therefore is 500 Hz, resulting in a typical Sampling Frequency of 1000 Hz, twice the cut-off frequency of pre-filtering. On the Lokomat , on the Haptic Walker and on the G-EO Systems the EMG signals were lowpass filtered at 500 Hz prior to sampling at 1000 Hz to avoid the aliasing phenomenon by the EMG analysis system. On the G-EO Systems the sampled data were further filtered by a Finite Impulse Response (FIR) filter of first order lowpass filter with Z-Transform

$$H(z) = \frac{1}{2}\frac{1z}{1+z} \tag{12}$$

The filter was intended for additional smoothing of the raw EMG signal for the following signal processing without affecting the useful information content in the signal band.

Additional signal filtering on the Haptic Walker was provided by a full wave rectification, followed by a highpass filtering to suppress measurement artifacts.

A full wave rectification converts the whole of the input signal to a signal of constant polarity at its output. The raw EMG signal has random variations between negative and positive peaks. By full wave rectification all negative amplitudes are converted to positive amplitudes, i.e. for a the raw EMG x(t) the full wave rectified output y(t) would be

$$y(t) = |x(t)| \tag{13}$$

The negative spikes are moved to positive values reflected on the baseline. Besides easier reading the main effect is that standard amplitude parameters like mean and area can be applied to the signal. The non rectified raw EMG has a mean value and area under signal of zero.

High-pass filtering of EMG signals is used to remove possible movement artifacts comprised in a low frequency range. Typical highpass filters for EMG signals start at a frequency between 10 and 20Hz.

2.4 Step determination and envelope calculation

The single steps were determined by the trigger signal provided by the foot switches of the EMG analysis system on the Lokomat and on the G-EO Systems.

For the Haptic Walker the trigger signal for determination of the single was provided by the gait robot itself. The reason for this choice was due to the end-effector principle. On the end-effector robots the feet have continuous contact to the footplate, i.e. the leg is supported by the robot not only during the stance phase but also during the swing phase. This would create an offset on the foot switches of the EMG analysis system for there would be easily some residual pressure on the foot switch. This would make it difficult for the analysis system to distinguish between the stance and the swing phase. Taking the data of the trigger signal directly from the gait robot bypassed the problem, furthermore it provided for stride

intervals of exactly the same duration between all the triggering peaks within the trigger signal.
Although the EMG analysis system used for the G-EO Systems was the same as for the Haptic Walker, the trigger signal was taken from the foot switches. The safety binding on the G-EO System allowed for more flexibility than the one of the Haptic Walker, resulting in less offset pressure on the foot switches. A further observation showed that the hemiparetic patients under test did not load the affected leg in the swing phase but loaded the non affected leg as much as possible. Under these considerations the trigger signal provided by the footswitches showed to be suitable for an analysis on an end-effector robot too.
After triggering the EMG signal the patterns for each stride had to be normalized in time. This had to be done in the case of the trigger signals taken by the foot switches, but not if the trigger signal was taken from the machine. The timing of the trigger peaks and the duration of the trigger intervals taken by the footswitches differed in a few milliseconds, resulting in a different number of samples associated to the single strides. On the Lokomat this was due to the fact that the ankle and the heel were not controlled by the gait robot, and on the G-EO Systems due to intra-subject variability of the strides made by the hemiparetic patients walking on the gait machine, although the machine provided for perfectly symmetrical walking.
Normalization was achieved by upsampling the single strides of the EMG signal and by resampling the upsampled strides to the same number of samples for each stride. Upsampling was made with the help of a cubic spline (Giakas & Baltzopoulos, 1997). A cubic spline was constructed of piecewise third-order polynomials which passed through a set of m control points. Weights were associated to the points to be connected by the third order polynomials. These coefficients bent the polynomials to pass through each of the data points without any erratic behavior or breaks in continuity. Considering a function of the form:

$$S(x) = \begin{cases} s_1(x) & if \;\; x_1 \leq x < x_2 \\ s_2(x) & if \;\; x_2 \leq x < x_3 \\ & \vdots \\ s_{n-1}(x) & if \;\; x_{n-1} \leq x < x_n \end{cases} \tag{14}$$

Where s_i was the third order polynomial defined as

$$s_i(x) = a_i\,(x - x_i)^3 + b_i\,(x - x_i)^2 + c_i\,(x - x_i) + d_i \tag{15}$$

for i = 1,..,n-1. The first and the second derivative of these n-1 equations were

$$s'_i(x) = 3a_i\,(x - x_i)^2 + 2b_i\,(x - x_i) + c_i \tag{16}$$

$$s''_i(x) = 6a_i\,(x - x_i) + 2b_i \tag{17}$$

for i = 1,..,n-1. The cubic spline needed to conform to the following:
1. The piecewise function S(x) had to interpolate all data points.
2. *S(x)* had to be continuous on the interval $[x_1, x_n]$
3. *S'(x)* had to be continuous on the interval $[x_1, x_n]$
4. *S''(x)* had to be continuous on the interval $[x_1, x_n]$

S(x) had to interpolate all of the samples, for i = 1,…, n-1

$$S(x_i) = y_i \tag{18}$$

Since $S(x_i) = y_i$ for all x_i in the closed interval $[x_i, x_{i+1}]$

$$y_i = s_i(x_i) \tag{19}$$

By substitution of (15) in (19)

$$y_i = d_i \tag{20}$$

The curve S(x) must be continuous in its entire interval, the subfunctions had to join at the samples

$$s_i(x_i) = s_{i-1}(x_i) \tag{21}$$

For i = 1,…,n. Letting $h = x_i - x_{i-1}$, the subfunction $s_{i-1}(x_i)$ was defined as

$$s_{i-1}(x_i) = a_{i-1}h^3 + b_{i-1}h^2 + c_{i-1}h + d_{i-1} \tag{22}$$

$$d_i = a_{i-1}h^3 + b_{i-1}h^2 + c_{i-1}h + d_{i-1} \tag{23}$$

The curve would only have been smooth across its interval only if the derivates were equal at the samples; that is

$$s_i'(x_i) = s'_{i-1}(x_i) \tag{24}$$

Solving for $s'_i(x_i)$ and $s'_{i-1}(x_i)$, considering again $h = x_i - x_{i-1}$

$$s'_i(x_i) = c_i \tag{25}$$

$$s'_{i-1}(x_i) = 3a_{i-1}h^2 + 2b_{i-1}h + c_{i-1} \tag{26}$$

By substitution of equation (25) in equation (26) c_i could be expressed for i = 2,…, n-1 as

$$c_i = 3a_{i-1}h^2 + 2b_{i-1}h + c_{i-1} \tag{27}$$

Solving equation (17) for $x = x_i$

$$s''_i(x_i) = 2b_i \tag{28}$$

For i = 2,…n-2.
Since $s''_i(x)$ had to be continuous across the interval, $s''_i(x_i) = s''_{i+1}(x_i)$ for i = 1,…,n-1. Considering this and equation (28) with $h = x_{i+1} - x_i$

$$s''_i(x_{i+1}) = 6a_i h + 2b_i \tag{29}$$

$$s''_{i+1}(x_{i+1}) = 2b_{i+1} \tag{30}$$

$$2b_{i+1} = 6a_i h + 2b_i \tag{31}$$

For easier notation $s''_i(x)$ was substituted by M_i. Expressing the equations (31) and (28) in terms of M_i and y_i resulted in the determination of the weights of the cubic spline a_i, b_i, c_i and d_i.

$$2b_{i+1} = 6a_i\, h + 2b_i \tag{31}$$

$$6a_i\, h = 2b_{i+1} - 2b_i$$

$$a_i = \frac{2b_{i+1} - 2b_i}{6h}$$

$$a_i = \frac{M_{i+1} - M_i}{6h} \tag{32}$$

$$s''_i(x_i) = 2b_i \tag{28}$$

$$M_i = 2b_i$$

$$b_i = \frac{M_i}{2} \tag{33}$$

$$d_i = a_{i-1}h^3 + b_{i-1}\, h^2 + c_{i-1}h + d_{i-1} \tag{23}$$

$$d_{i+1} = a_i h^3 + b_i\, h^2 + c_i h + d_i$$

$$c_i h = -a_i h^3 - b_i\, h^2 - d_i + d_{i+1}$$

$$c_i = \frac{-a_i h^3 - b_i\, h^2 - d_i + d_{i+1}}{h}$$

$$c_i = -a_i h^2 - b_i\, h + \frac{-d_i + d_{i+1}}{h}$$

$$c_i = \frac{y_{i+1} - y_i}{h} - \frac{M_{i+1} - M_i}{6h} h^2 - \frac{M_i}{2} h$$

$$c_i = \frac{y_{i+1} - y_i}{h} - \left(\frac{M_{i+1} + 2M_i}{6}\right) h \tag{34}$$

$$y_i = d_i \tag{20}$$

$$d_i = y_i \tag{35}$$

After upsampling and resampling all strides were of the same number of samples, but the information about the duration of the strides got lost. Normalization expressed the samples in relation to the gait cycle: A whole stride is considered as 100% of the gait cycle, every sample is put in relation to this gait cycle percentage. The gait cycle starts with the initial contact and ends at the subsequent initial contact. The gait cycle percentages ranging from 0% to 60% were considered as stance phase, the percentages from 60% to 100% were considered as swing phase.

Upsampling was not necessary for the Haptic Walker. The stride duration was exactly the same for all strides of the measurement, due to the trigger signal taken from the device. The EMG data were just normalized in relation to the gait cycle.

The envelope of the strides was determined with root mean square algorithms (Simons & Yang, 1991). The root mean square of the n samples a signal x_i, i = 1,…,n, is given by

$$RMS = \sqrt{\frac{\sum_{i=1}^{n} x_i}{n}} \tag{36}$$

For the Lokomat and the G-EO Systems the root mean square algorithm consisted in a 50-point root mean square, 150-point root mean square respectively. A k-point root mean square is defined as:

$$x_i = \sqrt{\frac{\sum_{l=i}^{i+k-1} x_l}{k}} \tag{37}$$

The sample x_i is determined not as the whole root mean square of the sampled signal, but as the root mean square of the ith sample and its following k-1 samples. This technique can be compared with a moving average filtering. Considering the signal x_i, with i = 1,…,n, for all samples of x_i where n-k+2 < i < n, the signal has to be replicated considering the samples from 1 to k-1 as the samples n+1 to n+k-1. The more samples are considered for the root mean square, the smoother the signal gets. For the Lokomat study the value chosen for k was 50, for the G-EO Systems 150. The final result of signal processing of the EMG signal in the Lokomat study therefore was more rippled than in the G-EO Systems study.

On the Haptic Walker the root mean square algorithm was based on a lowpass Bessel filer. A lowpass Bessel filter has a maximally flat group delay. Group delay is a measure of the time delay of the amplitude envelopes of the various sinusoidal components of a signal as a function of the frequency of each component. Analog Bessel filters are characterized by almost constant group delay across their passband, thus preserving the wave shape of signals filtered. The Laplace transform of the transfer function of a Bessel lowpass filter is expressed as (Barozzi, 2005):

$$H(s) = \frac{\vartheta(0)}{\vartheta(^{s}/_{\omega_0})} \tag{38}$$

where ω_0 is a pulsation chosen to give the desired cut-off frequency. The Bessel lowpass filter therefore has a low-frequency group delay of 1 / ω_0. Pulsation and frequency are closely related as:

$$\omega = 2\pi f \tag{39}$$

$\theta(s)$ is a reverse Bessel polynomial described by

$$\vartheta(s) = \sum_{k=0}^{n} \frac{(2n-k)!}{(n-k)!k!} \frac{s^k}{2^{n-k}} \tag{40}$$

with s expressed as a complex number $s = \sigma + j\omega$.

The final mean EMG patterns generated for the gait cycle of all three studies were computed for each subject by averaging all the individual stride cycles of the subject. If the EMG signal consists of k single strides, contained in the signal s(i) with i = 1,...k*n, the average signal samples S(i) with i = 1,…,n of k strides is given by

$$S(i) = \frac{1}{k} \sum_{l=1}^{k} s(l * i) \tag{41}$$

3. Conclusion

The present chapter highlighted the differences in the protocols and the different techniques in EMG signal processing of three studies on robotic gait machines. The results of the studies are not compared or discussed in this chapter, as the description of the methods showed differences which highlight how difficult a comparison would be.

The Lokomat study and the G-EO systems study had a similar signal processing strategy and a similar acquisition protocol. The G-EO Systems study in fact was inspired by the methods of the Lokomat study, but did not include healthy subjects, for the gait velocity provided by the G-EO Systems was too slow and a EMG signal analysis was already published for healthy subjects for the programmable foot plate concept taking in consideration the Haptic Walker. A comparison between the EMG signals of healthy subjects and stroke patients is difficult given the fact the muscle activation patterns of hemiparetic subjects differ considerably from healthy muscle activation patterns. Furthermore the individual patterns of hemiparetic patients vary considerably.

The Lokomat study and the Haptic Walker study both involved healthy subjects, but differed in the acquisition protocol and in the signal processing too. The Haptic Walker considered mostly just five strides during data acquisition and based its signal processing on different techniques, as explained in the previous sections.

The direct comparison between the Methods of the G-EO Systems study and the Haptic Walker study showed the use of the same design principle, the same data acquisition system, but different signal processing. The G-EO Systems study can be considered as an extension of the findings and the aims of the Haptic Walker study, but carried out with the Methods of the Lokomat study.

If looking for a comparison, the only way would be an analysis on these devices with the same protocol on a cluster of comparable patients with the same gait impairment. The acquired data should than be processed in the same way for the whole cluster of patients.

4. Acknowledgment

G-EO Systems was supported by a grant of the "Amt für Innovation, Landesregierung Südtirol", Italy. Scientific publication activities are also supported by the Landesregierung Südtirol, Italy and a grant of the Bundesministerium für Bildung und Forschung (BioFuture) of the German Government.

5. References

Barbeau, H. & Visintin, M. (2003). Optimal outcomes obtained with body-weight support combined with treadmill training in stroke subjects. *Archives of Physical Medicine and Rehabilitation,*Vol. 84, No. 10, (October 2003), pp. 1458-1465, ISSN 0003-9993

Barozzi G. (2005). *Matematica per ingegneria dell' informazione,* Zanichelli, ISBN 978-88-08-12546-0, Bologna, Italy

Colombo, G.; Joerg, M.; Schreier, R.; Dietz, V. (2000). Treadmill training of paraplegic patients using a robotic orthosis. *Journal of Rehabilitation Research and Development,* Vol. 37, No. 6, (November-December 2000) pp. 693-700, ISSN 0748-7711

Freivogel, S.; Mehrholz, J.; Husak-Sotomayor; T.; Schmalohr D. (2008). Gait training with the newly developed 'LokoHelp'-system is feasible for nonambulatory patients after stroke, spinal cord and brain injury. A feasibility study. *Brain Injury*, Vol. 22, No. 7, (July 2008), pp. 625-632, ISSN 1362-301X

Giakas, G. & Baltzopoulos V. (1997) A comparison of automatic filtering techniques applied to biomechanical walking data, *Journal of Biomechanics*, Vol. 30, No. 8, (August 1997), pp. 847–850, ISSN 0021-9290

Healthsouth Corporation. (2004). Powered gait orthosis and method of utilizing same. US Patent US2004/0143198

Hesse, S.; Bertelt, C.; Jahnke, M.; Schaffrin, A.; Baake, P.; Malezic, M.; Mauritz, K. (1995). Treadmill training with partial body weight support as compared to physiotherapy in non-ambulatory hemiparetic patients. *Stroke,* Vol. 26, pp. 976-981, ISSN 0039-2499

Hesse, S. & Uhlenbrock, D. (2000). A mechanized gait trainer for restoration of gait, *Journal of Rehabilitation Research and Development*, vol. 37, no. 6, (September 2000), pp. 701–708, ISSN 0003-9993

Hesse, S.; Waldner, A.; Tomelleri, C. Innovative gait robot for the repetitive practice of floor walking and stair climbing up and down in stroke patients. (2010) *Journal of NeuroEngineering and Rehabilitation*, Vol. 7, No. 30, (June 2010) pp. 1-10, ISSN 1743-0003

Hidler, J. & Wall, A. (2005). Alterations in muscle activation patterns during robotic-assisted walking. *Clinical Biomechanics* Vol. 20, (February 2005), pp. 184–193, ISSN 0268-0033

Hussein, S.; Schmidt, H.; Krüger, J. (2009) Adaptive control of an endeffector based electromechanical gait rehabilitation device, *Proceedings of the IEEE 11th International Conference on Rehabilitation Robotics, ICORR 2009*, pp. 366-371, ISSN 1945-7898, Kyoto, Japan, 23-26 June, 2009.

Jorgensen, H.; Nakayama, H.; Raaschou, H.; Olsen, T. (1995). Recovery of walking function in stroke patients: the Copenhagen stroke study. *Archives of Physical Medicine and Rehabilitation*, Vol. 76, No. 1, (January 1995), pp. 76: 27-32, ISSN 0003-9993

MPD Costruzioni Meccaniche. (2010). Robot motor rehabilitation device, World Patent WO 2010/105773

Oppenheim, A.; Willsky, A.; Nawab, S. (1996). *Signals & Systems*, Prentice Hall, ISBN 0-13-814757-4, Upper Saddle River, New Jersey, USA

Simons, W. & Yang K. (1991). Differentiation of human motion data using combined spline and least squares concept. *Journal of Biomechanical Engineering*, Vol. 113, (August 1991), pp. 348-351, ISSN 0148-0731

Schmidt, H.; Hesse, S.; Bernhardt, R.; Krüger, J, HapticWalker-a novel haptic foot device., (2005) ACM Transactions on Applied Perception, Vol. 2, No. 2, (April 2005), pp. 166-180, ISSN 1544-3558

Veneman, J.; Kruidhof, R.; Hekman. E.; Ekkelenkamp, R.; Van Asseldonk, E.; van der Kooij, H. (2007) Design and evaluation of the LOPES exoskeleton robot for interactive gait rehabilitation. IEEE Transactions on Neural Systems and Rehabilitation Engineering, Vol. 15, No. 3 (September 2007), pp. 379-86, ISSN 1534-4320

Yoon, J.; Novandy, B.; Yoon C;, Park, K. (2010) A 6-DOF Gait Rehabilitation Robot with Upper and Lower-Limb Connections that Allows Walking Velocity Updates on Various Terrains. *IEEE Transaction on Mechatronics*, Vol. 15, No. 2, (April 2010), pp. 201-215, ISSN1083-4435

3

Electromyography in the Study of Muscle Reactions to Vibration Treatment

Antonio Fratini[1], Mario Cesarelli[1], Antonio La Gatta[2], Maria Romano[1] and Paolo Bifulco[1]

[1]*Dept. of Biomedical, Electronic and Telecommunication Engineering, University of Naples "Federico II", Naples*

[2]*CNVR -Veneto Research Consortium, Saccolongo, Padua*

Italy

1. Introduction

Electromyography (EMG) is a common used technique to evaluate muscular activity. Analysis of EMG recordings is important for assessing muscle activation, its relationship to the force developed during specific tasks and for evaluating fatigue processes occurring in response to physical activity.

Electromyography can be performed using different types of electrodes, depending on the specific analysis: surface (or skin) electrodes or inserted electrodes (wire and needle); the first it is used to monitor the overall activity of a muscle while the second is generally used to reveal the electrical activity of a nerve root. (De Luca, 1997, Basmajan and De Luca, 1985)

Electrode types and configurations, as well as associated instrumentation, influence the quality of the EMG signal detected and displayed, recorded or processed (Merletti et al, 2001; Saitou et al, 2000; Rainoldi et al, 2004, Nishihara et al, 2008). Various studies have been dedicated to the matter and guidelines in EMG recording are available (Basmajan and De Luca, 1985, Hermens H.J. et al, 1999).

Surface electromyography (SEMG) analysis is a largely used EMG recording method as it is non-invasive, safe, it does not cause pain and it is simple to perform. Root mean square (RMS) of the surface EMG signals is often used as a concise quantitative index of muscle activity; indeed, electromyography devices often provide EMG RMS output.

SEMG is often used for the assessment of muscle activity occurring in response to physiological or to externally applied stimuli, i.e. vibratory stimulation.

Vibration stimulus is a mechanical muscle excitation, applied generally to a tendon, a muscle or to the body as a whole, aimed to activate muscles by eliciting stretch reflexes.

Local tendon vibrations induce activity of the muscle spindle Ia fibers, mediated by monosynaptic and/or polysynaptic pathways; the reflex muscle contraction that arises in response to such vibratory stimulus has been named Tonic Vibration Reflex (TVR). (Roll et al, 1989; Bongiovanni and Hagbart, 1990; Romaiguére et al, 1991; Person and Kozhina, 1992; Martin and Park, 1997)

As well as in other external stimulation, vibratory muscle activation can be examined by the analysis of electromyography recordings. Many studies report a significant increase of EMG RMS values in the lower body muscles during vibration training, these changes suggested

an increase in neuromuscular activity (Cardinale and Bosco, 2003; Verschueren et al, 2004). Specific WBV frequencies seem to produce a higher EMG RMS signal than others (Cardinale and Lim 2003).
However, as well as in every surface bio-potential recording, during local or whole body vibration treatment the EMG signal can be affected by artifacts.
Motion artifacts may in fact arise from relative motion between electrodes and skin and also between skin layers. The only skin stretch may result in a variation of electrode potential (Turker, 1993, De Talhouet and Webster, 1996; Ödman and Öberg, 1982, Searle and Kirkup, 2000, Tam and Webster, 1977).
In classical clinical EMG recordings (isokinetic, isotonic, gait, etc.), frequency content of motion artifact is considered below 10-20 Hz, then the general approach to motion artifact reduction is to apply a high-pass filter (e.g. with a cut-off frequency of 20 Hz).
During vibratory stimulation the artifact frequency contents, typically limited at vibratory frequency and its harmonics, extend within the EMG spectrum (Fratini et al, 2009) and standard high-pass filters are not suitable for filtering out this artifact.
In the majority of the cases appropriate filtering is used to remove motion artifacts before any signal analysis, while in some other they are used to characterize the mechanical response of the tissue to a specific stimulus (mechanogram) and its correlation to the stimulus itself (Person and Kozhina, 1992; Fratini et al, 2009).
With this chapter the authors aim to investigate the use and the efficacy of surface electromyography in the study of muscle response to vibration treatments. A review of vibration characterization and analysis is reported, SEMG recordings of Rectus Femoris , Vastus Medialis and Vastus Lateralis were collected and analyzed.
Specific artifacts were revealed and the role of those artifact was investigated and assessed. Since the use of vibratory stimulus produces peculiar EMG response a specific model was adopted to describe the EMG synchronization effect and its influence on the resultant recorded muscle activity (Person and Kozhina, 1992).

2. Vibratory stimulation

Different methods of vibratory stimulation have been reported in literature, however, the main are: local applied stimulus or whole body extended vibration.
Local stimulation is achieved by the use of vibrating devices directly applied on tendons of the muscle to be activated. The primary effect of this stimulation is a muscular reflex discharge of impulses some of which are locked with vibratory cycle.
Following the idea of stimulating muscle by using elicited reflex contraction like TVR, alternative methods have been proposed for vibration delivery.
Whole body vibration (vibration transferred to the body as a whole) is the most common used method of delivering vibration in the fields of sport medicine and exercise physiology for enhancing human performance.
In this mechanical stimulus delivery, individuals stand on an oscillating platform while vibrations transmit through the body to the target muscle depending on the subject posture.
Whole body vibration stimulations are produced in two main ways: by alternating rotation of a plate (tilting) or by vertical oscillation (see fig.1).
Alternative methods to deliver vibration are also reported in literature: vibratory modulation of loads during traditional dynamic exercise has also been applied to those typically seen in gymnasiums modified with a vibratory apparatus to produce localised

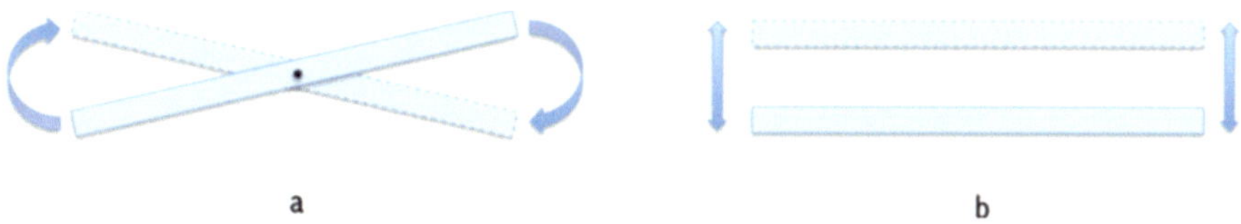

Fig. 1. Methods of whole body vibration stimulation. The figure depicts the two methods of platform oscillation: alternating rotation (a) and vertical oscillation (b).

vibrations to the body parts contacting the vibrating device (Cardinale and Bosco, 2003; Issurin et al, 1996; Yessis, 1992; Issurin and Tenenbaum , 1999; Nazarov and Spivak, 1987). However, in order to avoid misinterpretation in the communication of the experiments carried out by researchers, nomenclature has to be as standardized as possible (Lorenzen et al, 2008). Some few remarks are reported in the following paragraphs.

2.1 Magnitude of vibration

In whole body vibration studies, magnitude has been associated with displacement, amplitude, peak to peak displacement. (Lorenzen et al, 2008).

In the case of vibration, amplitude is the maximum displacement of a vibrating point from a mean position, while peak-to-peak displacement is used to describe the total vibration excursion of a point between its positive and negative extremes (see Figure 2).

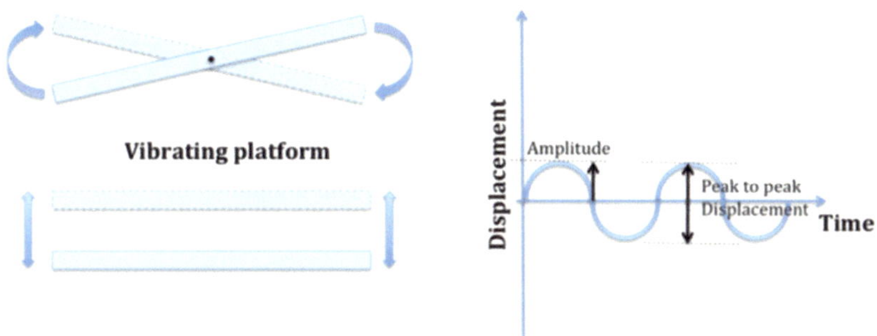

Fig. 2. Amplitude and peak to peak displacement of a vibrating object.

The movement of tilting and vertical oscillating platform can be assumed sinusoidal:

$$s(t) = A\sin(2\pi f) \tag{1}$$

where f is vibratory frequency, A is the amplitude.

In vertical oscillating platforms all the points will move approximately at the same way; they will have the same peak to peak displacement and the same maximal amplitude.

However, in tilting oscillating platform it is difficult to deduce the real acceleration or displacement to which the subject undergoes.

As shown in figure 3 feet distance from the rotation axis vary the magnitude of the stimulus delivered to the patient as well as the acceleration. It can be computed as the double derivatives of s(t):

$$a(t) = \frac{d^2 s(t)}{dt^2} = -A \cdot (2\pi f)^2 \cdot \sin(2\pi f) \tag{2}$$

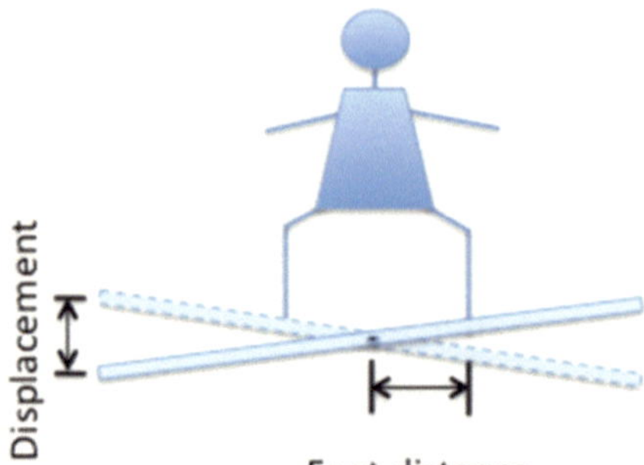

Fig. 3. Explanation of the variation in peak to peak displacement of platform fixed points depending on their distance from the axis.

2.2 Acceleration

Acceleration in not always reported as peak (maximal) acceleration, it depends on frequency and amplitude of the vibration (formula 2) and the maximal value (peak) can be easily computed by:

$$|a|_{\max} = A \cdot (2\pi f)^2 \tag{3}$$

Gravitational forces then, can be obtained by dividing the maximal acceleration by gravity g (9,81 [m][s]$^{-2}$). Therefore, an amplitude of 2.5 mm and a frequency of 25 Hz will produce a peak acceleration of a_{max} = 61.68 m s^{-2}. In Table 1 are shown some example of estimated maximal accelerations as a function of frequency and amplitude.

Amplitude [mm]	Frequency [Hz]	Acceleration [m][s]$^{-2}$
2	20	31,55
2	25	49,30
3	20	47,33
3	25	73,95
4	20	63,10
4	25	98,60

Table 1. Maximum acceleration produced for various amplitude and frequency.

Acceleration (maximum), amplitude and frequency are therefore the basic parameters to be reported in vibration studies. The use of the maximal acceleration will demonstrate to the reader the real vibration intensities applied to individuals.

3. Methods

3.1 Subjects & system set-up

Different individuals were involved in the study: twenty healthy subjects, ten males and ten females, not affected by any known neurological or musculoskeletal disorders, voluntarily participated in the study and gave their informed, written consent to participate. All of the subjects were not athletically trained.

A vibrating platform (XP Multipower - TSEM S.p.A., Padova - Italy) was used to deliver vibratory stimulation to the subjects.
Vibrations impressed by the platform were exclusively vertical (there was neither horizontal shift, nor pitch, roll or yaw); platform peak to peak displacement was set to 1.2 mm with a frequency ranging from 10 to 60 Hz. Being the peak-to-peak displacement constant, the maximum acceleration impressed to the patients depends on the square of the pulsation.

3.2 Data recording & processing

Before recording, the subjects were instructed about proper positioning on the platform (hack squat with a 110° knee flexion) and they were familiarized with the device. Signals from the Vastus Medialis (VM), Rectus Femoris (RF) and Vastus Lateralis (VL) of both of the legs were collected in accordance with SENIAM Project (Hermens et al, 1999) guidelines. In addition, a couple of supplementary electrodes was mounted on the patient's patella, supposing no EMG contribution at this site, to assess nature and magnitude of motion artifact on recordings. Signals were recorded using small disc Ag/AgCl electrodes (5 mm in diameter, inter-electrode distance of 20 mm arranged in the direction of the muscle fibres). Electrode skin areas were shaved and cleaned before the placement of electrodes and conductive paste was used. All the electrodes and cables were secured to prevent them from swinging and from causing induced artifact. EMG signals were amplified using a multi-channel, isolated biomedical signal amplifier (BM623 - Biomedica Mangoni, Pisa, Italy). The gain was set to 1000 V/V and a band pass filter (-3dB frequency 10 - 500 Hz) was applied; no notch filters were used. All signals were sampled at 2048 Hz. A set of consecutive 20-second vibrations at different frequencies: 15, 20, 25, 30, 35, 40, 45 Hz, spaced with 60 seconds rest intervals, was delivered to patient.
During rest intervals the patient stood up; five seconds before stimulus he reached the hack squat position. To minimize fatigue-related effects, the vibration frequencies order was randomized. Running RMS on each signal was estimated using 500 ms time window. RMS values were computed before and after artifact suppression to quantify motion artifact influence on EMG RMS.
Motion artifact components on recorded EMG signals were filtered out using a set of standard notch filters centred on the applied vibration stimulus frequency and its harmonics.
EMG power spectrum was computed using a standard FFT algorithm with a Hanning window of 2048 points. Noise (motion artifact) power was assessed considering only five narrow bands (1.5 Hz wide) centred at f0, 2f0, 3f0, 4f0, 5f0 where f0 is the applied vibration frequency. Artifacts filtering was achieved using sharp notch filter with a -3dB band of 3 Hz wide centred at f0, 2f0, 3f0, 4f0, 5f0.

3.3 EMG modelling

Surface electromyography signal acquired during a voluntary muscle contraction is assumed as summation of all the active Motor Units (MU) contributes (Basmajan and De Luca, 1985); it is largely dependent on the properties of MUs and their firing patterns as well as muscle innervation zones (Saitou et al, 2000).
The MUAP characteristics, i.e. shapes and distribution of amplitude and duration, are determined by morpho-functional properties of the activated muscle fibres and MUs,

together with passive and active bioelectric phenomena. The firing patterns reflect the motor control of the central nervous system and in particular situation, such as a vibratory stimulation, they may became correlated with the vibration frequency (Person and Kozhina, 1992, Lebedev and Polyakov, 1992).

3.3.1 MUAP shape

MUAPs shape was assumed biphasic and obtained by slightly modifying the type proposed by Lebedev and Polyakov described in the formula:

$$s_i(t) = a_i s(t) = \frac{a_i t}{(1.7t+1)^6} \tag{4}$$

where $s_i(t)$ represents the i-fibre MUAP waveform, t is the time variable expressed in ms and a_i corresponds to the MUAP amplitude. The formula was adapted to change independently either time-duration and amplitude variation for each phase, positive and negative (figure 4)

$$s_i(t) = a_i s(t) = \frac{a_i t}{((t*\tau)^6+1)} \tag{5}$$

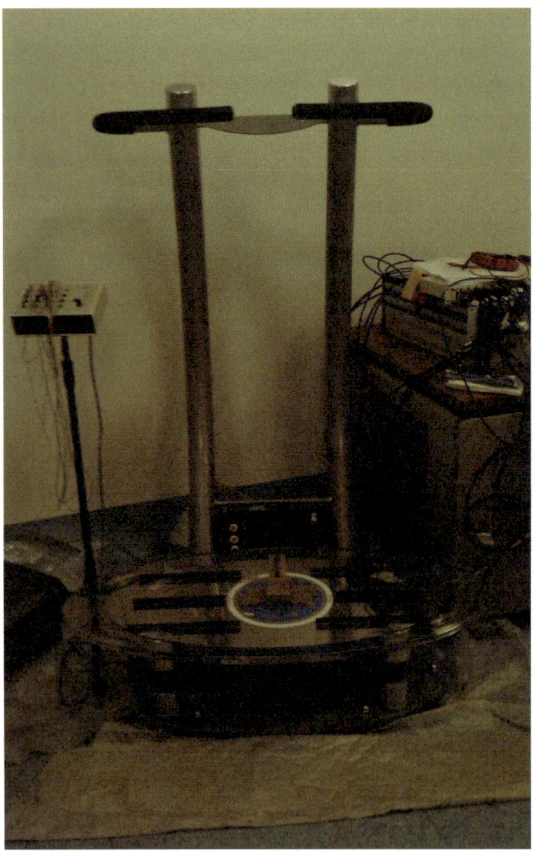

Fig. 4. Vibrating platform used to deliver vibratory stimulation (see text).

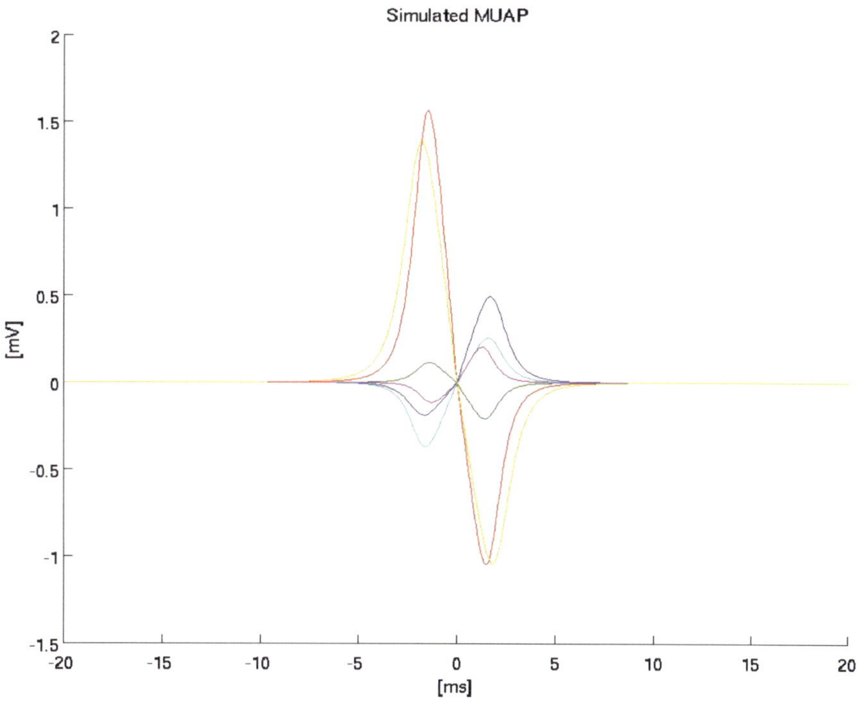

Fig. 5. Some of the different MUAPs obtained with the model.

The amplitude a_i was modeled as an uniform distribution in the range 0.01 to 0.5 mV to take in account the amplitude variability of the simulated signal.
The simulated EMG signal can be expressed as the summation of those MUAPTs:

$$e(t) = \sum_{i=1}^{N_{MU}} e_i(t) \tag{6}$$

where MUAPT, i.e. a summation of MUAPs of the same i-MU, $e_i(t)$, was described as follows:

$$e_i(t) = \sum_k s_i(t - t_k) \tag{7}$$

in which k is the number of pulses and t_k is the time instant of k-pulse of the i-MU.

3.3.2 Inter pulse interval

The general rule to describe the firing behavior of MUs is to consider their interpulse intervals (IPIs) as independent samples of a random variable.
The base distribution of the interpulse intervals, Δt_i ($t_{ki}-t_{(k-1)i}$) was then modeled as a normal distribution, with its probability density function (PDF) $g(\Delta t_i)$, with mean ΔT_i and standard deviation σ. Δt_i was considered as a random value uniformly distributed in the range 55-80 ms and σ equal to 12 ms in accordance to experimental data of Basmajian and De Luca (1985) on the Rectus Femoris.

However, different findings in literature have shown that when a vibratory stimulus is delivered to a tendon the firing rate became synchronous with the vibration cycle, that is t_{ki} is described by a specific PDF to that take into account this synchronization effect.
It is also known that, for vibration frequency under 60 Hz, the majority of MU (80 to 100%) are synchronous with the stimulus or its lower harmonics (Person and Kozhina, 1992).
The time interval between the vibratory stimulus and the activation of the i-MU (t_{cycle}) can also be characterized by a nearly Gaussian distribution $p(t_{cycle})$ with mean equal to half of the vibration period ($T_{vb}/2$) and variance (S_{cycle}) equal to 2 ms.

$$p(t_{cycle}) = Ae^{-\frac{(t_{cycle}-\frac{T_{vb}}{2})^2}{2S_{cycle}^2}} \tag{8}$$

with A is a normalizing factor and $0 < t_{cycle} < T_{vb}$
t_{cycle} is than correlated to the time variable t by:

$$\text{were n=1,2,3,...} \quad t = t_{cycle} + (n-1)T_{vb} \tag{9}$$

To provide simultaneously either the base variability of the interspike-intervals and the triggering effect modeled with $p(t_{cycle})$ distribution, a $h(t_{ki})$ PDF was built by multiplying the base PDF $g(\Delta t_i)$ with the $p(t_{cycle})$ PDF (these two distribution were assumed to be independent):

$$h(t_{ki}) = B \cdot g(t_{ki} - t_{ki-1}) \cdot p[-(n-1)T_{vb}] \tag{10}$$

where B is the normalization coefficient, and n is the number of cycle at which t_{ki} is referred to.
The initial value t_{1i} was generated from an uniform distribution in the range 0-ΔT_i; time of the kth discharge of the ith-MU t_{ki} was considered a random value, depending on the time of the preceding discharge t_{ki-1}.
If the effect of vibration is negligible, the PDF of the distribution of the IPIs would be close to $g(\Delta ti)$. However, in this work we assumed the majority of the MUs to be synchronous with vibration stimulus.

4. Results

Although prior to the stimulus onset the recorded signal resulted very low (subject were requested to maintain the hack squat position with a knee flexion of about 110°), after vibration start, the recorded EMGs grew, arising in amplitude.
Biopotential signals were recorded from VM, RF, VL and the patella and as it is possible to see from figure 6 a common behaviour was recognized. Patellar site was chosen for its negligible muscular contribution to the electrical potential recorded; however, its spectrum showed the same frequency components peaks of recorded EMGs (figure 7) and a first harmonic equivalent to the mechanical vibration frequency of the platform as already found in other studies (Fratini et al, 2009). Vibration-induced artifact appeared clearly visible in SEMG recordings (especially on VM, in the figure) after onset.
During vibration, power spectra clearly showed sharp peaks in correspondence to the mechanical frequency and its harmonics, similarly to those recorded onto the patella.

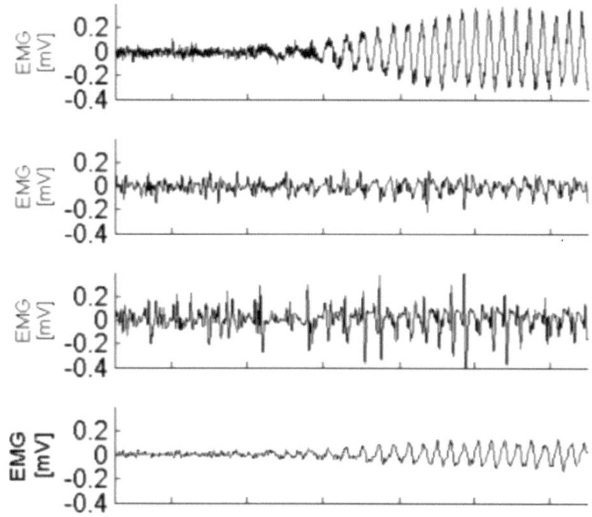

Fig. 6. Typical example of the recorded signals during a vibration onset. From the top to the bottom the first three signals represent VM, RF, VL SEMG respectively. The last is the recorded biopotential at the patellar site.

Presence of higher harmonics components could be an effect of non-linear mechanical behaviour of soft tissues.

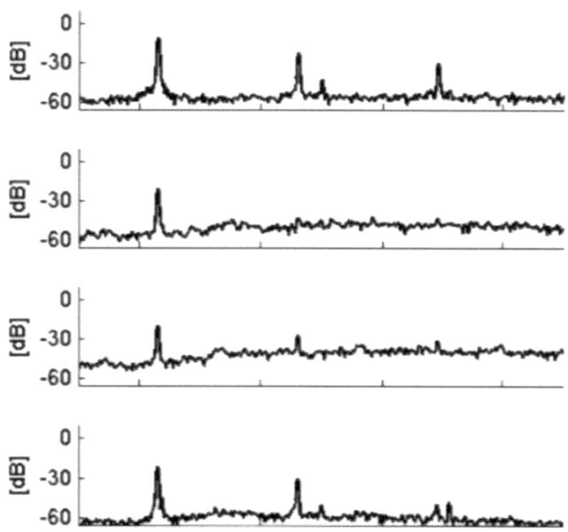

Fig. 7. Power spectrum of the previous SEMG and patella recordings, the first three signals represent VM, RF, VL SEMG spectra respectively while the last is spectrum of the biopotential recorded at the patellar site.

Previous results showed that the percentage of power content in artifacts bands represents less than 4% of total power (on average), while inter-subject standard deviation ranged from a minimum of 0.7% to a maximum 2.2% (on average) and as confirmed by our actual results after vibration onset, power related to the three to five considered bands raised significantly.

A typical SEMG response for RF muscle at different frequencies is depicted in figure 8; some frequencies seem to induce a higher myoelectrical activity. When subject held the hack squat position; the signal is supposed to contain only the spontaneous surface EMG, while a negligible contribution was recorded at the patellar site. However artifacts related to the vibration frequency and its harmonics laid within the standard surface EMG frequency band (a standard high-pass filter would be not suitable).

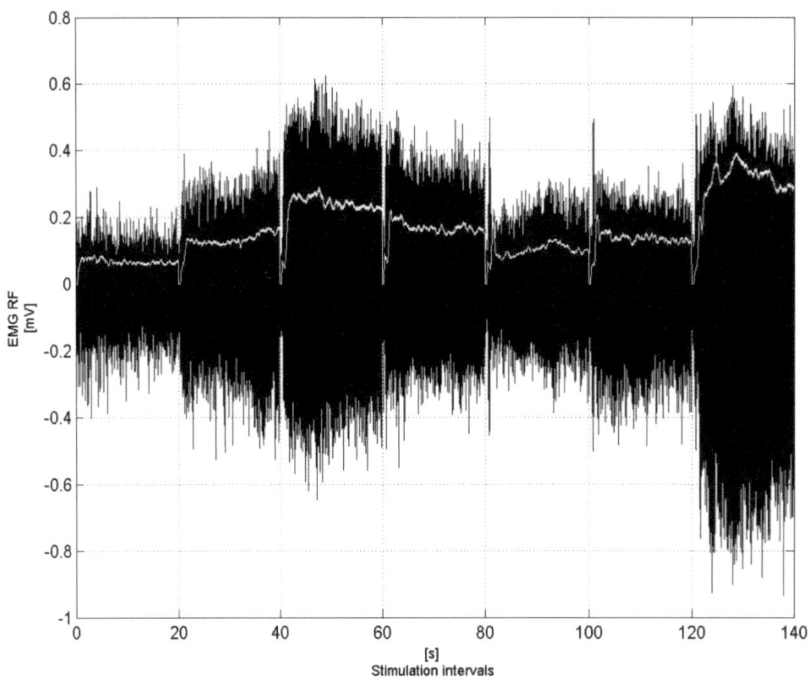

Fig. 8. Typical sequence of raw RF EMG recordings (only the stimulation phase is reported) at different stimulation frequency. A running RMS (white track) is also reported.

As previous study confirmed, the use of sharp notch filter can help in reduce uncertainty of muscle reaction analysis during vibratory stimulation.

After artifact removal signal changes significantly; results showed that the EMG RMS value computed on filtered signal (once motion artifact suppressed) can reduce up to 30% on average (up to 45% in some cases); this indicated that the power of motion artifact was not negligible with respect to SEMG activity.

The use of the considered model has helped in understanding of the behaviour of muscular complex response to vibratory stimulation: MUAP synchronization effect, distribution of IPI, etc. As result the simulated surface EMGs were very similar to those registered with surface electrodes from subjects under vibration.

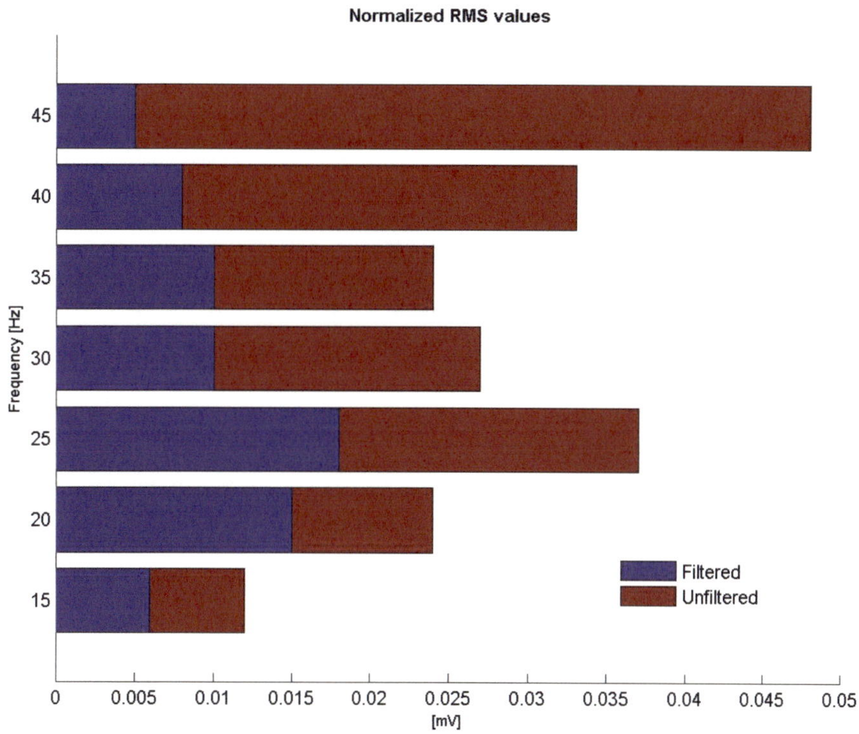

Fig. 9. Average RMS values of surface RF-EMG during vibration on all subjects: The diagram shows the difference of values between filtered (blue bars) and unfiltered signals (red bars). Signals were filtered using multiple notch to eliminate the artifact contribution (see text).

The example shown was obtained considering 600 active MUs and a 80% of them synchronous with a vibratory stimulation, and a random distance between electrodes and active end-plates. Vibration period in figure was set to 25 ms (40 Hz). As it can also be noticed from the figure, although none of the MUs is discharging at that frequency, there are peaks at 40 Hz and its multiples. It can be also noticed a slight increase of the spectrum at low frequencies, representative of the mean IPI (12-18 Hz).

Multiple test were conducted for each explored frequency, considering a random disposition of active end-plates. The power percentage of the spectrum, in a range of ±1.5 Hz around the vibration frequency and its first four superior harmonics, was estimated and on average less than 10% was found in those bands.

Various simulations were also conducted to determine the power percentage contained in the mentioned narrow bands without vibratory stimulation. The estimated power in those bands obviously decreases, in fact the first four multiples of 40 Hz had on average 5.38% of the total power with 0.95 standard deviation.

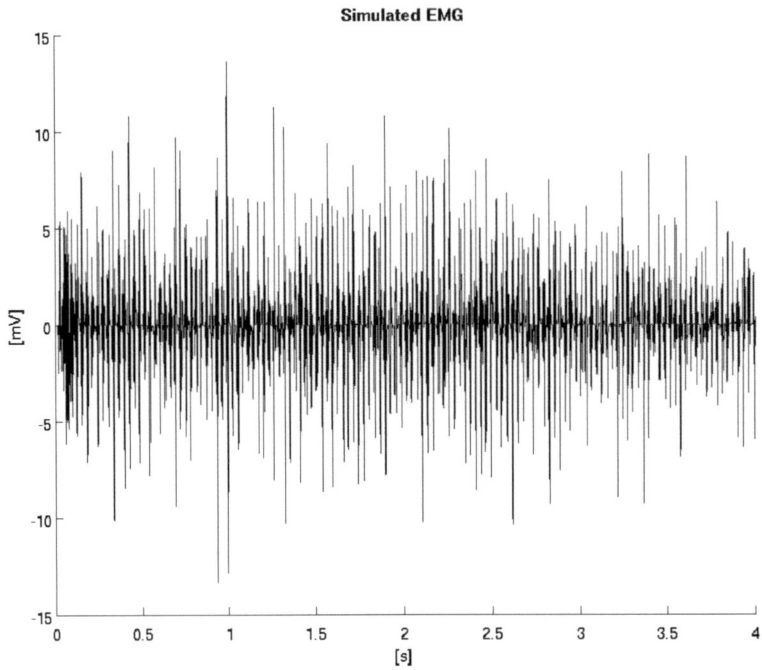

Fig. 10. An example of simulated SEMG signal obtained considering 600 active MUs and a vibratory stimulus at a frequency equal to 40 Hz.

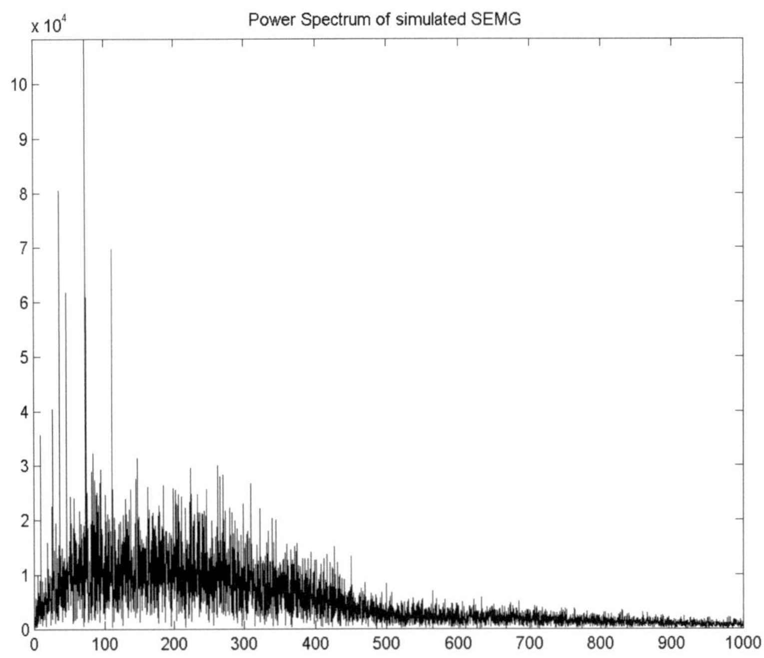

Fig. 11. An example of simulated SEMG signal obtained considering 600 active MUs and a vibratory stimulus at a frequency equal to 45 Hz.

5. Conclusion

Surface electromyography is a helpful technique for the analysis of muscle activity. However, its efficacy is related to the correct electrode positioning, the adequate skin preparation and opportune recording instrumentation. In addition, it is mandatory to recognize artifacts which may alter EMG signals and choose a particular filtering procedure before any additional analysis.

As confirmed by our results, vibrations generate peculiar, not negligible motion artifact on skin electrodes. The artifact appears in all the quadriceps muscles analysed (Vastus Medialis, Rectus Femoris and Vastus Lateralis) and in different amounts: artifact could depend on relative local muscle/electrode and skin layers motion.

Artifact spectrum only consists of the vibration frequency and its higher harmonics, its amplitude is unpredictable and depends on skin properties, electrode type and preparation, amplitude of vibration stimulus etc.

Artifact harmonics extend within the EMG spectrum, making classic high-pass filters unusable, however it is easy to get rid of the artifacts with a series of sharp notch filters centred at the vibration frequency and its superior harmonics applied to the raw EMG signal. Despite the presence of artifacts, some author consider the chance of a greater amount of true EMG appearing in the mentioned narrow frequency bands due to synchronous mechanical activation of muscles during vibration (Lebedev and Polyakov, 1992; Martin and Park, 1997).

Synchronization of motor unit (MU) during whole body vibration is a questionable argument. Surface EMG is formed by a summation of various MUAP components. Even not considering the contribution of the loosely-synchronized MU, all the MU synchronized with vibration must also be synchronized between each other in order to achieve a repeatable waveform.

Previous studies about the tonic vibration reflex concentrates on response of single motor unit (Romaiguère et al, 1991). A certain synchronization of some specific MUs, probably due to a monosynaptic reflex, has been found in response to vibration stimuli (taps) applied to proximal muscle tendon together with other much less synchronized MUs (probably polysynaptic reflexes) (Romaiguère et al, 1991). However, even the synchronized MUAP do not appear for each vibration pulse and also the latency from the tendon tap shows a standard deviation of about 1.4 ms (corresponding to a average of 22.7 ms) this implies a not exactly periodic signal. We have also pointed out differences between the case of delivery vibration stimuli directly to a specific muscle (often sequence of tapping of the distal tendon or muscle belly) and indirectly, i.e. from a sinusoidal vibrating plate (the vibration stimulus is mediated by a complex biomechanical chain before reaching a specific muscle).

The use of a specific EMG model in order to investigate and assess the actual muscle activity under vibratory stimulation was mandatory. The difference between simulated EMG signals and raw surface EMG recording, depending on the innervation zone, was found to be consistent, it can be reasonably justified by the presence of artifacts superimposed on the raw surface EMG.

However, results were find dependent on the relative position between electrodes and between electrodes and end-plates. In particular, a simulation of EMG recording considering MUAPs approaching only from a single direction would result in a much higher power percentage in the bands in which is also present the artifact contribution. However, according to our results, it is also true that the electrodes placed onto the patella showed an amount of power associated to the considered narrow bands comparable with that of the recorded EMG on quadriceps muscles. In conclusion, analysis of muscular activity during vibration based on unprocessed surface EMG recordings may significantly overestimate muscle response: filtering out the motion artifact would prevent misinterpretation of experimental results. It is our opinion however, that we cannot exclude a-priori that the true EMG power spectrum can show peak components at the vibration frequency and its harmonics.

6. Acknowledgment

Authors are grateful to TSEM S.p.A. for providing the vibration training device and customer hardware modifications.

7. References

Basmajian, J.V., De Luca, C.J. (1985). *Muscles alive* (5th ed.). Baltimore: Williams & Wilkins, ISBN 978-068-3004-14-4

Bongiovanni L.G. Hagbarth K.E. (1990). *TVR elicited during fatigue from maximal voluntary contractions in man*. Journal of Physiology (Lond) 423.

Burke D., Schiller, H.H. (1976). *Discharge pattern of single motor units in the tonic vibration reflex of human triceps surae*. Journal of Neurology, Neurosurgery & Psychiatry. Vol. 39, No. 8, pp 729-741.

Cardinale M., Bosco C. (2003). *The use of vibration as an exercise intervention*. Exercise & Sport Sciences Reviews. Vol. 31, No. 1, pp 3-7.

Cardinale M., Lim J. (2003). *Electromyography activity of vastus lateralis muscle during whole-body vibrations of different frequencies*. Journal of Strength & Conditioning Research. Vol. 17, No. 3, pp 621-624.

Clancy E.A., Morin E.L., Merletti R. (2002). *Sampling, noise-reduction and amplitude estimation issues in surface electromyography*. Journal of Electromyography and Kinesiology. Vol. 12, No. 1, pp 1-16.

De Luca, C.J. (1997). The use of surface electromyography in biomechanics, *Journal of Applied Biomechanics*, Vol.13, pp. 135-163

De Talhouet H., Webster J.G. (1996). *The origin of skin-stretch-caused motion artifact under electrodes*. Physiological Measurement. Vol. 17, No. 2, pp 81-93.

Fratini A, Cesarelli M., Bifulco P., Romano M. (2009). *Relevance of motion artifact in electromyography recordings during vibration treatment*. Journal of Electromyography & Kinesiology. Vol. 19, No.4, pp 710-718.

Hermens H.J., Freriks B., Merletti R., Stegeman D., Blok J., Rau G., Disselhorst-Klug C., Hägg G. (1999) European Recommendations for Surface ElectroMyoGraphy, *Results of SENIAM Project*. 8th ed. Enschede: Roessingh Research and Development

Issurin V.B., Tenenbaum G. (1999). *Acute and residual effects of vibratory stimulation on explosive strength in elite and amateur athletes.* Journal of Sports Sciences. Vol. 17, No. 3, pp 177-182.

Yessis M. (1992). *Vibrational devices.* Fitness and Sports Review International. Vol. 27, No. 2, pp 67.

Lebedev M.A., Polyakov A.V. (1992). *Analysis of surface EMG of human soleus subjected to vibration.* Journal of Electromyography & Kinesiology. Vol. 2, 1):26–35.

Lorenzen C., Mashette W., Koh M., Wilson C. (2008). *Inconsistent use of terminology in whole body vibration exercise research.* Journal of Science and Medicine in Sport, doi:10.1016/j.jsams.2008.06.008

Martin B.J., Park H.S. (1997). *Analysis of the tonic vibration reflex: Influence of vibration variables on motor unit synchronization and fatigue.* European Journal of Applied Physiology. Vol. 75, No. 6, pp 504–511.

Merletti R., Rainoldi A., Farina D. (2001). *Surface Electromyography for Noninvasive Characterization of Muscle.* Excercise and Sport Science Reviews. Vol.29, No.1,pp 20-25

Nazarov V., Spivak G. (1987). *Development of athlete's strength abilities by means of biomechanical stimulation method.* Theory and Practice of Physical Culture. Vol. 12, pp 37-39.

Nishihara K., Kawai H., Gomi T., Terajima M., Chiba Y. (2008). IEEE Transaction on Biomedical Engineering, Vol. 55, No. 2, pp 636-642

Ödman S, Åke Öberg P. (1982). *Movement-induced potentials in surface electrodes.* Medical and Biological Engineering and Computing. Vol. 20, No. 2, pp 159-66.

Person, R. ; Kozhina, G. (1992). Tonic vibration reflex of human limb muscles: Discharge pattern of motor units, *Journal of Electromyography and Kinesiology*,Vol.2, No. 1, pp. 1-9

Rainoldi A., Melchiorri G., Caruso I. (2004). *A method for positioning electrodes during surface EMG recordings in lower limb muscles.* Journal of Neuroscience Methods. Vol.34, pp 37-43

Roll J.P., Vedel J.P., Ribot E. (1989). *Alteration of proprioceptive messages induced by tendon vibration in man: a microneurographic study.* Experimental Brain Research. Vol. 76, No. 1, pp 213-22.

Romaiguère P, Vedel J.P., Azulay J.P., Pagni S. (1991). *Differential activation of motor units in the wrist extensor muscles during the tonic vibration reflex in man.* Journal of Physiology. Vol. 444, No. 1, pp 645-67.

Saitou K., Masuda T., Michikami D., Kojima R., Okada M. (2000). *Innervation zones of the upper and lower limb muscles estimated by using multichannel surface EMG.* Journal of Human Ergology. Vol.29, pp 35-52.

Searle A., Kirkup L. (2000). *A direct comparison of wet, dry and insulating bioelectric recording electrodes.* Physiological Measurement. Vol. 21, pp 271-83.

Tam H., Webster J.G. (1977) *Minimizing electrode motion artifact by skin abrasion.* IEEE Transactions on Biomedical Engineering. Vol. 24, No. 2, pp 134-39.

Turker KS. (1993). *Electromyography: some methodological problems and issues.* Physical Therapy. Vol. 73, No. 10, pp 698-710.

Verschueren S.M., Roelants M., Delecluse C., Swinnen S., Vanderschueren D., Boonen S. (2004). *Effect of 6-month whole body vibration training on hip density, muscle strength, and postural control in postmenopausal women: A randomized controlled pilot study.* Journal of Bone and Mineral Research. Vol. 19, No. 3, pp 352-359.

Part 2

Posture, Prevention of Falls and Robotics

4

The Role of Electromyography (EMG) in the Study of Anticipatory Postural Adjustments

William P. Berg[1] and Adam J. Strang[2]
[1]*Department of Kinesiology and Health, Miami University, Oxford, Ohio*
[2]*Consortium Research Fellows Program, Wright-Patterson AFB, Ohio*
USA

1. Introduction

Postural control and stability are critical to the execution of almost any voluntary movement. In fact, "posture is the foundation upon which movement rides" (Cram & Criswell, 2011, p. 182). Posture is actively controlled by the neuromuscular system in concert with somatosensory, visual and vestibular informational inputs. To maintain a desirable posture under a wide range of individual, task and environmental constraints, the central nervous system (CNS) minimizes deflections of the body from a desirable orientation through the use of postural adjustments that fall into two general categories, compensatory and anticipatory (Santos et al., 2010). *Compensatory postural adjustments* (CPAs) are feedback-based mechanisms that are initiated by sensory events following the loss of desirable posture (Alexandrov et al., 2005; Park et al., 2004). CPAs act to restore stability after a postural perturbation has occurred (Henry et al., 1998; Macpherson et al., 1989; Maki & McIlroy, 1996). For example, immediately after a trip, reflexive and/or consciously controlled CPAs could help prevent a fall.

The second category of adjustments, and the focus of this chapter, are *anticipatory postural adjustments* (APAs). APAs are feed-forward mechanisms elicited by expected postural disturbances that produce preemptive muscle responses that help maintain stability. For example, when reaching for an object such as a book on a shelf, muscles in the trunk and legs activate in advance of muscle activity and movement in the shoulder and arm (Aruin & Latash, 1995a). These contractions in trunk and leg muscles constitute APAs because they precede the principal (focal) movement of the arm[1].

APAs were first described in 1967 when Belen'kii et al. reported the existence of electrical activity in the sacrolumbar muscles of the trunk and upper leg prior to fast shoulder flexion in standing. The presumed functional roles of APAs are to predict the stability-perturbing forces to be generated by an imminent focal movement or external perturbation, and produce a preparatory muscular contraction (i.e., APA) to stabilize the body in advance of the perturbation (Aruin & Latash, 1995a; Bouisset & Zattara, 1987; Massion, 1992; Zattara & Bouisset, 1988). Research has demonstrated that APAs are tailored to specific characteristics

[1] There is a relationship between the anticipatory and compensatory components of postural control. Specifically, it has been proposed that the CNS attempts to optimize the use of APAs, when possible, in order to allow for a suitable "scaling-down" of compensatory activity (Santos et al., 2010).

of focal movements, such as the direction (Aruin & Latash, 1995a), load (Aruin & Latash, 1995b; Aruin et al., 2001), acceleration (Lee et al, 1987; Zattara & Bouisset, 1988), and velocity (Hodges & Richardson, 1999). APAs are also influenced by conditions such as Parkinson's disease (Aruin et al., 1996), stroke (Dickstein et al., 2004), low back injury (Hodges, 2001; Hodges et al., 2003; Hodges & Richardson, 1996; Hodges & Richardson, 1999), and muscle fatigue (Allison & Henry, 2002; Strang & Berg, 2007; Strang et al., 2008; Strang et al., 2009; Vuillerme et al., 2002). For example, fatigue in lower extremity, upper extremity, and trunk muscles has been shown to result in earlier APA onset during focal movements, compared to APA onset in the absence of fatigue (Allison & Henry, 2002; Kanekar et al., 2008; Strang & Berg, 2007; Strang et al., 2008; Strang et al., 2009; Vuillerme et al., 2002). It has been speculated that this effect represents a functional attempt by the CNS to limit additional postural disturbance resulting from the presence of muscle fatigue, when force-producing capabilities of muscles are likely compromised (Allison & Henry, 2002; Kanekar et al., 2008; Strang & Berg, 2007; Vuillerme et al., 2002). Strang et al. (2009) confirmed that fatigue-induced early APA onset is, indeed, a centrally mediated adaptation.

Compared to the role of APAs in self-induced stability perturbations - the focus of the discussion thus far - the role of APAs in externally-induced stability perturbations has received less attention. Externally-induced perturbations include those that can occur when catching an object or being knocked off balance while walking on a crowded sidewalk. There is evidence that APAs can occur in conjunction with catching an object, even though the stability perturbation is not self-induced (Eckerle et al., 2011; Kazennikov & Lipshits, 2010; Lacquaniti & Maioli, 1989a, 1989b; Shiratori & Latash, 2001). The function of APAs in catching is to predict the stability perturbing forces to be imposed by the object on the catcher, and to produce preparatory muscular activity in order to stabilize the limb/body in advance of the catch. It is also known that APAs occur in catching even when information about ball weight is unavailable (Kazennikov & Lipshits, 2010). In this case, the CNS appears to scale APA magnitude to afford the greatest chance of catching the ball, regardless of weight (Eckerle et al., 2011).

2. How are APAs studied?

Experiments intended to better understand APAs in self-induced stability perturbations require experimental tasks that when performed, reliably induce APAs. Many researchers have used rapid arm-raising/reaching tasks to produce postural perturbations in the anterior direction (Belen'kii et al., 1967; Benvenuti et al., 1997; Bouisset & Zattara, 1987; De Wolf et al., 1998; Friedli et al., 1984; Gantchev & Dimitrova, 1996; Latash et al., 1995; Shiratori & Latash, 2001; Slijper et al., 2002; Strang & Berg, 2007; Strang et al., 2008; Strang et al., 2009. In this task paradigm, research participants typically stand bipedally with arms at their sides, and respond to an auditory or visual stimulus by moving one or both arms forward and up in the saggital plane as quickly as possible using shoulder flexion exclusively (see Figure 1). This maneuver produces rapid forward-displacement of the center of mass (COM) and reliably elicits APAs in the lumbar paraspinal, abdominal, and hamstring muscles.

Experiments on the role of APAs in externally-induced stability perturbations have utilized moving platforms (Timmann & Horak, 2001), pendulums (Santos et al., 2010), and one-handed catching tasks (Eckerle et al., 2011; Kazennikov & Lipshits, 2010; Lacquaniti & Maioli, 1989a, 1989b; Shiratori & Latash, 2001). APAs are important in catching because the

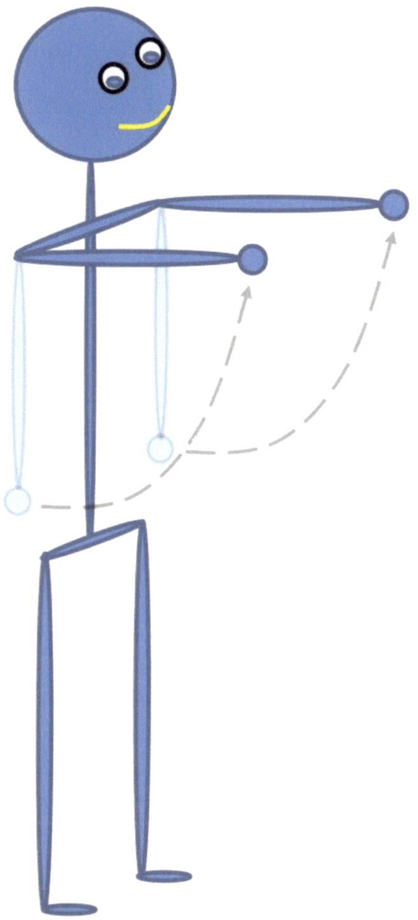

Fig. 1. Illustration of a rapid bilateral arm-raising maneuver (adapted from Strang et al., 2008).

compliance of the catching limb/hand needs to closely match the properties of impulsive impact. The properties of impact will vary depending on the weight of the object to be caught and the height from which the object is dropped. If limb compliance too high, the catching arm/hand could yield upon contact; whereas if limb compliance is too low, the object could rebound (Lacquaniti & Maioli, 1989a). In either case, arm/hand yielding or ball rebounding, a successful catch is unlikely. The catching maneuver depicted in Figure 2 produces rapid forward-displacement of the COM and the reliably elicits APAs in the wrist flexors, bicep brachii, anterior deltoid and lumbar paraspinal muscles.

Research participants have been asked to perform APA-inducing tasks, such as those described above, under various conditions that are determined by the research question under investigation. For example, Strang and colleagues have examined APAs under conditions of muscular fatigue (Strang & Berg, 2007; Strang et al., 2008; Strang et al., 2009). As for dependent variables, much of what has been learned about APAs has been acquired by recording electromyographic (EMG) signals from the muscles involved in both postural control and the focal movement (Rosenbaum, 2011). At any point in time, the surface EMG signal is a composite electrical sum of all active motor units in an observed muscle or muscle group (Robertson et al., 2004). The amplitude of the EMG signal is an indicator of the magnitude of muscle activity, and is produced by increases in the number of active motor units and the frequency of activation (Robertson et al., 2004). Naturally, EMG amplitude increases as the intensity of muscle contraction increases. However, the relationship between EMG amplitude and force frequently is nonlinear (Robertson et al., 2004).

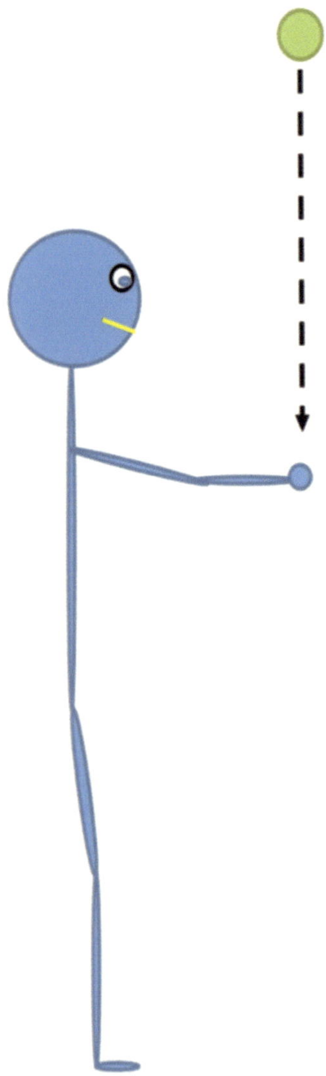

Fig. 2. Illustration of a one-handed catching task.

The purpose of EMG assessment is to document the activity of muscles under different conditions (Donaldson et al., 2003). As Basmajian (1967) stated, "electromyography is unique in revealing what a muscle actually does at any moment during movement and postures. Moreover, it reveals objectively the fine interplay or coordination of muscles: this is patently impossible by any other means" (p. 22). Regarding the study of APAs, EMG is commonly used to evaluate two fundamental properties of APAs, timing and magnitude.

3. Using EMG to ascertain the timing of APAs

Frequently, movement scientists are interested in determining when muscle electrical activity begins and/or ends, and this is especially true when studying APAs. Judging whether or not muscle activity qualifies as anticipatory requires a comparison of the onset of muscle activity to other temporal events, such as movement initiation or the activation onset of other muscles. The criteria used to identify muscle activity as anticipatory varies considerably in the literature. In most studies, however, muscle activity is considered anticipatory only when it occurs within a specified period of time - referred to as the APA timing-window (Allison, 2003). In studies on APAs resulting from self-induced postural perturbations, the APA timing-window has been established in reference to one of two events; 1) the onset of the focal movement (Aruin & Latash, 1995; Bleuse et al., 2006; Girolami et al., 2010; Mochizuki et al., 2004; Schmitz et al., 2002; van Dieën & de Looze, 1999), or 2) the onset of muscle activity in the prime mover (agonist) of the focal movement (De Wolf et al., 1998; Fujiwara et al., 2003; Jacobs et al., 2009; Kanekar et al., 2008; Lee et al., 2009; Mannion et al., 2008; Mezaour et al., 2010; Morris & Allison, 2006; Strang et al., 2007; Strang et al., 2008; Tsao & Hodges, 2007; Tsao & Hodges, 2008; van der Fits et al., 1999; van der Heide et al., 2003; Yiou et al., 2009). A common example of the latter reference event is the onset of anterior deltoid muscle activity during forward arm-raising (e.g., Fujiwara et al., 2003; Gantchev et al., 1996; Morrison & Allison, 2006; Nana-Ibrahim et al., 2008; Strang & Berg, 2007; Tsao & Hodges, 2007; Vuillerme et al., 2002). In either case, the reference event is referred to as time zero (T_0), and the APA timing-window is defined relative to T_0[2]. It is generally assumed that muscle activity occurring just before or very shortly after T_0 must be pre-programmed, and therefore qualifies as anticipatory - although there may be problems with this assumption, which will be addressed later in the chapter. In contrast, studies of externally-induced postural perturbations usually define T_0 as the onset of the perturbation (Eckerle et al., 2011; Kazennikov & Lipshits, 2010; Lacquaniti & Maioli, 1989a, 1989b; Li & Aruin, 2007; Santos & Aruin, 2008; Santos et al., 2010; Shiratori & Latash, 2001; Timmann & Horak, 1998).

APA researchers have used a variety of techniques for detecting the onsets of focal movements and externally-induced perturbations including accelerometers (Girolami et al., 2010), video/motion capture (Bleuse et al., 2006), force transducers (van Dieën & de Looze, 1999) switch mats (Strang et al., 2009), and photoelectric techniques (Eckerle et al., 2011). The only requirement is that these devices possess high levels of temporal resolution, accuracy and reliability, and that they be able to interface with an EMG recording system.

As for identifying the onset of muscle activity in a prime mover and/or postural control muscles, APA researchers typically use one of two general techniques. The first involves visually inspecting the EMG signal to identify the earliest detectable change in EMG activity

[2] One study, however, established the APA timing-window using both the onset of the focal movement and the onset of muscle activity in the prime mover of the focal movement (Strang et al., 2009).

beyond baseline (e.g., Allison & Henry, 2002; De Wolf et al., 1998; Hodges et al., 2001; Hodges & Richardson, 1996, 1998; Mannion et al., 2008; Mezaour et al., 2010; Strang & Berg, 2007; Strang et al., 2008; Strang et al., 2009; Tsao & Hodges, 2007, 2008). Although visual inspection of the EMG signal is subjective, this technique has been shown to be reliable (Hodges & Bui, 1996). Visual inspection requires that EMG readers have adequate training and experience, and that satisfactory inter and intra-reader reliability is achieved prior to the beginning of data reduction and analysis.

Alternative computer-based techniques utilize statistical algorithms to determine muscle EMG onset (e.g., Jacobs et al., 2009; Kanekar et al., 2008; van der Fits et al., 1999; van der Heide et al., 2003). The most common automated EMG onset detection technique is the standard deviation (SD) method (Hodges & Bui, 1996), also broadly referred to as Shewhart protocols (Allison & Eastwood, 2002; Stokes et al., 2000). Shewhart protocols use different thresholds as multiples of average baseline EMG amplitude during a target window, for example, two SD (Hodges & Richardson, 1996) and three or more SD (Di Fabio, 1987; Happee & Van der Helm, 1995; Hodges & Bui, 1996; Stokes et al., 2000; Studenski et al., 1991) above baseline EMG amplitude have been reported. The advantages of computer-based methods are increased objectivity, faster data reduction, and a reduced requirement for EMG reader experience. Regardless of the onset identification technique employed, a EMG sampling rate of at least 1000 Hz should be used to achieve satisfactory temporal resolution.

In comparing the applicability of visual inspection and computer-based muscle EMG onset detection techniques in the context of APAs, using computer-based methods is especially difficult because the detection algorithms need to be sensitive to very small increments beyond the baseline signal (Allison, 2003). The reason for this is that APA onset is followed immediately by significantly larger amplitude compensatory responses (Allison, 2003). Moreover, the SD method can be ineffective for identifying APA onset when there is significant noise and/or electro-cardiac (ECG) artifact, or when EMG activity increases slowly (Allison, 2003; Hodges & Bui, 1996). These issues may partly explain why visual detection methods are often preferred for detecting APA onset (Allison, 2003). Moreover, it is not uncommon for an automated method for identification of APA onset to be accompanied by a visual check of each trace against the computer-derived value to ensure that the onset is meaningful (Adkin et al., 2002).

Smoothing is typically done prior to analyzing EMG signals to reduce baseline noise or ECG artifact. However, excessive smoothing of the data results in a loss of information and inaccurate identification of muscle onset (Gabel & Brandt, 1994; Halbertsma & DeBoer, 1981; Soderberg & Cook, 1984). On the other hand, insufficient data smoothing results in delayed identification of muscle onset (Hodges & Bui, 1996). The low pass cut-off frequency that most accurately and consistently determined the muscle onset in a study by Hodges & Bui (1996) was 50 Hz. Other studies have incorporated filtration similar to this value (Di Fabio, 1987; Nashner et al., 1983).

To increase the likelihood of detecting genuine APA onsets, the only postural muscle onsets that qualify as anticipatory are those that occur within the defined APA timing-window. The use of the APA timing-window is based on physiological limits and expectations of response latencies (Allison, 2003). Muscle activity onsets that occur too long after T_0 are more likely to represent compensatory rather than anticipatory activity. Likewise, muscle activity that occurs too far in advance of T_0 may not be directly related to the focal movement.

There is tremendous variability in the literature regarding the definition of the APA timing-window. First, and as mentioned earlier, studies on self-induced APAs often differ as to how T_0 is defined, i.e., some researchers define focal movement onset as T_0 and some define the onset of EMG activity in the prime mover as T_0 . The impact of the discrepancy in defining T_0 as different motor events has not been discussed in the literature. However, this issue is important because for any given focal movement, these two events are unlikely to occur simultaneously. In fact, in most focal movements, there is a delay between the onset of EMG activity in the prime mover and the actual initiation of movement. The delay is referred to as motor reaction-time and is attributed to the contractile properties of muscle and spread of electrical activity across the muscle that is required to generate enough force to start a focal movement (Fischman, 1984; Weiss, 1965). Strang & Berg (2007) and Strang and colleagues (2009) showed that the delay in typical unilateral and bilateral arm-raising maneuvers was 70 ms and 140 ms, respectively[3]. From this, it is not only apparent that a significant delay exists between agonist EMG onset and movement initiation, but also that this lag is influenced by the nature of the focal task itself.

Finally, not only does the referent for establishment of the APA timing-window differ across studies, the establishment of the beginning and end of APA timing-windows also varies tremendously. Studies of self-induced APAs using onset of the focal movement as T_0 have employed APA timing-windows ranging from the 200 ms prior to T_0 (Mochizuki et al., 2004) to $T_0 \pm 50$ ms (Schmitz et al., 2002). $T_0 + 50$ ms is the most commonly used termination point for the APA timing-window. The rationale is that since a latency of $T_0 + 50$ ms marks the threshold for the monosynaptic reflex, i.e., the earliest any form of feedback can be used to produce movement adjustments (Aruin & Latash, 1995a, 1995b), $T_0 + 50$ ms reflects the latest point at which one can safely assume that only feed-forward activity (APA) is reflected in the EMG signal.

Studies of self-induced APAs using the onset of EMG activity in the prime mover as T_0 have utilized APA timing-windows ranging from 300 ms prior to T_0 to 50 ms after T_0 (Mezaour et al., 2010), to 100 ms proceeding T_0 to 200 ms after T_0 (De Wolf et al., 1998). The lack of standardization across studies in defining the APA timing-window means that postural muscle onsets that would be described as anticipatory in some studies would not be described similarly in other studies. As will be addressed in the next section, this methodological variation also impacts the measurement of APA magnitude. In studies of externally-induced APAs, where there has at least been agreement that external perturbation onset represents T_0, vastly different APA timing-windows have been employed as well, ranging from the 500 ms prior to T_0 (Kazennikov & Lipshits, 2010), to 100 ms before T_0 to $T_0 + 50$ ms (Aruin & Latash, 1995).

As an example of a study that focused on APA timing, Strang and Berg (2007) examined the fatigue-induced adaptive timing changes of APAs. APAs of 30 research participants were recorded before (baseline) and after (post-test) conditions of either rest (control group, n = 15) or fatigue (fatigue group, n = 15). Muscle fatigue was generated using a dead-lift exercise performed to exhaustion. Results showed that fatigue had no effect on postural stability during the focal movement, and yet caused earlier APA onsets in three of the six muscles evaluated. In spite of early APA activation, the APA EMG integrals of two of the three postural control muscles which exhibited fatigue-induced early APA onsets (T9 and L4

[3] Average motor reaction-times estimated from data collapsed across conditions shown in Table 1, p. 56 (Strang & Berg, 2007), and Table 3, p. 250 (Strang et al., 2009).

contralateral paraspinals) did not differ between baseline and post-test measures. The findings suggested that early APA onset may enhance postural stability by permitting a longer duration APA which can counteract fatigue-induced decreases in the force-producing capability of muscles that contribute to postural stability.

4. Using EMG to ascertain the magnitude of APAs

Researchers have relied on measures such as EMG integral (Aruin & Latash, 1995a, 1995b; Fujiwara et al., 2003; Strang & Berg, 2007), EMG Root Mean Square (RMS) amplitude (Lee et al., 2009; Tsao & Hodges, 2007), and EMG mean amplitude (van Dieën & de Looze, 1999; Van der Fits et al., 1999; van der Heide et al., 2003) to quantify the magnitude of muscle activity associated with APAs. In the following section, the nuances in the computations, interpretations, and applications of these measures are reviewed, along with a brief discussion of the EMG-force relationship within the context of APAs.

4.1 EMG integral

The most popular measure of APA magnitude has been the EMG integral, $\int EMG_{Integral}$ (Adkin et al., 2002; Aruin & Latash, 1995a, 1995b; Aruin et al., 1996; Aruin et al., 1998; De Wolf et al., 1998; Fujiwara et al., 2003; Girolami et al., 2010; Mochizuki et al., 2004; Nana-Ibrahim et al., 2008; Santos & Aruin, 2008; Strang & Berg, 2007; Xiaoyan & Aruin, 2007). This measure follows the basic formula, $\int EMG_{Integral} = \int EMG_{APA} - \int EMG_{Baseline}$ where $\int EMG_{APA}$ and $\int EMG_{Baseline}$ are the sum of rectified EMG amplitudes across timing-windows of equal duration. There are two noteworthy features regarding the computation of EMG integral for APAs, which are, 1) the EMG integral is an estimate of the total EMG activity associated with an APA relative to baseline EMG, and 2) estimates of the EMG integral require equivalent duration APA timing- and baseline timing-windows.

With regard to the first feature, there are both practical and theoretical reasons why EMG integrals for APAs are estimated relative to baseline EMG, rather than a more standard comparator, e.g., EMG obtained during maximal voluntary isometric contraction (MVIC). First, MVICs are difficult to obtain for lumbar and trunk muscles where APAs are often observed[4]. Second, APAs elicit EMG activity that is so small compared to that produced during voluntary isometric contractions[5], that relative comparisons would likely result in floor effects for integral estimates. Finally, while an APA can generally be considered a form of sub-maximal isometric muscle contraction, unlike MVICs, which are typically obtained during prolonged contraction following the slow development of muscle tension (Disselhorst-Klug et al., 2009), an APA exhibits a rapid onset, is involuntary, and take place over an extremely brief period of time (less than 150ms). These attributes of APAs make it difficult to estimate the force produced by APAs from EMG, since it is known that during rapid isometric contraction of relaxed muscles that force is not generated during the first 50-100ms of activation - this is because the muscle must first build intrinsic tension

[4] See McGill (1991) for a review of the difficulty in obtaining MVICs from lumbar and trunk muscles.

[5] See Figure 5, p. 402, of van Dieën & de Looze (1999) to view an example of how little EMG activity is associated with APAs relative to that produced during even sub-maximal voluntary isometric contractions of lumbar muscles.

(Disselhorst-Klug et al., 2009). Though speculative, this dilemma is why most researchers have refrained from attempting to draw direct inference about the force produced by APAs from APA magnitude measures.

For the most part, the APA timing-windows used for computing EMG integrals have been similar to those used for detecting APA onsets, and thus have been wildly diverse. What is unique in the case of EMG integral calculation is the requirement of an equivalent-duration baseline time-window, which has typically been set at some pre-established time period prior to T_0 (e.g., T_0 -800 ms to -650 ms; Strang & Berg, 2007) where muscles are assumed to be in a relaxed state[6]. It has also been common to obtain estimates of EMG baseline integrals in smaller timing-windows, e.g., 50 ms, and then multiply the integral estimate by a common factor, e.g., 2, to achieve equivalent-duration baseline integrals to that of the pre-defined APA timing-window (Aruin & Shiratori, 2003; Shiratori & Aruin, 2004).

Finally, it is worth noting that there is a practical concern for studies that compute the EMG integral while also defining T_0 as the beginning of the focal movement. APA onset in such cases could precede the established timing-window set for integral estimates. Put another way, it is possible that in some, or perhaps many cases, when T_0 is defined as focal movement initiation, that EMG activity indicative of an APA may not be included in the computation of the EMG integral. To illustrate this point, we re-examined data presented by Strang et al., (2009) that included reports of EMG onset of the prime mover (anterior deltoid), EMG APA onset in selected postural muscles (low back and hamstring), and focal movement initiation (reaction time). From these data it was discovered that if T_0 had been defined as focal movement initiation, as opposed to the onset of the prime mover as was the case, APA onsets would have preceded the established APA timing-window (T_0 -100ms to +50ms) by an average of 50ms. This means that a significant amount of EMG activity that potentially represented an APA would not have been included in EMG integral calculations had that measure been derived.

4.2 Normalizing the EMG integral

EMG integrals for APAs are not typically reported in standard units of voltage [e.g., millivolt/s, see Fujiwara et al., (2003)], but instead as normalized values. This is done to account for large within and between-subject variability typically seen in APA response across muscles. To accomplish this, two normalization techniques have been common. The first normalizes EMG integrals *within-trial* relative to baseline EMG, $\int EMG_{Integral} = \dfrac{\int EMG_{APA} - \int EMG_{Baseline}}{\int EMG_{Baseline}}$ where $\int EMG_{Integral}$ greater than 1 indicates increased APA activity in targeted muscles, and $\int EMG_{Integral}$ less than 1 indicates inhibition of APA activity (Aruin & Latash, 1995b; 1996; Latash et al., 1995; Mochizuki et al, 2004; Morris & Allison, 2006; Santos & Aruin, 2008; Strang & Berg, 2007; Xiaoyan & Aruin, 2007). This approach is satisfactory for within-subject designs because it accounts for changes in baseline EMG magnitude and noise within-trial and across conditions for individual

---

[6] Note that this statement is not true for studies in which the perturbation caused by the focal movement comes in the form of force unloading (e.g., dropping a held mass; Aruin & Latash, 1995b; Schmitz et al., 2002; Shiratori & Aruin, 2007). In these cases, baseline activity reflects low-level isometric contraction of APA muscles.

participants. For between-subject designs, EMG integrals haven been normalized *within-subject* according to, $\int EMG_{Integral} = \frac{\int EMG_{APA} - \int EMG_{Baseline}}{\int EMG_{APA}^{Max} - \int EMG_{Baseline}^{Max}}$, where $\int EMG_{APA}^{Max}$ is the highest APA integral value obtained across trials and condition and $\int EMG_{Baseline}^{Max}$ is the corresponding baseline EMG for that trial (Aruin, 2001; Girolami et al., 2010; Kanekar et al., 2008; Nana-Ibrahim et al., 2008; Schmitz et al., 2002; Shiratori & Latash, 2000; Shiratori & Aruin, 2007; Slipper & Latash, 2000; Xiaoyan & Aruin 2007). This approach restricts $\int EMG_{Integral}$ to a range of -1 to 1, where positive values indicate increased muscle activation in APA muscles and negative values corresponded to APA inhibition (Shiratori & Latash, 2000).

4.3 EMG mean amplitude and RMS

Because EMG mean amplitude is typically estimated after EMG amplitudes are rectified (van Dieën & de Looze, 1999), RMS and mean amplitude of EMG provide a similar quality of information, i.e., the central tendency of EMG amplitude response, despite subtle differences in mathematical computation. Also, it is worth mentioning that as long as the sampling rate of EMG is fixed, which was the case for every study reviewed for this chapter, EMG mean amplitude and EMG integral measures are equivalent for equal duration APA timing-windows. Finally, similar to EMG integral estimation, calculations of RMS and mean amplitude require an established APA timing-window. Researchers electing to use these alternative measures have mostly used timing-windows consistent with those described earlier (van Dieën & de Looze, 1999). The exceptions are two studies that calculated EMG mean amplitudes in adjacent epochs of 25ms (Lee et al., 2009) and 10ms (Tsao & Hodges, 2007) around T_0 to achieve higher resolution for description of changes in APA activity.

4.4 Limitations and caution for use of APA magnitude measures

Based on the information provide above, it is apparent that the accuracy of any estimation of APA magnitude is dependent on the reliability of EMG amplitude responses. However, there is ample reason to question the reliability of EMG when factors such as warm-up exercise, increased skin temperature (independent of exercise), and peripheral muscle fatigue are present. For example, peripheral muscle fatigue has been associated with both increases (Krogh-Lund, 1993) and decreases (Maton & Gamet, 1989) in EMG amplitude, compared to non-fatigued muscles. Bell (1993) demonstrated that increases in skin surface temperature, induced by blowing warm air directly onto the skin, elicited a decrease in EMG amplitude - thought to be caused by changes in fluid distribution within the muscle and/or nerve conduction velocity. Finally, Stewart and colleagues (2003) found that warm-up exercise caused a decrease in EMG amplitude during voluntary isometric contractions – thought to be caused by a rise in intramuscular temperature. Based on this, researchers seeking to examine the effects of muscle fatigue on APAs (Kanekar et al., 2008; Mezaour et al., 2010; Morris & Allison, 2006; Strang & Berg, 2007; Yiou et al., 2009), as well as those studies where experimental procedures might elicit changes in skin and/or muscle temperature following repeated experimental trials, should consider these effects when attempting to employ APA magnitude measures.

5. Conclusion

EMG has been, and will continue to be, an important tool for advancing understanding of anticipatory postural control. As this chapter has shown, the application of EMG in the study of APAs requires unique experimental methodologies, processing techniques, and statistical computations that accommodate both the behavioral constraints of the phenomenon within its observed context (e.g., self-induced or external perturbation) and the specific research question under examination. However, there is clearly more work needed that is focused on developing standard processing techniques (e.g., determination of the reference event for T_0 and the size of the APA timing-window) for the use of EMG in the study of APAs.

6. References

Alexandrov, A., Frolov, A., Horak, F., Carlson-Kuhta, P., & Park, S. (2005). Feedback equilibrium control during human standing. *Biological Cybernetics, 93,* 309–322.

Adkin, A., Frank, J., Carpenter, M., & Peysar, G. (2002). Fear of falling modifies anticipatory postural control. *Experimental Brain Research, 143,* 160-170.

Allison, G.T. (2003). Trunk muscle onset detection technique for EMG signals with ECG artifact. *Journal of Electromyography and Kinesiology, 13,* 209-216.

Allison, G.T., & Eastwood, P. (2002). Determining trunk muscle onsets in the presence of ECG artifact - alternatives to the Shewhart protocol. *In: 7th International Physiotherapy Congress, The Australian Physiotherapy Association,* Sydney.

Allison, G.T., & Henry, S.M. (2002). The influence of fatigue on trunk muscle responses to sudden arm movements: a pilot study. *Clinical Biomechanics, 17,* 414-417.

Aruin, A.S., Forrest, W.R., & Latash, M.L. (1998). Anticipatory postural adjustments in conditions of postural instability. *Electroencephalonography and Clinical Neurophysiology, 109,* 350-359.

Aruin, A.S., & Latash, M.L. (1995a). Directional specificity of postural muscles in feed-forward postural reactions during fast voluntary arm movements. *Experimental Brain Research, 103,* 323-332.

Aruin, A.S., & Latash, M.L. (1995b). The role of motor action in anticipatory postural adjustments studied with self-induced and externally triggered perturbations. *Experimental Brain Research, 106,* 291-300.

Aruin, A.S., & Latash, M.L. (1996). Anticipatory postural adjustments during self-initiated perturbations of different magnitude triggered by a standard motor action. *Electroencephalography and Clinical Neurophysiology, 101,* 497–503.

Aruin, A.S., Neyman, I., Nicholas, J.J., & Latash, M.L. (1996). Are there deficits in anticipatory postural adjustments in Parkinson's disease? *Neuroreport, 7,* 1794-1796.

Aruin, A., & Shiratori, T. (2003). Anticipatory postural adjustments while sitting: the effects of different leg supports. *Experimental Brain Research, 151,* 46-53.

Aruin, A., Shiratori, T., & Latash, M.L. (2001). The role of action in postural preparation for loading and unloading in standing subject. *Experimental Brain Research, 138,* 458-466.

Basmajian, J.V. (1967). Muscles alive: their functions revealed by electromyography, second edition. Baltimore, MD: Williams and Wilkins.

Belen'kii, V.Y., Gurnkel, V.S., & Pal'tsev, Y.I. (1967). Elements of control of voluntary movements. *Biofizika, 10,* 135–141.

Bell, D.G. (1993). The influence of air temperature on the EMG/force relationship of the quadriceps. *European Journal of Applied Physiology, 67,* 256-260.

Benvenuti, F., Stanhope, S.J., Thomas, S.L., Panzer, V.P., & Hallett, M. (1997). Flexibility of anticipatory postural adjustments revealed by self-paced and reaction time arm movements. *Brain Research, 761,* 59-70.

Bleuse, S., Cassim, F., Blatt, J.L., Labyt, E., Derambure, P., Guieu, J.D., & Defebvre, L. (2006). Effect of age on anticipatory postural adjustments in unilateral arm movement. *Gait and Posture, 24,* 203-10.

Bouisset, S., & Zattara, M. (1987). Biomechanical study of the programming of anticipatory postural adjustments associated with voluntary movement. *Journal of Biomechanics, 20,* 735–742.

Cram, J.F., & Criswell, E. (2011). *Introduction to surface electromyography.* Sudbury, MA: Jones and Bartlett Publishers.

De Wolf, S., Slijper, H., & Latash, M.L. (1998). Anticipatory postural adjustments during self-paced and reaction-time movements. *Experimental Brain Research, 121,* 7-19.

Di Fabio, R.P. (1987). Reliability of computerized surface electromyography for determining the onset of muscle activity. *Physical Therapy, 67,* 43-48.

Dickstein, R., Shefi, S., Marcovitz, E., & Villa, Y. (2004). Anticipatory postural adjustment in selected trunk muscles in post stroke hemiparetic patients. *Archives of Physical Medicine and Rehabilitation, 85,* 261-267.

Disselhorst-Klug, C., Schmitz-Rode, T., & Rau, G. (2009). Surface electromyography and muscle force: limits in sEMG-force relationship and new approaches for applications. *Clinical Biomechanics, 24,* 225-235.

Donaldson, S., Donaldson, M., & Snelling, L. (2003). SEMG evaluations: an overview. *Journal of Applied Psychophysiology and Biofeedback, 28,* 121-127.

Eckerle, J.J., Ward, R.M., & Berg, W.P. (2011). The effect of load uncertainty on anticipatory muscle activity in a one-handed catching task. *Journal of Sport and Exercise Psychology, 33 Suppl.,* 67.

Fischman, M. (1984). Programming time as a function of number of movement parts and changes in movement direction. *Journal of Motor Behavior, 16,* 405-423.

Friedli, W.G., Hallett, M., & Simon, S.R. (1984). Postural adjustments associated with rapid voluntary arm movements. 1. Electromyographic data. *Journal of Neurology, Neurosurgery and Psychiatry, 47,* 611–622.

Fujiwara, K., Toyama, H., & Kunita, K. (2003). Anticipatory activation of postural muscles associated with bilateral arm flexion in subjects with different quiet standing positions. *Gait and Posture, 17,* 254-263.

Gabel, R.H., & Brandt, R.A. (1994). The effect of signal conditioning on statistical analyses of gait EMG. *Electroencephalonography and Clinical Neurophysiology, 93,* 188–201.

Gantchev, G.N., & Dimitrova, D.M. (1996). Anticipatory postural adjustments associated with arm movements during balancing on unstable support surface. *International Journal of Psychophysiology, 22,* 117-122.

Gantchev, N., Viallet, F., Aurenty, R., & Massion, J. (1996). Impairment of posturo-kinetic coordination during initiation of forward oriented stepping movements in parkinsonian patients. *Electroencephalonography and Clinical Neurophysiology, 101,* 110-120.

Girolami, G.L., Shiratori, T., & Aruin, A.S. (2010). Anticipatory postural adjustments in children with typical motor development. *Experimental Brain Research, 205,* 153-165.

Halbertsma, J.M., & de Boer, R.R. (1981). On the processing of electromyograms for computer analysis. *Journal of Biomechanics, 14,* 431–435.

Happee, R., & Van der Helm, F.C. (1995). The control of shoulder muscles during goal directed movements, an inverse dynamic analysis. *Journal of Biomechanics, 28,* 1179-1191.

Henry, S.M., Fung, J., & Horak, F.B. (1998). Control of stance during lateral and anterior/posterior surface translations. *IEEE Transactions on Rehabilitation Engineering, 6,* 32–42.

Hodges, P.W. (2001). Changes in motor planning of feedforward postural responses of the trunk muscles in low back pain. *Experimental Brain Research,* 141, 261-266.

Hodges, P.W., & Bui, B.A. (1996). Comparison of computer based methods for determination of onset of muscle contraction using electromyography. *Electroencephalonography and Clinical Neurophysiology, 101,* 511-519.

Hodges, P.W., Cresswell, A.G., & Thorstensson, A. (2001). Perturbed upper limb movements cause short-latency postural responses in trunk muscles. *Experimental Brain Research, 138,* 243-50.

Hodges, P.W., Moseley, G.L., Gabrielsson, A., & Gandevia, S.C. (2003). Experimental muscle pain changes feedforward postural responses of the trunk muscles. *Experimental Brain Research, 151,* 262-271.

Hodges, P.W., & Richardson, C.A. (1996). Inefficient muscular stabilization of the lumbar spine associated with low back pain: a motor control evaluation of transversus abdominis. *Spine, 21,* 2460-2450.

Hodges, P.W., & Richardson, C.A. (1998). Delayed postural contraction of transversus abdominis in low back pain associated with movement of the lower limb. *Journal of Spinal Disorders, 11,* 46-56.

Hodges, P.W., & Richardson, C.A. (1999). Altered trunk muscle recruitment in people with low back pain with upper limb movement at different speeds. *Archives of Physical Medicine and Rehabilitation, 80,* 1005-1012.

Jacobs, J.V., Henry, S.M., & Nagle, K.J. (2009). People with chronic low back pain exhibit decreased variability in the timing of their anticipatory postural adjustments. *Behavioral Neuroscience, 123,* 455-458.

Kanekar, N., Santos, M.J., & Aruin, A.S. (2008). Anticipatory postural control following fatigue of postural and focal muscles. *Clinical Neurophysiology, 119,* 2304-2313.

Kazennikov, O., & Lipshits, M. (2010). Dependence of the anticipatory change in the grip force in the catching task on the result of the preceding trial. *Human Physiology, 36,* 370-371.

Krogh-Lund, C. (1993). Myo-electric fatigue and force failure from submaximal static elbow flexion sustained to exhaustion. *European Journal of Applied Physiology, 12,* 413–430.

Lacquaniti, F., & Maioli, C. (1989a). The role of preparation in tuning anticipatory and reflex responses during catching. *Journal of Neuroscience, 9,* 134-148.

Lacquaniti, F., & Maioli, C. (1989b). Adaptation to suppression of visual information during catching. *Journal of Neuroscience, 9,* 149-159.

Latash, M.L., Aruin, A.S., Neyman, I., & Nicholas, J.J. (1995). Anticipatory postural adjustments during self inflicted and predictable perturbations in Parkinson's disease. *Journal of Neurology, Neurosurgery and Psychiatry, 58*, 236-334.

Lee, W.A., Buchanan T.S., & Rogers, M.W. (1987). Effects of arm acceleration and behavioral conditions on the organization of postural adjustments during arm flexion. *Experimental Brain Research, 66*, 257–270.

Lee, L.J., Coppieters, M.W., & Hodges, P.W. (2009). Anticipatory postural adjustments to arm movement reveal complex control of paraspinal muscles in the thorax. *Journal of Electromyography and Kinesiology, 19*, 46-54.

Li, X., Zhou, P., & Aruin, A. (2007). Teager-Kaiser energy operation of surface EMG improves muscle activity onset detection. *Annals of Biomedical Engineering*, 35, 1532-1538.

Macpherson, J.M., Horak, F.B., Dunbar, D.C., & Dow, R.S. (1989). Stance dependence of automatic postural adjustments in humans. *Experimental Brain Research, 78*, 557-566.

Maki, B.E., & McIlroy, W.E. (1996). Postural control in the older adult. *Clinics in Geriatric Medicine, 12*, 635-658.

Mannion, A.F., Pulkovski, N., Schenk, P., Hodges, P.W., Gerber, H., Loupas, T., Gorelick, M., & Sprott, H. (2008). A new method for the non-invasive determination of abdominal muscle feedforward activity based on tissue velocity information from tissue Doppler imaging. *Journal of Applied Physiology, 104*, 1192-1201.

Massion, J. (1992). Movement, posture and equilibrium: interaction and coordination. *Progress in Neurobiology, 35*, 35–56.

Maton, B., & Gamet, D. (1989). The fatigability of two agonistic muscles in human isometric voluntary submaximal contraction: an EMG study. *European Journal of Applied Occupational Physiology, 58*, 369-374.

McGill, S.M. (1991). Electromyographic activity of the abdominal and low back musculature during the generation of isometric and dynamic axial trunk torque: Implications for lumbar mechanics. *Journal of Orthopaedic Research, 9*, 91-103.

Mezaour, M., Yiou, E., & Le Bozec, S. (2010). Effect of lower limb muscle fatigue on anticipatory postural adjustments associated with bi-lateral-forward reach in unipedal dominant and non-dominant stance. *European Journal of Applied Physiology, 110*, 1187-1197.

Mochizuki, G., Ivanova, T.D., & Garland, S.J. (2004). Postural muscle activity during bilateral and unilateral arm movements at different speeds. *Experimental Brain Research, 155*, 352-361.

Morris, S.L., & Allison, G.T. (2006). Effects of abdominal muscle fatigue on anticipatory postural adjustments associated with arm-raising. *Gait and Posture, 24*, 342-348.

Nana-Ibrahim, S., Vieilledent, S., Leroyer, P., Viale, F., & Zattara, M. (2008). Target size modifies anticipatory postural adjustments and subsequent elementary arm pointing. *Experimental Brain Research, 184*, 255-260.

Nashner, L.M., Shumway-Cook, A. & Marin, O. (1983). Stance posture control in select groups of children with cerebral palsy: deficits in sensory organization and muscular coordination. *Experimental Brain Research, 49*, 393–409.

Park, M.C., Belhaj-Saïf, A., & Cheney, P.D. (2004). Properties of primary motor cortex output to forelimb muscles in rhesus macaques. *Journal of Neurophysiology, 92*, 2968–2984.

Robertson, G., Caldwell, G., Hamill, J., Kamen, G., & Whittlesay, S. (2004). *Research methods in biomechanics*. Champaign, IL: Human Kinetics.

Rosenbaum, D.A. (2011). *Human motor control: second edition*. Boston, MA: Academic Press.

Santos, M.J., & Aruin, A.S. (2008). Role of lateral muscles and body orientation in feedforward postural control. *Experimental Brain Research, 184*, 547-559.

Santos, M.J., Kanekar, N., & Aruin, A.S. (2010). The role of anticipatory postural adjustments in compensatory control of posture: 2. Biomechanical analysis. *Journal of Electromyography and Kinesiology, 20*, 398-405.

Schmitz, C., Martin, N., & Assaiante, C. (2002). Building anticipatory postural adjustment during childhood: a kinematic and electromyographic analysis of unloading in children from 4 to 8 years of age. *Experimental Brain Research, 142*, 354-364.

Shiratori, T., & Aruin, A.S. (2004). Anticipatory postural adjustments associated with rotational perturbations while standing on fixed and free-floating supports. *Clinical Neurophysiology, 115*, 797-806.

Shiratori, T., & Aruin, A.S. (2007). Modulation of anticipatory postural adjustments associated with unloading perturbation: effect of characteristics of a motor action. *Experimental Brain Research, 178*, 206-215.

Shiratori, T., & Latash, M.L. (2000). The roles of proximal and distal muscles in anticipatory postural adjustments under asymmetrical perturbations and during standing on roller skates. *Clinical Neurophysiology, 111*, 613-23.

Shiratori, T., Latash, M.L. (2001). Anticipatory postural adjustments during load catching by standing subjects. *Clinical Neurophysiology, 112*, 1250–1265

Slijper H., & Latash, M. (2000). The effects of instability and additional hand support on anticipatory postural adjustments in leg, trunk, and arm muscles during standing. *Experimental Brain Research, 135*, 81-93.

Slijper, H., Latash, M.L., & Mordkoff, J.T. (2002). Anticipatory postural adjustments under simple and choice reaction time conditions. *Brain Research, 924*, 184-197.

Soderberg, G.L., & Cook, T.M. (1984). Electromyography in biomechanics. *Physical Therapy, 64*, 1813-1820.

Stewart, D., Macaluso, A., & DeVito, G. (2003). The effect of an active warm-up on surface EMG and muscle performance in healthy humans. *European Journal of Applied Physiology, 89*, 509-513.

Stokes, I.A.F., Gardner-Morse, M., Henry, S., & Badger, G.J. (2000). Decrease in trunk muscular response to perturbation with preactivation of lumbar spinal musculature. *Spine, 25*, 1957–1964.

Strang, A.J., & Berg, W.P. (2007). Fatigue-induced adaptive changes of anticipatory postural adjustments. *Experimental Brain Research, 178*, 49-61.

Strang, A.J., Choi, H.J., & Berg, W.P. (2008). The effect of exhausting aerobic exercise on the timing of anticipatory postural adjustments. *Journal of Sports Medicine and Physical Fitness 48*, 9-16.

Strang, A.J., Berg, W.P., & Hieronymus, M. (2009). Fatigue-induced early onset of anticipatory postural adjustments in non-fatigued muscles: support for a centrally mediated adaptation. *Experimental Brain Research, 197*, 245-254.

Studenski, S., Duncan, P.W., & Chandler, J. (1991). Postural responses and effector factors in persons with unexplained falls: results and methodologic issues. *Journal of the American Geriatric Society, 39*, 229-234.

Timmann, D., & Horak, F.B. (1998). Perturbed step initiation in cerebellar subjects. 1: Modifications of postural responses. *Experimental Brain Research, 119*, 73–84.

Tsao, H., & Hodges, P.W. (2007). Immediate changes in feedforward postural adjustments following voluntary motor training. *Experimental Brain Research, 181*, 537-546.

Tsao, H., & Hodges, P.W. (2008). Persistence of improvements in postural strategies following motor control training in people with recurrent low back pain. *Journal of Electromyography and Kinesiology, 18*, 559-567.

van der Fits, I.B.M., Otten, E., Klip, A.W.J., van Eykern, L.A., & Hadders-Algra, M. (1999). The development of postural adjustments during reaching in 6- to 18-month-old infants: evidence for two transitions. *Experimental Brain Research, 126*, 517-528.

van der Heide, J.C., Otten, B., van Eykern, L.A., & Hadders-Algra, M. (2003). Development of postural adjustments during reaching in sitting children. *Experimental Brain Research, 151*, 32-45.

van Dieen, J.H., & de Looze, M.P. (1999). Directionality of anticipatory activation of trunk muscles in a lifting task depends on load knowledge. *Experimental Brain Research, 128*, 397-404.

Vuillerme, N., Nougier, V., & Teasdale, N. (2002). Effects of lower limb muscle fatigue on anticipatory postural adjustments during arm motions in humans. *Journal of Sports Medicine and Physical Fitness, 42*, 289-294.

Weiss, A.D. (1965). The locus of reaction time change with set, motivation and age. *Journals of Gerontology, 20*, 60-64.

Xiaoyan, L., & Aruin, A.S. (2007). The effect of short-term changes in the body mass on anticipatory postural adjustments. *Experimental Brain Research, 181*, 333-346.

Yiou, E., Heugas, M., Mezaour, M., & LeBozec, S. (2009). Effect of lower limb muscle fatigue induced by high-level isometric contractions on postural maintenance and postural adjustment associated with bilateral forward-reach task. *Gait and Posture, 29*, 97-101.

Zattara, M., & Bouisset, S. (1988). Posturo-kinetic organization during the early phase of voluntary upper limb movement. 1. Normal subjects. *Journal of Neurology, Neurosurgery and Psychiatry, 51*, 956–965.

5

Application of Surface Electromyographic Signals to Control Exoskeleton Robots

R. A. R. C. Gopura[1] and Kazuo Kiguchi[2]
[1]*University of Moratuwa*
[2]*Saga University*
[1]*Sri Lanka*
[2]*Japan*

1. Introduction

The electromyographic signals abbreviated as EMG, represent the amount of electrical potential generated by the muscle cells when they contract or when they are at rest. Basically, EMG signals can be classified into two types according to the place where they are extracted. The EMG signals detect from inside of the muscles are called as intramuscular EMG whereas EMG signals detect from skin surface of the muscles are called surface EMG. The extraction procedure of intramuscular EMG signals is invasive. The intramuscular EMG signals are difficult to use practically, since the invasive procedure of extraction. EMG signals of human muscles are important biological signals to understand the motion intention of human. Therefore, the EMG signals can be used as input information to control robotic systems (Farry *et al.*, 1996; Kiguchi *et. al.*, 2001). The surface EMG signal is commonly used for this purpose since it can be extracted easily without applying a non-invasive method (Farry *et al.*, 1996).
The exoskeleton robot is a device which can be worn by the human operator as an orthotic device (Perry & Rosen, 2007). The same system operated in different modes can be used for different fundamental applications: power-assist device, human-amplifier, rehabilitation device, and haptic interface (Perry & Rosen, 2007). The skin surface EMG signals of the muscles can be used as input information of the controllers of exoskeleton robot (Kiguchi *et al.*, 2001). The EMG signals vary from person to person. In addition, it differs for the same motion even with the same person. The physical conditions such as tiredness, sleepiness, *etc.* (Kiguchi *et al.*, 2007). Therefore, characteristics of the EMG signals should be carefully considered when developing a control method for exoskeleton robot using EMG signals as input information. Since the surface EMG signals can directly reflect the human motion intention they can be used as main input information to the controller of exoskeleton robot to realize automatic control for the physically weak persons without manipulating any other equipment. Such kind of control is especially important for the system used by elderly, injured, or physically weak persons.
This chapter presents an experimental study of upper-limb surface EMG signals and two cases of applying surface EMG signals to control an upper-limb exoskeleton robot. The applied method to process surface EMG signals to use as input information to the control method is also explained. At first, surface EMG signal extraction method and processing

method are presented in this chapter. Then, the upper-limb muscle activities during daily upper-limb motions have been studied to enable exoskeleton robots to estimate human upper-limb motions based on EMG signals of related muscles. The muscle combinations are identified to separate some motions of upper-limb. Minimum number of muscles to extract signals to control frequent daily upper-limb motions has been identified. In the next step, EMG signal of identified muscles are used to control two upper-limb exoskeleton robots. A three degree of freedom (DOF) exoskeleton robot (W-EXOS) for the forearm pronation/supination, wrist flexion/extension and ulnar/radial deviation are controlled by applying the surface EMG signals of six muscles. Surface EMG signals of upper-limb muscles are applied as input information to control a 6DOF exoskeleton robot (SUEFUL-6). In each case of applying EMG signals experiments have been carried out to evaluate the effectiveness of the EMG based control method.

In the next section, the detection and processing of surface EMG signals are presented. The experimental study of upper-limb surface EMG is explained in section 3. Application of EMG signals to control the W-EXOS is described in section 4. Section 5 explains the EMG based control of the SUEFUL-6. The discussion in section 6 is followed by the conclusion in the section 7.

2. Detection and processing of surface EMG signals

Detection methods of the EMG signals vary according to its type. Since almost all of the EMG-based control methods use surface EMG signals, the surface EMG signal detection and processing procedure is discussed in this subsection.

2.1 Detection of surface EMG signals

Detection procedure of surface EMG signals is illustrated in Fig. 1. First step of the EMG signal detection procedure is attaching the surface electrodes [e.g., NE-101A, Nihon Kohden Co., Japan] on the skin surface of the muscles. The electrode and the skin should be cleaned well before adhering on the skin. Usually, alcoholic liquid is used for the cleaning. In this study, ethanol is used. A conductive ionic paste is applied between the skin and the electrode to get rid of static electric insulation of dry skin. In this study, EEG paste [Z-181JE, Nihon Kohden Co., Japan] is used as the conductive ionic paste. Usually, a pair of surface electrodes is adhered on the skin surface of the muscle with a separation of 1cm (Luca, 2002). Additionally, a reference electrode is attached on electrically unrelated tissue. Detected EMG signals are then passed to an input box. Input box consists of input channels for several electrodes and a reference electrode. The input box [JB-620J, Nihon Kohden Co., Japan] used in this study has eight input channels for eight electrodes and another one for the reference electrode. From the input box EMG signals are passed to multi-channel amplifier. The gain of the multi-channel amplifier [MEG-6108, Nihon Kohden Co., Japan] is set to 50 µV/V in this study. Amplified EMG signals are then passed to a computer via an interface card [e.g., JIF-171-1, JustWare Co., Japan] by converting to digital signals. EMG signals are processed on the computer for feature extraction.

2.2 Feature extraction of raw EMG signals

Since raw EMG data is difficult to be dealt as input information for the controller of exoskeleton robots, the features have to be extracted from the raw EMG data. Several feature extraction methods are available for this purpose (Hudgins, 1993). Some of them are mean

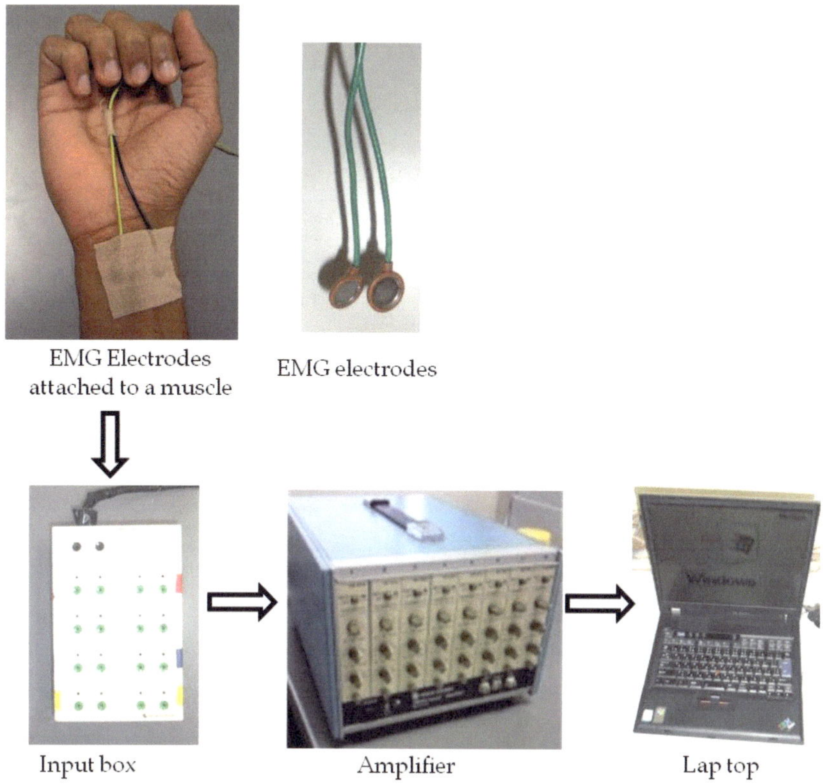

Fig. 1. Detection procedure of surface EMG signals.

absolute value, mean absolute value slope, waveform length, zero crossings, and root mean square value. The features of raw EMG data have to be extracted in real time to use EMG as input information for the controllers of exoskeleton robots. Considering the advantage of ability of real time feature extraction, Root Mean Square (RMS) method is applied to extract features of raw EMG in this study. RMS value can be stated as follows.

$$\mathrm{RMS} = \sqrt{\frac{1}{N}\sum_{i=1}^{N} v_i^2} \tag{1}$$

where, v_i is the voltage value at the ith sampling and N is the number of samples in a segment. The number of sample is set to be 100 and the selected sampling frequency is 2 kHz in this study. Figure 2 shows an example for a raw EMG signal and its RMS value. The RMS value of EMG is used as input information for the exoskeleton robot controller.

3. Experimental study of upper-limb surface EMG signals

Human upper-limb consists of several degrees of freedoms (DOF); basically 3DOF in the shoulder joint, 2DOF in the elbow joint and 2DOF in the wrist joint. The basic motions of upper-limb can be categorized into eight individual motions (Rosen *et al.*, 2005); shoulder vertical flexion/extension, shoulder horizontal flexion/extension, shoulder adduction/ abduction, shoulder internal/external rotation, elbow flexion/extension, forearm

Motion	Activated Muscles
Shoulder vertical flexion (SVF)	Coracobrachialis, Deltoid (anterior), Pectoralis major
Shoulder vertical extension (SVE)	Deltoid (posterior), Teres major, Latissimus dorsi
Shoulder horizontal flexion (SHF)	Pectoralis major (calvicular part)
Shoulder horizontal extension (SHE)	Deltoid (posterior)
Shoulder adduction (SAD)	Coracobrachialis, Latissimus dorsi, Teres major, Pectoralis major
Shoulder abduction (SAB)	Deltoid, Supraspinatus
Shoulder internal rotation (SIR)	Deltoid (anterior), Subscapularis, Latissimus dorsi, Teres major
Shoulder external rotation (SER)	Deltoid (posterior), Infraspinatus, Teres minor
Elbow flexion (EF)	Biceps brachii, Brachioradialis, Brachialis
Elbow extension (EE)	Anconeus, Triceps brachii
Forearm supination (FS)	Supinator, Biceps brachii (long head)
Forearm pronation (FP)	Pronator quadratus, Pronator teres
Wrist flexion (WF)	Flexor carpi radialis, Flexor carpi ulnaris, Palmaris longus
Wrist extension (WE)	Extensor carpi radialis longus, Extensor carpi radialis brevis, Extensor carpi ulnaris
Wrist ulnar deviation (WUD)	Flexor carpi ulnaris, Extensor carpi ulnaris
Wrist radial deviation (WRD)	Extensor carpi radialis longus, Extensor carpi radialis brevis, Flexor carpi radialis

Table 1. Activated muscles for upper-limb motions.

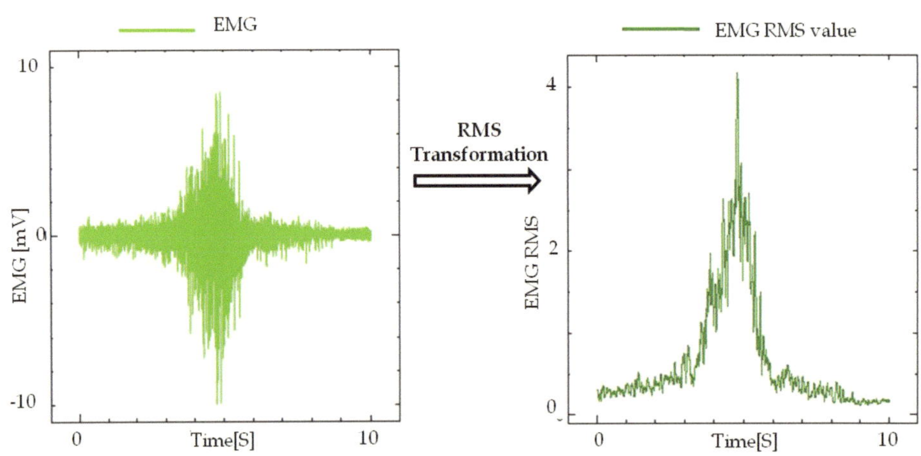

Fig. 2. Example of a raw EMG signal and its RMS value.

supination/pronation, wrist flexion/extension, and wrist ulnar/radial deviation. The daily upper-limb motions are the combination of these basic motions. Additionally fingers also have several DOF.

Human upper limb is activated by many kinds of muscles. Some of them are bi-articular muscles and the others are uni-articular muscles. In the upper-limb agonist-antagonist muscles activate shoulder, elbow and wrist. The upper-limb motions and the related muscles for the motions (Martini *et al.*, 1997) are shown in Table 1.

3.1 Procedure of experimental study

In order to obtain the relationships between the human upper-limb motions and activities of related muscles, the experiments were performed with 26 and 28 years old healthy male subjects (subject A and B, respectively). In the experiment, the basic motions and the selected daily activities of upper-limb were performed three times by each subject. Figure 3 shows the initial position and motion range of each basic motion in the experiments. The daily activities were performed in either standing or sitting posture in accordance with the nature of the daily activity. Initial and final postures of the daily activities are shown in Fig. 4. The angles of each joint of the upper-limb during the daily activities were measured by the motion capture system (Vicon MX+, 2009). Reflective markers were attached to subjects at key anatomical locations as shown in Fig. 5. Considering the muscle characteristics, sixteen muscles; Ch.1: Deltoid (anterior), Ch.2: Deltoid (posterior), Ch.3: Pectoralis major (calvicular part), Ch.4: Teres major, Ch.5: Pectoralis major, Ch.6: Infraspinatus, Ch.7: Biceps brachii, Ch.8: Triceps brachii, Ch.9: Brachialis, Ch.10: Supinator, Ch.11: Pronator teres, Ch.12: Pronator quadratus, Ch.13: Extensor carpi radialis brevis, Ch.14: Extensor carpi ulnaris, Ch.15: Flexor carpi radialis and Ch.16: Flexor carpi ulnaris, were selected for analysis in this study. Additionally another EMG electrode is attached on the skin of the abdomen as ground electrode. EMG signals of selected muscles were measured for each activity. The locations of EMG electrode are shown in Fig. 6. Subscapularis, teres minor, and anconeus are neglected in this analysis since they are overlapped with other muscles (Martini *et al.*, 1997). Since the palmaris longus is a weak flexor (Martini *et al.*, 1997), it is not taken into account. Only extensor carpi radialis brevis is taken for analysis from extensor muscle group. The brachialis is selected from the brachialis and brachioradialis since both seem to act for the elbow flexion motion. EMG signals are processed using the procedure given in the previous section.

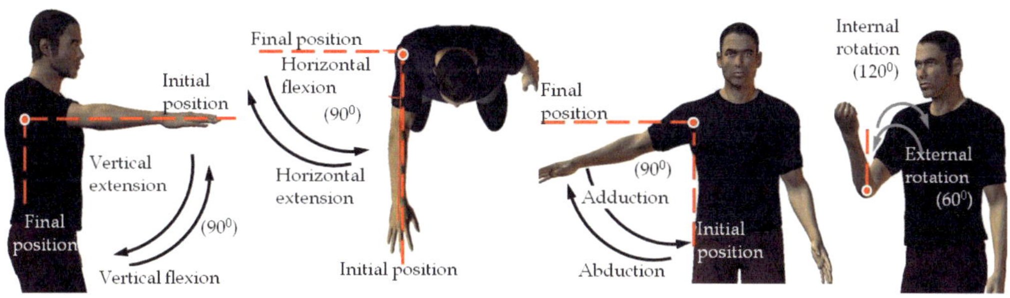

(a) Shoulder motions

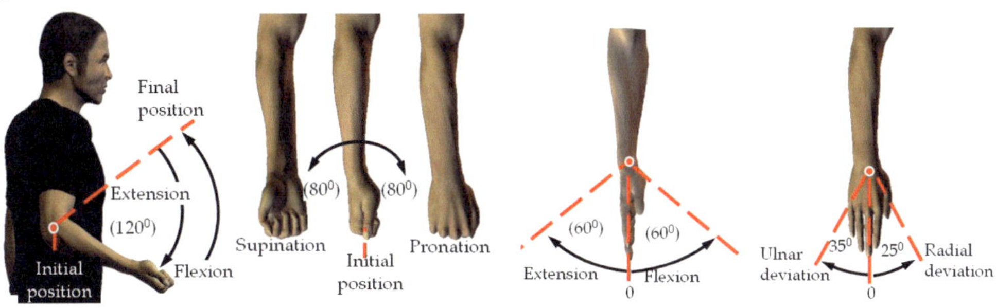

(b) Elbow and forearm motions (c) Wrist motions

Fig. 3. Initial positions and motion ranges of experimental motions.

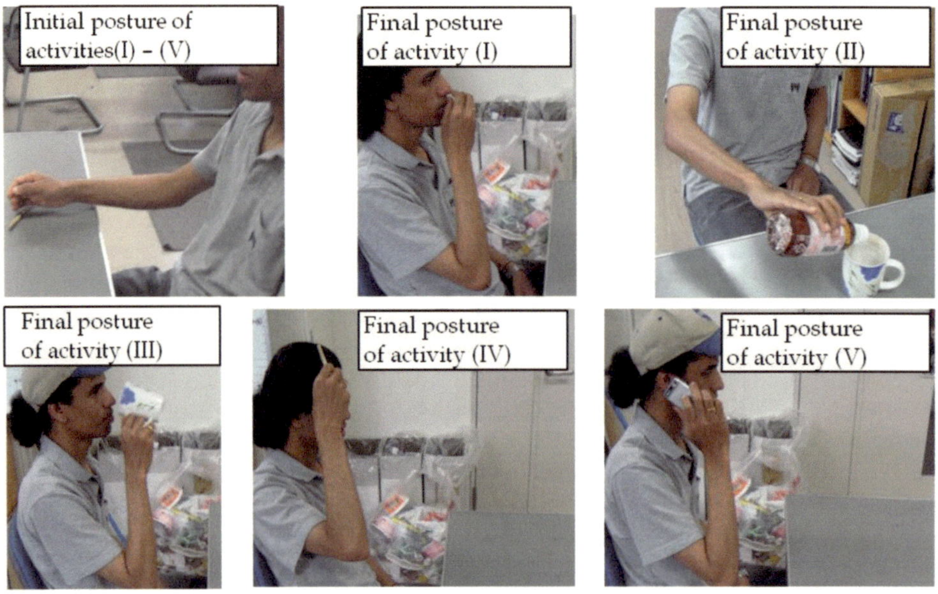

Fig. 4. Initial and final positures of selected daily activities.

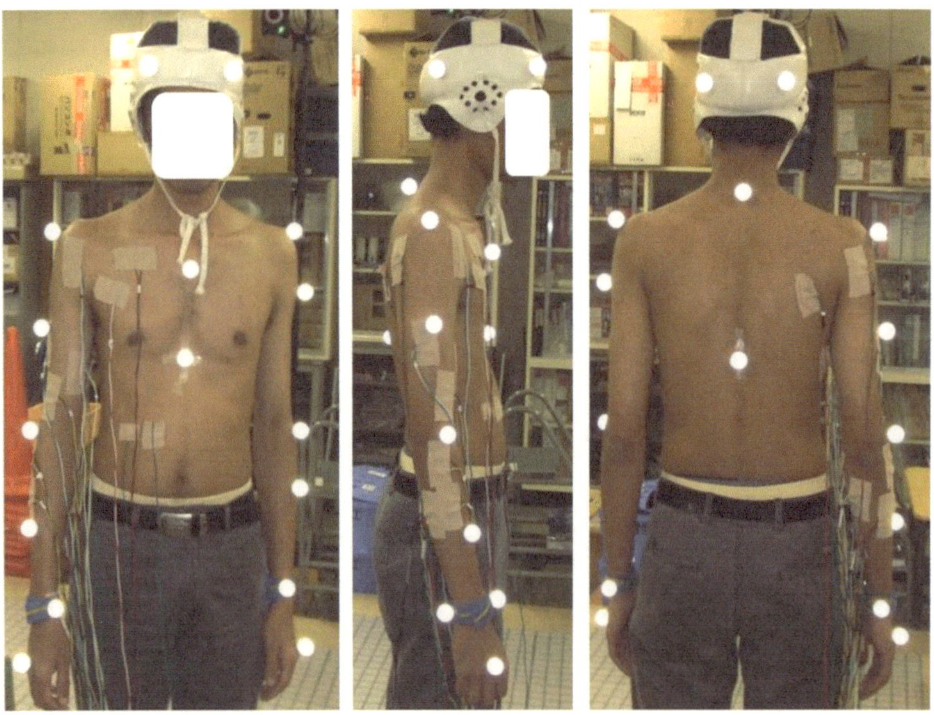

(a) (b) (c)

Fig. 5. Locations of markers. (a) Anterior view (b) Lateral view (c) Posterior view.

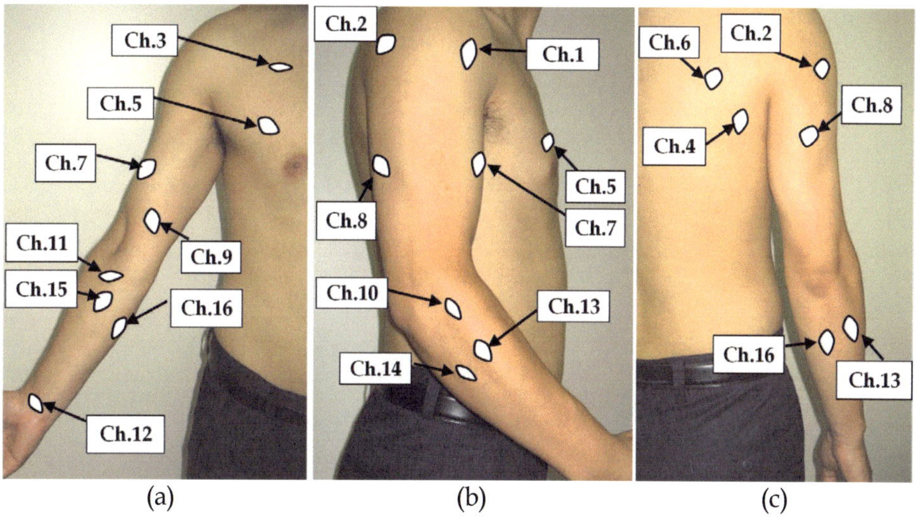

Fig. 6. Locations of EMG electrodes. a) Front view, (b) Side view, (c) Rear view.

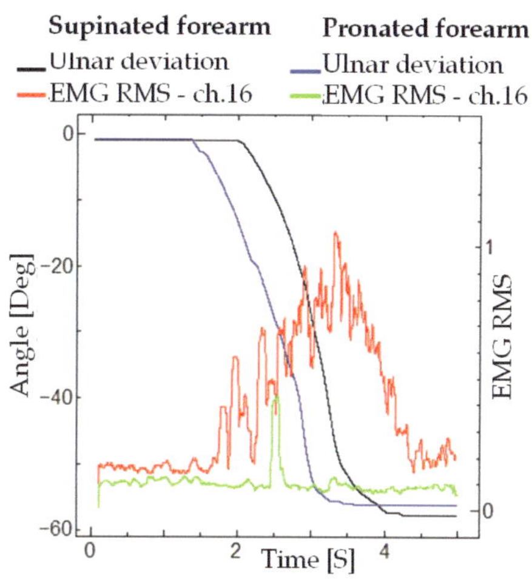

Fig. 7. EMG RMS for Ulnar deviation.

3.2 Analysis of results

It can be identified that the EMG activity levels related to the basic upper-limb motions (see Fig. 3) depend on the joint angles and the upper-limb posture (Gil Coury *et al.*, 1998). As an example, the experimental result of the full range ulnar deviation shown in Fig. 7 indicated that EMG RMS values for ulnar deviation are different in the supinated forearm posture and pronated forearm posture. Figure 8 shows the relationship of activity level of extensor carpi radialis brevis for wrist extension and radial deviation. Although some muscles are not bi-articular muscles, they act for a few motions (see Fig. 8). From Fig. 8, it can be seen that extensor carpi radialis brevis is activated for both wrist extension and radial deviation. Figure 9 shows the relationship between EMG RMS values of muscles and wrist motions. The extensor carpi ulnaris is activated for both wrist extension and ulnar deviation (see Fig. 9). Flexor carpi radialis is activated for both wrist flexion and radial deviation.

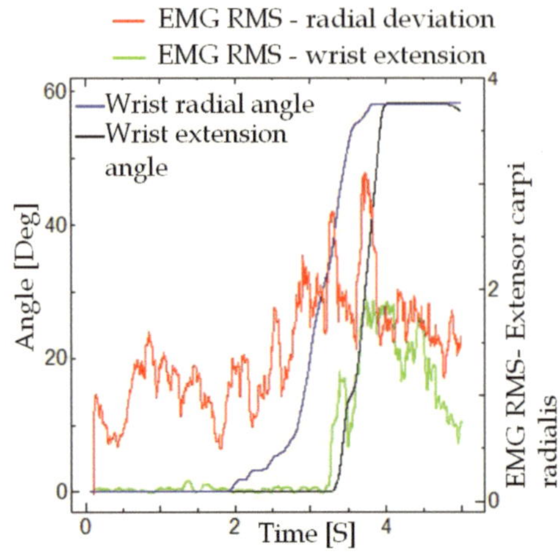

Fig. 8. EMG RMS- extensor carpi radialis brevis.

Although the flexor carpi ulnaris is not bi-articular muscle, it is activated for both wrist flexion and ulnar deviation. By analyzing results of the experiments, it can be seen that some basic upper-limb motions within the motion ranges used in the experiments can be separated by using the combinations of related muscles. Although many muscles are involved in wrist motions, each basic wrist motion can be uniquely identify in any forearm posture by considering simultaneous activation of two of muscles. Although the extensor carpi radialis longus, extensor carpi radialis brevis and extensor carpi ulnaris generate the wrist extension, the extensor carpi radialis brevis and extensor carpi ulnaris can be used to separately identify the wrist extension [see Fig. 9(b)]. Simultaneous activation of both muscles generates wrist extension in any forearm posture even though extensor carpi radialis brevis also activates the wrist radial deviation and extensor carpi ulnaris also activates the wrist ulnar deviation. Similarly, simultaneous activation of flexor carpi radialis and flexor carpi ulnaris generates wrist flexion even though they generate wrist radial and ulnar deviations, respectively [see Fig. 9(a)]. Therefore, wrist flexion motion can be separated by considering simultaneous activation of the flexor carpi radialis and flexor carpi ulnaris. Similarly, simultaneous activation of extensor carpi radialis and flexor carpi radialis generates wrist radial deviation [Fig. 9(c)]. Thus, those muscles can be used to separate wrist radial deviation. Simultaneous activation of extensor carpi ulnaris and flexor carpi ulnaris separates the wrist ulnar deviation from the other wrist motions [see Fig. 9(d)]. Even though supinator and biceps brachii activate the forearm supination motion, biceps brachii works only if elbow flexion angle is about 90 degrees. Activation of only supinator can estimate forearm supination (Gopura *et al.,* 2010). The activation of pronator teres or pronator qudratus can be used to identify forearm pronation motion although both activate the motion (Martini *et al.,* 1997). Figure 10 depicts the relationship of EMG RMS values of activated muscles and elbow and shoulder motions. When performing the basic elbow motions shown in Fig. 10, the shoulder angles was maintained about 0 degrees.

The elbow flexion is generated by the biceps brachii, brachialis, and brachioradialis. However, from the analysis, it was found that even only the brachialis can be used to identify the motion [see Fig. 10(a)]. Although several muscles activates for shoulder motions, activation of one/two muscles can be used to identify each shoulder motion. As shown in Fig. 10(e), activation of infraspinatus and/or deltoid-posterior can be used to

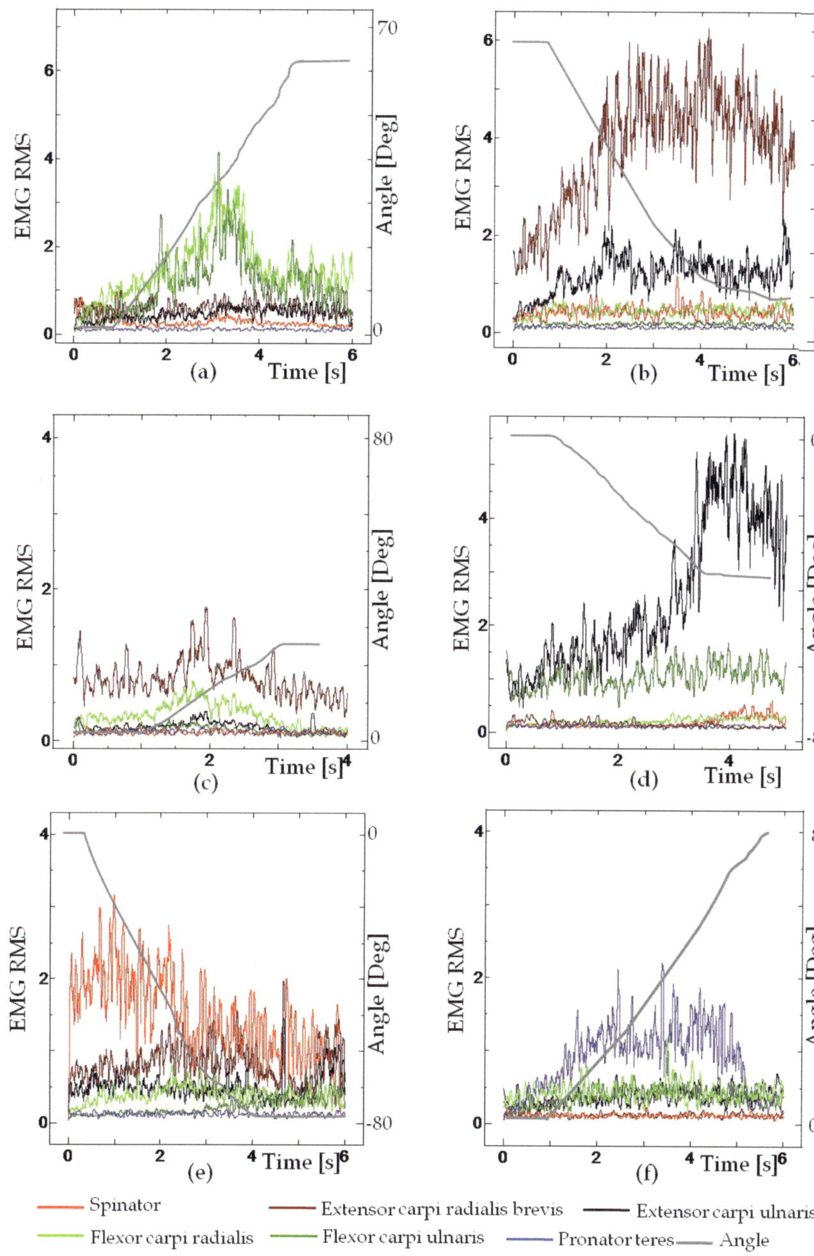

Fig. 9. Relationship of EMG RMS and basic wrist motions. (a) Wrist flexion. (b) Wrist extension. (c) Radial deviation. (d) Ulnar deviation.

identify external rotation within the experimental motion ranges. Activation of the whole deltoid muscle (*i.e.*, anterior and posterior) can be used to recognize the shoulder abduction [see Fig. 10(b)] within the experimental motion range. When the shoulder internal rotation is not activated, teres major and pectoralis major simultaneously generate shoulder adduction

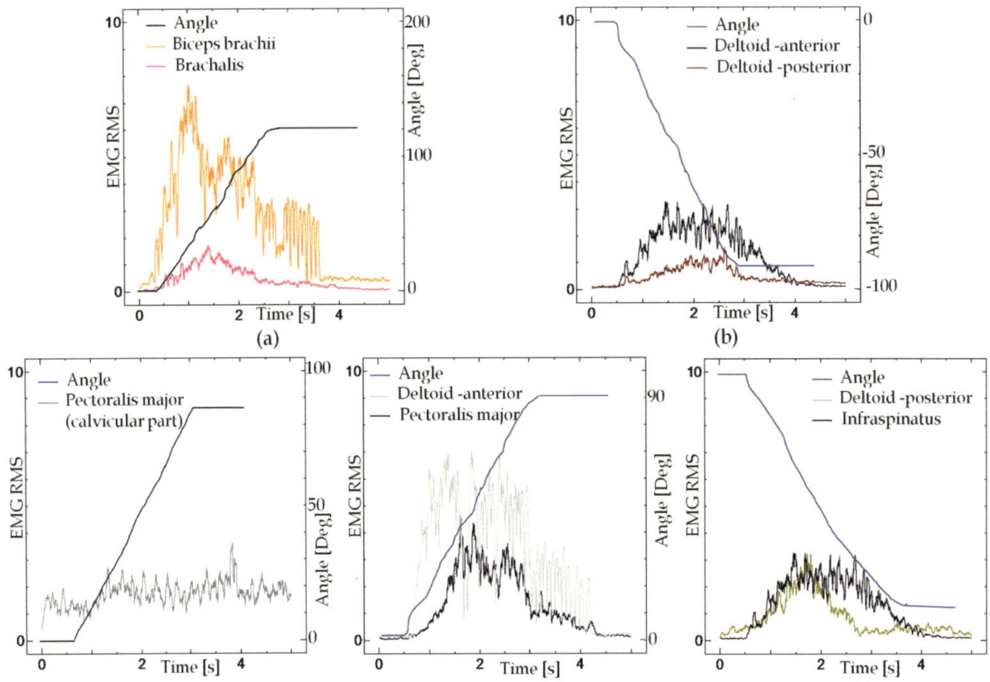

Fig. 10. Relationship of EMG RMS and basic elbow and shoulder motions. (a) Elbow flexion. (b) Shoulder abduction. (c). Shoulder horizontal flexion. (d) Shoulder vertical flexion. (e) Shoulder external rotation.

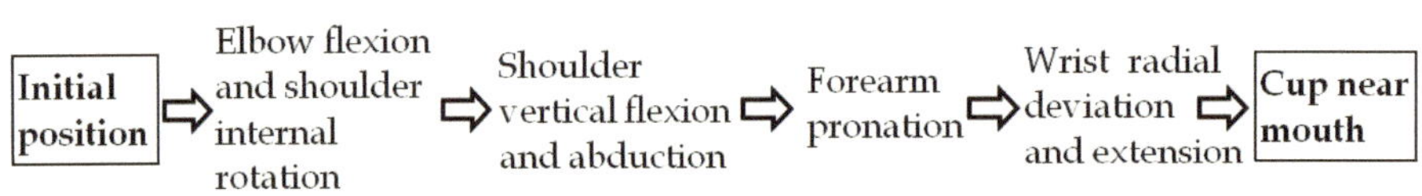

Fig. 11. Sequence of joint motion activation by the subject-A for moving the upper-limb for drinking from cup.

in the experimental motion range. When shoulder vertical motion angle is within 0 to 90 degrees, pectoralis major-calvicular part can be used [see Fig. 10(c)] to identify shoulder horizontal flexion. As identified from Fig. 10(d), deltoild-anterior and pectoralis major can be used to identify shoulder vertical flexion.

Every daily activity of upper-limb is a combination of basic upper-limb motions. Therefore, the relationship between each basic motion angle and related muscle activities are analyzed. A daily activity is explained in detail here as an example. In the activity of moving the upper-limb for drinking from a cup, initially the hand was kept near the cup on the table as shown in Fig. 11. The final position of the hand was near the mouth. In the activity, each upper-limb joint motion of subject-A were generated as follows. At first elbow flexion and the shoulder internal rotation were carried out at the same time. Then, shoulder was vertically flexed and adducted. When the cup came near the mouth, forearm pronation was carried out. Finally, wrist flexion and radial deviation were carried out. However, forearm

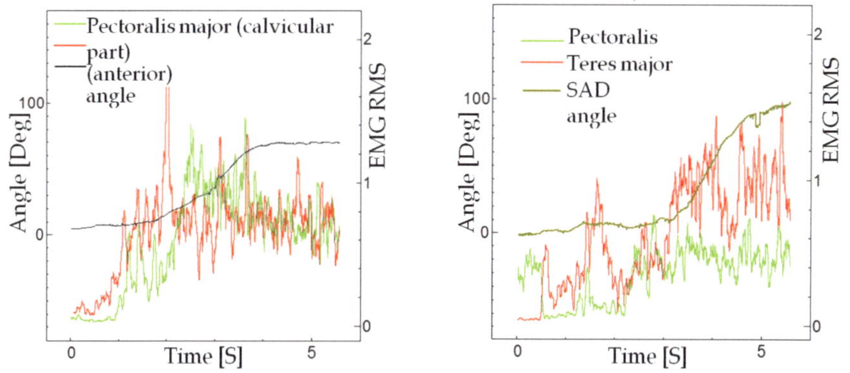

(a) (b)

Fig. 12. Relationships between muscle activities and motion angles for moving upper-limb for drinking from cup. (a) Shoulder vertical flexion (SV) angle. (b) Shoulder adduction (SAD) angle.

Motion	Identified Muscles for Motion
SVF	Deltoid -anterior, Pectoralis major-calvicular part
SVE	Deltoid -posterior, Teres major
SHF	Pectoralis major-calvicular part
SHE	Deltoid-posterior
SAD	Teres major, Pectoralis major
SAB	Deltoid -anterior, Deltoid -posterior
SIR	Deltoid-anterior, Teres major
SER	Infraspinatus,
EF	Biceps brachii, Brachialis
EE	Triceps brachii
FS	Supinator
FP	Pronator teres
WF	Flexor carpi radialis, Flexor carpi ulnaris
WE	Extensor carpi radialis brevis, Extensor carpi ulnaris
WUD	Flexor carpi ulnaris, Extensor carpi ulnaris
WRD	Extensor carpi radialis brevis, Flexor carpi radialis

Table 2. Identified muscles to generate upper-limb motions.

and wrist motions were minimal. The relationship between the shoulder vertical flexion angle and EMG RMS levels of the related muscle are shown in Fig. 12(a). As shown in Fig. 12(a), the shoulder vertical flexion motion of this activity can be identified considering the simultaneous activation of pectoralis major-calvicular part and deltoid-anterior. The shoulder adduction of the activity can be identified from the activation of pectoralis major and teres major [see Fig. 12(b)]. Some other experimental results and details of this study can be found in (Gopura *et al.*, 2010).

By analysing the experimental results following conclusions are derived. Although several muscles activate to generate upper-limb motions, sixteen upper-limb muscles can be used to estimate the upper-limb motions. Simultaneous activation of two muscles involved in wrist motions can uniquely identify the basic wrist motions. The identified muscles to generate basic upper-limb motions (only in the experimental motion range) are listed in Table 2. The combinations of the EMG signals of identified muscles can be used as input information to the controllers of upper-limb exoskeleton robot.

4. Application of EMG signal to control 3DOF exoskeleton robot

A 3DOF exoskeleton robot, W-EXOS is shown in Fig. 13. It has been developed to assist forearm pronation/supination, wrist flexion/extension and ulnar/radial deviation (Gopura & Kiguchi, 2008a). The original feature of the design is the axes offset of wrist joint, which was not considered in any other design. Therefore, undesired pain of the user's wrist joint can be avoided. In addition, the hand-robot interface has been designed so as not to disturb the finger motions. The axes offset of wrist joint is important for a wrist exoskeleton robot, since the wrist joint is sensitive to change in position and torque (Perry & Rosen, 2007). The W-EXOS mainly consists of forearm motion support part and wrist motion support part. The forearm motion support part consists of two links (upper-arm link and forearm link), a direct current (DC) motor, a drive and driven spur gear pair (gear ratio 1:3), a wrist holder, a forearm cover and torque sensors. The wrist motion support part consists of a link attachment, two DC motors, two drive and driven bevel gear pairs (gear ratio-1:2), a palm holder, a three axis force sensor and a link (wrist link) which connects the

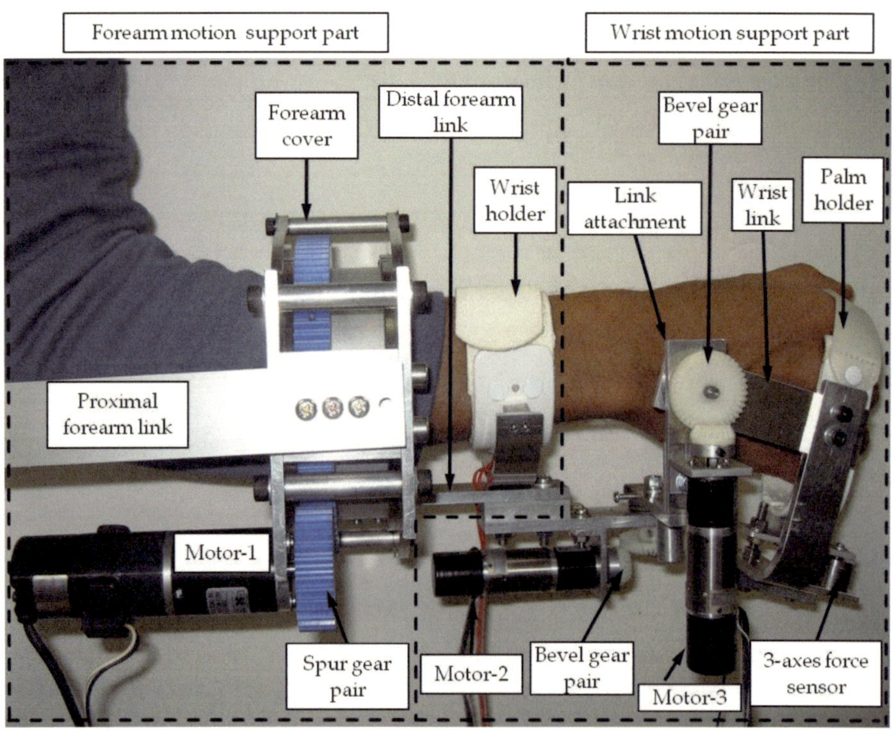

Fig. 13. 3DOF upper-limb exoskeleton robot (W-EXOS).

palm holder and link attachment as shown in Fig. 13. Proximal end of the Link-1of the W-EXOS can be attached to the upper-limb exoskeleton robot which is installed on a mobile wheel chair that can be used by many physically weak persons. Therefore, the user does not feel the weight of the exoskeleton robot at all. The details about the design and the mechanism of the W-EXOS can be referred in (Gopura & Kiguchi, 2008a). Since the W-EXOS is directly in contact with the human user, safety is essential. Mechanical stoppers are attached for each motion to prevent the exceeding of the movable range. The robot does not include any sharp edges in its mechanical construction and mechanical stoppers. Furthermore, each motor has an individual switch and there is an emergency stop switch beside the exoskeleton robot.

4.1 EMG-based control of the W-EXOS

The W-EXOS is controlled based on EMG signals as main input information to its controller. Additionally, the force/torque sensor signals of the W-EXOS are used as secondary input information. Hand force is the measured force from the three axes force sensor when the robot user performs wrist flexion/extension and/or radial/ulnar deviation. Forearm torque is measured with the torque sensor when the robot user performs the forearm supination/pronation. In the control method, the power assist is carried out based on the EMG activity levels and/or the hand force/forearm torque according to the fuzzy rules of the controller. EMG signals of six muscles are measured to control the motions of the W-EXOS. The muscles are selected according to the experimental results explained in the previous section. Monitored muscles are Ch.10: supinator (SP), Ch.11: pronator teres (PT) Ch.13: extensor carpi radialis brevis (ECRB), Ch.14: extensor carpi ulnaris (ECU), Ch.15: flexor carpi radialis (FCR) and Ch.16: flexor carpi ulnaris (FCU). In the control method, movable ranges of forearm supination/pronation and wrist flexion/extension are divided into three sections each and expressed by membership functions (Gopura & Kiguchi, 2008c). Therefore nine movable range combinations are available for forearm supination/pronation and wrist flexion/extension. By expressing the range of each section with membership functions, the controller can be gradually switched to membership functions of each section according to angles of the motions. The movable range of wrist radial/ulnar deviation is not divided into sections, since its range is comparatively narrow. In each movable range combination, a fuzzy-neuro controller has been designed. Therefore, nine fuzzy-neuro controllers are designed altogether for forearm supination/pronation and wrist flexion/extension. Another fuzzy-neuro controller is designed for wrist radial/ulnar deviation.

The structure of the control method of the W-EXOS is shown in Fig. 14. It consists of nine fuzzy-neuro controllers for the forearm motion and the wrist flexion/extension. Another fuzzy-neuro controller is deployed for wrist radial/ulnar deviation. Input information for the nine fuzzy-neuro controllers is the RMS values of six muscles (Ch.10, Ch.11, Ch.13-Ch.16), the force sensor signal, and the torque sensor signal. In addition to the RMS values of EMG signals and force/torque sensor signals, angles of forearm motion and wrist flexion/extension are given as additional input information to the nine controllers for switching the required controller according to the angles of forearm and wrist flexion/extension. Input information for the wrist radial/ulnar fuzzy-neuro controller is the RMS value of EMG signals obtained at four muscles (Ch.11, Ch.13-Ch.15), the force sensor signal and the torque sensor signal. In the controller, generated hand force/forearm torque is considered to be more reliable when the user of the exoskeleton robot slightly activates the muscles (*i.e.*, the EMG activity levels of the user are low), and the EMG signals are

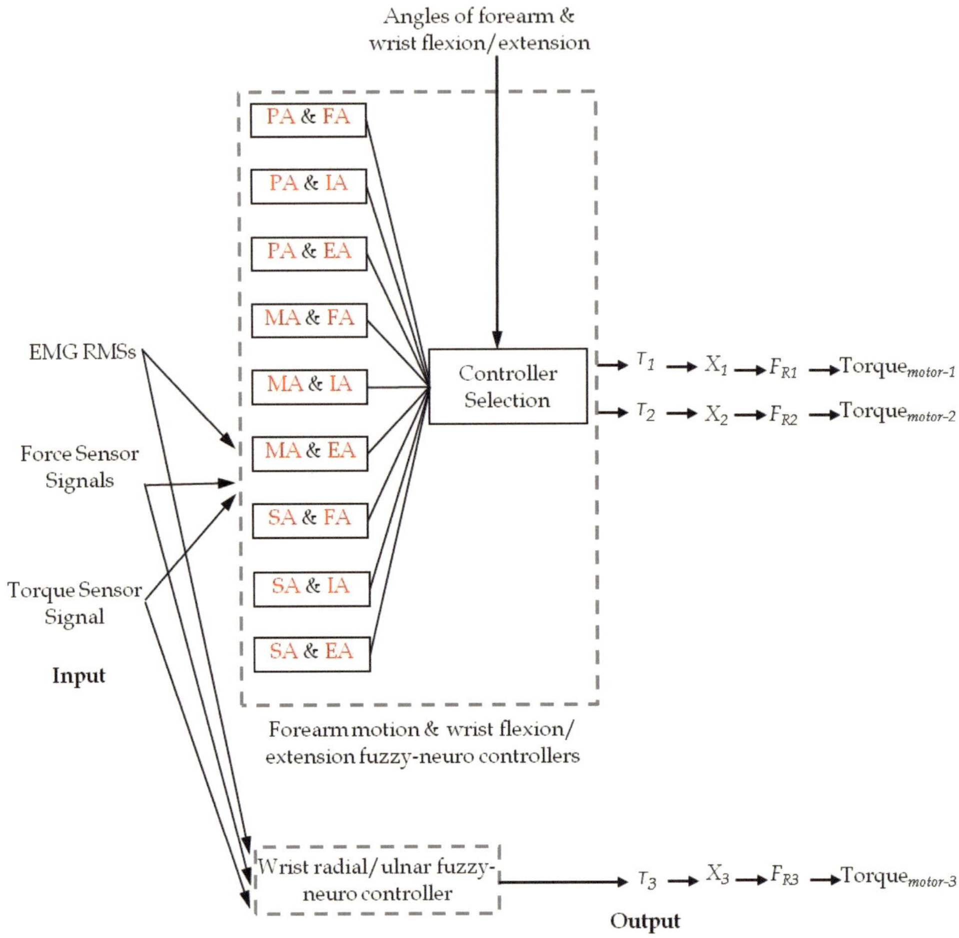

Fig. 14. Structure of the controller of the W-EXOS. PA & FA is the controller which is defined for the forearm pronated region and wrist flexed region. Other controllers are also defined for the relevant regions indicated by their names (Gopura & Kiguchi, 2008c).

more reliable when the user considerably activates the muscles (*i.e.*, the EMG activity levels of the user are high). Therefore, the exoskeleton robot is controlled based on the generated hand force/forearm torque when the EMG activity levels of the user are low, and the exoskeleton robot is controlled based on the EMG signals when the EMG activity levels of the user are high. Consequently, the exoskeleton robot can be controlled in accordance with the user intention.

The initial fuzzy if-then control rules have been designed based on preliminary experiment (Gopura & Kiguchi, 2008a) which was performed to find out the activity patterns of EMG signals of the muscles used for the forearm and wrist motions. In the experiment, EMG patterns have been identified for different motions and different torques of wrist and forearm. Fuzzy rules are designed to provide torque commands according to the EMG RMSs of six muscles and force/torque sensor signals. Defined fuzzy rules are listed in Table 3 and Table 4 (Gopura & Kiguchi, 2008a). Then the defined fuzzy rules are transferred to a neural network to implement in a fuzzy-neuro controller. Therefore, nine fuzzy rule

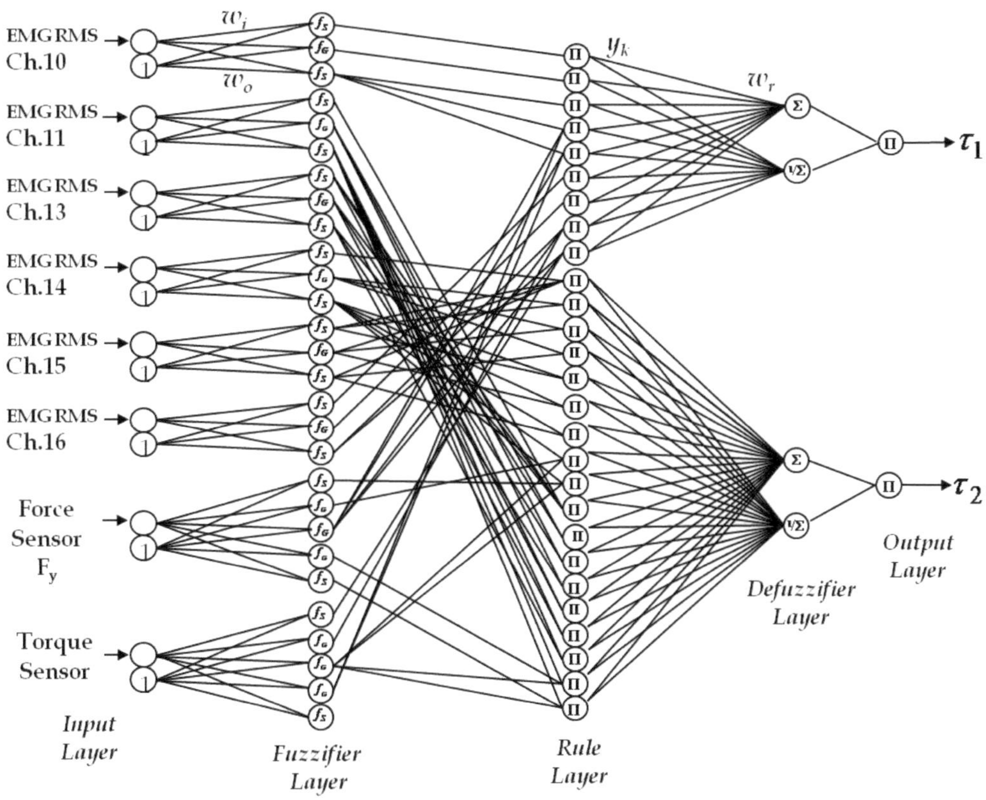

Fig. 15. Architecture of fuzzy-neuro controller.

structured neural network (fuzzy-neuro) controllers are designed in total for the forearm motion and wrist flexion/extension. For wrist radial/ulnar deviation, another fuzzy-neuro controller is designed considering movable range of wrist radial/ulnar deviation as one section. The architecture of one fuzzy-neuro controller is shown in Fig. 15 as an example. The architectures of the other controllers are also similar to the shown controller except the changes in the connection between the fuzzifier and rule layers, since the fuzzy rules are different. Each fuzzy-neuro controller consists of five layers: input layer, fuzzifier layer, rule layer, defuzzifier layer, and output layer.

4.1.1 Input layer
EMG RMS values and force/torque sensor signals are input to the input layer (see Fig. 14) of each fuzzy-neuro controller. Six EMG RMS values, a force sensor signal [Fx], and a torque sensor signal are applied to each forearm motion and wrist flexion/extension fuzzy-neuro controller. Four EMG RMS values, a force sensor signal [Fz], and a torque sensor signal are applied to wrist radial/ulnar deviation fuzzy-neuro controller. Fx and Fz are the force sensor signals for x and z axis, respectively.

4.1.2 Fuzzifier layer
Input information is then fuzzified in the fuzzifier layer. Three fuzzy linguistic variables (ZO: Zero, PS: Positive Small and PB: Positive Big) are prepared for each EMG RMS and five

variables (NB: Negative Big, NS: Negative Small, ZO: Zero, PS: Positive Small and PB: Positive Big) are prepared for each sensor signal and torque command. The nonlinear functions f_G and f_S are applied to express the membership of the fuzzy linguistic variables. f_G is the Gaussian function and f_S is the Sigmoid function which are expressed in the following equations.

$$f_S(u_S) = \frac{1}{1+e^{-U_S}} \tag{2}$$

$$u_S(x) = w_o + w_i x \tag{3}$$

$$f_G(u_G) = e^{-U_S^2} \tag{4}$$

$$u_G(x) = \frac{w_o + x}{w_i} \tag{5}$$

where w_o is the threshold value, w_i is the weight value, and x is the input value. w_o and w_i is calculated using membership functions of fuzzy linguistic variables.

4.1.3 Rule layer

In the rule layer, defined fuzzy if-then rules are applied. For the wrist radial/ulnar fuzzy-neuro controller, eighteen fuzzy rules are applied (see Table 3). Number of applied fuzzy

Rule	If	Then
01	Ch.11 = ZO and Ch.14 = ZO or Ch.14=PS or Ch.14=PB	T3= ZO
02	Ch.11 = PS and Ch.14 = ZO	T3= ZO
03	Ch.11 = PS and Ch.14 = PS	T3= PS
04	Ch.11 = PS and Ch.14 = PB	T3= PS
05	Ch.11 = PB and Ch.14 = ZO	T3= ZO
06	Ch.11 = PB and Ch.14 = PS	T3= PS
07	Ch.11 = PB and Ch.14 = PB	T3= PB
08	Ch.11! = PB and T=ZO and Fz=NS	T3=PS
09	Ch.11! = PB and T=ZO and Fz=NB	T3=PS
10	Ch.13 = ZO and Ch.15 = ZO or Ch.15=PS or Ch.15=PB	T3= ZO
11	Ch.13 = PS and Ch.15 = PS	T3= NS
12	Ch.13 = PS and Ch.15 = ZO	T3= ZO
13	Ch.13 = PS and Ch.15 = PB	T3= NS
14	Ch.13 = PB and Ch.15 = ZO	T3= ZO
15	Ch.13 = PB and Ch.15 = PS	T3= NS
16	Ch.13 = PB and Ch.15 = PB	T3= NB
17	Ch.13! = PB and T = ZO and Fz=PS	T3=NS
18	Ch.13! = PB and T = ZO and Fz=PB	T3=NS

Table 3. Fuzzy if-then control rules for wrist radial/ulnar deviation. NB, NS, ZO, PS and PB are fuzzy linguistic variables. In Table 3; Chi- Channel i, i =11, 13,14, 15; Fz=Force sensor signal for Z-axis; T=Torque sensor signal; T3 =Torque command for wrist radial/ulnar motor.

Rule	If	Then
01	Ch.10 = ZO	T1= ZO
02	Ch.10= PS	T1= PS
03	Ch.10 = PB	T1= PB
04	Ch.10! = PB and Fx! = ZO and T = PS	T1= PS
05	Ch.10! = PB and Fx! = ZO and T = PB	T1= PB
06	Ch.16 = ZO	T1= ZO
07	Ch.16 = PS	T1= NS
08	Ch.16! = PB and Fx! = ZO and T = NS	T1= NS
09	Ch.16! = PB and Fx! = ZO and T = NB	T1= NB
10	Ch.14 = ZO and Ch.15 = ZO or Ch.15=PS or Ch.15=PB	T2= ZO
11	Ch.14 = PS and Ch.15 = ZO	T2= ZO
12	Ch.14 = PS and Ch.15 = PS	T2= NS
13	Ch.14 = PS and Ch.15 = PB	T2= NS
14	Ch.14 = PB and Ch.15 = ZO	T2= ZO
15	Ch.14 = PB and Ch.15 = PS	T2= NS
16	Ch.14 = PB and Ch.15 = PB	T2= NB
17	Ch.14! = PB and T = ZO and Fx=NS	T2= NS
18	Ch.14! = PB and T = ZO and Fx=NB	T2= NS
19	Ch.11 = ZO and Ch.13 = ZO or Ch.13=PS or Ch.13=PB	T2= ZO
20	Ch.11 = PS and Ch.13 = ZO	T2= ZO
21	Ch.11 = PS and Ch.13 = PS	T2= PS
22	Ch.11 = PS and Ch.13 = PB	T2= PS
23	Ch.11 = PB and Ch.13 = ZO	T2= ZO
24	Ch.11 = PB and Ch.13 = PS	T2= PS
25	Ch.11 = PB and Ch.13 = PB	T2= PB
26	Ch.11! = PB and T = ZO and Fx=PS	T2= PS
27	Ch.11! = PB and T = ZO and Fx=PB	T2= PS

Table 4. Fuzzy if-then control rules for one of the forearm motion and wrist flexion/extension fuzzy-neuro controllers (PA & FA controller). In Table 4; Chi- Channel i, i =10, 11, 13, 14, 15, 16; Fx=Force sensor signal for X-axis; T=Torque sensor signal; Tk =Torque command for motor k, k=1, 2; '!=' represents "not equal".

control rules is different in each of the forearm motion and wrist flexion/extension fuzzy-neuro controller. Fuzzy if-then rules for one of forearm motion and wrist flexion/extension fuzzy-neuro controllers, PA & FA controller are shown in Table 4 as an example. In rule layer, Π is the multiplicand of the fuzzified inputs.

4.1.4 Defuzzifier layer and output layer

The defuzzification is carried out in the defuzzifier layer. Σ is summation of inputs of defuzzifier layer. The following equation is used to calculate the outputs of the fuzzy-neuro controllers, since the process of the fuzzy-neuro controller is same as that of an ordinal fuzzy controller.

$$\text{Output} = \frac{\sum_{i=1}^{N} w_{ri} y_{ki}}{\sum_{i=1}^{N} y_{ki}} \tag{6}$$

$$\text{Torque}_{motor\ j} = (\text{Output}) \times X_j + F_{Rj} \tag{7}$$

where, y_{ki} is the degree of fitness of ith rule, w_{ri} is the weight for ith rule, N is number of rules for the particular motion, X is the assist rate, F_R is the friction compensation, and j = 1, 2, 3. The outputs of the forearm motion and wrist flexion/extension fuzzy neuro controllers are the torques of forearm supination/pronation and wrist flexion/extension. They are represented as τ_1 and τ_2 in the output layer of the fuzzy-neuro controller respectively [see Fig. 13]. The output, τ_3 of wrist radial/ulnar fuzzy-neuro controller is the torque of the wrist radial/ulnar deviation motor. Controller outputs are multiplied by the power-assist rate and the friction compensation value is added to obtain the torque commands of three motors as in equation (7).

4.2 Controller adaptation

The adaptation of the controllers to the conditions of the robot user is important (Kiguchi *et al.*, 2001), since the EMG signal is a biological signal that varies according to the person and also to the physical and psychological conditions of the same person even for the same motion. The adaptation of fuzzy-neuro controllers is carried out by adjusting each weight values of the fuzzy-neuro controller to minimize an evaluation function. In this study, error back-propagation learning algorithm has been applied to minimize the squared error function given below.

$$E = \tfrac{1}{2}\left((\theta_d - \theta)^2 + a\sum (RMS_d - RMS)^2 \right) \tag{8}$$

where θ_d is desired joint angle indicated by a motion indicator (*i.e.*, a teaching device), θ is the joint angle of the robot, a is the rate of EMG adaptation, and RMS_d is the desired EMG RMS level. Certain percentage of the maximum value of each related EMG RMS are modeled as sinusoidal function at the beginning and the ending of the motions and taken as RMS_d. This modeling eliminates the undesired errors of the RMS_d at the beginning and the ending of the motions. In the middle of the motions, the same percentage of the maximum value of EMG RMS is taken as RMS_d. More details of controller adaptation can be referred in (Kiguchi *et al.*, 2004).

4.3 Evaluation of EMG-based control method

The experiments have been performed with three young healthy male subjects (subject A, B, and C) to evaluate the effectiveness of the EMG-based control method. The experimental set-up is shown in Fig. 16. In the first experiment, subject-A performed individual and cooperative motions of wrist and forearm with and without power-assist of the W-EXOS. Forearm and wrist motions have been performed with assist of the W-EXOS for three different power-assist rates: lower rate, medium rate, and higher rate. If the exoskeleton robot properly assists the motions the muscle activation levels should be reduced with the

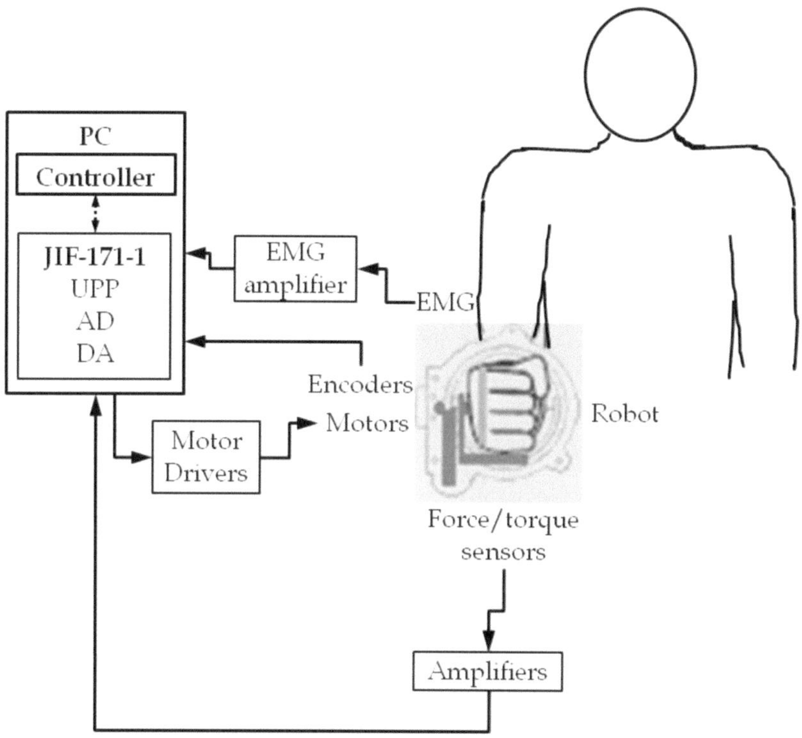

Fig. 16. Experimental set-up.

power-assist. In the second experiment, subject-B and C performed wrist and forearm motions with and without power-assist of the exoskeleton robot.

EMG RMS levels of extensor carpi ulnaris and extensor carpi radialis brevis of subjects-A for combined wrist radial deviation and wrist extension are shown in Fig. 17. 20% power-assist ratio was applied when the motion was carried with power-assist. The power-assist ratio indicates percentage of power supplied from the robot and required power for the motion. Figure 17 shows that the average value of EMG RMS of extensor carpi radialis brevis has reduced from 3.17 to 2.58 when applied the power-assist of the W-EXOS with the EMG-based control method. The EMG RMS value reduction is by 18.61%. The reduction of average value of EMG RMS of extensor carpi ulnaris is by 18.68% for the same motion. Therefore, with the EMG-based control method the W-EXOS has assisted the motion approximately equal assist rate that has been set in the program (20%). Figure 18 shows the experimental result for wrist flexion/extension. From Fig. 18, it can be seen that the activation level of ECRB and FCR is reduced with power-assist (assist rate-20%) of the W-EXOS when applied the EMG-based controller. The activation level the flexor carpi ulnaris for wrist flexion is shown in Fig. 19. The result shows that the raw EMG level of FCU is reduced with the power-assist. From the results it is concluded that EMG can effectively be applied to control the exoskeleton robot. Further, the results show that the EMG-based control method can be used to effectively assist human wrist and forearm motions.

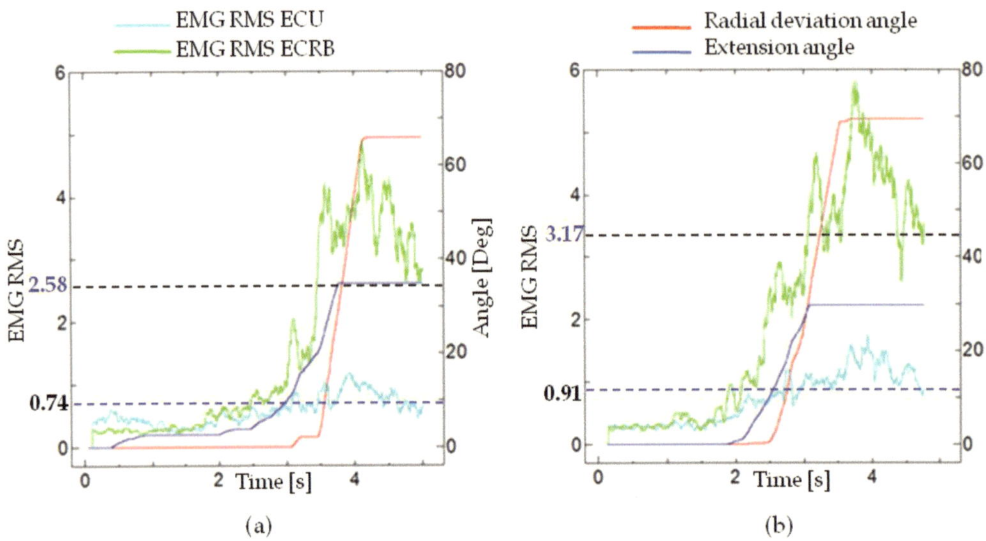

Fig. 17. Experimental results of subject-A for wrist extension and radial deviation. (a) With 20% power-assist. (b) Without power-assist.

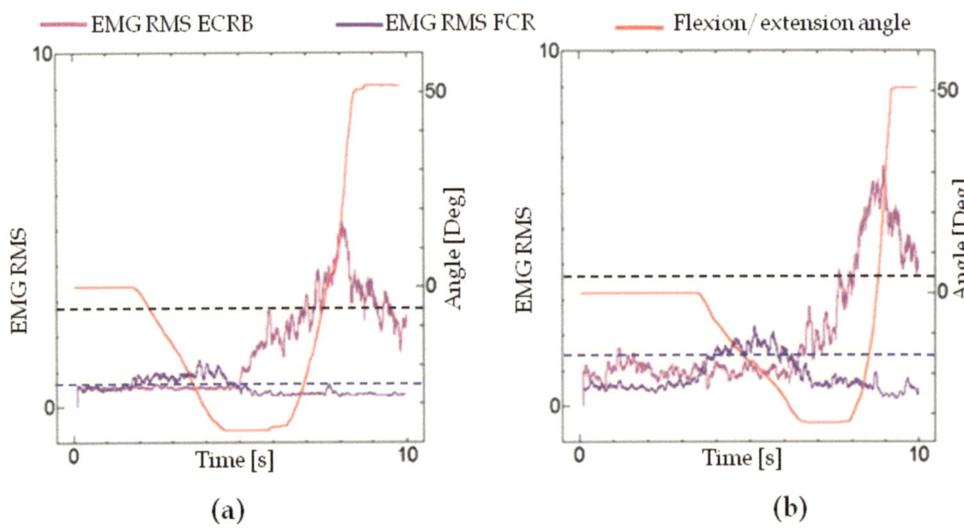

Fig. 18. Experimental results of subject-B for wrist flexion/extension. (a) With 20% power-assist. (b) Without power-assist.

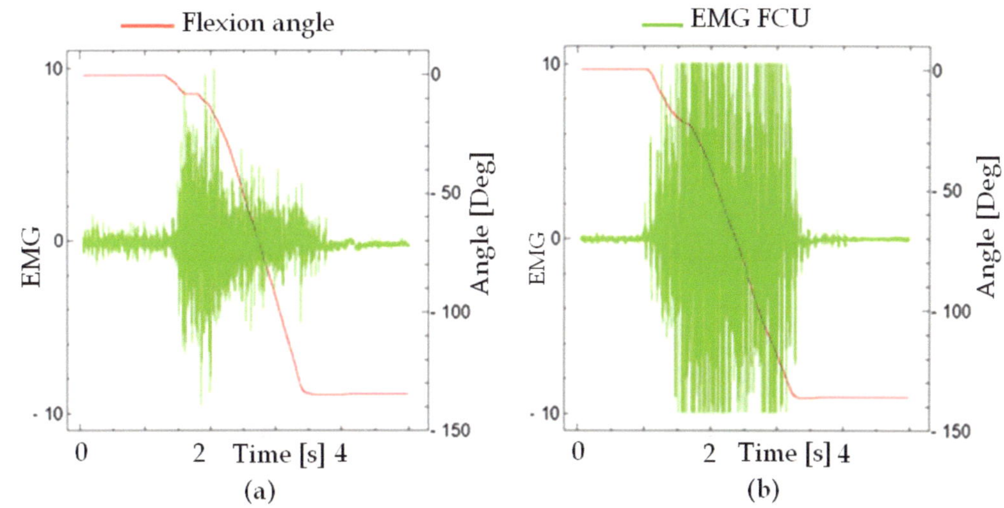

Fig. 19. Experimental results of subject-C for wrist flexion. (a) With 20% power-assist. (b) Without power-assist.

5. EMG-based control of a 6DOF exoskeleton robot

The 6DOF exoskeleton robot, SUEFUL-6 (Gopura & Kiguchi, 2008b) has been designed to be worn by a right upper-limb as shown in Fig. 20. Considering that most physically weak persons use wheel chairs, the SUEFUL-6 is designed to be installed on a wheel chair of physically weak persons. Therefore, the user does not feel the weight of the robot. The SUEFUL-6 mainly consists of a shoulder motion support part, an elbow motion support part, a forearm motion support part and a wrist motion support part. Figure 21 depicts the six axes of the SUEFUL-6. The shoulder motion support part of the SUEFUL-6 consists of an upper-arm link, driven pulleys for shoulder horizontal flexion/extension motion and shoulder vertical flexion/extension motion, potentiometers, an arm holder, a slider and the mechanism for moving center of rotation (CR). The rotational motions generated in the motors are transferred to the shoulder driven pulleys of the SUEFUL-6 through cable drives. The arm holder is attached to upper-arm link as shown in Fig. 20. The arm holder is made of thin flexible plastic with magic tape ribbon to hold the user's upper-arm. The distance between the arm holder and the CR of the shoulder joint of the exoskeleton is moderately adjusted automatically in accordance with the shoulder motion, in order to cancel out the ill effects caused by the position difference between the CR of the robot shoulder and the human shoulder (Kiguchi *et al.*, 2008). The distal end of the upper-arm link is attached to the elbow joint. The 1DOF elbow motion assist part of the exoskeleton robot consists of the proximal forearm link, a pulley, and a potentiometer. The motor pulley acts as driven pulley to generate elbow flexion/extension motion. The motor for the elbow flexion/extension motion have been fixed in the separate location of the frame of the robot. The rotational motion generated in the motor is transferred to the elbow driven pulleys of the SUEFUL-6 through a cable drive. The forearm motion support part and wrist motion support part are same as the W-EXOS. Only different is the attachment of forearm force sensor between proximal forearm link and distal forearm link as shown in the Fig. 20. The motor for supination/pronation (motor-D) is attached in the outer housing of the forearm cover. The distal forearm link is attached to the inner frame of the

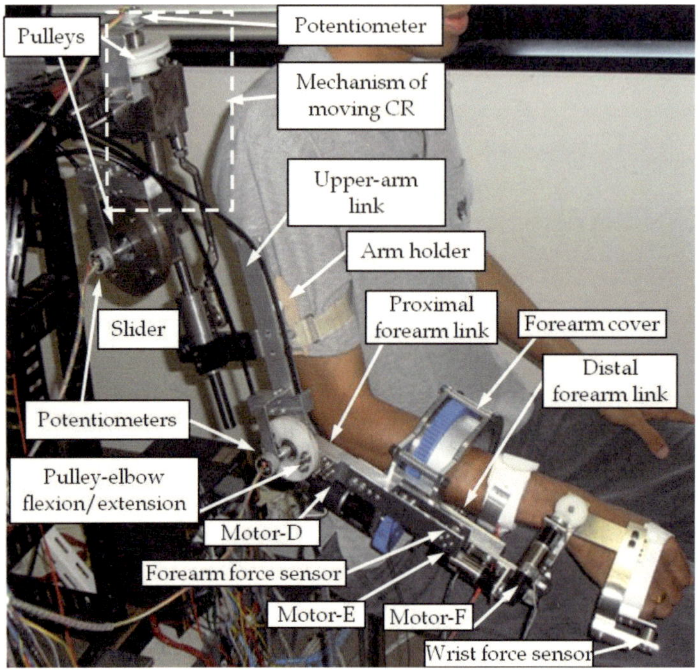

Fig. 20. 6DOF upper-limb motion power-assist exoskeleton robot (SUEFUL-6).

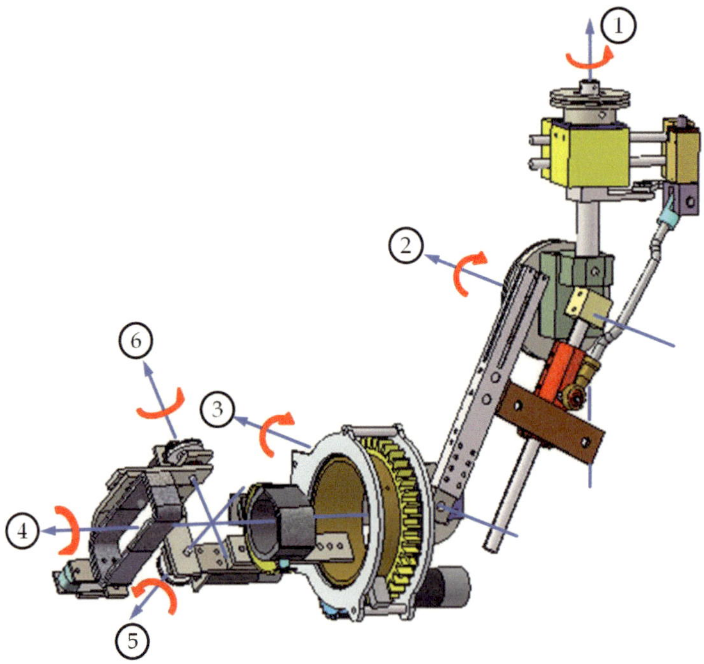

Fig. 21. CAD model of the SUEFUL-6 with axes of rotation. Number 1 to 6 indicates the axis for shoulder horizontal and vertical flexion/extension, elbow flexion/extension, forearm supination/pronation, wrist flexion/extension and radial ulnar deviation, respectively.

forearm cover. The wrist holder can be worn to the forearm of the user. The motor for wrist flexion/extension (motor-E) is fixed on the distal forearm link. The link attachment holds the motor (motor-F) for the wrist radial/ulnar deviation. More details of SUEFUL-6 can be referred in (Gopura & Kiguchi., 2008b).

5.1 EMG-based control method

EMG signals are used as main input information to control the SUEFUL-6 according to the user's motion intention. As in the EMG-based control method of the W-EXOS, the force/torque sensor signals of the sensors of the SUEFUL-6 are used as subordinate input information. The forearm force/torque and hand force are used as input information for the controller. When the user activates the muscles little (*i.e.,* EMG signal level is low) the forearm force/torque and hand force are used to control the SUEFUL-6. When the user activates the muscle a lot (*i.e.,* EMG signal level is high) EMG signals are used to control the SUEFUL-6. When the users muscle activation level is medium EMG signal, forearm force/torque and hand force are used to control the robot. By using input information as above, the error motions cause by the little EMG signal levels and the unexpected motion cause by the external forces affecting the user's upper-limb can be avoided. In order to identify the 6DOF upper-limb motions, the EMG signals of fourteen locations: (see Fig. 6 for locations of muscles) deltoid-anterior part, deltoid-posterior part, pectoralis major-clavicular part, teres major, biceps-short head, biceps-long head, triceps-long head, triceps-lateral head, pronator teres, supinator, extensor carpi radialis brevis, extensor carpi ulnaris, flexor carpi radialis and flexor carpi ulnaris are monitored.
Applying the monitored muscle signals fuzzy if-then control rules were designed. Basically the fuzzy-rules designed for the W-EXOS (Gopura & Kiguchi, 2008a) and 3DOF exoskeleton robots (Kiguchi *et al.,* 2008) were used with the modifications. Ten fuzzy if-then control rules were designed for the shoulder motions (Kiguchi *et al.,* 2008). An additional eleven fuzzy if-then control rules were designed for the elbow motion (Kiguchi *et al.,* 2008). For the forearm and wrist motions the control rules designed for the EMG-based controller of the W-EXOS is basically used (explained in section 4) with the modification to eliminate the effect of shoulder and elbow motion muscles. As an example, the modified fuzzy if-then rules for supination are shown in the Table 5. The fuzzy rules related to the shoulder and elbow motions are transferred to the fuzzy-neuro controller as explained in (Kiguchi *et al.,* 2008). The fuzzy rules related to the forearm and wrist motions are transferred to the fuzzy-neuro controller as explain in section 4. To eliminate the improper motion assist that might occur in the case of cooperative motion of the elbow and forearm (*i.e.,* simultaneous elbow flexion/extension and forearm supination/pronation) the RMS of the pronator teres

Rule	If	Then
01	Ch.10 = ZO and Ch.7=ZO	T1= ZO
02	Ch.10 = PB and Ch.7!=ZO	T1= PB
03	Ch.10! = PB and Ch.7!=ZO and Fx! = ZO and T = PS	T1= PS
04	Ch.10! = PB and Ch.7!=ZO Fx! = ZO and T = PB	T1= PB

Table 5. Some modified fuzzy if-then control rules. In Table 4; Fx=Force sensor signal for X-axis; T=Torque sensor signal; T1 =Torque command for forearm motor; '!=' represents "not equal".

(*i.e.*, a muscle common to both elbow flexion/extension and forearm pronation/supination) was used as an input variable to adjust the weight in the consequent part of the fuzzy control rules for the supination (Kiguchi *et al.*, 2005).

5.1.1 Training of the controller

The training (adaptation) of fuzzy-neuro controllers is carried out by adjusting each weight values of the fuzzy-neuro controller to minimize evaluation functions. In this study, error back-propagation learning algorithm has been applied to minimize the squared error functions. The error function is the same in (8). The adaptation of the controllers to the conditions of the robot user is important, since the EMG signal is a biological signal that varies according to the person and also to the physical and psychological conditions of the same person even with the same motion. The desired joint angle is indicated by a motion indicator (*i.e.*, a teaching device).

5.2 Evaluation of EMG-based controller SUEFUL-6

The experiments are performed with healthy male subjects (subject A-29 years, subject B-27 years) to evaluate the effectiveness of power-assist of the EMG-based control method. Human subjects performed daily activities of upper-limb without and with power-assist of the SUEFUL-6. The experimental set-up is basically similar to the set-up shown in Fig. 16.

The EMG levels of the related muscles were measured for both cases. When the motions are performed without power-assist, sensor signal based control was applied to the exoskeleton robot to perform natural upper-limb motions without any disturbance. If the SUEFUL-6 assists the motions properly from the EMG-based control method, the EMG levels of related muscles should be reduced when the robot assist the motions. The experimental results of subject-A for drinking motion (bringing a cup from table to near the mouth) is shown in Fig. 22. When the drinking motion was carried out with power-assist of 20% the maximum EMG

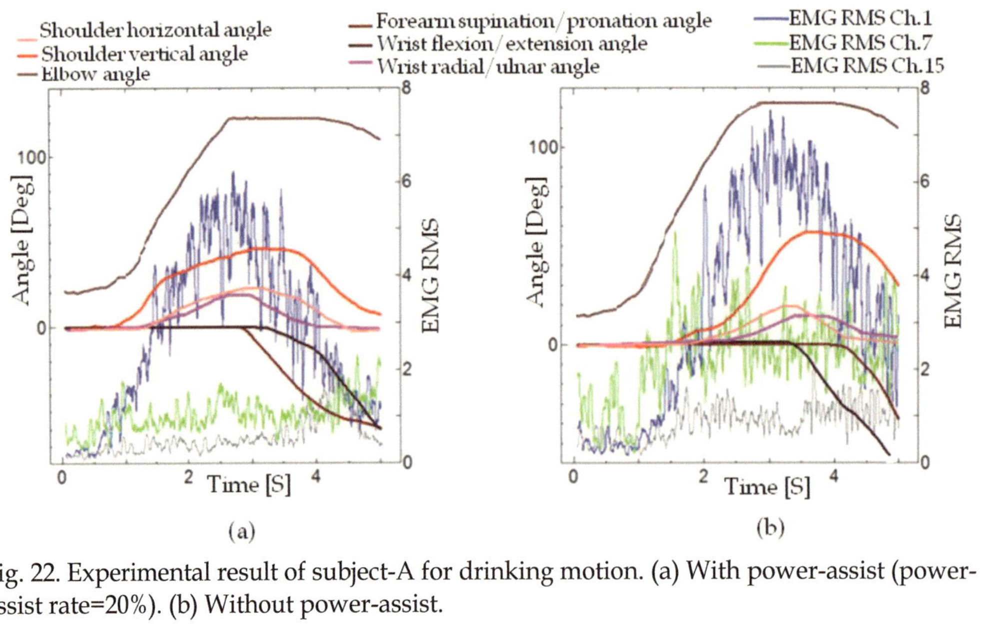

Fig. 22. Experimental result of subject-A for drinking motion. (a) With power-assist (power-assist rate=20%). (b) Without power-assist.

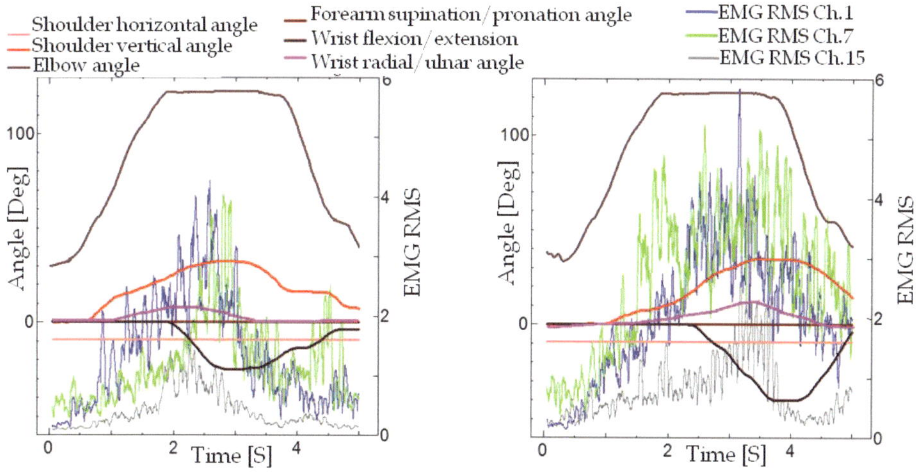

Fig. 23. Experimental result of subject-B for cooperative motions of upper-limb. (a) With power-assist (power-assist rate=45%). (b) Without power-assist.

RMS level of deltoid-anterior part (Ch.1) has reduced, where as it was higher without power-assist. The experimental result of subject-B for the cooperative motions of upper-limb is depicted in Fig. 23. In the experiment, when the motion was carried out with power-assist 45% power-assist is applied. Figure 23 shows that EMG RMS levels of related muscles have been reduced for the with power-assist motion. From the results it can be concluded that EMG can effectively be applied to control the SUEFUL-6. Further, the results show that the EMG-based control method can be used to effectively assist human upper-limb motions.

6. Conclusion

This chapter presents the application of surface EMG signals to control exoskeleton robots. At first the applied method to detect and process the surface EMG signals is explained. Then, the upper-limb muscle activities during daily upper-limb motions have been experimentally studied to enable exoskeleton robots to estimate human upper-limb motions based on EMG signals of related muscles. In the experimental study, minimum number of muscles to extract signals to control daily upper-limb motions has been identified. Then two case studies of application of EMG signals to control exoskeleton robots were presented. In the case studies EMG-based control methods and their evaluation is explained. From the evaluation results it is identified EMG signals can be used to control upper-limb exoskeleton robot. Further, the evaluation results verified that presented EMG-based control methods can be used to effectively assist human upper-limb motions.

7. Acknowledgment

The authors gratefully acknowledge the partial support provided for this research by Japan Society of Promotion of Science (JSPS) Grant-in-Aid for Scientific Research (C, 19560258). The authors would also like to extend their sincere gratitude to Prof. Etsuo Horikawa, Manoj Liyanage, Hui He and Dr. Nirosha Agalawatta for their cooperation to the research.

8. References

Farry, K. A.; Walker I. D. & Baraniuk R. G. (1996). Myoelectric Teleoperation of a Complex Robotic Hand. *IEEE Transaction on Robotics and Automation*, Vol.12, No. 5, pp. 775-788.

Gil Coury, H.; Kumar, S. & Narayan, Y. (1998). An Electromyographic Study of Upper Limb Adduction Force with Varying Shoulder and Elbow Postures. *Journal of Electromyography and Kinesiology* Vol. 8, pp. 157-168.

Gopura, R. A. R. C.; Kiguchi, K. & Horikawa, E. (2010). A Study on Human Upper-Limb Muscles Activities during Daily Upper-Limb Motions. *International Journal of Bioelectromagnetism*, Vol.12, No. 2, pp. 54-61.

Gopura, R. A. R. C. & Kiguchi, K. (2008a). An Exoskeleton Robot for Human Forearm and Wrist Motion Assist- Hardware Design and EMG-Based Controller. *International Journal of Advanced Mechanical Design, Systems, and Manufacturing*, Vol. 2, No. 6, pp. 1067-1083.

Gopura, R. A. R. C. & Kiguchi, K. (2008b). Development of a 6DOF Exoskeleton Robot for Human Upper-Limb Motion Assist. *Proceedings of International Conference on Information and Automation for Sustainability*, pp. 13-18, Colombo, Sri Lanka.

Gopura, R. A. R. C. & Kiguchi, K. (2008c). A Human Forearm and Wrist Motion Assist Exoskeleton Robot with EMG-Based Fuzzy-Neuro Control. *Proceedings of IEEE RAS/EMBS International Conference on Biomedical Robotics and Biomechatronics*, pp. 550-555, Scottsdale, Arizona, USA.

Hudgins, B.; Parker, P. & Scott, R. N. (1993). A New Strategy for Multifunction Myoelectric Control. *IEEE Transactions on Biomedical Engineering*, Vol. 12, No. 1, pp. 82-94.

Kiguchi, K.; Rahman, M. H.; Sasaki, M. & Teramoto, K. (2008). Development of a 3DOF Mobile Exoskeleton Robot for Human Upper Limb Motion Assist. *Robotics and Autonomous Systems*, Vol. 56, No. 8, pp. 678-691.

Kiguchi, K.; Imada Y. & Liyanage, M. (2007). EMG-Based Neuro-Fuzzy Control of a 4DOF Upper-Limb Power-Assist Exoskeleton", *Proceedings of International Conference on the IEEE Engineering in Medicine and Biology Society*, pp. 3040-3043.

Kiguchi, K.; Esaki, R. & Fukuda, T. (2005). Development of a Wearable Exoskeleton for Daily Forearm Motion Assist. *Advanced Robotics*, Vol. 00, No. 0, pp. 1-21.

Kiguchi, K.; Tanaka, T. & Fukuda, T. (2004). Neuro-Fuzzy Control of a Robotic Exoskeleton with EMG Signals. *IEEE Transactions on Fuzzy Systems*, Vol. 12, No. 4, pp. 481-490.

Kiguchi, K.; Kariya, S.; Watanabe, K,; Izumi, K. & Fukuda, T. (2001). An Exoskeletal Robot for Human Elbow Motion Support-Sensor Fusion, Adaptation, and Control. *IEEE Transaction on System Man Cybernetics. B*, Vol. 31, No. 3, pp. 353-361.

Luca, C. J. D. (2002). *Surface Electromyography: Detection and Recording*, Delsys Inc.

Martini, F. H.; Timmons M. J. & Tallitsch R. B. (1997) *Human Anatomy*, Pearson Education Inc., ISBN:0-13-049178-0, New Jersey.

Perry, J. C. & Rosen, J. (2007). Upper-Limb Powered Exoskeleton Design. *IEEE/ASME Transaction on Mechatronics*, Vol. 12, No. 4, pp. 408-417.

Rosen, J.; Perry, J. C.; Manning, N.; Burns, S. & Hannaford, B. (2005). The Human Arm Kinematics and Dynamics During Daily Activities-Toward a 7 DOF Upper Limb Powered Exoskeleton. *Proceedings of International Conference on Advanced* Robotics, pp. 532-539.

Vicon MX+, In: *Vicon Products*, 13.06.2011, Available from http://www.vicon.com/

6

Trunk Muscle Activity Affects the Level of Performance in Human Body

Satoru Kai
Faculty of Allied Health Sciences, Kansai University of Welfare Sciences, Japan

1. Introduction

1.1 To attain an excellent body performance level

In rehabilitation practices, we therapists often offer support to patients so they can perform the very basic operations smoothly, such as getting up, standing up and walking. A decrease in daily life activity after a fall-caused fracture among senior citizens has now become an object of public concern in rapidly graying societies. Various approaches to fall prevention have therefore been tried, particularly from the viewpoint of preventive medicine. We also lend support to precisely those seniors with decreased body performance so as to improve that very performance level. We shall clarify in what follows how excellent body performance levels can be attained by activating the trunk muscle activity.

1.2 Why we focus on the deep muscle of the trunk

Lower trunk, or abdominal-dorsal part of the spine supports the body, has the following support system. The back is supported by the spine, the front is protected by rectus abdominal muscle between the ribs and pubic bone, and the lateral abdomen on each side is covered by three muscles, i.e., the external oblique muscle, the internal oblique muscle, and the transversus abdominis muscle (Fig. 1). The pelvis serves as the trunk's lower border, while the upper part, or abdominal cavity, is demarcated by the diaphragm. Transversus abdominis muscle, a deep muscle, plays a role of a corset together with the lumbodorsal fascia of the back.

In more details, anterolateral abdominal muscles and the muscles that form the roof (diaphragm), floor (pelvic floor muscles) and posterolateral (quadratus lumborum and psoas) aspects of the abdominal cavity contribute the control of the lumbar spine and pelvis (Richardson et al., 2004). Transversus abdominis muscle, the deepest of the abdominal muscles, arises from the thoracolumbar fascia between the iliac crest and the twelfth rib at the lateral raphe, the internal aspects of the lower six costal cartilages, where it interdigitates with the diaphragm, the lateral third of the inguinal ligament and the anterior two-thirds of the inner lip of the iliac crest (Richardson et al., 2004). Internal oblique muscle forms the middle layer of the lateral abdominal wall, with a muscular attachment to the lateral two-thirds of the inguinal ligament, the anterior two-thirds of the iliac crest and the lateral raphe of the thoracolumbar fascia in a band 2-3cm wide, attaching to fibers of the deep lamina arising from the L3 spinous process (Richardson et al., 2004). External oblique muscle is the

most superficial of the lateral abdominal muscles. It arises via eight digitations from the external surface of the lower eight ribs (Richardson et al., 2004).
The global muscles such as the obliques, rectus abdominis, erector spinae and superficial multifidi are designed for movement but not for stability (Lee, 2004). The trunk stability is important for trunk mobility. Stability is achieved through motion, not rigidity (Lee, 2004). The transversus abdominis muscle, or trunk stabilizer muscle, is controlled by voluntary contraction, because it is a skeletal muscle. It is therefore important to keep transversus abdominal muscle ready for action at any given time. Transversus abdominis muscle is also an anticipatory muscle for stabilization of the lower back and is recruited prior to the initiation of any movement of the upper or lower extremity (Lee, 2004).

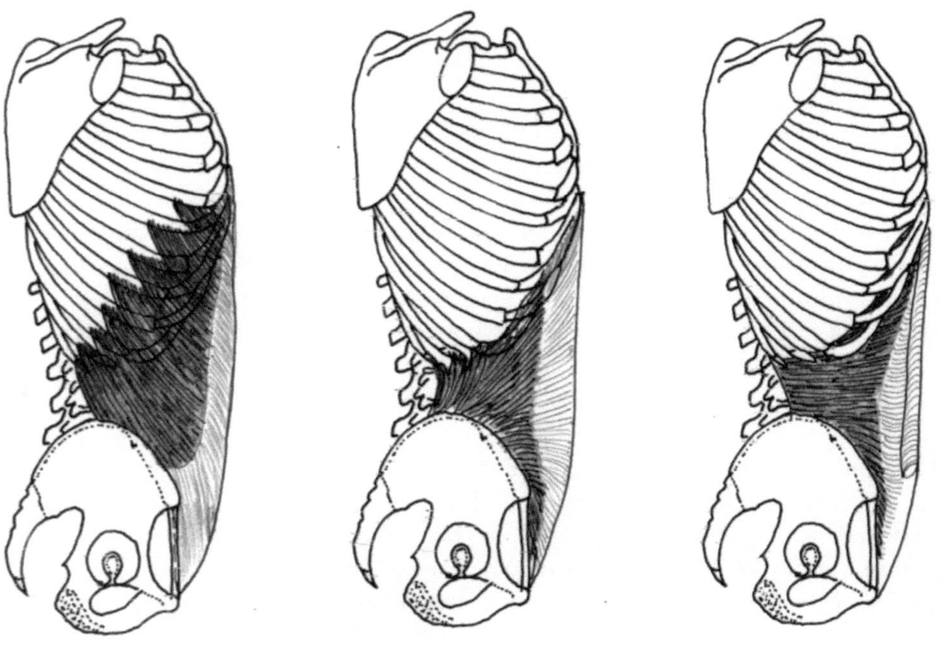

Fig. 1. Lateral abdominal muscles.
a. External oblique muscle: superficial layer
b. Internal oblique muscle: middle layer
c. Transversus abdominis muscle: deep layer

2. Health science research making use of electromyography

We have continued to examine body performance levels in terms of electromyography (Kai et al., 2008a, 2008b). Electromyographic waves can shed light on various phenomena through frequency analysis and wavelet transform, among others. Surface electrodes have proved to be a useful non-invasive tool to measure body performance levels. A fair number of researchers have argued, however, that once electrodes are detached after a measurement, the very conditions that have given the readings are lost, reducing the reliability of the data considerably. That may well be one of the limits of the analysis of body functions by means of electromyographs. (We are dealing with living human bodies after all.) There is a method of regularizing the myogenic potential, however, if one takes into account the amount of muscle activity at the time of its maximum isometric contraction. One may still argue that there is a possibility that the amount of muscle activity at maximum isometric contraction may change through long-term intervention. Real changes in the performance level may not be caught by the %MVC evaluation over time. To address this weakness in the research protocol directly, we have devised a system whereby the intervention effect is measured and evaluated on the same day.

3. To improve standing balance

3.1 Trunk muscle activity while moving from two-leg to one-leg standing in healthy elderly adults (Kai et al., 2008b)

Standing balance ability covers static and dynamic balancing. When a subject is moving, such as in walking, dynamic balancing is needed for him to fulfill the needed capacity of balance. We have singled out anticipatory postural adjustment for examination from among the various factors that figure in the balance ability. Anticipatory postural adjustment refers to an adjustment made in a subject's posture in which his weight gathers in the left, for instance, before he raises the right leg while standing. We have analyzed the muscle activity of the trunk and the hip joint while he shifts from two-leg to one-leg standing. Electromyographic activities were recorded of left internal oblique, left multifidus, left gluteus medius, and right iliopsoas muscles by surface-type electromyography (Fig. 2). No differences in muscle activity were found between young subjects and healthy elderly adults. We therefore concluded that healthy elderly adults in general have kept the muscle activity level necessary for anticipatory postural adjustments.

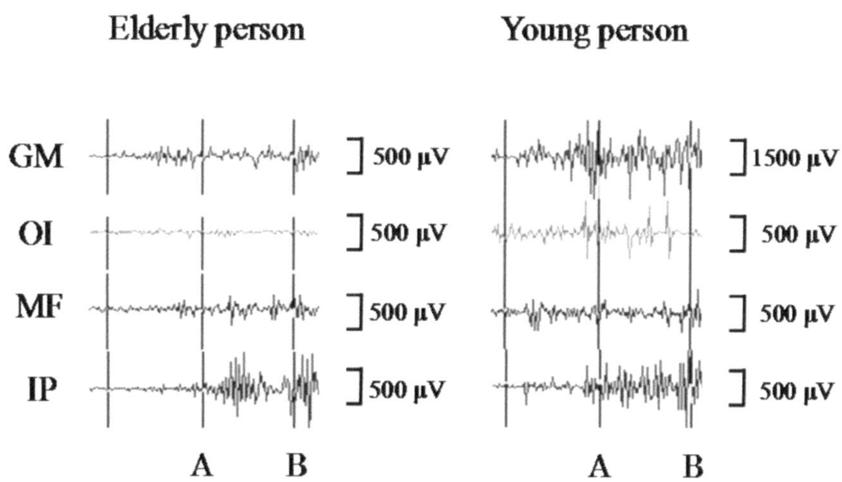

Abbreviations, GM, gluteus medius muscle; OI, internal oblique muscle (obliquus internus abdominis); MF, multifidus muscle; IP, ilio-psoas muscle;

(Reproduced with permission from Kai et al., 2008b, p.78.)

Fig. 2. Representative EMG of GM, OI, MF and IP.
A: 500 ms before the start of raising the right foot.
B: just before the start of raising the right foot.

3.2 Immediate effect of trunk muscle training in healthy elderly adult (Kai et al., 2008a)

We are also doing research on fall prevention among the elderly. Specifically, we are examining how they can improve their body performance by activating trunk muscles for posture control. We have focused on just those elderly people with rather poor balance while standing and examined their postural adjustment before and after a training session in activating internal oblique muscle. We found that % integrated electromyography and the coefficient of variation of internal oblique muscle decreased significantly, and % integrated electromyography of multifidus muscle decreased under action. In gluteus medius muscle, on the other hand, no changes were observed before and after the training (Table 1). Based on these results, we suggest that the training method adopted here may prove useful in activating a series of smooth activities of lower trunk muscles during action.

Muscle	OI		MF		GM	
	%iEMG	CV	%iEMG	CV	%iEMG	CV
Pre-training	19.08±2.43	37.57±10.06	5.14±1.04	32.24±16.20	6.99±1.41	25.99±15.01
Post-training	15.61±2.42*	19.38±10.16*	3.93±0.55*	21.41±12.73	6.33±1.36	26.18±11.13

*p<0.01: pre-training vs post-training
Mean ± standard deviation
Abbreviations, OI, internal oblique muscle (obliquus internus abdominis); MF, multifidus muscle; GM, gluteus medius muscle; CV, coefficient of variation.

(Reproduced with permission from Kai et al., 2008a, p.64.)

Table 1. Average %iEMG and coefficient of variation of 10 intervals before and after the training.

3.3 Immediate effect of trunk muscle training in young healthy people

We shall describe what effect trunk muscle training had among young healthy people in their ability of one-leg standing balance. Though they are no doubt needed, trunk muscles of the abdomen are not used very much in daily life. In healthy young women in Japan in particular, physical training is not part of their lifestyle to begin with. In the present study, we shall clarify how activation of trunk muscles can lead to alleviation of unsteadiness in their center of gravity during one-leg standing. Eighteen healthy adult women (average age 21.5 years old; range 20-23 years old) participated in the study. Unsteadiness of their center of gravity during one-leg standing was measured before and after a seat sitting balance exercise. While the subjects gazed forward while standing first on the right leg, the total tracks length was measured for 30 seconds; and then the same was repeated on the left leg. In the seat sitting balance exercise, the subjects gazed forward with both legs off of the floor and both arms hung loosely down, and they maintained the seat sitting for 2 minutes on a balance cushion (Fig.3). Results were that those women poor in balance with 100cm or more in total tracks length before the exercise (Group A, and less than 100cm in total tracks length is Group B) showed significant decreases in the total tracks length (Fig. 4). The finding suggests that trunk muscle training was effective in improving one-leg standing balance ability. We also suggest that activation of trunk muscles does influence balance taking while standing.

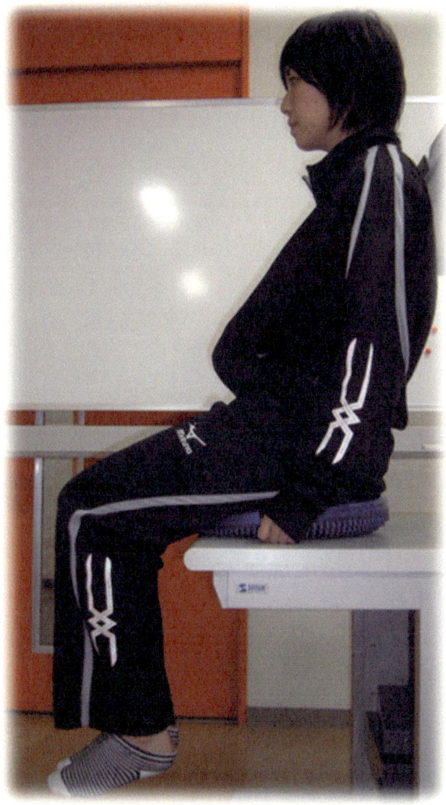

Fig. 3. The seat sitting balance exercise.

Group A*

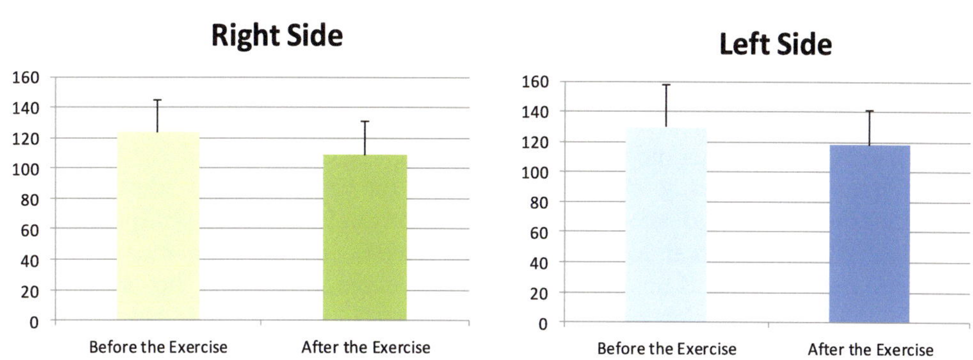

Fig. 4. (Continued)

Group B

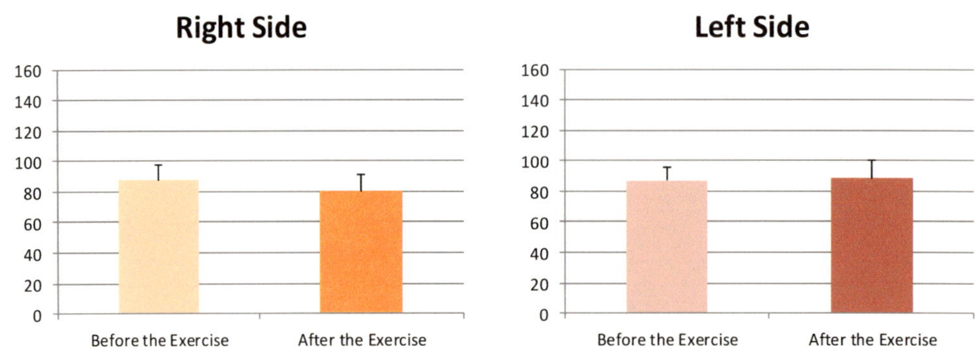

Unit: cm
Group A: 100cm or more in total tracks length before the exercise
Group B: less than 100cm in total tracks length before the exercise
*p<0.05: before the exercise vs. after the exercise

Fig. 4. Total tracks length while one-leg standing for 30 seconds before and after the exercise.

4. To improve general reaction in human body

4.1 Whole body reaction time and muscle activity in jump action

Whole body reaction time is used as a measurement of the body performance. Jump action is generally used for the measurement of the whole body reaction time. We have focused on trunk muscle activity in jump action. We then clarified the relationship between whole body reaction time and muscle activity in trunk muscles and leg extensor muscle in vertical jump action (Tanabe et al., 2010). Twelve healthy men (average 22.3±0.8 years old; range 21-24 years old) participated. When a red light, placed 2m ahead, lit, a subject jumped vertically as quickly as possible. And the time from light stimulus to both feet aloft was measured and recorded 5 times each for the following muscles in the order given: right gastrocnemius muscle, right biceps femoris muscle, right internal oblique muscle, and right multifidus muscle by surface electromyograph. Fig.5 shows the results. Average whole body reaction time was 291.8±37.2 msec, while significance was found only in internal oblique muscle ($r=0.80$, $p<0.05$) in the relationship between whole body reaction time and muscle contraction inception time (Fig.6). We suggest that a person capable of using his internal oblique muscle can start the foot-off action more quickly, and that the trunk muscles took part in whole body agility.

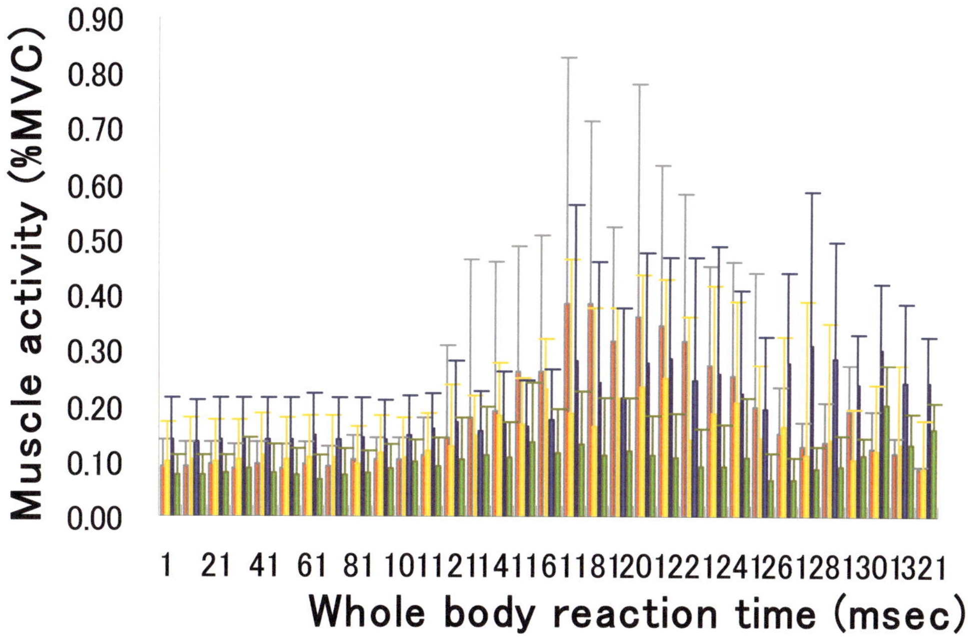

Red label: gastrocnemius muscle
Yellow label: biceps femoris muscle
Blue label: Internal oblique muscle
Green label: multifidus muscle

Fig. 5. EMG during jump action.

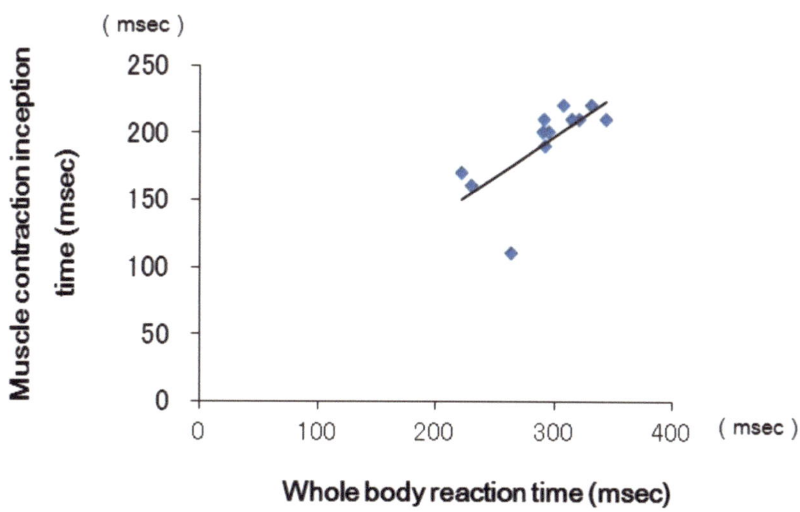

Fig. 6. Relationship between whole body reaction time and muscle contraction inception time.

4.2 Improving general reaction by expiration muscle training

Having clarified the relationship between quick jump action and internal oblique muscle, we went on to determine how to train this particular muscle to shorten the whole body reaction time. Internal oblique muscle was activated by using expiration muscle training. Ten healthy men (average 21.6±0.7 years old; range 20-22 years old) participated. The jump action given them was the same as in 4.1 above. Muscle activity was recorded from right internal oblique muscle. There was a significant shortening in whole body reaction time before and after the training (Fig.7). We have thus verified an effect of trunk muscle training, and internal oblique's role in the shortening of the whole body reaction time.

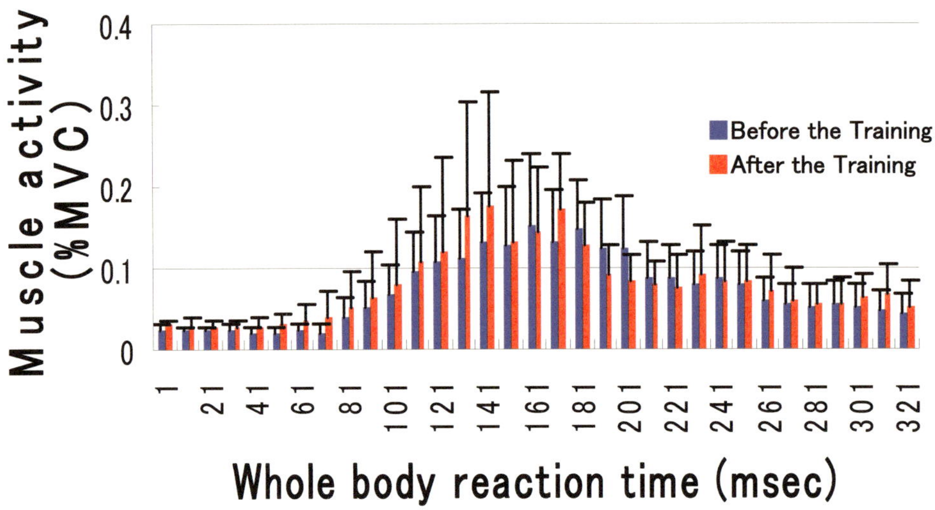

Fig. 7. Whole body reaction time before and after the training.

5. Body performance and trunk muscle activity

5.1 Improving trunk muscle output after breath training

We have demonstrated a positive effect of effort expiratory training on the shortening of whole body reaction time. Rectus abdominis, internal and external oblique, transversus abdominis, transversus thoracis, and internal intercostalis muscles are known as muscles that act in effort expiration. The four abdominal muscles work as a group in expiration to bend the chest, and to depress both the rib cage and the sternum. The intra-abdominal pressure is then indirectly raised, and the diaphragm is pushed forcefully up in the thoracic cavity via compression of the organs in the thorax. The action of transversus thoracis and internal intercostalis muscles in expiration is to depress the rib, which in turn decreases the amount of the thoracic cavity content. Rapid expiration, if needed, is done thanks to the action of these muscles. We then confirmed muscle activity in effort expiration before trying to determine whether stimulating the expiration muscles would improve the trunk muscles' muscular power. Six healthy men (average 22.3±0.5 years old; range 21-23 years old) participated. The muscular power of the trunk muscles was compared before and after an effort expiration action using a spirometer. Surface electromyogram was used to trace the muscle activity under measurement. Internal oblique, rectus abdominis, multifidus, and erector spinae muscles were chosen for recording. The muscular power of the flexor and extensor muscles of the trunk was measured twice each by isokinetic movement of 60°/sec. There was a significant increase ($p<0.05$) in average power value of the extensor muscle. All the subjects showed an increase in the activity of internal oblique muscle while using a spirometer. These results suggest that the approach to the inner, or core, muscles comes to influence the stability of the trunk, facilitating the work of the outer muscles.

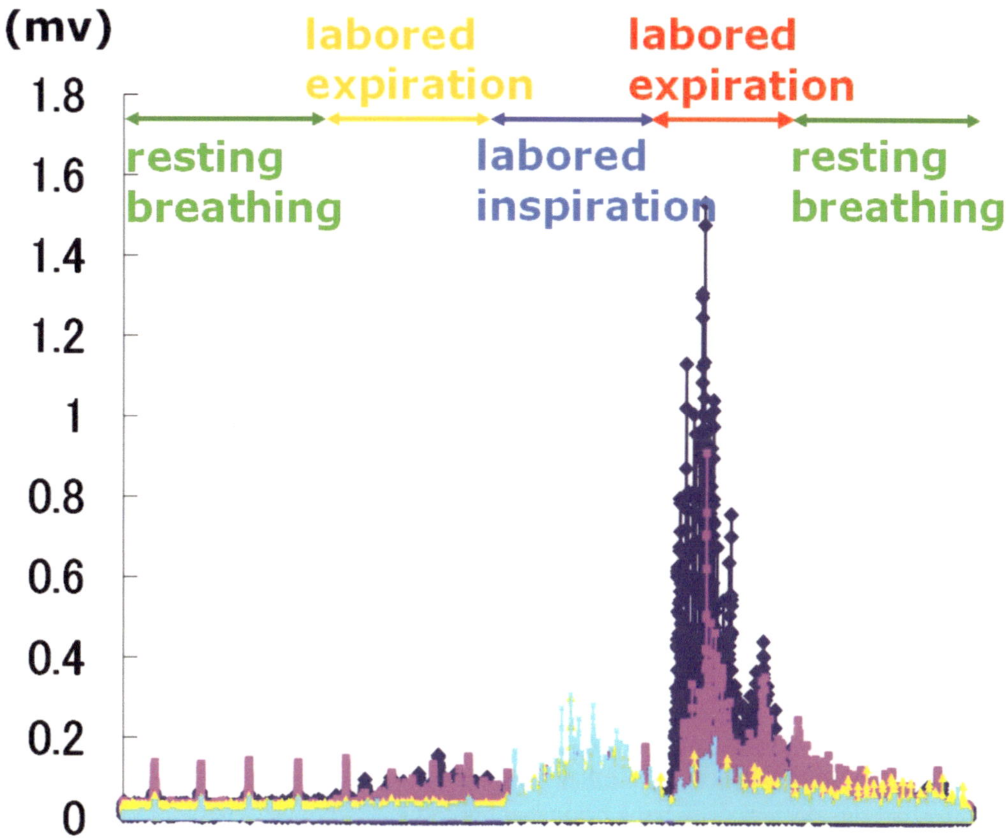

Fig. 8. EMG during labored respiration.

EMG black line: Internal oblique muscle, pink line: Rectus abdominis muscle, yellow line: Multifidus muscle, light blue line: Erector spinae muscle

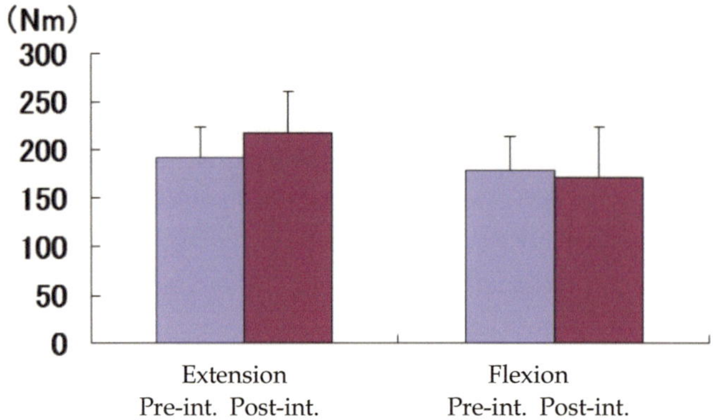

Fig. 9. Maximum torque value of the pre- and post-intervention.

5.2 Relationship between posture and trunk muscle activity – research by means of electromyography and ultrasound imagery

We have a number of research projects focusing on the relationship between body trunk muscles and body performance. There now exists a variety of trunk muscle training methods, including machine-assisted exercise regimens in the gym. In general, however, trunk muscles are not used all that much in an average person's daily life, so that even a simple home exercise routine can prove effective in the strengthening of trunk muscles. That being the case, we tried to determine, using surface electromyography and ultrasound imagery, whether keeping a posture for a certain length of time would enhance activation of the trunk muscles. Ten healthy adult men (average 21.5±0.5 years old; range 21-22 years old) participated in this program. The measurement postures were i) resting supine position (rest), ii) on knee-elbow position (knee-elbow), iii) elbow setting up lateral decubitus position (side-lying bridge), and iv) two legs bent and raised supine position (supine). An electrode was attached to external oblique muscle between ribs and to internal oblique muscle on the bottom of the abdomen. Ultrasound imagery was taken from a part of the abdominal side so that we could confirm all three layers (external oblique, internal oblique, and transversus abdominis muscles). Results showed that internal oblique muscle worked more actively in the side-lying bridge than in the rest of the positions by ultrasound imagery research. This fact should in passing be incorporated into an effective trunk muscle training program.

EMG results showed that external oblique (EO) muscle activity in side-lying bridge was higher than in other positions, but internal oblique/external oblique ratio (IO/EO ratio) of muscle activity was lower than in other positions (Fig. 10). The outcome prompted us to assume that this posture (side-lying bridge) enhanced the muscular activity of outer muscle more markedly than that of inner muscle. In supine position, in contrast, internal oblique (IO) and IO/EO ratio of muscle activity were higher than in other positions, which means that inner muscle is promoted more in muscle activity than in outer muscle (also Fig. 10).

Changes of muscle thickness taken by ultrasound imagery showed an increase in the transverse diameter of a muscle, which was indicative of sustained muscular contraction (Fig. 11). Because of a 1.5-fold increase in IO/EO ratio in both knee-elbow and side-lying bridge positions in outer muscle thickness, we suggest that inner muscle is definitely easier to grow in muscle thickness in both these positions (Fig. 12).

EMG showed higher IO and IO/EO ratio in supine position than in other positions, but that was not the case in ultrasound imagery study. The relationship between the two awaits clarification in the future.

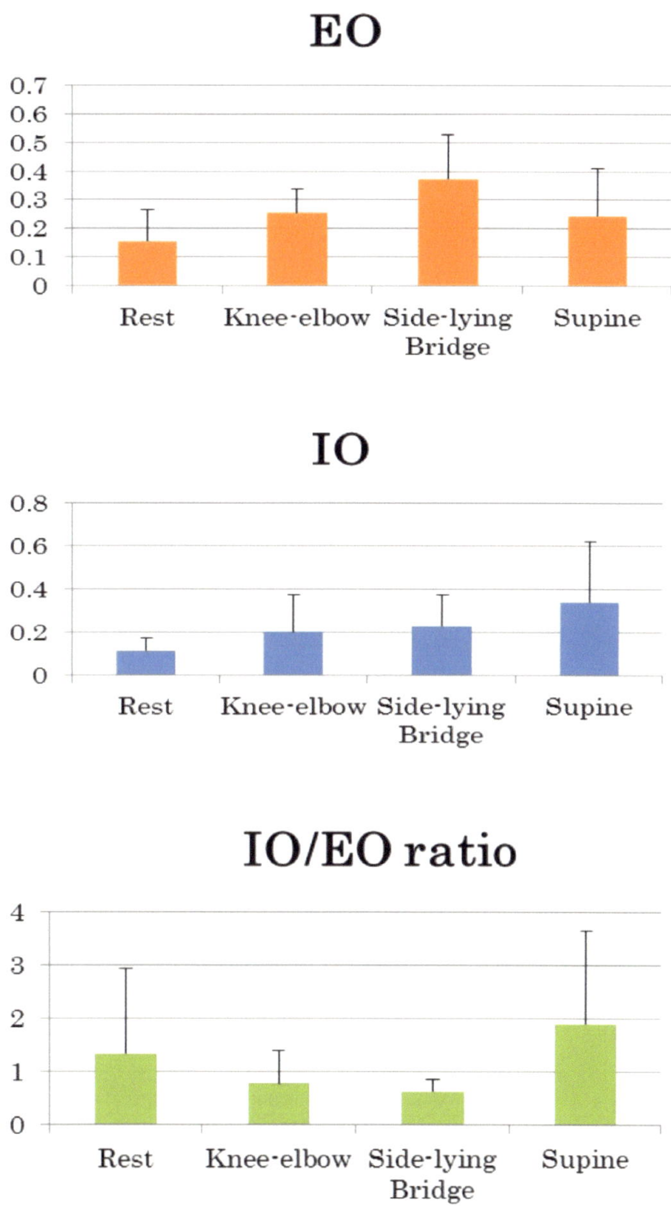

Abbreviations, EO, external oblique muscle; IO, internal oblique muscle; IO/EO ratio, internal oblique muscle/external oblique muscle ratio;

Fig. 10. EMG of EO, IO, and IO/EO ratio in each position.

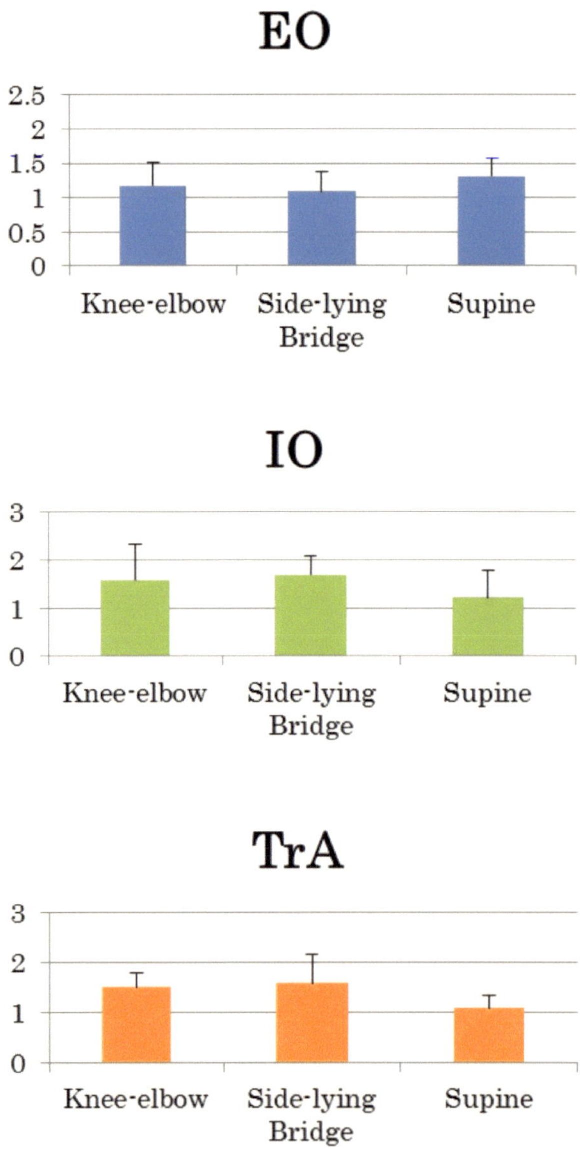

Abbreviations, EO, external oblique muscle; IO, internal oblique muscle; TrA, transversus abdominis muscle;

Fig. 11. Muscle contracted-rest thickness of EO, IO, and TrA in each position.

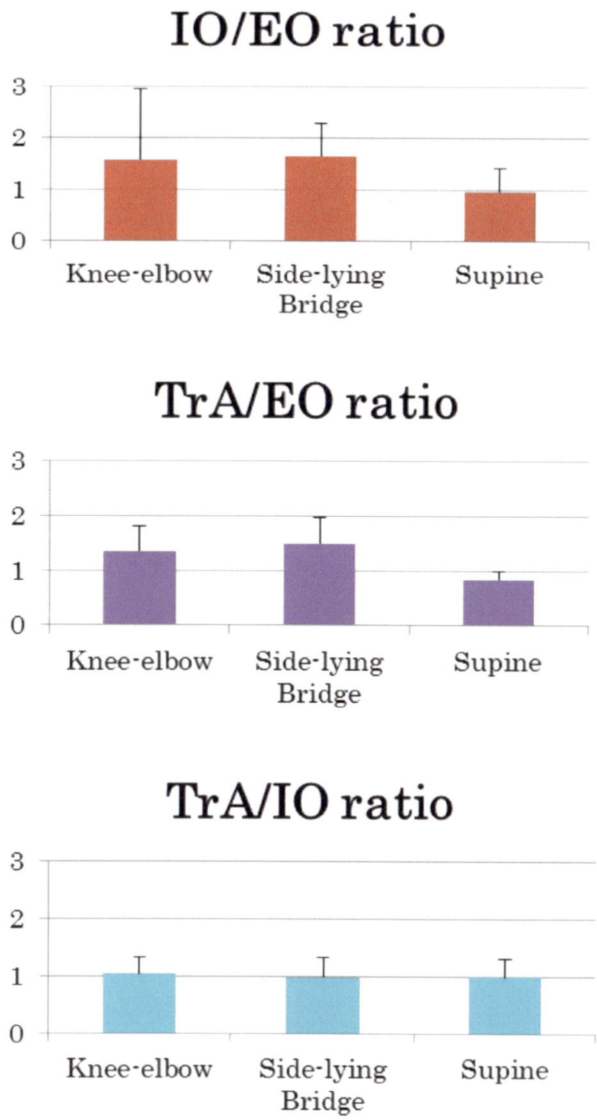

Abbreviations, IO/EO ratio, internal oblique muscle/external oblique muscle ratio;
TrA/EO ratio, transversus abdominis muscle/external oblique muscle ratio;
TrA/IO ratio, transversus abdominis muscle/internal oblique muscle ratio;

Fig. 12. Muscle contracted-rest thickness of IO/EO, TrA/EO, and TrA/IO ratios in each position.

6. Conclusion

A patient is referred to us physical therapists for an evaluation and treatment of his/her condition, we come up with a list of signs and symptoms, and we try to determine how best to proceed. We know that by increasing the patient's strength and endurance we will often see a decrease (or disappearance) in some of those signs and symptoms, ostensibly curing the patient. We hope to have shown that electromyography is a means that is highly useful, therefore important, in the evaluation of the conditions of a patient's trunk muscle activity.

7. Acknowledgements

This study was supported in part by The Japan Health Foundation for the Prevention of Chronic Diseases and the Improvement of QOL of Patients.

8. References

Kai, S.; Yoshimoto, R.; Nakahara, M.; Murakami, S.; Watari, K.; Takahashi, S. (2008a). Change of the muscular activity by activation training of the lower trunk muscle in two-leg to one-leg standing shift of an elderly man, *J. Phys. Ther. Sci.*, vol. 20, pp. 63-66

Kai, S.; Yoshimoto, R.; Nakahara, M.; Murakami, S.; Watari, K.; Takahashi, S. (2008b). Trunk muscle activity in two-leg standing to one-leg standing in healthy elderly adults, *J. Phys. Ther. Sci.*, vol. 20, pp. 77-80

Lee, D. (2004). The pelvic girdle, 3rd ed, Elsevier

Richardson, C.; Hodges, P.; Hides, J. (2004). Therapeutic exercise for lumbopelvic stabilization, 2nd ed, Elsevier

Tanabe, T.; Yamamoto, H.; Ariyoshi, Y.; Matsumoto, A.; Momii, Y.; Koga, M.; Yoshino, C.; Kai, S.; Takahashi, S. (2010). Whole body reaction time and muscle activity in jump action, *The 45th Congress of JPTA.*, vol. 37, pp. 1521

7

EMG in People with Different Heel Height Condition

Xiaoxiang Su[1] and Yaodong Gu[2]
[1]School of Engineering, Liverpool John Moores University, Liverpool
[2]Faculty of Sport Science, Ningbo University, Ningbo
[1]UK
[2]China

1. Introduction

It has been reported that a prevalence proportion of foot problems in women were associated with wearing high-heeled shoes [1]. Women's walking pattern and the biomechanical behavior of the foot could be altered significantly by raising the heel height [2, 3]. Biomechanical studies showed that walking in high-heeled shoes may alter lower-extremity joint function [4], raise the peak pressure in the forefoot [5], and alter the load distribution on the media foot region [6]. Some of these biomechanical changes can be detrimental to the foot structure, such as increasing the metabolic cost of gait, accelerate on of muscle fatigue [7], high inner stress level of metatarsal bones [8]. In Latin dancing, partners perform tightly choreographed routines in which they must project energy and passion. The pair's appearance, including costuming and shoes, is important to the success of the routine. A detailed biomechanical study of different types of human movement such as walking, dancing, etc. would help to improve the understanding of the biomechanics and provide important data for design optimization to reduce the adverse effects associated with high heeled shoes.

The detailed diagnosis and correction of pathologic states of human mobility is mainly limited by an incomplete knowledge of the musculoskeletal system and the detailed and quantitative description of the activity of the individual muscles in the synergistic patterns which combine to produce different human movement. Commonly used techniques which employ myolectric, force plate and kinematic gait pattern acquisition only provide a representation of the external manifestations of the underlying muscle physiology. At present, there is no exist research equipment to study the actions of the involved muscles non-invasively. A model of the musculoskeletal system could, in principle, given kinematic data and with assumptions to mitigate muscle redundancy, predict individual muscle behavior. Surface electromyography (SEMG), has been used in both research and clinical applications for non-invasive neuromuscular assessment in several different fields such as sport science, neurophysiology and rehabilitation. Different variables, related to different aims, can be monitored: muscle activation intervals are useful to evaluate motor coordination and treatment efficacy [9]; myoelectrical manifestations of fatigue [10] can be used to assess EMG signal modifications in pathologies such as exercise [11], back pain [12] and neurological diseases [13]. Previous EMG study in high heel gait found out the low back EMG increased significantly while walking with high-heeled shoes, which successfully explained the reason why high heel wearers always complained of lumber back pain [14]. But there is very limited study of the high-heeled state of muscle activity in a high intensity movement such as dancing. Female dancers have to wear high-heeled shoes during routine exercise and competitions, while passively raised heel could greatly increased the foot injury probability [5]. The objective of this study is to investigate the lower limb muscles' surface SEMG activity during Latin dancing with different heel height shoes.

2. Methods

The study involved 10 professional female dancers to participate in the biomechanical tests and data collection. The mean age of the subjects was 22.8years (S.D. 2.3 years), the mean weight of the subjects was 49.5kg (S.D. 5.2 kg), and the mean height of the subject was 163.6cm (S.D. 2.5 cm). Each participant has more than five years' dancing history. The subjects' feet/lower limb was clinically checked to ensure that there was no recent injury phenomenon or medical conditions that may affect their performances. The shoes used in this study have a similar structure apart from the heel height. Typical dancing conditions included four shoes with a heel height of 1.0cm, 4.5cm, 7.5cm and 10cm, designated as flat, low heel, medium high heel and high heel shoes, respectively.

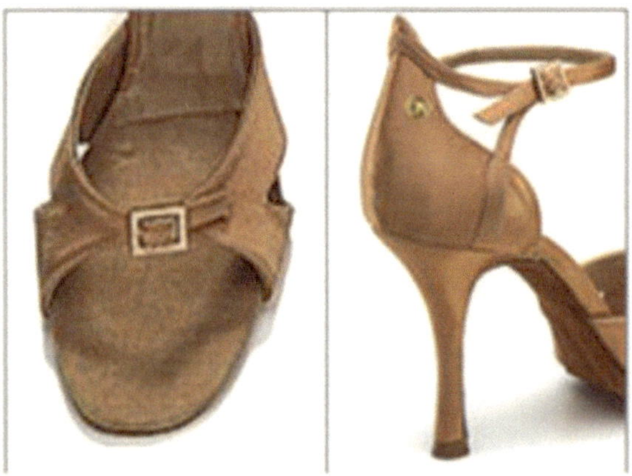

Fig. 1. The structure of typical dancing shoes.

Typical dancing shoes are made of leather, women's Latin dance shoes are lightweight, flexible and have suede soles, which provide the right blend of grip and slide while moving across the floor (Fig.1). In the study, shoes of different heel heights (1.0cm, 4.5cm, 7.5cm and 10cm) were randomly assigned to the participants. Each participant walked 5 minutes before the test in order to habituate to each heel height shoes, and took a 20-min rest in-between dance to prevent body fatigue. All the subjects were required to perform a similar warm up exercise before the test, and the Latin basic motion *visk* step (basic crossing step, Fig.2) was selected as experiment motion, concomitance with the dancing music.

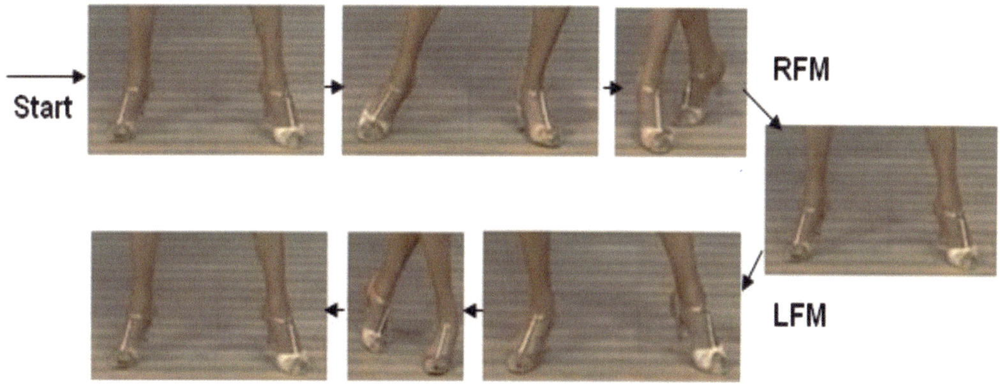

Fig. 2. Illustration of *visk* (crossing) step in the latin dancing: RFM (right foot move); LFM (left foot move).

SEMG activities of the tibialis anterior (TA), medial and lateral sides of gastrocnemius (MG and LG), soleus (SO) and biceps femoris (BF) were obtained using self-adhesive pairs of disposable Ag/AgCl surface electrode pairs with an electrode diameter of 10mm and an inter-electrode spacing of 20mm. Low impedance at the skin-electrode interface was obtained by skin preparation procedure of shaving, light abrasion and cleaning. For electrode placement, the SENIAM [15] recommendations for SEMG were followed (Fig.3). Furthermore, the electrode placement was confirmed by palpations of muscle bulk during brief maximal isometric contraction. The raw SEMG signal was recorded at the sampling rate of 1000Hz using a device (ME6000, Mega Electronics, Finland). The average EMG (aEMG) for the five muscles were calculated which using the rectified signal with a 512ms window, and used for further analysis.
Statistical data analysis was conducted with the statistical software package SPSS (version 13.0). Analysis of variance was employed to study the effects of heel height, and Turkey's HSD test was used for post hoc comparison. The level of significance was set at the 5% level.

3. Results

Fig.4 illustrated the comparison of aEMG data in five lower limb muscles during dancing under different heel height. It was clearly shown that all the muscles aEMG values except BF were significantly increased in heightened heel shoes comparing to wearing the flat heel height dancing ($p<0.05$). The largest increasing value of aEMG between flat and low heel height was appeared in LG, which was up to 36%. Differences were not found in LG, MG and SO among low, medium and high heel height.
Meanwhile, it was interesting to find that the aEMG value was quite close between the low and medium heel height in LG. Also, in BF the muscle activity was not changed a lot between the medium and high heel height. Although the mean value of aEMG data increased from low to high heel height, the significant difference only appeared at TA in which the high heel height was larger than the value in both low and medium heel height.

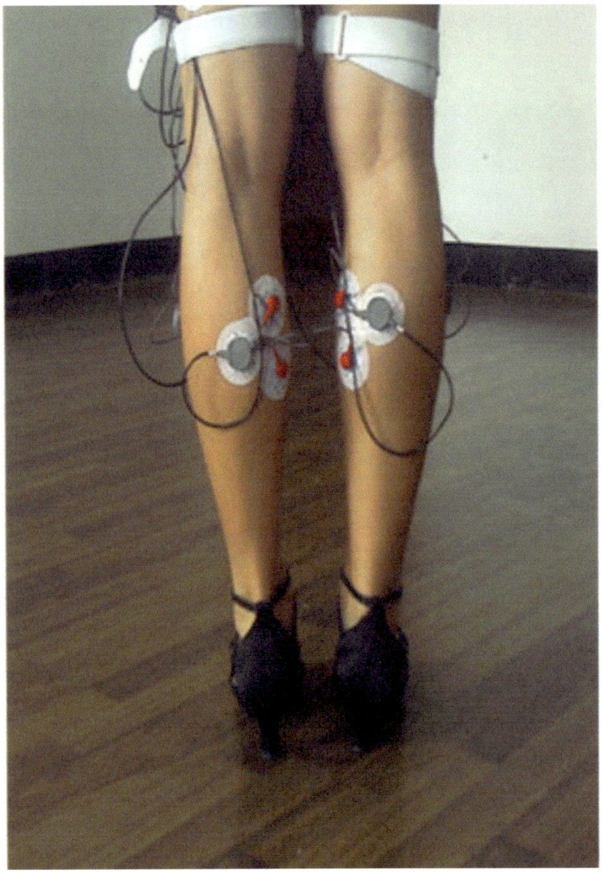

Fig. 3. Electrode placement methods.

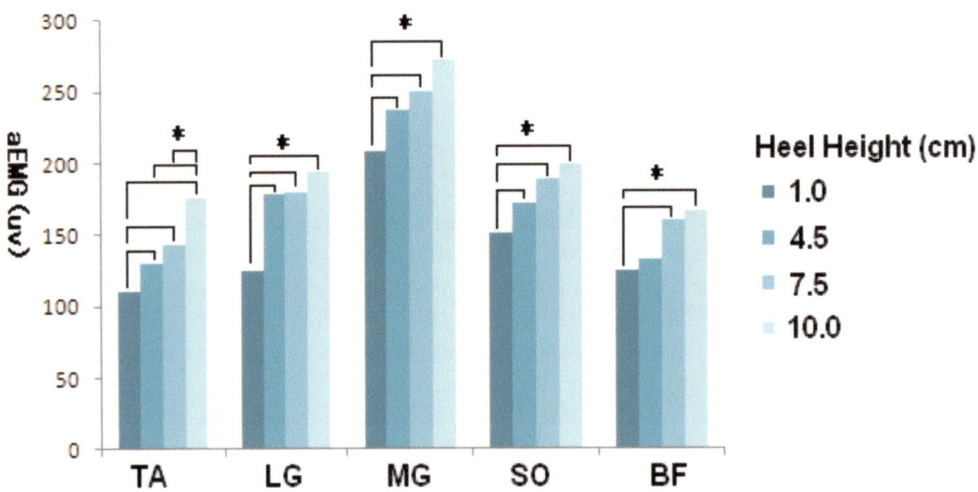

Fig. 4. Comparison of aEMG data in five muscles of lower limb during different heel heights dancing (Significant change *p<0.05).

Another interesting finding in these dancing testing subjects, in which 70% are found have a certain extent deformation in the first metatarsal-phalangeal joint (Fig.5, should to further think about the muscles activity to cause joint deformation.

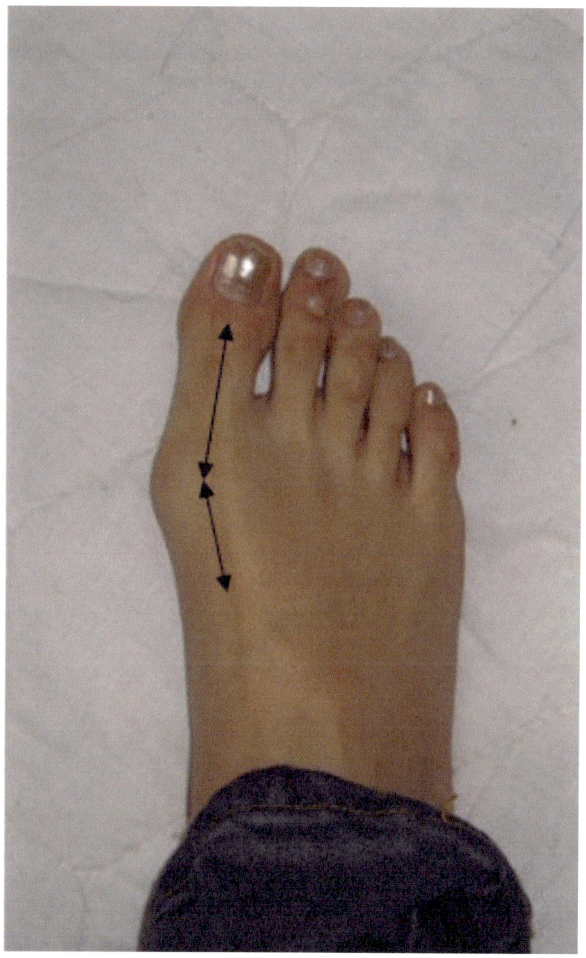

Fig. 5. The certain extent deformation in the first metatarsal-phalangeal joint of the testing subject.

4. Discussion

The results of this study showed that increasing heel height caused increases in SEMG activity in lower limb muscles during dancing. Although previous studies in high heel gait reported similar trend [16, 17], to the authors' knowledge, no studies of heeled dancing movement have evaluated at lower limb muscles activity. It's interesting to find the SEMG activity of the TA was seemed as the most vulnerable part to the heel height increasing. While the heel height increased to 10cm, the aEMG data of TA significantly higher than both 4.5cm and 7.5cm heel height. Due to the function of TA was to adjust dorsiflexion of the foot, acting as a stabilizer of the ankle, this implies that dancing with high heel shoes would consume more energy to control the balance. The trend of activity of LG increased more versus that of MG in heel height increased from flat to low. This different response of the two sides of the gastrocnemius under different heel height was close to one other study conducted by Gefen et al. [18]. The increased muscle acitivity would apparently cause higher loads on the shoe's front part and accelerate its damage or worn out that correlates well with failure analysis of dancing shoes after a long time of training (Fig. 6).

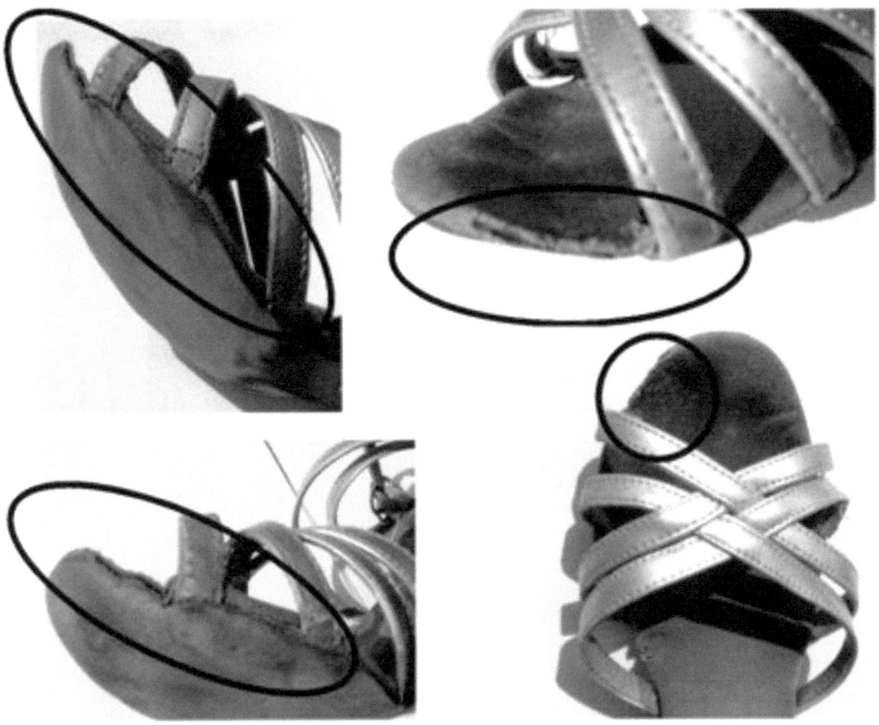

Fig. 6. Damage part in shoe's front part after a long time of training.

There are limitations to the current study, which could be developed further. The lack of kinematic and kinetic data means that confounding variables may be present. In addition, all participants who took part in this study were experienced high heel wearers. Muscle response to heel height may difference between regular and non-regular wearers of high-heeled shoes.

5. References

[1] Lee KH, Shieh JC, Matteliano A et al. (1990) Electromyographic changes of leg muscles with heel lifts in women: therapeutic implications. Arch Phys Med Rehabil 71: 31-33.

[2] Rong M, Wang YX, Gu YD (2009) Plantar pressure distribution character in the Latin dance. Footwear Science 1: 36-37.

[3] Speksnijder CM, Munckhof RJ, Moonen SA et al. (2005) The higher the heel the higher the forefoot pressure in ten healthy women. The foot 15: 17-21.

[4] Esenyel M, Walsh K, Walden JG et al. (2003) Kinetics of high-heeled gait. J Am Podiatr Med Assoc 93: 27-32.

[5] Mandato MG, Nester E (1999) The effects of increasing heel height on forefoot peak pressure. J Am Podiatr Med Assoc 89: 75-80.

[6] Eisengardt JR, Cook D, Pregler I et al (1996) Changes in temporal gait characteristics and pressure distribution for bare feet versus heel various heel height. Gait Posture 12: 280-286.

[7] Snow RE, Williams KR, Holmes GB (1992) The effects of wearing high heeled shoes on pedal pressure in women. Foot Ankle 13: 85-92.

[8] Gu YD, Li JS (2005) Finite element analysis of the instep fatigue trauma in the high-heeled gait. WJMS 1: 117-122.

[9] Benedetti M (2001) Muscle activation intervals and EMG envelope in clinical gait analysis. IEEE Eng Med Biol Mag 20: 33-34.

[10] Merletti R, Knaflitz M, De Luca CJ (1990) Myoelectric manifestations of fatigue in voluntary and electrically elicited contractions. J Appl Physiol 69:1810–1820.

[11] Casale R, Rainoldi A, Nilsson J et al (2003) Can continuous physical training counteract aging effect on myoelectric fatigue? A surface electromyography study application. Arch Phys Med Rehabil 84:513–517.

[12] Mannion AF, Dumas GA, Stevenson JM et al (1998) The influence of muscle fiber size and type distribution on electromyographic measures of back muscle fatigability. Spine 23:576–584.

[13] Zwarts MJ, Drost G, Stegeman DF (2000) Recent progress in the diagnostic use of surface EMG for neurological diseases. J Electromyogr Kinesiol 10:287-291.

[14] Lee CM, Jeong EH, Freivalds A (2001) Biomechanical effects of wearing high-heeled shoes Int J Ind Ergon 28:321-326.

[15] Hermens HJ, Freriks B, Merletti R. et al. (1999) Seniam 8: European recommendations for surface electromyography. Roessingh Research and Development, Netherlands

[16] Stefanyshyn DJ, Nigg BM, Fisher V et al. (2000) The influence of high heeled shoes on kinematics, kinetics and muscle EMG of normal female gait. J Appl Biomech 16: 309-319.

[17] Lee CM, Jeong EH, Frievalds A (2001) Biomechanical effects of wearing high-heeled shoes. Int J Ind Ergon 28: 321-326.

[18] Gefen A, Megido-Ravid M, Itzchak Y et al. (2002) Analysis of muscular fatigue and foot stability during high heeled gait. Gait & Posture 15: 56-63.

8

Muscle Activation Patterns During Level Walking and Stair Ambulation

Maria Grazia Benedetti[1], Valentina Agostini[2], Marco Knaflitz[2] and Paolo Bonato[3]
[1]*Movement Analysis Laboratory, Rizzoli Orthopaedic Institute, Bologna*
[2]*Dipartimento di Elettronica, Politecnico di Torino, Torino*
[3]*Department of Physical Medicine & Rehabilitation, Harvard Medical School, Boston MA,*
[1,2]*Italy*
[3]*USA*

1. Introduction

Dynamic electromyographic (EMG) data recorded using surface electrodes is commonly used to measure muscular activity during the performance of motor tasks and investigate normal and pathological motor strategies (Frigo & Crenna, 2010; Ferdjallah, 1998). In clinical gait analysis, the determination of the timing of muscle activation ("on-off") is of paramount importance (C.J. De Luca, 1997; Shiavi, 1985). The evaluation of the "on-off" pattern of one or more muscles, particularly when examined together with kinematics (joint angles) and kinetics (joint moments and powers), provides an insight into the performance of muscles and their role in accomplishing a motor task (Gage, 1992; Benedetti et al., 1999; Davis, 1997). The relevance of considering the muscle activation timing is supported by several publications demonstrating its usefulness in orthopaedics (Andriacchi et al., 1982; Winter, 1984), treatment of cerebral palsy (Rose et al., 1999; Lyons et al., 1983; P.A. De Luca et al., 1987), and a number of other clinical applications (C.J. De Luca, 1997). More specifically, the timing of activation of muscles ("on-off" pattern) is the only reliable information that can be obtained from surface EMG signals recorded during dynamic contractions. In fact, the amplitude of the EMG signal is not only influenced by the actual electrical activation level of the muscle, but also by the electrical characteristics of the tissue between the active muscle fibers and the surface electrodes. Furthermore, since the relationship between electrical activity level and muscle force is non-linear, caution has to be taken in the interpretation of the EMG amplitude as an indicator of the muscle force output when data are recorded in dynamic conditions (C.J. De Luca, 1997). Unfortunately, this approach does not allow one to investigate completely the advanced control features of the central nervous systems, since muscle activation is simplified considering a muscle either "on" or "off". However, in a great number of the clinical queries, the muscle activation timing represents the information of interest for the clinician, provided that reliable data are obtained for the activation intervals.

Methods proposed in literature to determine the onset and offset of muscle activation intervals generally rely on an arbitrary choice of the threshold value that discriminates background noise from the signal generated by the active muscles (Hodges & Bang, 1996; Winter & Yack, 1987). The main drawbacks of these methods are: (1) the estimated activation patterns strongly depend on the subjective decision of such threshold value thus resulting in unreliable estimates and large variability (Bonato et al., 1998); and (2) these methods do not allow for the appraisal of the likelihood of false positive (specificity) and false negative (sensitivity) detections. In order to overcome these limitations, a double-threshold detector of muscle activation, based on the statistical properties of the EMG signal was developed (Bonato et al., 1998).

In a recent study this method was applied to obtain a paediatric reference data-set of muscle activation patterns during gait (Agostini et al., 2010).

The aim of the present work is to provide a reliable reference data set, referred to an adult population, of the muscular activation timing during common activities of daily living - such as level walking and stair ambulation - for clinical and research use. To this purpose, raw surface EMG signals from trunk and lower limb muscles were recorded in a sample population of healthy young volunteers and processed by means of the above-mentioned double-threshold detector. The main problems encountered during data collection and processing are herein discussed to provide suggestions for further improvements to be accomplished in future work.

2. Materials and methods

Sixteen young subjects were recruited in this study, 9 males and 7 females, age 27.7±2.6 years (mean and standard deviation), weight 67.4±10.5 kg and height 171.6±8.8 cm. They had no history of locomotor disturbances or injuries. Subjects walked barefoot, along a 15m-walkway, at a self-selected speed of progression (Table 1). Two force platforms (Kistler Instruments, Switzerland) were mounted in the walkway to measure ground reaction force and detect the occurrence of stance and swing phases.

	Mean	SD
Walking (cm/s)	125.6	16.8
Stair ascending (cm/s)	43.9	6.6
Stair descending (cm/s)	48.1	1.7

Table 1. Speed of progression.

The same group of subjects was tested while walking up and down a flight of stairs barefoot at a self-selected speed of progression (Table 1). The staircase was made in wood, its dimensions were chosen according to the architectural normative in use in Italy. It was composed of three steps, each with a tread depth of 28 cm , a width of 86 cm, and a riser of 16 cm. The first and the third steps were connected to the two Kistler force platforms. During stair ascent, the stride cycle was defined by the right foot, beginning at foot contact on the first step and ending at subsequent contact of the foot on the third step. During stair descent the stride cycle was defined by the right foot beginning at foot contact on the third step and ending at subsequent contact of the same foot on the first step.

2.1 Muscles investigated

Eight muscles were considered for the right side of each subject: ipsilateral and contralateral erector spinae at lumbar site, gluteus medius, rectus femoris, medial hamstrings, lateral hamstrings (biceps femoris, long head), gastrocnemius (medial head), and tibialis anterior.

2.2 Electromyographic instrumentation and methodology

The surface EMG signal was detected using active clip-type probes connected to adhesive disposable electrodes made of Ag/AgCl for paediatric electrocardiographic application. The inter-electrode distance was 20 mm, center to center. The signal was amplified using an eight-channel system (TELEMG, BTS, Milan, Italy). Sampling rate was 500 Hz, low and high cut-off frequencies of the amplifier were 40 Hz and 200 Hz, respectively. Three repetitions were gathered for each subject.

The location and orientation of the electrodes for each muscle were identified according to the literature (Delagi & Perotto, 1981). The skin under the electrodes was shaved and cleansed with alcohol.

2.3 Statistical double-threshold detector for muscle on-off timing

EMG signals were processed using a statistical detector designed and implemented as briefly summarized in the following. The complete description and full characterization of the algorithm is provided in a previous work (Bonato, 1998).

The raw EMG signal was first processed using an adaptive whitening filter. Then an auxiliary time-series was derived by squaring and summing adjacent samples. The amplitude of the auxiliary time-series was therefore χ^2 distributed. Based on a background noise sample, we determined the characteristics of the χ^2 distribution of the data for intervals when muscles were silent. A window of 5 samples was slid through the auxiliary time-series. A double-threshold strategy was applied to the samples within the window to determine whether the signal reflected a silent or active status of the monitored muscle. A first threshold was set on the amplitude of the samples of the auxiliary time-series. A second threshold was set on the number of samples within the sliding window that needed to be above threshold to result in a detection of muscular activity. Moreover, through the definition of receiver operating characteristics derived via simulation, the user is provided with means to choose the operating point defined by sensitivity and false alarm probability with more degrees of freedom than what traditional approaches would provide. This allows the user to adapt the behaviour of the detector as a function of the signal characteristics (e.g. signal-to-noise ratio). This strategy was applied to the EMG signal together with a post-processor that rejected transitions shorter than 30 ms. The combination of the two techniques provided us with means to detect muscle activation intervals with probability of false alarm smaller than 2 % and sensitivity higher than 85 % for a signal-to-ratio (SNR) as low as 6 dB. Fig. 1 shows an example of application of the double-threshold detection algorithm to an EMG signal. As suggested in the literature (Perry, 1992; Bogey et al., 1992) we defined the minimum period of muscle inactivity between contractions as 5% of the gait cycle. When the duration of "on" intervals was less than 5% of the gait cycle, the muscle was considered as silent, i.e. the short detected activation between two silent periods was considered a false detection and corrected. Similarly, when "off" intervals shorter than 5 % were detected, the muscle was considered as active, i.e. the short silent period between intervals of muscle activity was considered a false negative and corrected.

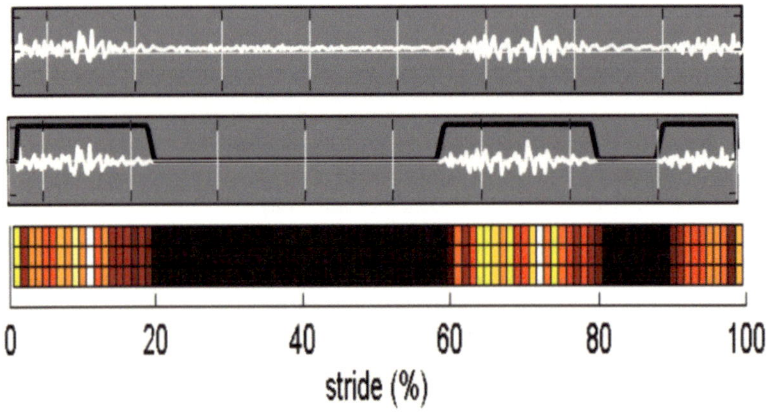

Fig. 1. Example of raw EMG signal (upper plot), whitened EMG signal and on-off detection of muscle activations (middle plot), and representation of the amplitude of the EMG signal using five discrete levels of intensity represented by different colors (lower plot).

3. Results

In order to give a global representation of the muscle activation intervals on the entire population we considered, for each percent of the gait cycle, the percentage of subjects in which a specific muscle is active. Fig. 2 shows the on-off muscle activation intervals of the population during level walking, Fig. 3 represents the on-off intervals during stair ascending, while Fig. 4 represents the on-off intervals during stair descending. In Figs. 2-3-4, vertical bars reaching 100% mean that all the subjects have a specific muscle active at the percent of the stride considered. On the contrary, null vertical bars (0%) mean that all the subjects have their muscle silent at the specific percent of the stride considered.

3.1 Level walking

Right Erector Spinae. In all subjects, the ipsilateral erector spinae muscle was active around initial contact and between terminal stance and pre-swing (Fig. 2).

Left Erector Spinae. The activation pattern of the contralateral muscle is very similar to that of the ipsilateral one. Synergic lumbar paraspinal muscles function consists of decelerating the forward trunk rotation at heel strike and toe off. A further activity of this muscle is present, in a certain number of patients, during midstance, aimed to sustain the swinging limb on the coronal plane and tilting the trunk on the support limb.

Gluteus Medius. In all the subjects the activity begins at terminal swing, in preparation to heel strike, and it continues throughout the first half of the stance phase.

Rectus Femoris. The rectus femoris resulted to be active, in all the subjects, during the terminal swing and during the first part of the gait cycle, thus stabilizing the knee under loading. In a small percentage of subjects, in accordance with previous findings (Nene, 1999), we detected activity at toe off.

Lateral Hamstrings. The long head of the biceps femoris begins to be active in the last part of swing phase - decelerating hip flexion and knee extension, and preparing the lower limb to heel strike and load absorption - and continues during initial stance phase, extending the

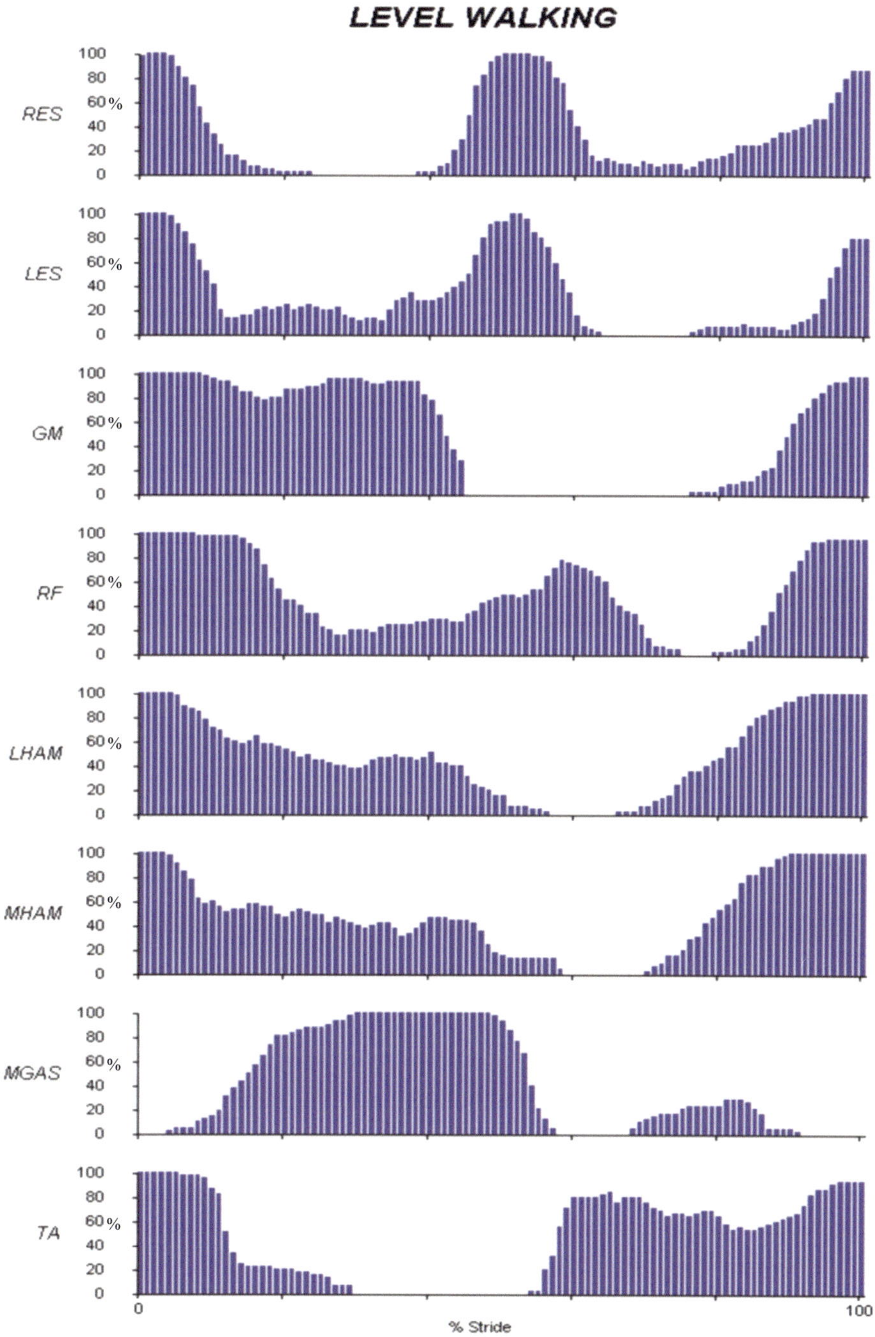

Fig. 2. On-off muscle timing during level walking, as a function of the percentage of the gait cycle. For each muscle, the muscular activity is presented as percentage of subjects whose muscle is active at the specific percent of the stride considered. RES: right erector spinae, LES: left erector spinae, GM: gluteus medius, RF: rectus femoris, MHAM: medial hamstrings, LHAM: lateral hamstrings, MGAS: medial gastrocnemius, TA: tibialis anterior.

hip and stabilizing the knee in co-contraction with the rectus femoris. In agreement with Shiavi (Shiavi, 1981) a further period of activity was present, in 50 % of the subjects, during terminal stance, to lead into the unloading response of preswing when inertia is not sufficient to flex the knee.

Medial Hamstrings. Semitendinosus and semimembranosus activity during gait is generally similar to the lateral hamstrings activity.

Medial Gastrocnemius. The gastrocnemius muscle begins its activity during initial stance and ends its activity at terminal stance in accordance with literature (Shiavi et al., 1983). In a small percentage of the examined subjects we detected also a short burst of activity in the middle of the swing phase, as previously already observed (Basmajian, 1978).

Tibialis Anterior. The tibialis anterior activity begins at the toe off and continues throughout the swing phase with decreased amplitude during mid swing in most of the subjects. This muscle is active at heel strike and continues to be active during the loading response phase, until the foot is completely in contact with the floor.

3.2 Stair ascending

Erectors Spinae. No comparable data are available in the literature for these muscles during stair climbing. The muscle contralateral to the supporting limb is active throughout the stance phase. Its activity helps the climbing limb to swing over the next step thus elevating the pelvis on this side. Vice versa, the ipsilateral erector spinae is generally active at initial stance, controlling the limb loading, and during midstance, as fixators of pelvis during contralateral swing (Fig. 3).

Gluteus Medius. As for walking, the gluteus medius is active in the first half of the stance phase of the supporting limb.

Rectus Femoris. Results obtained in our subjects are consistent with data previously published by others (Andriacchi et al., 1980), reporting activity of this muscle in the first half of the stance phase. Nevertheless, there is only partial agreement with findings by Perry (Perry, 1992), who documented a pattern marked by two activation intervals during initial stance and mid swing.

Hamstrings. The activity of these muscles starts at the end of the swing phase to continue during initial stance, extending the hip. The activity continues, in most subjects, during midstance, fixing the hip under loading. Furthermore all subjects, approximately at toe off, activate the hamstrings to flex the knee for the next step over. Data previously published (Lyons et al., 1983) reports similar activation patterns.

Medial Gastrocnemius. Gastrocnemius is active for most of the stance phase. This finding is not in agreement with what reported in the literature (Andriacchi et al., 1980). In fact, in our recordings, the onset of the gastrocnemius activity occurs earlier, at heel strike. However, this pattern can be justified, from a kinesiological point of view, since the initial support during stair ascending is on the forefoot.

Tibialis Anterior. The tibialis anterior muscle is active during the swing phase, providing adequate foot clearance. Its activity continues, in most of the subjects, after the ground contact in order to control the foot landing. Moreover, a certain activity is present in many subjects throughout stance. It is worthwhile to emphasize the role of the tibialis anterior in the control of foot inversion-eversion, a very important motion for balance control in the coronal plane during single limb support.

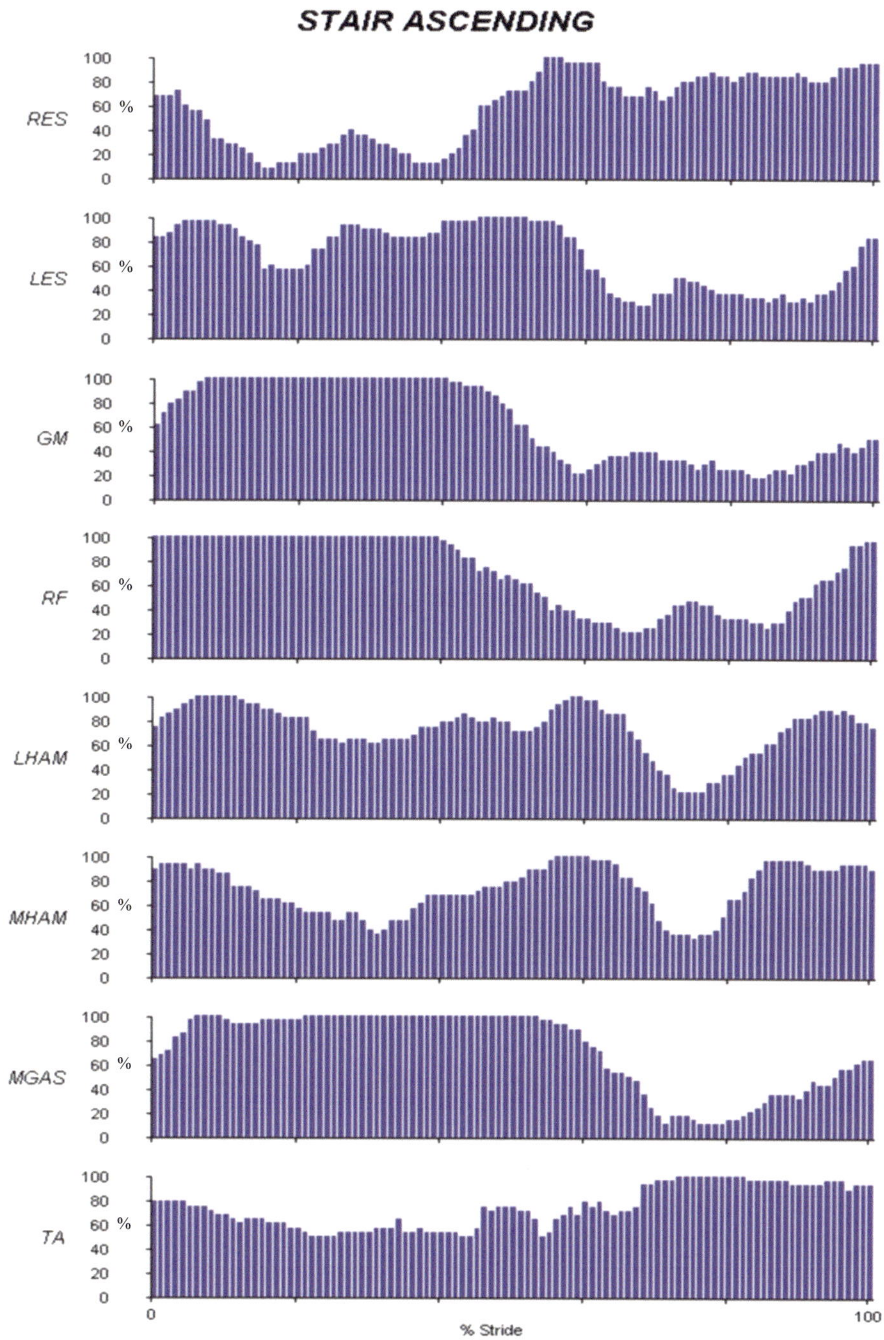

Fig. 3. On-off muscle timing during stair ascending, as a function of the percentage of the gait cycle. For each muscle, the muscular activity is presented as percentage of subjects whose muscle is active at the specific percent of the stride considered. RES: right erector spinae, LES: left erector spinae, GM: gluteus medius, RF: rectus femoris, MHAM: medial hamstrings, LHAM: lateral hamstrings, MGAS: medial gastrocnemius, TA: tibialis anterior.

3.3 Stair descending

Right Erector Spinae. In the large majority of subjects, the onset of this muscle is found twice, at heel strike and toe off. These two activations are likely to be related to the control of the trunk forward momentum. Furthermore, this muscle presents activity, in many subjects, during the swing phase, probably controlling the fall down of the pelvis due to the descending limb. No references are available for this muscle in the literature (Fig. 4).

Left Erector Spinae. In the examined group of subjects this muscle shows a continuous activity during the stance phase, aimed at controlling the obliquity of the pelvis, while subjects swing the limb to reach a lower step of the stair.

Gluteus Medius. In the majority of the subjects, this muscle is active throughout the stance phase. All subjects show a first muscle activation interval during the loading response, likely to be associated with the stabilization of the pelvis in the coronal plane while the weight is transferred to the ipsilateral limb. The large majority of subjects show also a second activation interval associated to the contralateral foot contact. No reference data are available for this muscle.

Rectus Femoris. This muscle is active during stance, controlling knee flexion, and in mid and terminal swing, contributing to knee extension and preparing the landing limb to load transfer.

Hamstrings. There is hamstrings activity at the beginning of the stance phase, to extend the hip controlling inertia, and at toe off, to flex the knee. Furthermore, this muscle shows activity, in the majority of the population, at mid swing, in opposite phase with respect to the activity of rectus femoris, aimed to reduce knee extension and to prepare the limb loading. The hamstrings are also active at the end of the swing phase. This activity is observed in all the subjects in preparation to limb loading.

Medial Gastrocnemius. Similarly to what was observed for stair ascending, we detected an activation onset of medial gastrocnemius around heel strike, that is, hence, anticipated in comparison to what was found by others in the past (Andriacchi et al., 1980). This finding is consistent with the forefoot initial contact during stair descending. The activity of the gastrocnemius muscle lasts until terminal stance. This muscle is active again at the end of the swing phase preparing foot landing.

Tibialis Anterior. The activity observed in the population for this muscle is spread throughout the stance phase. Subjects typically show muscle activation at initial stance, probably controlling foot inversion-eversion. Furthermore, it can be observed muscle activity, common to most of the subjects, at initial swing, to sustain the foot during the landing on the lower step, and before initial contact.

4. Discussion

Procedures previously adopted for the on-off pattern detection were generally based on single-threshold methods (Bekey et al., 1985). These methods have been shown to be strongly dependent on the arbitrary choice of the threshold value. Different threshold values may lead to dramatically different estimates of the EMG activation intervals (Winter & Yack, 1987). The double-threshold statistical detector used in the present study outperforms single-threshold methods (Staude, 2001). For a given value of false alarm probability, it leads to higher detection probability. The increase in sensitivity provided by the double-threshold approach depends on the SNR and it is dramatic for relatively low values of SNR and low values of false alarm probability.

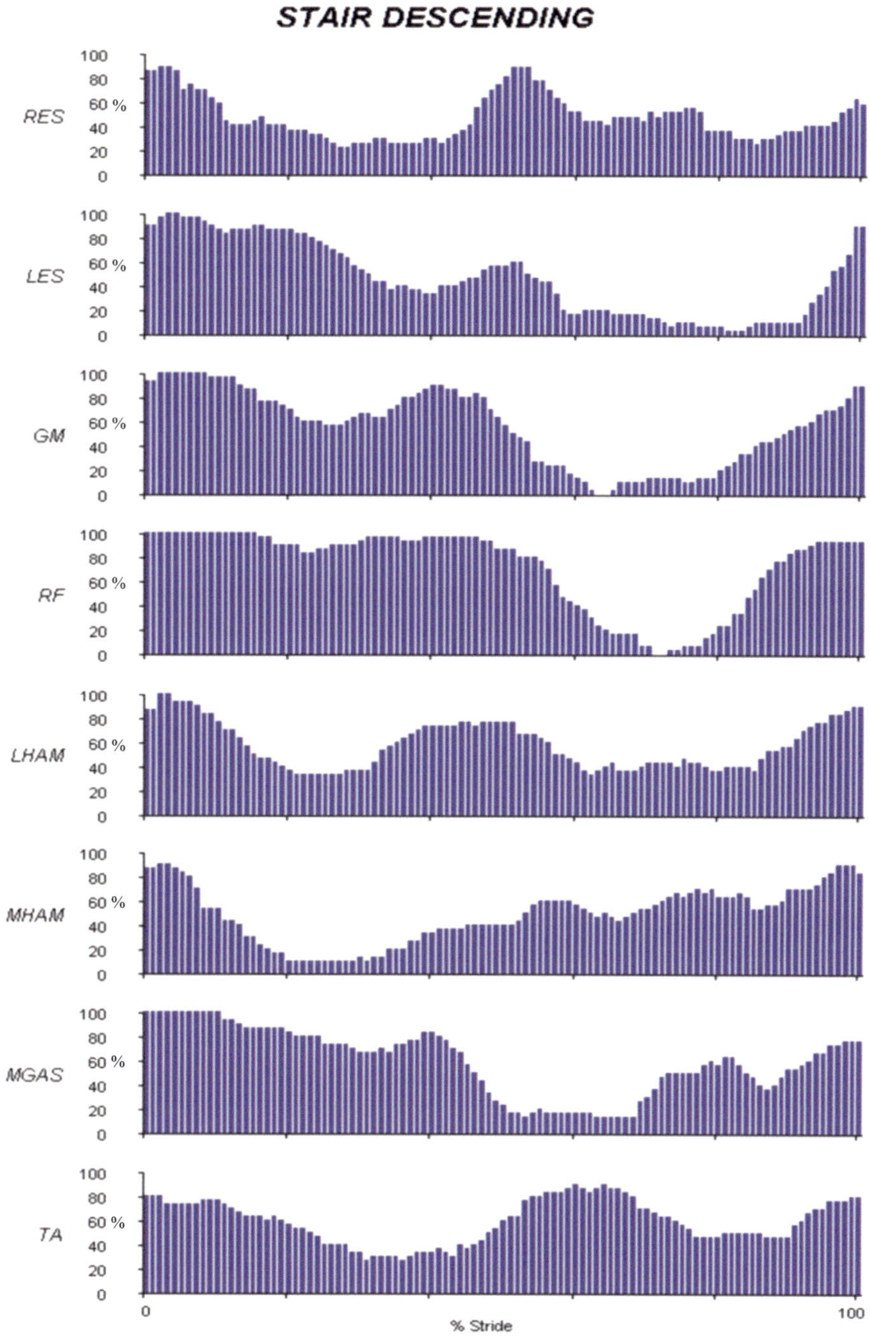

Fig. 4. On-off muscle timing during stair descending, as a function of the percentage of the gait cycle. For each muscle, the muscular activity is presented as percentage of subjects whose muscle is active at the specific percent of the stride considered. RES: right erector spinae, LES: left erector spinae, GM: gluteus medius, RF: rectus femoris, MHAM: medial hamstrings, LHAM: lateral hamstrings, MGAS: medial gastrocnemius, TA: tibialis anterior.

The application of the statistical detector to the large number of EMG trials collected in this study was completely automatic, once the parameters of the algorithm were tuned on the characteristics of the EMG signals. Detected phases of activity of the examined muscles were in most of the cases comparable with previous work for level walking at self-selected speed (Arsenault et al., 1986; Basmajian, 1978; Battye & Joseph, 1996; Kadaba et al., 1989; Yang & Winter, 1985; Perry, 1992; Wootten et al., 1990) and, when available, for stair ascending /descending (Basmajian, 1978; Joseph & Watson, 1967; Powers et al., 1997; Shiavi, 1981; Shinno, 1971; Townsed et al., 1978). Only in a few cases our results appeared to be different from previous findings by others (Andriacchi et al., 1980). The detection of the rectus femoris activity is problematic when one uses surface electrodes, as the activity of other heads of quadriceps muscle appears to affect the signal recorded from the rectus femoris (Perry, 1992; Nene et al., 1999).

Results for the gastrocnemius muscle appear to be consistent with the biomechanics of motion even if different from results previously reported in the literature. The activity that we detected at heel strike during stair ambulation is consistent with the need to control the forward momentum of the trunk. In interpreting the results for stair ambulation, it must be taken into account that differences with respect to previous studies may depend on external factors such as the staircase set-up.

Problems related to the presence of crosstalk were encountered in some cases. In the EMG signals recorded for the present study, cross-talk affected particularly the signals relative to the gastrocnemius and the tibialis anterior muscles at the beginning of the stride, during mid stance, and during the swing phase. If detected during the acquisition session, cross-talk could be reduced by decreasing the inter-electrode distance or by using electrode arrays such as the double differential electrode (C.J. De Luca & Merletti, 1988). When cross-talk is unavoidable during the signal acquisition, and evident from the shape and the timing of the burst, it is manually rejected from the on-off detection.

The clinical relevance of the analysis of muscle activation intervals has been established. Nevertheless, the use of a detector limited to the determination of the muscle activation onset and offset, disregarding the relative magnitude of the EMG signal, fails to recognize as pathological a muscle activation with correct timing but inappropriate intensity. In order to overcome this restriction, it was decided to perform also a gross amplitude quantification in five levels of intensity. Hence Fig. 5 shows, for various muscles, the mean amplitude values over the population. In this representation, amplitude values are color-coded. The black color represents high-intensity muscle activation, while the white color represents a condition in which the muscle is silent.

The purpose of this added information is mainly to provide a qualitative evaluation of the location of the peak of the EMG activity and of its sharpness in the gait cycle. According to Perry (Perry, 1992), this information could be of relevance for clinical applications.

A limit of this study is that the results presented here refer only to the most frequent pattern of activation of each muscle, leaving out less frequent patterns that may be observed. This is a point often disregarded by traditional approaches, though it may be of relevance in interpreting clinical data. In fact, during a continuous and cyclical motor task - such as gait or stair ambulation – each subject typically shows different muscular patterns of activation. This means that, during subsequent cycles of the same motor task, a specific muscle shows a different number of activations, possibly with different timing. This was demonstrated for level walking in a population of 100 children (Agostini, 2010). Recording and processing a considerable amount of cycles (tens to hundreds) for each subject makes it possible having a

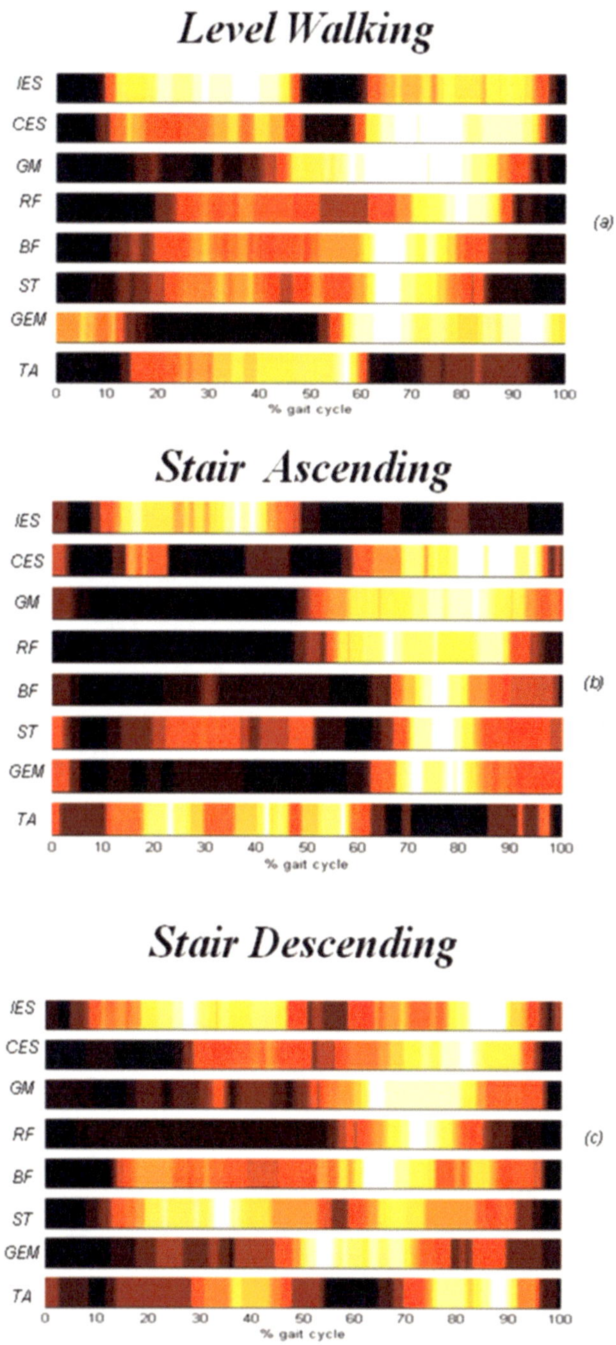

Fig. 5. Muscle timing during (a) level walking, (b) stair ascending and (c) stair descending. The EMG amplitude is color-coded with five colors that roughly codify the amplitude of the envelope of the EMG signal, with the purpose of allowing for the location of the peak amplitude occurring within each signal burst and of providing a rough estimate of its shape.

statistical description of the muscle activation patterns during performance of a motor task. Hence, one can calculate in which percentage of cycles a certain muscle pattern is observed. This allows one to capture more accurately the characteristics of the subject motor control and abilities. As an example, Fig. 6 reports the results obtained from the gait analysis of an adult volunteer who walked for 160 s. The figure refers to the EMG patterns obtained from the rectus femoris muscle during walking. The left plot of Fig. 6 reports the histogram of the number of activations observed during all the observed strides. In 54% of the strides there are three activations (most frequent pattern), in 22% of the strides there are only two activations, while in 21% of the strides there are four activations. The right plot of Fig. 6 shows the activation patterns for the three main activation modalities. When the muscle is active, the amplitude of the signal is color-coded using three levels: red means high activation amplitude (greater than 66% of the maximum root-mean-square value observed during walking), green means medium activation amplitude (between 33% and 66%) and yellow represents low activation amplitude (lower than 33%). The root-mean-square value of the signal is computed over subsequent windows lasting 50 ms.

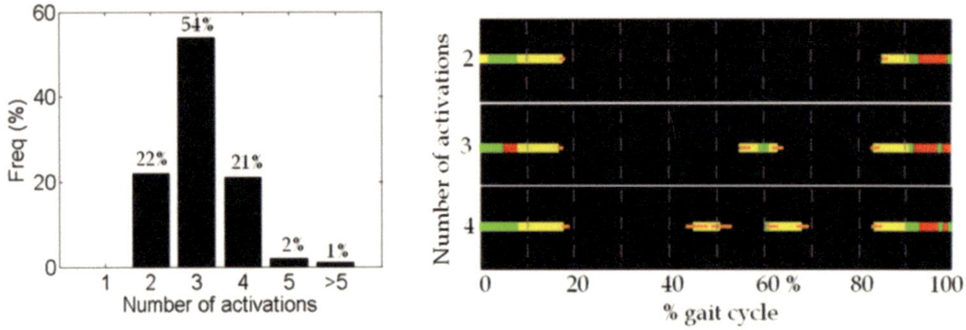

Fig. 6. Analysis of 80 strides recorded during level walking in a healthy adult subject. Left plot: histogram of the number of activations observed in the rectus femoris. Right plot: muscle activation patterns for each activation modality.

5. Conclusion

In order to define what is "pathological" it is necessary to have previously defined what is "normal". This was the aim of the study and the reason why we collected a reference dataset from healthy subjects. Due to the statistical properties of the EMG signal, detecting "on" and "off" timing of muscle activity is a challenging task, particularly when dealing with signals having poor SNR, as those often seen in clinical practice. The application of the double-threshold statistical algorithm has provided a reliable documentation of "normal" muscle timing during the motor tasks explored. The adaptive properties of this technique with respect to the variations of the SNR allowed us to estimate muscle activation intervals from all the EMG recordings.

Results obtained from this study can be relevant both to basic research, as reference for motor control pattern studies, and to clinical research, in order to document pathological patterns of muscle activation and their consistencies with kinematics and kinetics findings.

In future studies, the methodology herein explored may become a valuable tool for investigating the causes of motor impairment and for allowing an objective evaluation of the outcome of therapeutic approaches.

6. Acknowledgment

The authors are grateful to Prof. Silvano Boccardi for suggestions and critical review of the manuscript.

7. References

Agostini, V. ; Nascimbeni, A.; Gaffuri, A.; Imazio, P.; Benedetti, M.G. & Knaflitz, M. (2010). Normative EMG activation patterns of school-age children during gait. *Gait & Posture*, Vol.32, pp. 285–289

Andriacchi, T.P.; Andersson, G.B.J.; Fermier, R.W.; Stern, D. & Galante, J.O. (1980). A study of lower-limb mechanics during stair-climbing. *J Bone Joint Surg*, Vol.62A, pp. 749-757

Andriacchi, T.P.; Galante, J.O. & Fermer, R.W. (1982). The Influence of total Knee-replacement Design on walking and Stair-Climbing. *J Bone Joint Surg*, Vol.64A, pp. 1328-1335

Arsenault, A.B.; Winter, D.A. & Marteniuk, R.G. (1986). Is there a "normal" profile of EMG activity in gait? *Med Biol Eng Compu*, Vol.24, pp. 337-343

Basmajian J.V. (1978). *Muscles Alive*, Baltimore: The William and Wilkins Co.

Battye, C.K. & Joseph, J. (1996). An investigation by telemetering of the activity of some muscles in walking. *Med & Biol Eng*, Vol.4, pp.125-135

Bekey, G.A.; Chang, C.W.; Perry, J. & Hoffer M.M. (1985). Pattern Recognition of Multiple EMG Signals Applied to the Description of human Gait. *IEEE Proc*, Vol.65, pp. 674-681

Benedetti, M.G.; Bonato, P.; Catani, F.; D'Alessio, T.; Knaflitz, M.; Marcacci, M. & Simoncini, L. (1999). Myoelectric Activation Pattern During Gait in Total Knee Replacement: Relationship with Kinematics, Kinetics, and Clinical Outcome. *IEEE Trans Rehab Eng*, Vol.7, pp. 140-149

Bogey, R.A., Barnes, L.A. & Perry J. (1992). Computer Algorithms to Characterize Individual Subject EMG Profiles During Gait. *Arch Phys Med Rehabil*, Vol.73, pp. 835-851

Bonato, P.; D'Alessio, T. & Knaflitz, M. (1998). A Statistical Method for the Measurement of Muscle Activation Intervals from Surface Myoelectric Signal During Gait. *IEEE Trans Biomed Eng*, Vol.45, pp. 287-299

Davis, R.B. (1997). Reflections on Clinical Gait Analysis. *J Electromyogr Kinesiol*, Vol.7, pp. 251-257

De Luca, P.A.; Davis, R.B.; Ounpuu, S.; Rose, S. & Sirkin, K.R. (1987). Alterations in surgical decision making in patients with cerebral palsy based on three dimensional gait analysis. *J Pediatr Orthop*, Vol.17, pp. 608-614

De Luca, C.J. (1997). The use of Surface Electromyography in Biomechanics. *J Appl Biomech*, Vol.13, pp. 135-163

De Luca, C.J. & Merletti, R. (1988). Surface EMG crosstalk among muscles of the leg. *Elettroen Clin Neur*, Vol.69, pp. 568-575

Delagi, E.F. & Perotto, A. (1981). *Anatomic Guide for the Electromyographer*, Springfield: C Thomas Pub.

Ferdjallah, M. & Wertsch, J.J. (1998). Anatomical and technical consideration in surface electromyography. *Phys Med Rehabil Clin N Am*, Vol.9, pp. 925-931

Frigo, C. & Crenna, P. (2009). Multichannel SEMG in clinical gait analysis: a review and state-of-the-art. *Clin Biomech*, Vol.24, pp. 236–245

Gage, J.R. (1992). Clinical use of kinetics for gait pathology in cerebral palsy. *Gait & Posture*, Vol.2, pp. 36-37

Hodges, P.W. & Bang, H.B. (1996). A comparison of computer-based methods for the determination of onset of muscle contraction using electromyography. *Electroen clin Neur*, Vol.10, pp. 511-519

Joseph, J. & Watson, R. (1967). Telemetering electromyography of muscles used in walking up and down stairs. *J Bone Joint Surg*, Vol.49B, pp. 774-780

Kadaba, M.P.; Ramakrishnan, H.K.; Wootten, M.E.; Gainey, J.; Gorton, G. & Cochran, G.V.B. (1989). Repeteability of Kinematic, Kinetic, and Electromyographic data in Normal Adult Gait. *J Orthop Res*, Vol.7, pp. 849-860

Lyons, K.; Perry, J.; Gronley, J.K.; Barnes, L. & Antonelli, D. (1983). Timing relative intensity of hip extensor and abductor muscles action during level and stair ambulation. An EMG study. *Phis Ther*, Vol.63, pp. 1597-1605

Nene, A.; Mayagoitia, R. & Veltink, P. (1999). Assessment of rectus femoris function during initial swing. *Gait & Posture*, Vol.9, pp. 1-9

Perry, J. (1992). *Gait Analysis, Normal and pathological function*, NewYork: Slack Inc.

Powers, C.M.; Boyd, L.A.; Torburn, L. & Perry, J. (1997). Stair ambulation in person with transtibial amputation: An Analysis of the Seattle LightFoot. *J Rehabil Res Dev*, Vol.34, pp. 9-18

Rose, J.; Martin J.G.; Torburn, L.; Rinsky, L.A. & Gamble, J.G. (1999). Electromyographic differentiation of diplegic cerebral palsy from idiopatic toe walking involuntary coactivation of the quadriceps and gastrocnemius. *J Pediatr Orthop*, Vol.19, pp. 677-682

Shiavi, R. (1981). Variability of Electromyographic Patterns for Level-Surface Walking through a Range of Self-Selected Speeds. *Bull Prosth Res*, Vol.18, pp. 5-14

Shiavi, R. & Griffin, P. (1983). Changes in Electromyographic Gait Patterns of Calf Muscles with Walking Speed. *IEEE Trans Biomed Eng*, Vol.30, pp. 73-76

Shiavi, R. (1985). Electromyographic patterns in adult locomotion: A comprehensive review. *J Rehabil Res Dev*, Vol.22, pp. 85-98

Shinno, N. (1971). Analysis of knee function in ascending and descending stairs. In: *Medicine and Sport*, Vol.6: Biomechanics II, pp. 202-207, Basel: Karger

Staude, G.; Flachenecker, C.; Daumer, M. & Wolf, W. (2001). Onset detection in surface electromyographic signals: a systematic comparison of methods. *EURASIP JAppl Signal Process*, Vol.2, pp. 67–81

Townsed, M.A.; Lainhart, S.P.; Shiavi, R. & Caylor, J. (1978). Variability and biomechanics of synergistic patterns of some lower limb muscles during ascending and descending stairs and level walking, *Med. & Biol Eng and Comput*, Vol.16, pp. 681-688

Winter, D.A. (1984). Pathologic Gait Diagnosis with Computer-Averaged Electromyographic Profiles. *Arch Phis Med Rehabil*, Vol.65, pp. 393-398

Winter, D.A. & Yack, H.J. (1987). EMG profiles during normal human walking: stride-to-stride and inter-subject variability. *Electroen clin Neur*, Vol.67, pp. 402-411

Wootten, M.E.; Kadaba, M.P. & Cochran, G.V.B. (1990). Dynamic Electromyography. II Normal patterns during gait. *J Orthop Res*, Vol.8, pp. 259-265

Yang, J.F. & Winter, D.A. (1985). Surface EMG profiles during different walking cadences in Humans. *Electroen Clin Neur*, Vol.60, pp. 485-491

Part 3

Back Care

9

Experimentation and Structural Modeling of Stimulus-Evoked Electromyography in Muscles During Electrically-Elicited Fatigue Process

Shao-Hsia Chang[1] and Nan-Ying Yu[2]
[1]*Department of Occupational Therapy,*
[2]*Department of Physical Therapy,*
I-Shou University, Kaohsiung City,
Taiwan

1. Introduction

Functional electrical stimulation (FES) has been adopted to induce muscle contraction to provide functionally useful movements in spinal cord injured (SCI) individuals. It was described as electrical stimulation of muscle deprived of nervous control with a view of providing muscular contraction and providing a functionally useful movement. The term FES is applied to systems which attempt to restore lost or impaired neuromuscular function, such as standing and walking in cases of paraplegia. By the application of electrical pulses to neural pathways or, but less often, directly to muscles. It is also sometimes known as Functional Neuromuscular Stimulation or FNS. Figure 1 shows the demonstration of general applications of FES for the restoration of limb functions. Among all the limiting factors in the application of FES, muscle fatigue that can directly discontinue the application is considered the most important [1]. Many researchers have studied electrically elicited muscle fatigue of paralyzed limb muscles from the biomechanical, metabolic and electrophysiological aspects [2, 3, 4]. During electrical stimulation, the decline of torque values during isometric contraction is usually observed which exhibited a sigmoid-like curve consisting of a main slope and two plateaus [5, 6, 7]. Researchers reported that the first plateau represents the status before fatigue and the major slope indicates the exhausted expenditure of easily-fatigued (type II) MUs. Following the quick fatigue process, the final plateau represents the activation of the residual fatigue-resistant (type I) MUs [8].
From the electrophysiological aspect, the evoked EMG or compound muscle action potential (CMAP) of the stimulated muscle has been studied during the fatiguing process. The close correlation between muscle force and stimulus-evoked EMG peak to peak (PTP) amplitude indicates that the stimulus EMG amplitude could directly provide information for monitoring FES-induced muscle force and as control signals for compensating the decrease of muscle force due to fatigue [9, 10]. In addition to PTP, the other characteristics of CMAP, such as temporal features including latency, rise time to peak (RTP), and PTP duration (PTPd) as well as frequency characteristics have also been used to quantify the muscle fatigue process [11, 12]. Both temporal and frequency features were presumably related to

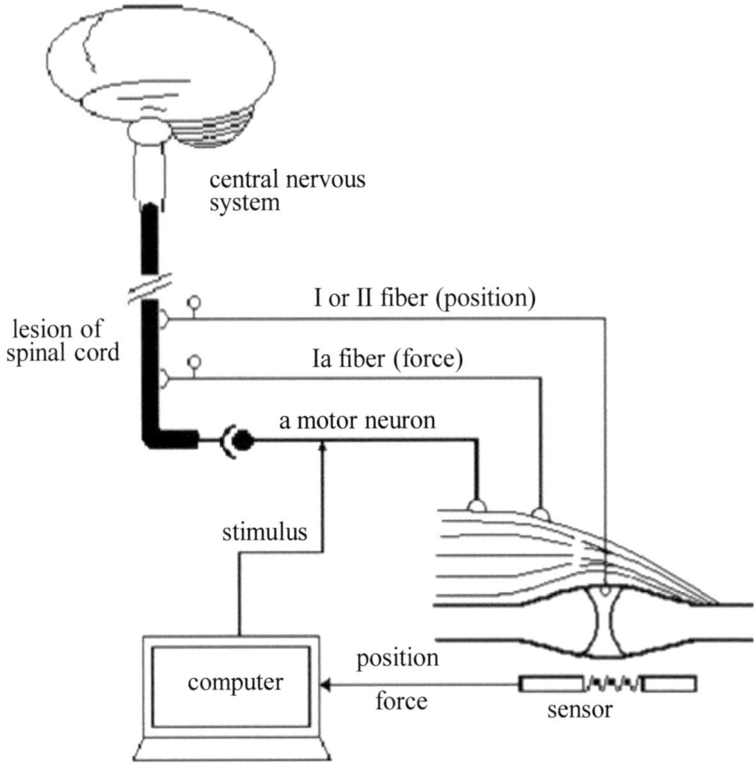

Fig. 1. Illustration of functional electrical stimulation. Arrowed lines show the interface of electrical stimulation and neuromuscular system.

the propagation velocity of motor unit action potential (MUAP) in muscle fibers. Most of the results showed decrease in muscle fiber conduction velocity and reduction in mean/median frequency during the muscle fatigue process [13].

Several studies confirmed that the lengths of stimulated muscle could affect the spectral, temporal, and amplitude features of evoked EMG [13, 14, 15]. Our previous study indicated that the amplitudes of the evoked EMG of the quadriceps muscle in electrically elicited muscle contractions were significantly different when the knee angle was varied [16]. Other studies also indicated that surface EMG features might vary due to the change in relative location between the electrodes and the muscle fibers during stimulation in different muscle lengths which should be taken into consideration for the measurement of evoked EMG [17]. These studies revealed the necessity of electrophysiological studies to illuminate the fatigue characteristics of muscles stimulated in different lengths.

Although studies of the length effects on the fatigue characteristics of stimulated muscles have been proposed, experimental designs to explain some of the intrinsic factors, such as the changes in CMAP amplitude or duration in different muscle fiber types during muscle fatigue process as well as those under different measurement configurations (e.g. varied muscle lengths) are intractable. Thus, a simulation EMG model becomes necessary in describing the meanings of the parameters derived from an evoked EMG, and then verifying their relationships with the fatigue process. For EMG modeling, Fuglevand et al.

developed a structural MUAP model to investigate the influence of electrode size and spacing [18]. The model of MUAPs has been expanded by Farina et al. in order to consider the effects of electrode configuration, electrode size and the inclination of the fibers with respect to the detection system [14, 19].

The study aim is to combine the experimental design and modeling technique from which the electrophysiological changes of stimulated paralyzed muscle during fatigue process can be interpreted from the amplitude and temporal features of CMAP and its muscle fiber constituents. This study first compared the changes in amplitude and temporal features of CMAP and torque output between the shortened and lengthened paralyzed muscles. Due to the lack of a MUAP model dedicated to SCI paralyzed muscles, we modified the structural MUAP model developed by Fuglevand et al. [18], by incorporating the viable parameters obtained from paralyzed muscles, mainly on the different distributions in MU types and their simulation parameters. Based on the modified structural CMAP model, the stimulus-evoked EMG can be modeled by summing up all the MUAPs together with the parameters representing the characteristics of slow-twitch (type I) and fast-twitch (type II) motor units.

2. Methods

2.1 Experimental protocol

Six spinal cord injured subjects (5 males and 1 female) with mean ± SD age of 38.6±7.5 yr were recruited for this experiment. The average time post-injury was 6.3±0.45 years. The neurological levels of the subjects are between C7 and T11 and with little or no spasticity in the lower limb muscles. All subjects had no musculoskeletal problems in their lower extremities. All subjects signed an informed consent form approved by National Cheng Kung University Hospital, Tainan, Taiwan.

During the muscle fatigue study, stimulation electrodes (5cm×10cm) were placed to the distal and proximal ends of the quadriceps muscle bellies. The anode was placed 5 cm above the upper border of the patella. The cathode was placed 20 cm proximal to the placement of anode. During the experiment, the subject was seated in the chair of an electrodynamometer (Cybex 6000, Lumex, Inc., NY, USA), with his or her hip joint fixed in an 80° flexion. The muscle group was stimulated by a constant current stimulator with a monophasic waveform at 20 Hz and pulse duration of 300 μsec for 120 seconds. Figure 2 shows the apparatuses for the experiment and data acquisition. Muscle fatigue study was performed at two knee flexion angles at a selected stimulation intensity when the torque output of stimulated muscle reached a stable plateau or when the intensity reached the maximum of 120 mA. The two knee flexion angles were 30° (short length) and 110° (long length) with reference to knee full extension at 0°. In this arrangement, the muscles can be stimulated in both comparatively short and long positions. In addition to the stimulus-evoked EMG, the generated torque was also recorded during isometric tests. Adequate rest (at least 24 hours) was required to avoid a possible carry-over effect due to a short recovery time after muscle fatigue [1].

To detect the stimulus-evoked EMG, active bipolar surface electrodes with preamplifiers (Motion Control Co., Salt Lake City, Utah, USA) were placed on the RF muscle belly. The recording electrodes were placed inside the stimulation electrodes and mid-way between the anterior superior iliac spine (ASIS) and the upper border of the patella [20]. The interelectrode distance was 20 mm and the electrode position was marked between sessions and maintained in each subject throughout the experiments. Figure 3 shows the placement

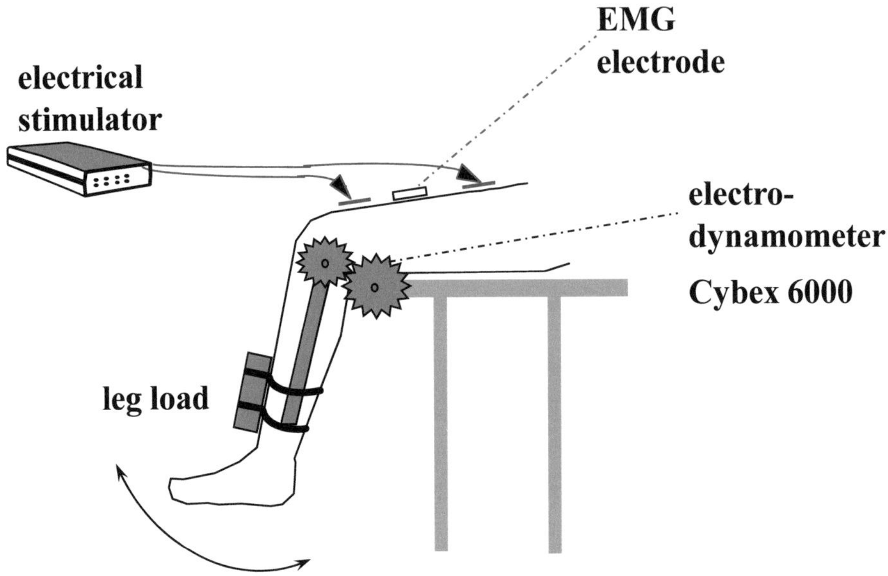

Fig. 2. Apparatuses for stimulation and data recording (knee extension torque and EMG).

of detecting and stimulating electrodes. Before the application of measurement electrodes, the skin was abraded carefully to reduce skin-electrode impedance. To suppress the stimulus artifact, the output stage of the stimulator was grounded immediately after the stimulus pulse was generated which was followed by artifact suppression algorithm [21]. The signal was differentially amplified with a gain of 380. After artifact suppression and amplification, the stimulus-evoked EMG was sampled through an analogue-to-digital converter with 5 kHz sampling rate after an anti-aliasing filter at 2.5 kHz. The measured data were directly saved to a hard disk for later analysis using Matlab (Mathwork Co., Natick, Mass., USA) signal processing software.

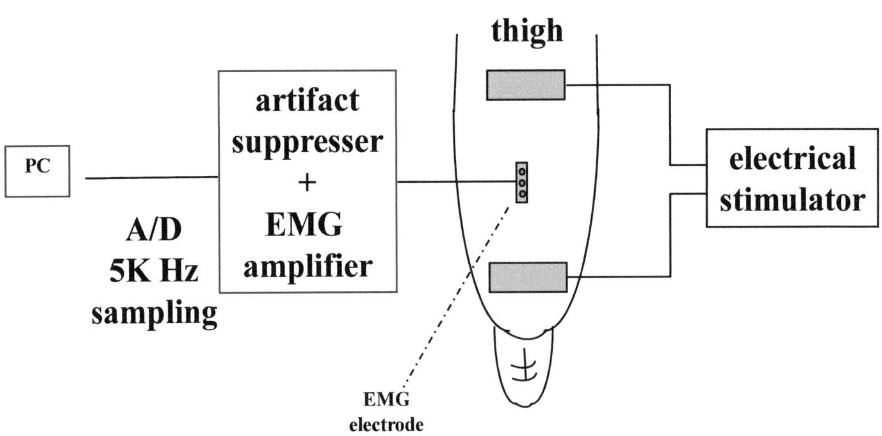

Fig. 3. The placement of EMG and stimulating electrodes.

2.2 Analysis of fatigue process from features of evoked EMG

Both amplitude and temporal features are commonly used to characterize the waveform of the stimulus-evoked EMG. In a succession of sustained muscle contractions, the change in the amplitude parameter can be divided into the first plateau, a decaying slope, and the residual asymptotic level. Conversely, the changes of temporal parameters with inverted manifestation to the frequency parameter can be divided into an initial lower plateau, a rising slope, and the maximal asymptotic level. Our interest is in observing the rising and decaying processes of the CMAP parameters and the torque output during the fatigue process, rather than in making a direct comparison of their values. Thus, the data collected from the same session were first normalized to their initial value and then fitted using the hyperbolic function, which could also alleviate the inter-subject variations and muscle-length discrepancies.

To characterize the fatigue process, a hyperbolic tangent equation, generally used for the description of empirical data with a sigmoid-like curve, was adopted to fit both the parameters of the CMAP and the torque output [8]:

$$Y = a \times \tanh(b \times t - c) + d \tag{1}$$

where Y is the measured parameter of the CMAP or the generated torque as a function of time, t. The parameters a, b, c and d are estimated by using the least-square error method [8]. The inflection time and time constant, representing the time to reach 50% of the change range and its changing rate, can be obtained from c/b and $1/b$, respectively. Derived from the parameters, $d-a$ and $d+a$ represent the initial plateau and the asymptotic value respectively. The total change of the parameter (the difference between maximum and minimum values) is $2a$. The value of $(d+a)/(d-a)$ represents the relative asymptotic value.

With the extracted parameters, muscle fatigue tests were performed in each lower limb at two different muscle lengths of all six SCI subjects, making a total of 24 experimental specimens of the stimulus EMG and torque. Since the normalization was performed, the effect of muscle length on the fatigue process was analyzed by comparing the time constant, inflection time and relative asymptotic value of the four measures including torque output, PTP, RTP, PTPd, between the two lengths (30° and 110° knee flexion). Paired t tests were utilized to test the length effect. The significant level was defined as $\alpha<0.05$. Data are reported as means ± SD within the text and the table.

2.3 Analysis of fatigue process from muscle fiber components of evoked EMG

Compared to the ordered recruitment of MUs in voluntary EMG, the CMAP is considered as the summation of the MUAPs simultaneous firing from different types of muscle fibers near the detecting electrode (Figure 4). Thus, the measured CMAP can be decomposed into the MUAPs with slow-twitch (type I) or fast-twitch (type II) characteristics. Figure 5 illustrates the propagation characteristics of MUAPs from type I or type II units. However, the technique to estimate the muscle fibers components from its summation, i.e. the CMAP, belongs to an inverse problem which requires a model to simulate the CMAP (called forward modeling) and an optimization technique to measure the goodness of resulting modeling parameters (called backward optimization). For the CMAP modeling, the generation of MUAP is adopted from structural EMG modeling of Fuglevand *et al.* [18] with some modifications to take in account of parameters for different muscle fiber types. Figure 6 depicts the schematic diagram of the CMAP signal generation mechanism which consists of slow-twitch and fast twitch fibers during electrically elicited contractions. To simplify the computational process, each motor unit territory area was crossed by a number of semicircular layers with an increment of 0.5 mm (equivalent to about 9 average fiber diameters), where each MU at the same layer is assumed to contribute the same potential to the detecting electrode.

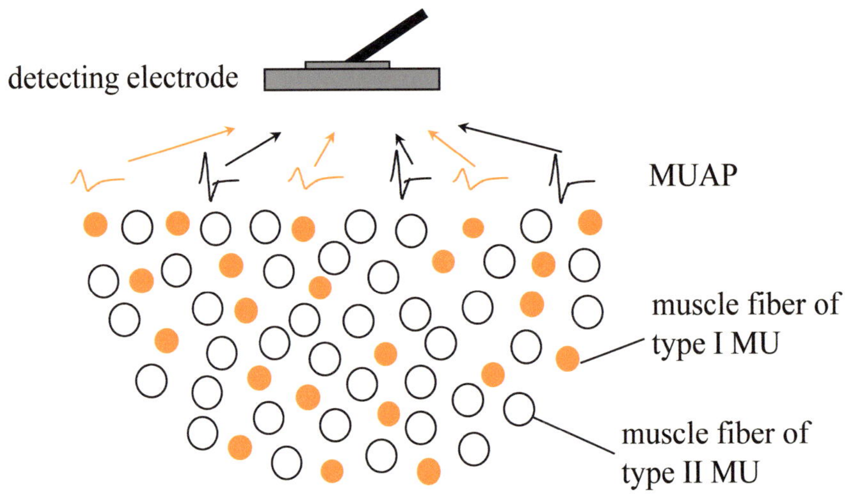

Fig. 4. The CMAP is composed of MUAPs simultaneously firing from the muscle fibers near the detecting electrode.

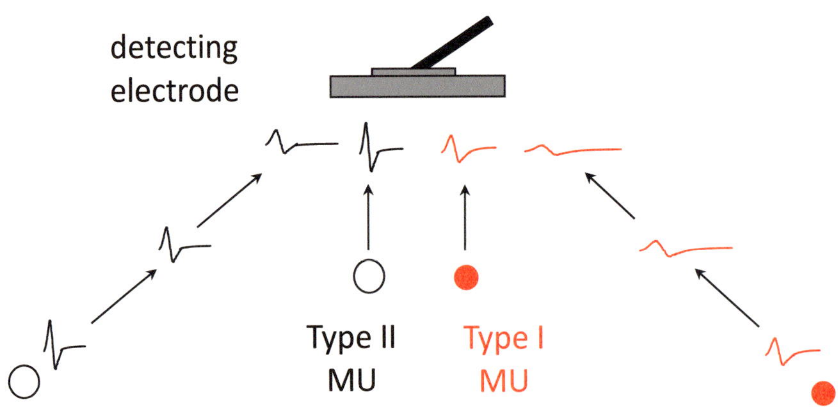

Fig. 5. Waveforms of MUAP at different distances from signal source.

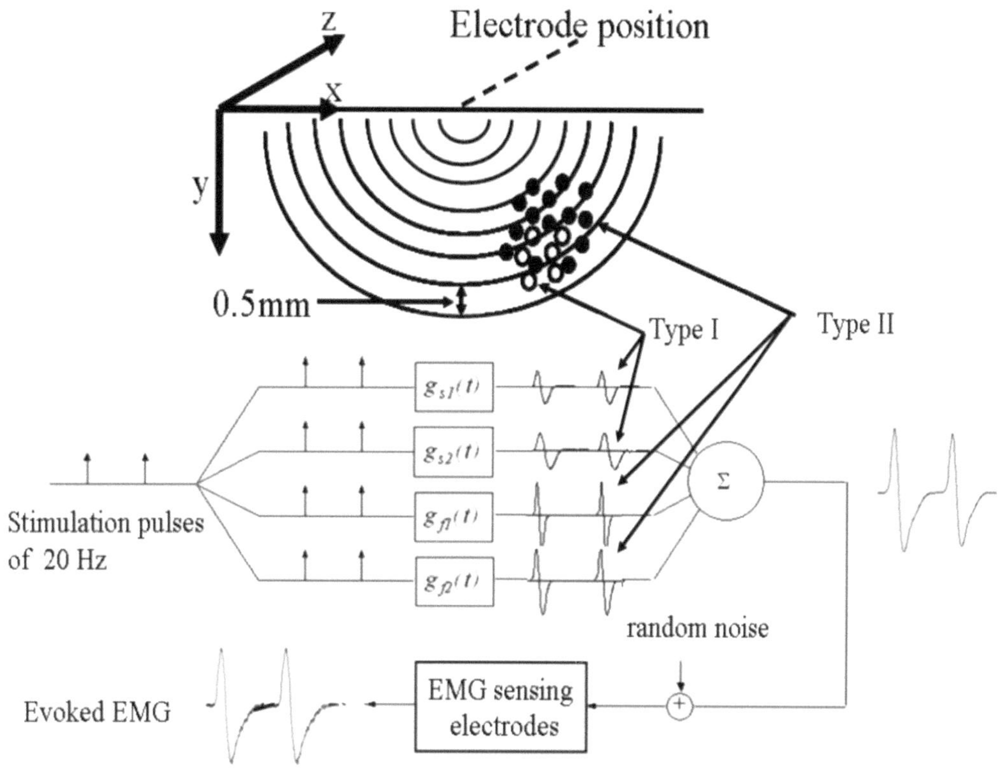

Fig. 6. Schematic diagram of the measured stimulus EMG can be modeled as the sum of MUAPs, with type I (slow-twitch) or type II (fast-twitch) characteristics, simultaneously firing from the muscle fibers randomly distributed within the detection range of surface EMG electrode. The generation of MUAP is based on structural EMG modeling developed by of Fuglevand *et al.* with some modifications to include two muscle fiber types of slow-twitch, $g_s(t,)$ and fast twitch, $g_f(t)$. It is known that type I muscle fibers have smaller amplitude and slower conduction velocity with wide duration, compared with those of type II. In addition, type I muscle fibers (o) are located deeper and have lower distribution percentages (30 % type I vs. 70 % type II) than those of type II muscle fibers (•) in chronic SCI subjects.

The function of a CMAP which comprises m type I MUs and n type II MUs can be formulated as:

$$G(t) = \sum_{i=1}^{m} k_s e^{-t_{si}/\tau} g\left(b_{si} \cdot (t - t_{si})\right) + \sum_{i=1}^{n} k_f e^{-t_{fi}/\tau} g\left(b_{fi} \cdot (t - t_{fi})\right) \quad (2)$$

where g is an MUAP function with m fibers from slow-twitch MUs and n fibers from fast-twitch ones. Figure 7 shows the model of CMAP composed of type I and type II MUAPs. Parameters k_s and k_f are amplitude gains of type I and type II MUs respectively. The exponential term in equation 2 represents the amplitude gain of each MUAP which is inversely and exponentially proportional to the time delays t_{si} and t_{fi} with a fixed decaying time constant τ. The temporal coefficients b_{si} and b_{fi} are used to determine the duration of i-th MUAP. The propagation time along the muscle fiber determines the time delay and the duration of an MUAP which are directly related to the conduction distance of the MUAP. Therefore, MUAPs from different distances have different amplitudes, durations and time delays which are all functions of the electrode-motor unit territory distance (ETD). When a conduction distance along the muscle fiber is longer, the amplitude of the evoked EMG decreases and the duration increases due to the desynchronization of single motor unit potential arrivals at the recording site [22]. Therefore, both amplitude and temporal coefficients are functions of the ETD, the simulation model can hence be formulated as:

$$G(d) = \sum_{r=1}^{d} \mathrm{A(r)} e^{-r/\lambda} \left(\mathrm{k}_s g_s(r) + \mathrm{k}_f g_f(r) \right) \tag{3}$$

where $g_s(r)$ and $g_f(r)$ represent the MUAPs of slow twitch (type I) and fast twitch (type II) muscle fibers from a distance of r, i.e. they are functions of ETD. The r in equation 3 represents the radius of each semicircular layer, with the same origin at the center of the detecting electrode. Equation 3 comprises a number of functions which represent the MUAPs generated from their corresponding isopotential layers. The area of the r-th isopotential layer $A(r)$ is $\frac{1}{2}\pi(2r-1)$.

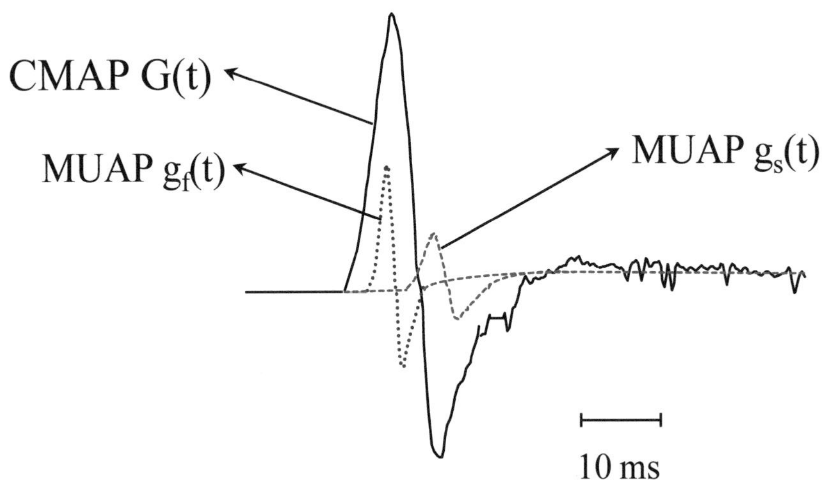

Fig. 7. Illustration of the Model of CMAP.

The generation of MUAP function g can be obtained from the parameters provided by Fuglevand et al. [18] with some modifications to include slow-twitch and fast-twitch MUs. The ranges of the assigned parameters for the modeling of evoked-EMG from two types of muscle fibers are listed in Table 1.

Muscle fiber types	Type I (slow twitch)	Type II (fast twitch)
Percentages of distribution	30 %	70 %
Amplitude	Small	Large
Initial value for gain coefficients before fatigue	k_s =[0.03 0.09]	k_f =[0.05 0.15]
Propagation velocity	1.5-3.0 m/s	4.5-9.0 m/s
Initial value for temporal coefficients before fatigue	b_s =[2.0 3.5]	b_f =[1.0 1.5]

Table 1. Parameters for the simulation of MUAPs for type I and type II muscle fibers.

First, researchers have shown that the distribution percentages of muscle fibers are around 30% (type I) versus 70 % (type II) in chronic SCI cases, different from those of normal subjects with percentages of 52% (type I) versus 48 % (type II) [23]. The proportion of MU type was fixed but the gain values, k_s and k_f, were varied according to the general consensus that type I muscle fibers are smaller in amplitude and are located deeper than the type II muscle fibers. The ranges for k_s and k_f are listed in Table 1.

Second, the average conduction velocity for all fiber types, 4 m/s, was assigned in previous structural EMG model [18], which was divided into 1.5-3.0 m/s for type I and 4.5-9.0 m/s for type II muscle fibers [22]. In addition to elongated duration because of lower conduction velocity, the type I muscle fibers are usually located deeper which results in smaller amplitude in the surface recording. By identifying the relationship between the two pairs of temporal coefficients, the estimation process can be simplified to assess either b_{si} and b_{fi} or t_{si} and t_{fi}. This is because the time delay t_{si} and t_{fi} are related to the anisotropic conduction velocity of muscle fiber, whereas the coefficients b_{si} and b_{fi}, used for determining the duration of an MUAP, are directly related to the longitudinal conduction velocity. The radial conduction velocity of muscle fiber is about one sixth of the longitudinal conduction velocity, therefore the values of t_{si} and t_{fi} can be assumed to depend on those of b_{si} and b_{fi}. The assigned values for b_{si} and b_{fi} are inversely proportional to the physiological ranges of conduction velocity for Type I and Type II muscle fibers, as listed in Table 1. The estimation of the above parameters was obtained by fitting the measured data to the simulated function.

Among the structural EMG parameters, k_s and k_f are amplitude gain features of type I and type II muscle fibers respectively. Another set of important features are the temporal coefficients b_{si} and b_{fi} which were used to determine the duration of every MUAP. The estimation of the above parameters was obtained by fitting the measured data to the simulated function. A nonlinear curve fitting technique was used to find the optimal parameters such that the error could be reduced to a minimum by using the Nelder-Mead simplex algorithm [24]. The parameters derived from the evoked-EMG during fatigue process of two different positions were compared.

3. Results

3.1 Characteristics of muscle fatigue at different knee angles

Figures 8 shows the representative CMAP (dotted lines) measured from the shortened and lengthened muscles from the beginning of stimulation (10th second) and the fatigue situation (120th second), respectively. We can clearly observe that CMAPs before fatigue have a greater amplitude and more compact waveform compared to those with smaller amplitude and broader waveform measured from the 120th second. Comparing the CMAPs with different muscle lengths, the amplitude decreased and the duration of CMAP was elongated extensively in the lengthened muscles, as shown in Fig. 8(b).

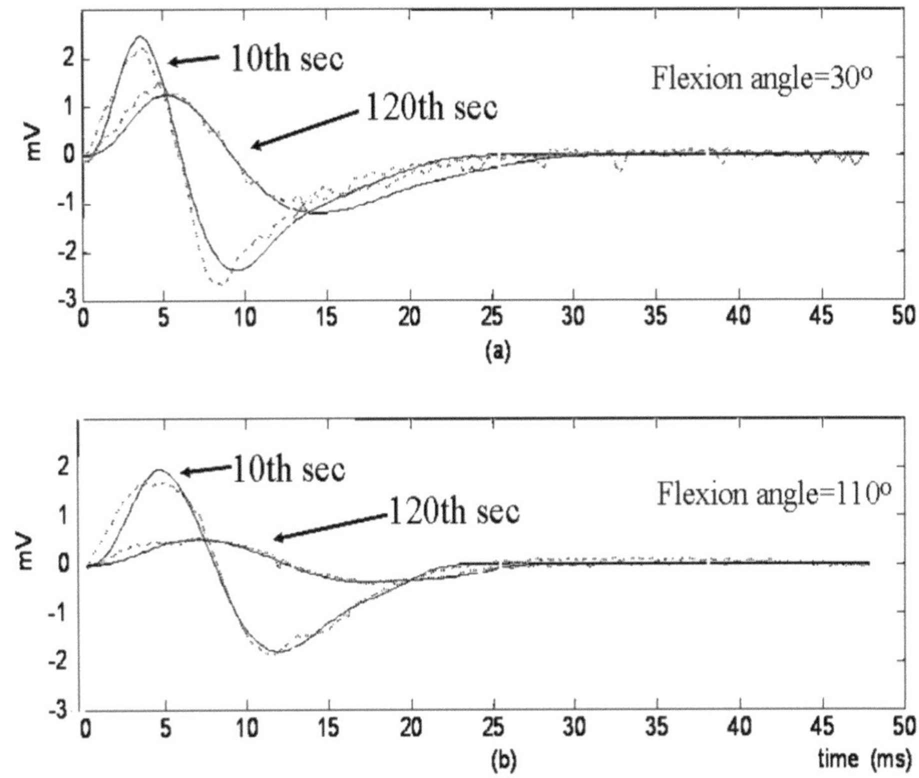

Fig. 8. Representative CMAP signals (dashed line) measured at the 10th and 120th seconds at (a) shortened and (b) lengthened positions. Compared to those measured in the 120th sec, CMAPs have higher amplitude and shorter duration before fatigue. In addition, CMAPs measured at shorter muscle length have short peak-to-peak duration in comparison with those of lengthened one. The solid lines represent the fitted curves which were generated from a structural EMG model consisting of two muscle fibers types.

The influence of muscle lengths on torque and EMG features can be observed from the measurements of isometric contractions measured at two different knee angles. The EMG amplitude (PTP) and torque output were normalized with respect to their maximum, but the EMG RTP and PTP duration were normalized with respect to their minimum. Figure 9 shows the means and standard deviations of the normalized torque output and the EMG features of the six SCI subjects for muscles stimulated at 30° (-o-) and 110° (-x-) of knee flexion. The corresponding parameters for fitting the sigmoid function to the curves are listed in Table 2.

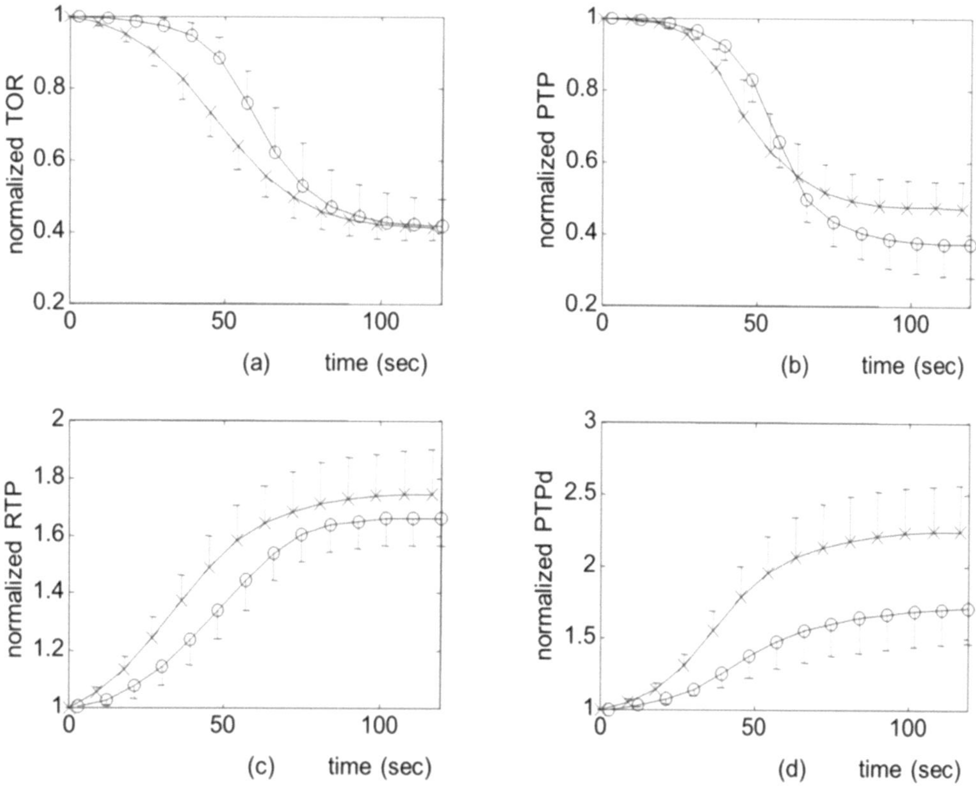

Fig. 9. The measurements of torque output (TOR) and EMG features after amplitude normalization are averaged for isometric contractions at knee flexion at 30° (-o-) and 110° (-x-), with standard deviations shown in vertical bars. The (a) torque output and (b) EMG PTP amplitude show decreasing trends while the (c) EMG RTP and (d) EMG PTP duration exhibit increasing trends during muscle fatigue. All the measurements are fitted to hyperbolic functions with parameters summarized in Table 2.

The torque measured in this process is used to assess when the stimulated-muscle reached the fatigue level, i.e. a plateau at a relatively lower torque output. Figure 9(a) shows that the torques in 30° knee flexion (muscles in shortened length) has an initial plateau and then decreases at a fast rate to a lower plateau with a relative asymptotic value of 0.41, derived from d+a/d-a. Torques from lengthened muscles (110° knee flexion) show no obvious initial plateau but decrease earlier at a slower rate to a similar asymptotic value of 0.39. These observations can be confirmed from the significant differences in time constant (20.79±4.43 s vs. 29.83±9.63 s) and inflection time (61.15±9.69 s vs. 49.12±8.83 s) in torque output between the two flexion angles (Table 2).

Similarly, in EMG PTP amplitude, the significantly smaller inflection time of a 110° flexion angle (48.53±8.70 s compared to 55.13±4.03 s at 30°) indicates that the lengthened muscle fatigues earlier than the shortened muscle. A relatively close time constant and asymptotic

	Time constant (1/b) (sec)	Inflection time (c/b) (sec)	Relative asymptotic value (d+a)/(d-a)
TOR_{30}	20.79(4.43)*	61.15(9.69)*	0.41(0.10)
TOR_{110}	29.83(9.63)*	49.12(8.83)*	0.39(0.05)
PTP_{30}	15.87(9.54)	55.13(4.03)*	0.39(0.14)
PTP_{110}	15.56(4.87)	48.53(8.70)*	0.45(0.13)
RTP_{30}	35.33(9.92)	48.44(11.93)*	1.64(0.31)
RTP_{110}	30.39(7.48)	35.49(6.41)*	1.75(0.63)
$PTPd_{30}$	32.03(9.57)*	46.39(9.55)*	1.77(0.54)*
$PTPd_{110}$	24.71(8.12)*	36.40(12.63)*	2.23(0.74)*

PTP = peak to peak amplitude, RTP = rise time to peak, PTPd = peak to peak duration. The subscript '30' and '110' denote the knee flexion angles. The '*' denotes the difference ($\alpha < 0.05$) between the parameters measured at two knee flexion angles.

Table 2. Summary of hyperbolic fit parameters for the fatigue process during isometric contractions at two knee flexion angles (30° and 110°). The values in brackets are the corresponding standard deviations.

value can be observed in the PTP amplitudes of the two flexion angles (Table 2 and Fig. 9(b)). Our results also show that both the RTP and PTPd of the lengthened muscles increase earlier (with a shorter inflection time of 35.49±6.41 and 36.40±12.63, respectively) than those of shortened muscles (48.44±11.93 and 46.39±9.55, respectively), as depicted in Fig. 9(c) and 9(d). The relative asymptotic value of PTPd in lengthened RF muscle is higher than that in the shortened position (2.23±0.74 vs. 1.77±0.54), as shown in Fig. 9(d).

3.2 Analysis of fatigue process based on muscle fiber components

To estimate the amplitude and temporal coefficients form the CMAP, the initial values of amplitude gains (k_s and k_f) and temporal coefficients (b_s and b_f) were initially assigned according to the physiological values, as listed in Table I. In general, the slow twitch muscle fibers have smaller amplitude (smaller k_s) and lower conduction velocity (greater b_s), compared to those of fast twitch muscle fibers [22]. After the assignment of initial values, the nonlinear curve fitting technique was used to estimate those values from each CMAP measured during fatigue process. As shown in Fig. 8, the estimated MUAP waveforms (solid lines) closely resemble to the measured ones (dotted lines) with an average relative error smaller than 5 % of the measured MUAP.

Feature extraction of muscle fiber components was performed with the curve fitting technique on the measured CMAP for duration of 120 s. The averages of amplitude coefficients of slow-twitch (k_s) and fast-twitch (k_f) for shortened and lengthened muscle positions are shown in Fig. 10, where the dashed and solid curves show the changes of k_s and k_f respectively. At the beginning of stimulation, amplitude coefficients of fast twitch are greater than those of slow twitch, which is even evident in RF muscle in a shortened condition (Fig. 10(a)). With the time elapse of stimulation, both of the coefficients in the shortened muscle increased first then decreased into a residual value (Fig. 10(a)). In the lengthened muscle, both the coefficients decreased near monotonically to a lower residue value as shown in Fig. 10(b). When comparing their decreasing speeds, the amplitude coefficient in type II MU dropped abruptly into a lower plateau at around 40 seconds after the beginning of stimulation (Fig. 10(b)). Although the declining curve was not so steep in the shortened muscles, the apparent drops of the amplitude coefficients in the type II MU can also be noted. In addition, the amplitude gains of type I MU dropped to 33 % and 30 % for shortened and lengthened muscles. In contrast, those of type II MU dropped to 15 % and 13 % of their original values. The amplitude gain coefficients of slow twitch became larger than those of fast twitch, at the last period of stimulation around 80th s in shortened position and after 40th s in lengthened position.

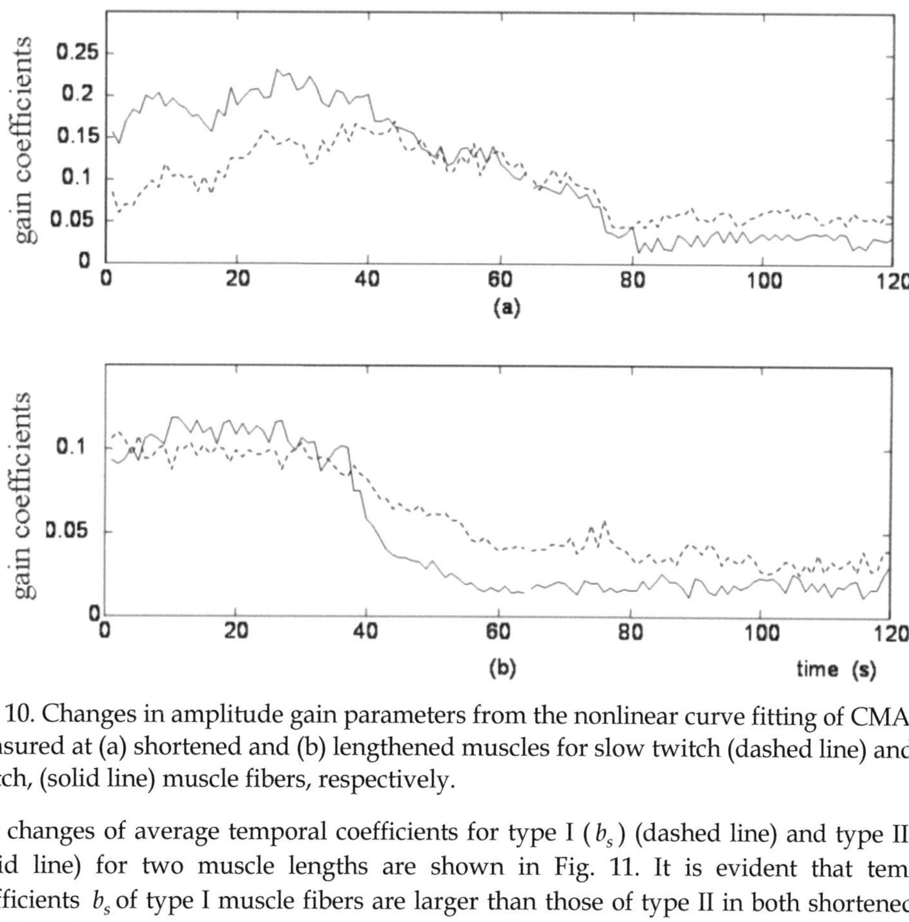

Fig. 10. Changes in amplitude gain parameters from the nonlinear curve fitting of CMAP measured at (a) shortened and (b) lengthened muscles for slow twitch (dashed line) and fast twitch, (solid line) muscle fibers, respectively.

The changes of average temporal coefficients for type I (b_s) (dashed line) and type II (b_f) (solid line) for two muscle lengths are shown in Fig. 11. It is evident that temporal coefficients b_s of type I muscle fibers are larger than those of type II in both shortened and lengthened positions. In shortened muscles, the b_s and b_f coefficients started at around 1.9 and 1.1 which increased monotonically into an upper plateau around 2.9 and 1.8, respectively, Similar observations can be found in lengthened muscles which increased from 2.2 to 5.0 for b_s and from 1.5 to 3.8 for b_f, respectively. In addition, the increasing rate of b_s and b_f is higher for lengthened muscles, compared to that of shortened one. However, the increasing speed of two temporal coefficients at a same flexion angle does not show significant difference.

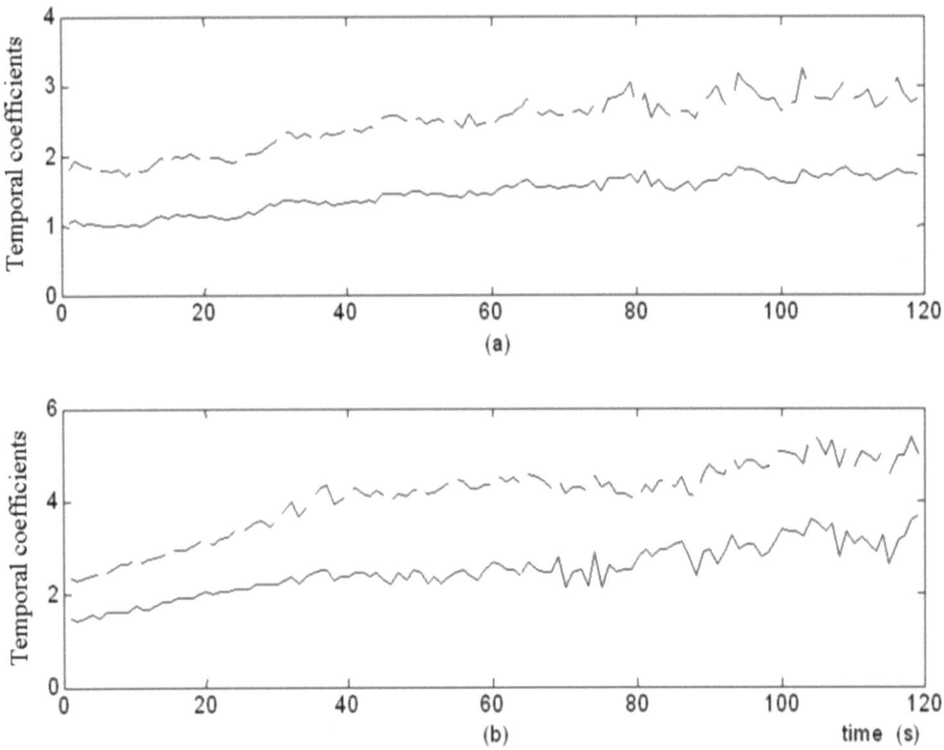

Fig. 11. The extraction of temporal coefficients from the measured CMAP of (a) shortened and (b) lengthened muscles during 120 seconds of fatigue process. Increasing trend in the temporal coefficients for slow twitch (b_s, dashed line) and fast twitch (b_f, solid line) muscle fibers can be observed.

4. Discussion

4.1 Effect of muscle length on the fatigue process

Under continuous stimulation, the EMG PTP amplitude exhibited a decreasing trend which exhibited a sigmoid-like curve with a main slope and two plateaus during muscle fatigue. Concurrently with the reduction in EMG PTP amplitude, the increase in RTP and PTP duration denotes a broadening of the CMAP, which is commonly explained by the reduction of the muscle fiber's conduction velocity during the fatigue process [7].

Among the amplitude and temporal parameters, our results showed a larger inflection time for the four measured features in shortened muscles, compared to those in lengthened muscles (Table 2). Previous studies on the effect of muscle length on temporal features revealed differences in conduction velocity estimates in muscles with different lengths [13, 17]. Differences in amplitude features were also found at different muscle lengths [16]. When a muscle is shortened, assuming no or little change in the volume of muscle fibers, the conduction velocity must be increased because of the larger diameter of muscle fibers with lower conducting impedance [13]. Action potentials propagating along muscle fibers with faster conduction velocities are detected more nearly simultaneously, causing the CMAP to appear larger and more compressed. During the fatigue process, the conduction velocity in T-tube and sarcoplasmic reticulum is reduced such that the propagation time in the muscle fiber is further prolonged [25]. The longer the muscle fiber, the more difficult the propagation in the muscle fibers, resulting in earlier and faster fatigue. Researchers have also indicated that the fatigue-resistant characteristics can be found in shortened muscles of healthy subjects [26]. These phenomena were interpreted that a reduced force in shortened muscles reflects a reduced number of cross-bridge interactions and a lower total ATP turnover. Other researchers studied the effects of length on the change of contractile properties [27] and stimulation frequency on the fatigue properties [25]. They found similar fatigue properties in shortened muscles and high frequency stimulation, and attributed the phenomena to the failure of sarcolemmal action potential propagation in the transverse tubules of shortened muscles.

4.2 Physiological implications of muscle fiber components during muscle fatigue

It is known that different types of MU have their own features in the electrically-elicited myoelectric signal [28, 29]. The action potential propagation velocity in muscle fiber is known to be related to the type and diameter of muscle fiber [29], to the extracellular potassium concentration, and to the pH of intracellular or interstitial fluid [30]. Research has shown that fast-twitch MUs display a marked reduction in amplitude and the integrated area, whereas the slow-twitch MUs shows little or no change in surface action potential during muscle fatigue [28]. Other studies indicated that the decreasing curves of the EMG amplitude could be the reflection of the activation of the residual fatigue-resistant MUs, which have small amplitude in MUAPs [7]. Thus, the distinct components in the rising sigmoid curve of the temporal features of CMAP might not only denote the reduction in the conduction velocity but also indicate which type of MU is predominating during the muscle fatigue process. Our analysis of fatigue process from the muscle fiber components supported this observation.

The amplitude gains in the shortened muscle increased first then decreased monotonically. It seems that the electrical activity of both types of MUs were initially potentiated and then released gradually in the shortened muscle. This phenomenon could be ascribed to a process of synchronized MUAPs which matches the early plateau observed in the aspects of both torque output and the EMG PTP (Fig. 9(a) and (b)). Contrary to the shortened muscles, the lengthened muscles exhibited a slow decrease in amplitude gain at a prolonged duration during the first 40 second of stimulation. After that, the amplitude gain coefficients of type II MU dropped abruptly into a lower plateau, especially in when the muscles were stimulated in the lengthened positions. These results implied that early fatigue in lengthened muscles might be due to the quick depletion of the type II MUs. Through making a comparison between the two types of MU, the more intense decline of the amplitude coefficient of type II MU especially in lengthened muscle (Fig. 10(b)) indicates its contribution to the early muscle fatigue. From the slower declining speed of the amplitude coefficient of type I MU, the greater amplitude gain implying more dominant contribution from the fatigue-resistant muscle fibers could be noted in the late period of stimulation (Fig. 10).

The temporal coefficients b_s and b_f of two muscle lengths show steady increase during the fatigue process, differently from the amplitude coefficients. The increasing rate of b_s and b_f

is higher for lengthened muscles (Fig. 11(b)), compared to that of shortened one (Fig. 11(a)). An increase in temporal coefficient means the elongated duration of the CMAP and the decrease in conduction velocity during muscle fatigue in both muscle types. The changes of temporal coefficients in type I and type II MUs (Fig. 11) of two muscle lengths exhibited similar characteristics when compared with the temporal PTPd features of the CMAP (Fig. 9 (d)), which showed a higher increasing rate with lower time constant and higher relative asymptotic value for lengthened muscle (Table 2).

Our results supported that the sigmoid-like curves in the CMAP features might correlate with the changed contributions of two MU types. The smaller RTP and PTP duration in the first plateau (Fig. 9(c) and (d)) and larger amplitude coefficients (Fig. 10) in fast twitch muscle fibers indicate that type II MUs with larger diameter muscle/nerve fibers and fast conduction velocity are those predominantly activated in early electrical stimulation period. By contrast, type I MUs with lower conduction velocities are more resistant to fatigue and might, therefore, be predominant in the EMG signal when muscle fatigue progresses [31]. This predominance tends to decrease the average muscle fiber conduction velocity, and then to elevate the curves of the temporal features to the final plateau. These phenomena can also be observed from larger amplitude coefficient and higher residual values for type I MUs (Fig. 10) during muscle fatigue at the end of stimulation period.

5. Conclusions

The hyperbolic curve fit of CMAP features as well as the extracted coefficients of muscle fiber components were used to observe muscle fatigue induced by continuous electrical stimulation at two different muscle lengths. Our results showed that RF muscle is more easily fatigable when lengthened than when shortened, which can be observed from shorter inflection times of CMAP features and from abrupt decreasing trend in gain coefficient of type II MUs. Compared to type II MUs, the amplitude gain coefficients of type I MUs started at smaller values but slowly dropped to a plateau level which was higher than those of fast twitch ones. These observations correlate well with the predominance of fast twitch type II MUs at the beginning of stimulation but the fatigue resistant type I MUs predominate the fatigue process at the end of stimulation period. . The higher increasing rate and larger final values of temporal coefficients in lengthened muscles, compared to that of shortened one, exhibited similar characteristics to the temporal PTPd features of the CMAP during fatigue process. However, our estimation of muscle fiber components was based a structural EMG model of Fuglevand *et al.* by adding additional parameters to specify the numbers, amplitude, and temporal coefficients for two different types of MUs. With more information acquired from the configuration and proportion of the MU types in paralyzed limb, constructing a sophisticated model of CMAP consisting for varied distributions of muscle types will be a challenge for future works. The interpretation from the distribution of muscle fiber components during fatigue process might become feasible by integrating the experimental design and evoked-EMG modeling.

6. References

[1] J. Mizrahi, "Fatigue in muscles activated by functional electrical stimulation," Crit. Rev. Phys. Rehabil. Med., vol. 9, pp. 93-129, 1997.

[2] Y. Giat, J. Mizrahi, and M. Levy, "A model of fatigue and recovery in paraplegic's quadriceps muscle subjected to intermittent FES," J. Biomech. Eng., vol. 118, pp. 357-366, 1996.

[3] M. Levy, T. Kushnir, J. Mizrahi, and Y. Itzchak, "In vivo ^{31}P NMR studies of paraplegics' muscles activated by functional electrical stimulation. Magn. Res. Med., vol. 29, pp.53-58, 1993.

[4] J. Mizrahi, M. Levy, H. Ring, E. Isakov, and A. Liberson, "EMG as an indicator of fatigue in isometrically FES-activated paralyzed muscles," IEEE Trans. Rehab. Eng., vol. 2, pp. 57-65, 1994.

[5] B. K. Boom, A. J. Mulder, and P. H. Veltink, "Fatigue during functional neuromuscular stimulation," Progr. Brain Res., vol. 97, pp.409-418, 1993.

[6] E. Rabischong and F. Ohanna, "Effects of functional electrical stimulation on evoked muscular output in paraplegic quadriceps muscle," Paraplegia, vol. 30, pp. 467-473, 1992.

[7] E. Rabischong, "Surface action potential related to torque output in paraplegics electrically stimulated quadriceps muscle," Med. Eng. Phys., vol. 18, pp.538-547, 1996.

[8] E. Rabischong and D. Guiraud, "Determination of fatigue in the electrically stimulated quadriceps muscle and relative effect of ischemia," J. Biomed. Eng., vol. 15, pp.443-450, 1993.

[9] W. Girsch, M. Bijak, G. Heger, R. Koller, H. Lanmuller, W. Mayr, H. Thomas, and U. Losert, "Monitoring of FES-induced muscle-activity by continuous EMG-recording," Int. J. Artif. Org., vol. 18, pp.340-244, 1995.

[10] J. Winslow, P. L. Jacobs, and D. Tepavac, "Fatigue compensation during FES using surface EMG," J. Electromyogr. Kinesiol., vol. 13, no. 6, pp.555-568, 2003.

[11] M. Bilodeau, J. Houck, T. Cuddeford, S. Sharma, and N. Riley, "Variations in the relationship between the frequency content of EMG signals and the rate of torque development in voluntary and elicited contractions," J. Electromyogr. Kinesiol., vol. 12, no. 2, pp. 137-145, 2002.

[12] N. C. Chesler and W. K. Durfee, "Surface EMG as a fatigue indicator during FES-induced isometric muscle contractions," J. Electromyogr. Kinesio., vol. 7, pp. 27-37, 1997.

[13] R. Merletti, L. R. Lo Conte, C. Cisari, and U. Massazza, "Effect of ankle joint position on electrically evoked surface myoelectric signals of the tibialis anterior muscle," Arch. Phys. Med. Rehabil., vol. 74, pp. 501-506, 1993.

[14] D. Farina, M. Fosci, and R. Merletti, "Motor unit recruitment strategies investigated by surface EMG variables: An experimental and model based feasibility study," J. Appl. Physiol., vol. 92, pp. 235-247, 2002.

[15] W. Muhammad, O. Meste, H. Rix, and D. Farina, "A pseudo joint estimation of time delay and scale factor for M-wave analysis," IEEE Trans. Biomed. Eng. Vol. 50, no. 4, pp. 459-468, 2003.

[16] J. J. Chen and Y. N. Yu, "The validity of stimulus-evoked EMG for studying muscle fatigue characteristics of paraplegic subjects during dynamic cycling movement," IEEE Trans. Rehab. Eng., vol. 5, pp. 170-178, 1997.

[17] D. Farina, R. Merletti, M. Nazzaro, and I.Caruso, "Effect of joint angle on EMG variables in leg and thigh muscles: what influence does muscle length and

electrode location have on EMG signals during dynamic tasks?," IEEE Eng. Med. and Bio., vol. 20, pp. 62-71, 2001.
[18] J. Fuglevand, D. A.Winter, A. E. Patla, and D. Stashuk, "Detection of motor unit action potentials with surface electrode size and spacing," Biol. Cybern., vol. 67, pp. 143-53, 1992.
[19] D. Farina and R. Merletti, "A novel approach for precise simulation of the EMG signal detected by surface electrode," IEEE Trans. Biomed. Eng., vol. 48, pp.637-646, 2001.
[20]] E. F. Delagi and A. Perotto, Anatomic guide for the electromyographer: the limbs. 2nd ed., Thomas, Springfield, 1980.
[21] J. Minzly, J. Mizrahi, N. Hakim, and A. Liberson, "A stimulus artifact suppresser for EMG recording during FES by a constant-current stimulator," Med. Biol. Eng. Comput., vol. 31, pp.71-75, 1993.
[22] Y. Okajima, N. Chino, A. Tsubahara, and A. Kimura, "Waveform analysis of compound nerve action potentials: A computer simulation," Arch. Phys. Med. Rehabil., vol. 75, pp.960-964, 1994.
[23]] R. Scelsi, "Skeletal muscle pathology after spinal cord injury: our 20 year experience and results on skeletal muscle changes in paraplegics, related to functional rehabilitation," Basic Appl. Myol., vol. 11, no.2, pp.75-85, 2001.
[24] J. C. Lagarias, J. A. Reeds, M. H. Wright, and P. E. Wright, "Convergence properties of the Nelder-Mead simplex method in low dimensions," SIAM Journal on Optimization, vol. 9, no. 1, pp. 112-147, 1998.
[25] P. Sacco, D. B. McIntyre, and D. A. Jones, "Effects of length and stimulation frequency on fatigue of the human tibialis anterior muscle," J. Appl. Physiol., vol. 77, pp.1148-1154, 1994.
[26] R. D. Kooistra, C. J. de Ruiter, and A. de Haan, "Muscle activation and blood flow do not explain the muscle length-dependent variation in quadriceps isometric endurance," vol. 97, pp. 1693–1701, J. Appl. Physiol., vol. 98, pp.810-816, 2005.
[27]] N. Place, N. A. Maffiuletti, Y. Ballay, and R. Lepers, "Twitch potentiation is greater after a fatiguing submaximal isometric contraction performed at short vs. long quadriceps muscle length," J. Appl. Physiol., vol. 98, pp.429-436, 2005.
[28] K. Hainaut and J. Duchateau, "Muscle fatigue, effects of training and disuse," Muscle Nerve, vol. 12, pp.660-669, 1989.
[29] M. Knaflitz, R. Merletti, and C. J. DeLuca, "Inference of motor unit recruitment order in voluntary and electrically elicited contractions," J. Appl. Physiol., vol. 68, pp.1657-1667, 1990.
[30] C. Juel, "Muscle action potential propagation velocity changes during activity," Muscle Nerve, vol. 11, pp. 714-719, 1988.
[31] L. Arendt-Nielsen, K. R. Mills, and A. Forster, "Changes in muscle fiber conduction velocity, mean power frequency, and mean EMG voltage during prolonged submaximal contractions," Muscle Nerve, vol. 12, pp. 493-497, 1989.

10

Assessment of Low Back Muscle by Surface EMG

Adalgiso Coscrato Cardozo and Mauro Gonçalves
São Paulo State University
Brazil

1. Introduction

Surface electromyography (EMG) is wide used to analyze back muscle activity. This tool is a non-invasive technique that allows the evaluation of muscle activity. Extensive researches were made to understand the surface EMG techniques and its application to the analysis of low back muscles for classifying healthy subjects and low back pain (LBP) patients, trained and non-trained subjects, subjects under rehabilitation treatments, as well as to access the muscle activity during labor tasks, sports practice or daily life activities.

So, the development of biomechanical tests that enable identifying standards of muscular activity characteristic of a fatigue process, one of the causes for spine muscular-skeletal lesions, which emerges through the task repetitiveness and overload, may be a possibility of preventing lumbar lesions.

The aim of this chapter is to provide a global understand of EMG parameters used to access low back muscle. For this it will be presented some issues that affect the surface EMG for low back muscle as: the reliability of low back muscle EMG; the behavior of low back muscle EMG during isometric contractions by means the analysis of the root mean square (RMS), median frequency (MF) and mean power frequency (MPF); the biomechanical parameter to identify the fatigue threshold known as Electromyographic Fatigue Threshold (EMG_{FT}); the used of surface EMG to the assessing low back pain; and the influence of the manual load lifting to the EMG signal in low back muscle.

2. Reliability of low back muscle EMG

EMG has been used to study physiological aspects of muscle activity. The reliability of the EMG spectral parameters in low back muscles has been analyzed by different authors (Bouillard et al., 2011, van Dieën & Heijblom, 1996, Dolan et al., 1995, Ng & Richardson, 1996). This reproducibility refers to the consistency in the measurement tool used, where a reproducible method is one that has a small measurement error (Elfving et al., 1999). When evaluating different methods of exercise, the reproducibility of the experiment is very important, and the test/re-test methodology is used to estimate the variability of the measures in repeated tests (Dedering et al., 2000).

Tools commonly used for analysis of reproducibility are the Standard Error of the Measurement (SEM) and the Intra-class Correlation Coefficient (ICC), which appear to be complementary of each other (Elfving et al., 1999). The first can be used to check the size of the error relative to the size of the changes in the variables analyzed while the second can be used to consider the size of the error related to differences between measures (Keating & Matyas, 1998).

The ICC rang from 0.00 to 1.00, were the perfect reliability is 1.00 and the poorest is 0.0. A high ICC reflects a small within-subject variance compared to the between-subjects variance. There are different ways to calculate the ICC depending on the experimental design and the composition of the group being tested (Keating & Matyas, 1998), therefore, we must be careful when comparing it in different groups, and extrapolates it to heterogeneous populations.

Low back muscles EMG parameters are not easily comparable between studies of reproducibility, since the methodology often varies. In several studies (van Dieën & Heijblom, 1996, Dolan et al., 1995, Ng & Richardson, 1996) the number of subjects varies between 4 and 28, mostly males. Also, different locations of electrodes, test positions and levels of muscle contraction are used by different authors in testing low back muscles (Elfving et al., 1999).

The EMG signal is generally obtained in two locations ranging between T10 and L5 vertebrae. The positions of the test usually used are: prone (Mannion & Dolan, 1994, Moffroid, 1993, Ng & Richardson, 1996, Coleman et al., 2011), sitting (Carpenter & Nelson, 1999, van Dieën & Heijblom, 1996, Elfving et al., 2003) and standing (Cardozo & Gonçalves, 2010, Cardozo et al., 2011). The time between test and re-test ranging from 5 to 60 minutes in a comparison intra-day and 1 to 6 days in a comparison of day (Elfving et al., 1999).

Several authors have made studies to verify reliability of surface EMG methods. Spector (1979) found correlation coefficients ranging from 0.73 and 0.97, while Komi & Buskirk (1970) achieved a test-retest reliability of 0.88 for surface electrodes.

Danneels et al. (2002) have reported an excellent within-day ICC for EMG parameters performed at the maximum voluntary contraction (MVC) for both healthy and LBP subjects.

During a sub-maximal protocol Dedering et al. (2000) have shown good reliability for EMG parameters, corroborating with study performed by Fleiss (1986), who also demonstrated good reliability for low back muscles. In his study he found ICCs ranging from 0.443 to 0.727 for the initial MF, and ranging from 0.273 to 0.734 for the MF slope. These better results to the initial values comparing to the slope values is supported by study of Peach et al (1998) performed to analyze back muscle fatigue.

Another measure of reproducibility of EMG parameters is intra and inter-subject coefficient of variation (CV), where lower values represent greater repeatability (Knutson et al., 1994). The CV reflects the dispersion of data around the mean and it is calculated by the root square of the standard deviation divided by the mean. The high or low values are not considered good or bad. Some degree of variability is necessary to demonstrate reproducibility. A low CV suggests homogeneity of the group, which allows creating a diagnostic or a model that can be compared to other assessments. This is the basis on which the average dynamic electromyography has been considered as a normalization value when studying dynamic events.

Since EMG analysis have been an alternative to check the resistance of low back muscles due to the contraction time, the reproducibility of these measures becomes paramount. According to the studies presented in the current chapter, it is possible to note that during isometric contractions surface EMG can access low back muscles with good reproducibility.

3. Low back muscle fatigue during isometric contractions

The possibility of preventing overload-associated lumbar lesions caused by the practice of sports, daily activities and especially at work may come from the development of tests aimed at allowing identifying muscular activities patterns characteristic of a fatigue state, which is one of the evident causes of muscular-skeletal lesions in the spine, once this type of injury is established due to the task repetitiveness and overload.

The EMG spectral analysis is widely used to control the development of the localized muscular fatigue. Fatigue promotes changes on the EMG signal frequencies usually evidenced by the analysis of the MF and MPF (Kumar et al., 1998).

These changes on the spectral values are associated with physiological changes as the waveform of the motor units action potentials affected by alterations on the muscular fibers conduction velocity. This velocity decreases due to changes on the muscular pH that in turn, changes in function of the accumulation of the lactate generated in the muscle (Cardozo & Gonçalves, 2010, DeLuca, 1997). This promotes an increase on the low frequencies and a decrease on the high frequencies making the spectral parameters to change and the MF and MPF parameters to decrease (Figure 1).

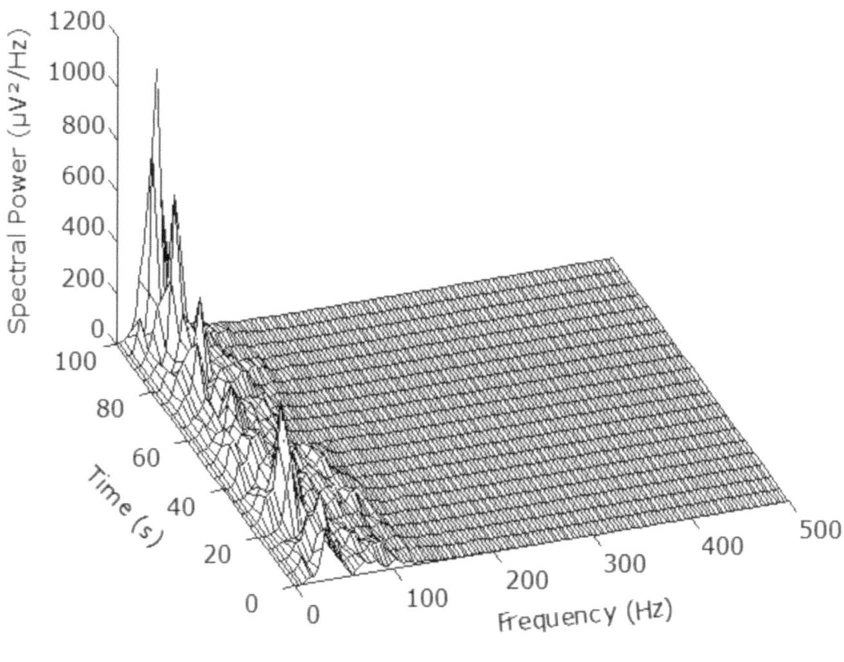

Fig. 1. EMG spectral analysis over time.

But the use of the MF and MPF reflects the global behavior of spectral parameters, and not specific frequencies, which can be important to the analysis of back muscle. With this in mind Dolan et al. (1995) developed an alternative protocol called "Frequency Banding. In their study thirty-five health volunteers pulled upward with constant force on a handlebar attached to the floor while the EMG signal from the erector spinae was recorded at the levels T10 and L3. The power spectra were divided into 10 frequency bands between 5Hz and 300Hz (5-30 Hz, 30-60 Hz, 60-90 Hz etc. up to 300 Hz), as shown in figure 2.

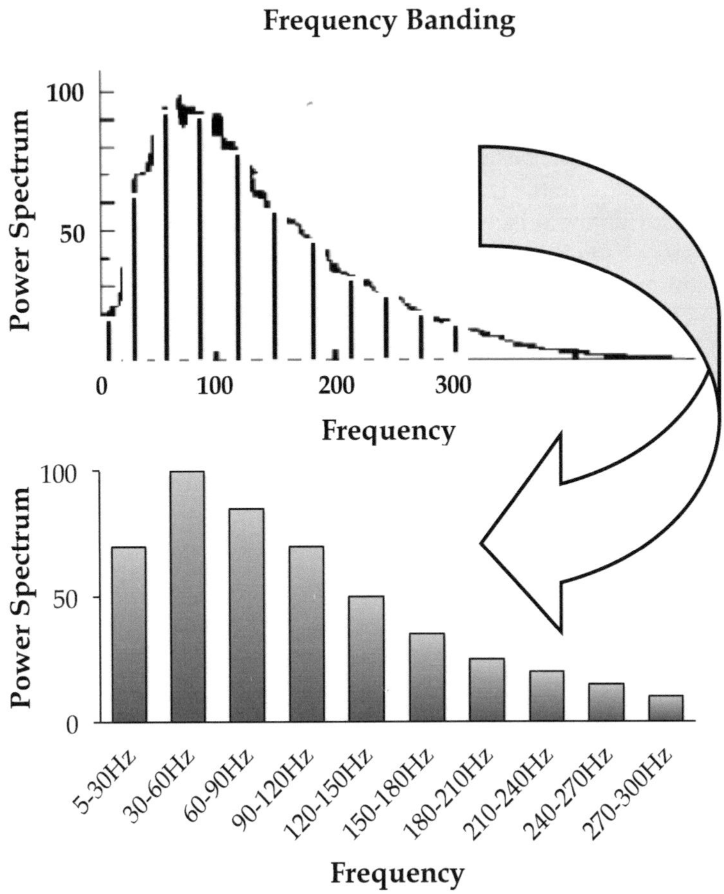

Fig. 2. Frequency Banding technique.

The authors affirm that this range was choose because preliminary tests showed that most of the signal above 300Hz was noise, and signal below 5Hz was most susceptible to movement artifact. They compared changes in these frequency bands of the EMG power spectrum with changes in MF and total power during sustained isometric contractions of the back muscles and found that changes in the lowest frequency band (5 to 30Hz) were the most reliable index of fatigue. They also found that changes in this band correlated best with the measured endurance time.

More recently Cardozo et al. (2011), using the frequency banding technique, found that the signal in the low frequency part of the EMG power spectrum increases with fatigue in a load-dependent manner. Also, they found that the rate of change in low frequency power may be a useful indicator of fatigue rate or "fatigability" in back muscles and may provide a useful tool for assessing changes in muscle function in patients in response to rehabilitation and muscle training regimes, and that changes in low frequency power are more evident than changes in the MF.

Another methodology aimed at observing the muscular fatigue process through EMG is the RMS value taken as indicative of the muscular activity variation both in the fire rate and in the amplitude, once this value is directly associated to the behavior of the motor units involved.

Most skeletal muscles respond to fatiguing submaximal contractions with an increase on the EMG signal amplitude (Cardozo & Gonçalves, 2003). However, some studies report that during trunk extension exercises, the back muscles respond differently, as a decrease or no change on the EMG signal (Hermann & Barnes, 2001). It is likely that these contradictions are due to differences of protocols between studies. Studies performed with high load levels have reported decreases on the EMG signal with the fatigue (Hermann & Barnes, 2001), however, other studies involving contractions with low load levels did not presented this decreasing RMS behavior in function of time (van Dieën et al., 1993, Morlock et al., 1997, Ng et al., 1997). Another potential explanation for these conflicting results in back muscles is related with the type of exercise, once these muscles are configured at several directions in the spine (Haldeman, 1999), pure trunk extension exercises may present different results in relation to those using rotation exercises or even combined extension and rotation exercises.

4. Electromyographic fatigue threshold for low back muscle

To evaluate the muscular conditions biomechanically and to obtain an index that allows instructing activities, postures and even exercises to improve the general physical conditions, becomes the main justification to develop a protocol in order to evaluate the development of the fatigue process of back muscle in isometric tasks by means EMG with the objective of obtaining and evaluating a fatigue threshold.

In the fatigue state, differences in EMG activity for agonists' muscles have been suggested (Tesch et al., 1983). Several protocols have been developed for the identification of muscular fatigue, most of them is based in the methodology described by DeVries (1982) that analyze the RMS with the time (Graef et al., 2008, Kendall et al., 2010, Matsumoto et al. 1991, Oliveira et al., 2007, Pavlat et al. 1995, Smith et al., 2007, Viitasalo et al. 1985) at different perceptual of load, allowing to determine the index called Electromyographic Fatigue Threshold (EMG_{FT}).

The EMG_{FT} correspond the higher intensity of load that the subject can maintain without starting the process of neuromuscular fatigue. In this intensity, the EMG activity does not change with the progress of the exercise (Moritani et al. 1993).

To the determination of the EMG_{FT}, DeVries et al. (1982) proposed a methodology in which the subjects performed an incremental protocol in a cycle-ergometer. The EMG signals were obtained from quadriceps muscle in different loads and, in each load, it was performed a linear regression between the EMG signal and time to obtain the slope (Figure 3-A). After that, a new linear regression was performed between the slope and its corresponding load, been the intercept of the line considered the EMG_{FT} (Figure 3-B).

Pavlat et al. (1995) adapted the protocol of DeVries et al. (1982) and proposed to determinate the EMG_{FT}, the use of predictive loads with fixed duration of 1 minute, and 12 consecutives sets of EMG signs with 5 seconds of duration each. This author performed this protocol to avoid the increase of temperature, which can reduce the amplitude of EMG signs.

Housh et al. (1995) utilized the EMG_{FT} of vastus lateralis (VL), vastus medialis (VM) and rectus femoris (RF) muscles in the cycle-ergometer during loads from 200 to 400W and concluded that EMG_{FT} of RF was smaller than VL, suggesting that there is a dissociation in the characteristics of superficial muscles of quadríceps femoris.

About the reproducibility DeVries et al. (1987) verified a correlation of 0,94 between test and re-test. Pavlat et al. (1993) determined the EMG_{FT} of VL muscle and obtained a correlation of 0,65 between test and re-test. This author also found no differences between values.

Several researchers have attempted to develop testing protocols that allow the evaluation of muscle behavior, but all these protocols were performed for limb muscles. The first study

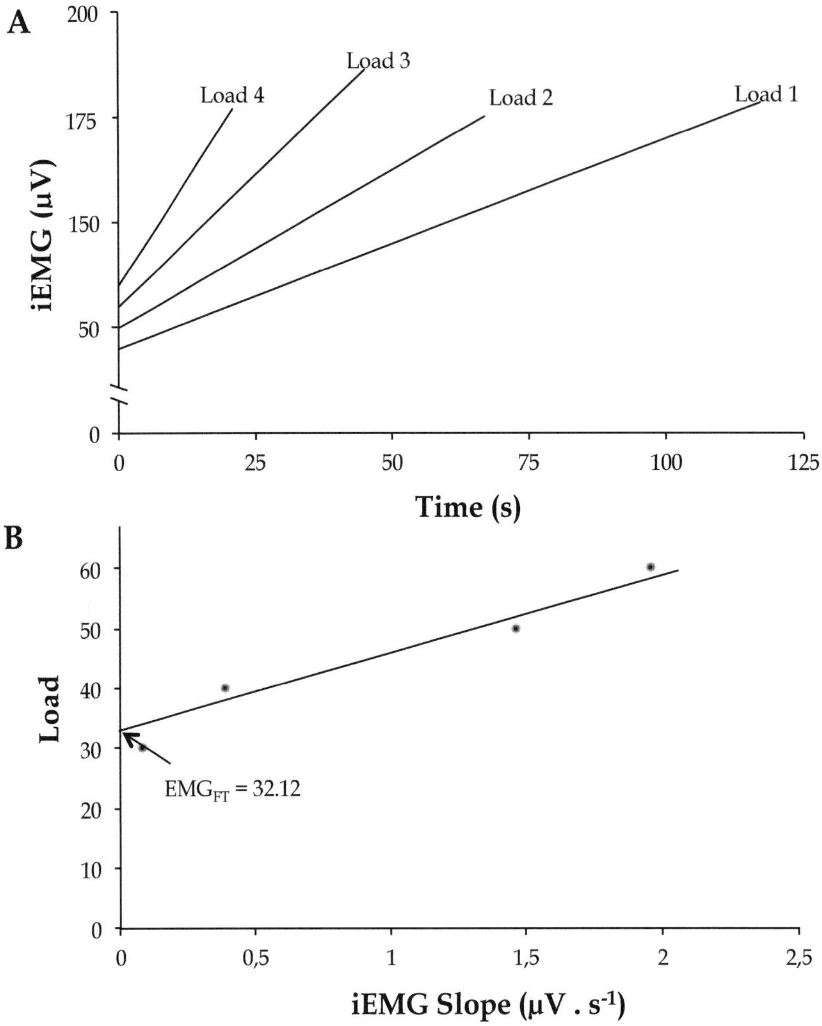

Fig. 3. Determination of the Electromyographic Fatigue Threshold (EMG_{FT}) by DeVries et al. (1982) protocol. A: linear regression between the EMG signal and time to obtain the slope; B: linear regression performed between the slope and its corresponding load (the intercept of the line is considered the EMG_{FT}).

developed to identify the EMG_{FT} for back muscle was accomplished by Cardozo & Gonçalves (2003). Based on the protocol proposed by DeVries *et al.* (1982), they developed a specific protocol for the determination of the EMG_{FT}, particularly for the erector spinae muscles and observed that the attainment of this index is possible for low back muscles.

But, these protocols were performed by means of the signal amplitude, but the changes on the RMS values as the fatigue process develops are related to mechanical-physiological alterations in the muscle with the increase on the fire rate and the recruitment of new motor units (Gonçalves, 1998). Also, to the determination of the EMG_{FT} it is necessary a linear positive behavior of the RMS values in function of time. In studies involving fatiguing tests for back muscle not always it is observed this kind of behavior. Several studies have found linear negative behavior of the RMS with the fatigue process development (Cardozo & Gonçalves, 2003), and others have found non-linear behavior of the RMS in function of time (Clark et al., 2003), what would make impossible the EMG_{FT} identification by this parameter. However, the changes on the MF values are related to physiological changes as the wave shape of the action potential of motor units affected by alterations on the conduction velocity of muscular fibers.

With this in mind Hendrix et al. (2009) found that the EMG_{FT} can also be obtained by spectral parameters of the EMG signal, using an adopted protocol based on DeVries work (Figure 4).

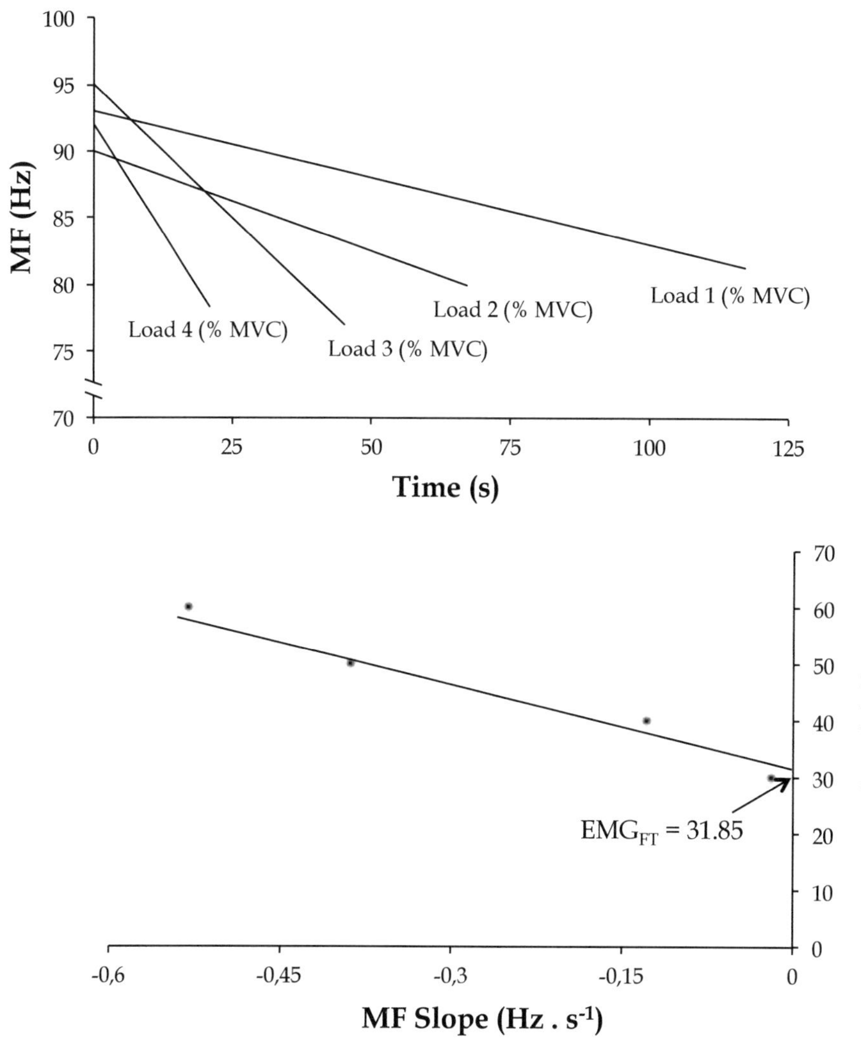

Fig. 4. Determination of the Electromyographic Fatigue Threshold (EMG_{FT}) by Hendrix et al. (2009) protocol.

Even the EMG_{FT} has been wide used over years, its usefulness is still discussed. Recently Bouillard et al. (2011) found an inability to detect an EMG_{FT} by means the RMS values in

most of the subjects. To achieve this threshold the author established three criteria: (i) significant positive linear regression between load and slope, (ii) a coefficient of determination greater than 0.85, and (iii) a standard error for the EMG_{FT} below 5% of MVC. Their results show the possibility to determine the EMG_{FT} in only nine of the 37 subjects by means the RMS values. The EMG_{FT} by means the MF values allowed the determination of 27 out of the 37 subjects, but with a weak reproducibility, concluding that the EMG_{FT} is not a valid tool to assess muscle function.
So, more studies must be performed to understand the significance of this parameter and its application to access low back muscle by means surface EMG.

5. EMG in assessing low back pain

LBP causes an socio-economic impact promoting many day lost in work. It is a multifaceted problem and because of this nature the extend contribution in causation of the problems is not ascertainable. Most are the factors that has relation with de LBP: history of back pain, psychological and work related factors, heavy physical work, prolonged sitting, lifting, trunk rotation, pushing/pulling, vibrations and factors genetic, muscle strength, physical fitness and one of the most important related to musculoskeletal disorders is the fatigue due the repetition of movement or intensity of work.
In order to create a methodology that could be used to evaluate isometric resistance of low back muscles, as well as to analyze disorders of the lumbar spine, Biering-Sorensen (1984) proposed a test called "Sorensen Test."
In this test the subjects are positioned prone on a test table where the legs are fixed by belts and the arms are folded across the chest touching the contralateral shoulder. In this position, subjects were instructed to keep the trunk in a horizontal position and parallel to the ground by means of isometric contractions held until exhaustion (Figure 5).

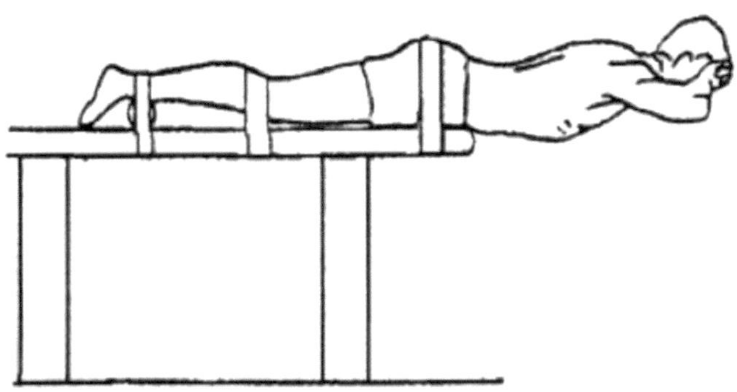

Fig. 5. Sorensen Test.

The isometric endurance time (IRT), defined as the time to maintain the proposed approach to exhaustion, was recorded. The results showed that men with a history of LBP, but without the presence of this symptom at the time of testing, had an IRT average of 176 seconds, while men without the presence of LBP at the time of the test and no history of this symptom had an IRT average of 198 seconds.
This test is considered safe for both healthy people and for people with LBP (Alaranta et al., 1995, Biering-Sorensen, 1984, Moffroid, 1997, Peltonen et al., 1998), whereas perform maximal contractions may not be safe for this second group (Moffroid et al., 1993).

Luoto et al. (1995) also showed that subjects with IRT less than 58 seconds are three times more likely to develop LBP after one year follow-up than men with IRT greater than 104.
Other studies using the approach proposed by Biering-Sorensen (1984) (Kankaanpää et al., 1998, Mannion & Dolan, 1994, Sparto et al. 1997) or by deploying the test relation to the original form of execution (Seidel et al., 1987), were able to produce similar results. From these results, researchers began to suggest that fatigue of low back muscles might represent a risk factor for the development of LBP.
However, the analysis only the IRT is a procedure that is highly dependent on the subjects' motivation for its validity (Mannion & Dolan, 1994), because it requires a certain level of strength to maintain the exercise for as long as possible. For this reason, EMG analysis of certain parameters, such as the decline in MF and MPF, and their initial values, which cannot be voluntarily controlled by subjects, have been used to assess the isometric strength of low back muscles.
The observation of the MF behavior may yet have clinical applications as those reported in the study of Ng & Richardson (1996) and Roy et al. (1995), who performed an EMG spectral analysis of the back muscles in patients with LBP during the rehabilitation, where the results were analyzed in order to determine if the EMG procedures are capable of: (i) distinguishing patients with LBP from normal individuals; (ii) to control changes on the muscular function after rehabilitation from lumbar lesion. One concluded that the procedures adopted allowed distinguishing patients with LBP from healthy individuals and those subjects presented decreased fatigability after rehabilitation, according to the EMG spectral analysis. Therefore, this procedure may be useful in the LBP rehabilitation process.
Furthermore, when comparing EMG parameters with spinal mobility and trunk strength from athletes with LBP, Klein et al. (1991) found that the recovery of the EMG is better than the others parameters, showing its usefulness to evaluate training and rehabilitation programs.
Some authors have found that the greater is the load the lower is the spectral value (Dedering et al. 2002; Mannion & Dolan, 1996). These authors explain this behavior by the fact that to sustain high loads it is necessary to the recruitment of type II muscle fibers, which in the lumbar muscles, unlike appendicular muscles, have a smaller diameter than type I fibers (Mannion & Dolan, 1996; Roy et al., 1989). With this smaller diameter fiber that has a lower conduction velocity, thus contributing to the reduction in MF values when increasing the initial charge level. Therefore this variable can even identify the muscle fiber composition (Biedermann et al., 1991).
Also, higher initial value for MF is related to higher concentration of type I fibers and lower values are associated with higher concentrations of type II fibers. People with LBP may develop atrophy of type II fibers in the muscles of the spine and consequently have a higher concentration of type I fibers.
So, EMG parameters seems to be related to muscle composition and might be useful to measure muscle ability in a noninvasively way.

6. Low back muscle EMG during manual load lifting

The act of load lifting is included in many movements that we do during the day and we perform many times automatically and unconscious of necessaries mechanisms to lift this load or to maintain it.

This continued load lifting has brought one important percentage of all LBP result from bad mechanics and postural habits and the majority of LBP is localized at level L4/L5 and L5/S1. This fact can be justified because the occupational activities are designed to meet occupational demands and not to optimize biological compatibility (Kumar, et al., 2001).

Chaffin & Anderson (1984) claim that NIOSH (The National Institute for Occupational Safety and Health) found that rates of muscle-skeletal injuries, even though the number of injuries per hour/men in the work and rate of severity, and the numbers of hours lost due to injuries per hour/men at work increased when: heavy and dense objects were lifted from the ground, with high rates of lifting, position of load relationship with the body and duration of activity. These can promote a significant increase of injuries risk and fatigue for some people if they aren't carefully trained for the tasks of lifting.

The load lifting causes a great lost time in industrial injuries and high stress in the muscle skeletal system (Frievalds et al., 1984). Many of industrial accidents cause injuries in the lumbar column. The LBP has been the most common cause of work absenteeism and also a significant factor in functional disability and is the most common cause of activity limitation among people in many countries, having a general agreement that mechanical stresses to spine is related to the development of degenerative disc disease and this problem is significant yet.

During the manual load lifting many variables interfere in this action and can influence in its efficiency such as: (i) joint posture before and after the load lift (Kumar & Garand, 1992); (ii) the magnitude of the mechanical load (Chaffin & Park, 1973); (iii) the type of contractions used where dynamic strengths are significantly lower than isometric strengths (Kumar & Garand, 1992); and (iv) the maximal capability of any individual varies with posture (Kumar & Garand, 1992).

An important factor that interferes in an EMG activity during load lift is the velocity of execution and a significant difference between static and dynamic strength has been also reported by MacGill & Norman (1985) and Kumar (1994).

The muscle activity during the load lifting has been correlated between posture of trunk (Kumar et al., 1996), distance of load of body (Cook & Neumann, 1987), the velocity of lifting (Winters & Woo, 1990), different plans (Seroussi & Pope, 1987), high of handles (Andersson et al., 1975), and the initial position of load (Gracovetsky, 1988),

Studies about accessories to help the load lifting and to protect the worker have been interests particularly about the use of pelvic belt. The experience in the use of this accessory associate at kind of breath can modify the activity of rectus abdominis, obliquos extern abdominis and erectors spinae during load lifting (Udo & Yoshinaga, 1997) as well as increasing the intra-abdominal pressure (Lander et al., 1992). In sports as the squat, when a belt is used, the movements were faster than without the use of it, however, the EMG activity of the erector spinae and obliquos externus muscles decrease with the use of the belt.

Many occupational activities have been realized repetitively and employ many muscles. Asymmetric motions are very frequently and muscles can also be differently loaded promoting differences amounts of fatigue and the rate with which they fatigue may also be different (Kumar et al., 2001).

Several researchers have attempted to develop testing protocols that allow for the evaluation of muscle behavior in this extremely demanding activity.

The literature contains several proposals for test protocols, some of which include the use of manual load lifting accessories such as pelvic belts, which have been found to reduce EMG activity but to interfere little in the development of the fatigue process (Gauglitz et al., 2003).

7. Conclusion

This chapter presented the basic concepts of surface EMG techniques and its application to the assessment of low back muscle. It was shown that the surface EMG has a good reliability in its parameters, and is a good tool to access muscle fatigue. We can also note that it is possible to obtain an index to verify the fatigue state, by means the EMG_{FT}, as well to identify LPB noninvasively.

8. Acknowledgment

The authors would like to thank the Biomechanics Laboratory of the Department of Physical Education-IB (São Paulo State University).

9. References

Alaranta H, Luoto S, Heliövaara M & Hurri H. Static back endurance and the risk of low-back pain. *Clin Biomech* 1995; 10(6): 323-324.

Andersson BJG, Herberts P & Örtengren R. (1975). Myoelectric back muscle activity in standardized lifting postures, In: *Biomechanics,* Paavo Komi (Ed.), Baltimore, University Park Press.

Biedermann, H. J. et al. Power spectrum analyses of electromyographic activity: Discriminators in the differential assessment of patients with chronic low back pain. *Spine* 1991: 16(10): 1179-84.

Biering-Sorensen F. Physical measurements as risk indicators for low back pain trouble over a one-year period. *Spine* 1984; 9(2): 106-19.

Bouillard K, Guével A & Hug F. The electromyographic fatigue threshold is not a valid tool to assess muscle function. *J Electromyogr Kinesiol* 2011; 21: 229-3.5

Cardozo AC, Gonçalves M & Dolan P. Back extensor muscle fatigue at submaximal workloads assessed using frequency banding of the electromyographic signal. *Clin Biomech* 2011; 20. [Epub ahead of print]

Cardozo AC & Gonçalves M. Effect of load level on the EMG spectra of longissimus thoracis muscle during isometric fatiguing contractions. *Electromyogr Clin Neurophysiol.* 2010; 50(2): 75-85.

Cardozo AC & Gonçalves M. Electromyographic fatigue threshold of erector spinae muscle induced by muscular endurance test in health men. *Electromyogr Clin Neurophysiol* 2003; 43: 377--80.

Carpenter DM & Nelson BW. Low back strengthening for the prevention and treatment of low back pain. *Med Sci Sports Exerc* 1999; 31(1): 18-24.

Chaffin DB, Park KS. A longitudinal study of low-back pain as associated with occupational weight lifting factors. *Am Ind Hyg Assoc J* 1973; 34(12): 513-25.

Chaffin DB & Andersson GBJ (1984). *Ocupational Biomechanics.* John Wiley e Sons, New York.

Clark BC, Manini TM & Ploutz-Snyder LL. Derecruitment of the lumbar musculature with fatiguing trunk extension exercise. *Spine* 2003; 28: 282--287.

Coleman JL, Straker LM, Campbell A, Izumi H & Smith A. Biering-Sorensen test performance of Japanese young males: comparison with other ethnicities and relationship to electromyography, near-infrared spectroscopy and exertion ratings. *Ergonomics* 2011; 54(7): 636-55.

Cook TM & Neumann DA. The effects of load placement on the EMG activity of the low back muscles during load carrying by men and women. *Ergonomics* 1987; 30(10): 1413-23.

Danneels LA, Coorevits PL, Cools AM, Vanderstraeten GG, Cambier DC, Witvrouw EE & De CH. Differences in electromyographic activity in the multifidus muscle and the iliocostalis lumborum between healthy subjects and patients with sub-acute and chronic low back pain. *Eur Spine J* 2002; 11(1): 13–9.

Dedering A. et al. Electromyography and ratings of lumbar muscle fatigue using a four-level staircase protocol. *Clin Biomech* 2002; 17(3): 171-6.

Dedering A, Roos af Hjelmsäter M, Elfving B, Harms-Ringdahl K & Németh G. Between-days reliability of subjective and objective assessments of back extensor muscle fatigue in subjects without lower-back pain. *J Electromyogr Kinesiol* 2000; 10(3): 151-8.

DeLuca CJ. The use of surface electromyography in biomechanics. *J Appl Biomech* 1997; 13: 135-63.

deVries HA, Moritani T, Nagata A & Magnussen K. The relation between critical power and neuromuscular fatigue as estimative from electromyographic data. *Ergonomics* 1982 25: 783-91.

deVries HA, Tichy MW, Housh TJ, Smyth KD, Tichy AM & Housh DJ. A method for estimating physical working capacity at the fatigue threshold (PWCFT). *Ergonomics* 1987; 30(8): 1195-204.

Dolan P, Mannion, AF & Adams MA. Fatigue of the erector spinae muscles. A quantitative assessment using "frequency banding" of the surface electromyography signal. *J Biomech* 1995; 20(2): 149-59.

Elfving B, Ne´meth G, Arvidsson I & Lamontagne M. Reliability of EMG spectral parameters in repeated measurements of back muscle fatigue. *J Electromyogr Kinesiol* 1999; 9: 235–43.

Elfving B, Dedering A & Nemeth G. Lumbar muscle fatigue and recovery in patients with long-term low-back trouble--electromyography and health-related factors. *Clin Biomech* 2003; 18(7): 619-30.

Fleiss, J.L. (1986). *The design and analysis of clinical experiments.* John Wiley and Sons. United States.

Gauglitz ACF, Gonçalves M, Cardozo AC, Malagodi BM & Silva SRD. Análise eletromiográfica do levantamento de carga durante o movimento repetitivo com e sem o uso do cinto pélvico. *Rev IMES Bras Ciên Saú* 2003, 1: 28-32.

Gonçalves M. Variáveis biomecânicas analisadas durante o levantamento manual de carga. *Motriz* 1998; 4: 85-8.

Gracovetsky S, Farfan HF & Lamy C. The mechanism of the lumbar spine. *Spine* 1988; 6: 249-62.

Graef JL, Smith AE, Kendall KL, Walter AA, Moon JR, Lockwood CM, Beck TW, Cramer JT & Stout JR. The relationships among endurance performance measures as estimated from VO2PEAK, ventilatory threshold, and electromyographic fatigue threshold: a relationship design. *Dyn Med* 2008; 10: 7-15.

Haldeman S. Low back pain: current physiologic concepts. *Neur Clin,* 1999;17(1):1-15.

Hendrix CR, Housh TJ, Johnson GO, Mielke M, Camic CL & J.M. Zuniga JM *et al.* A new EMG frequency-based fatigue threshold test, *J Neurosci Methods* 2009; 181: 45–51.

Hermann KM, Barnes WS. Effects of eccentric exercise on trunk extensor torque and lumbar paraspinal EMG. *Med Sci Sports Exerc* 2001; 33(6): 971–7.

Housh TJ, deVries HA, Johnson GO, Housh DJ, Evans SA, Stout JR, Evetovich TK & Bradway RM. Electromyographic fatigue thresholds of the superficial muscles of the quadriceps femoris. *Eur J Appl Physiol Occup Physiol* 1995; 71(2-3): 131-6.

Kankaanpãã, M. et al. Back and hip extensor fatigability in chronic low back pain patients and controls. *Arch Phys Med Rehabil* 1998; 79(4): 412-7.

Keating J & Matyas T. Unreliable inferences from reliable measurements. *Aust J Physiother* 1998; 44(1): 5-10.

Kendall KL, Smith AE, Graef JL, Walter AA, Moon JR, Lockwood CM, Beck TW, Cramer JT & Stout JR. Validity of electromyographic fatigue threshold as a noninvasive method for tracking changes in ventilatory threshold in college-aged men. *J Strength Cond Res* 2010; 24(1): 109-13.

Klein, A. B. et al. Comparison of spinal mobility and isometric trunk extensor forces with electromyographic spectral analysis in identifying low back pain. *Phys Ther* 1991; 71(6): 445-54.

Knutson LM, Soderberg GL, Ballantyne BT & Clarke WR. A study of various normalization procedures for within day electromyographic data. *J Electromyogr Kinesiol* 1994; 4(1): 47-59.

Komi PV & Buskirk ER. Reproducibility of electromyographic measurements with inserted wire electrodes and surface electrodes. *Electromyography* 1970; 10(4): 357-67.

Kumar S & Garand D. Static and dynamic lifting strength at different reach distances in symmetrical and asymmetrical planes. *Ergonomics* 1992; 35(7-8): 861-80.

Kumar S, Narayan Y & Zedka M. An eletromyographic study of unresisted trunk rotation with normal velocity among healthy subjects. *Spine* 1996; 21(13): 1500-12.

Kumar S, Narayan Y & Zedka M. Trunk strength in combine motions of rotation and flexion extension in normal adults. *Ergonomics* 1998; 41(6): 835-52.

Kumar S, Narayan Y, Stein RB & Snijders C. Muscle fatigue in axial rotation of the trunk. *Int J Ind Erg* 2001; 28: 113-25.

Kumar S. The epidemiology and functional evaluation of low back pain: a literature review. *Eur J Phys Med and Rehab* 1994; 4: 15-27.

Lander EJ, Hundley JR & Simonton RL. The effectiveness of weight-belts during multiple repetitions of the squat exercise. *Med Sci Sports Exercise* 1992; 24: 603-9.

Luoto S, Heliövaara M, Hurri H. et al. Static back endurance and the risk of low-back pain. *Clin Biomech* 1995; 10: 323-4.

Manion AF & Dolan P. The effects of muscle length and force output on the EMG power spectrum of the erector spinae. *J Electromyogr Kinesiol* 1996; 6(3): 159-68.

Mannion AF & Dolan P. Electromyographic median frequency changes during isometric contraction of the back extensors to fatigue. *Spine* 1994; 19: 1223-9.

Matsumoto T, Ito K & Moritani T. The relationship between anaerobic threshold and electromyographic fatigue threshold in colleague women. *Eur J Appl Physiol* 1991; 63: 1-5.

McGill SM & Norman RW. Dynamically and statically determined low back moments during lifting. *J Biomech* 1985; 18(12): 877-85.

Moffroid MT, Haugh LD, Haig AJ, Henry SM & Pope MH. Endurance training of trunk extensor muscles. *Phys Ther* 1993; 73(1): 10-7.

Moffroid MT. Endurance of trunk muscles in persons with chronic low back pain: assessment, performance, training. *J Rehabil Res Dev* 1997; 34(4): 440-7.

Moritani T, Takaishi T & Matsumoto T. Determination of maximal power output at neuromuscular fatigue threshold. *J Appl Physiol* 1993; 74(4): 1729-34.

Morlock MM et al. Trunk muscle fatigue and associated EMG changes during a dynamic iso-inertial test. *Eur J A O Physiol* 1997; 76(1):75-80.

Ng JK & Richardson CA. Reliability of electromyographic power spectral analysis of back muscle endurance in healthy subjects. *Arch Phys Med Rehabil* 1996; 77(3): 259-64.

Ng JK, Richardson CA & Jull GA. Electromyographic amplitude and frequency changes in the iliocostalis lumborum and multifidus muscles during a trunk holding test. *Phys Ther* 1997; 77(9): 954-61.

Oliveira AS, Cardozo AC, Barbosa FS & Gonçalves M. Electromyographic fatigue threshold of the biceps brachii: the effect of endurance time. *Electromyogr Clin Neurophysiol* 2007; 47(1): 37-42.

Pavlat DJ, Housh TJ, Johnson GO & Eckerson JM. Electromyographic responses at the neuromuscular fatigue threshold. *J Sports Med Phys Fitness* 1995; 35: 31--37.

Pavlat DJ, Housh TJ, Johnson GO, Schmidt RJ & Eckerson JM. An examination of the electromyographic fatigue threshold test. *Eur J Appl Physiol Occup Physiol* 1993; 67(4): 305-8.

Peach JP, Gunning J & McGill SM. Reliability of spectral EMG parameters of healthy back extensors during submaximum isometric fatiguing contractions and recovery. *J Electromyogr Kinesiol* 1998; 8: 403–10.

Peltonen JE, Taimela S, Erkintalo M, Salminen JJ, Oksanen A & Kujala UM. Back extensor and psoas muscle cross-sectional area, prior physical training, and trunk muscle strength--a longitudinal study in adolescent girls. *Eur J Appl Physiol Occup Physiol* 1998; 77(1-2): 66-71.

Roy SH et al. Spectral electromyographic assessment of back muscles in patients with low back pain undergoing rehabilitation. *Spine* 1995; 20(1): 38-48.

Roy SH, DeLuca C & Casavant D. Lumbar muscle fatigue and chronic low back pain. *Spine* 1989; 14(9): 992-1001.

Seidel H, Beyer H & Brauer D. Electromyographic evaluation of back muscle fatigue with repeated sustained contractions of different strengths, *Eur J A Physiol* 1987; 56(5): 592-602.

Seroussi RE & Pope MH. The relationship between trunk muscle electromyography and lifting moments in the sagittal and frontal planes. *J Biomech* 1987; 20(2): 135-46.

Smith AE, Walter AA, Herda TJ, Ryan ED, Moon JR, Cramer JT & Stout JR. Effects of creatine loading on electromyographic fatigue threshold during cycle ergometry in college-aged women. *J Int Soc Sports Nutr* 2007; 26: 4-20.

Sparto PJ et al. Spectral and temporal responses of trunk extensor electromyography to an isometric endurance test. *Spine* 1997; 22(4): 418-26.

Spector B. Surface electromyography as a model for the development of standardized procedures and reliability testing. *JMPT* 1979; 2(4): 214.

Tesch PA, Komi PV, Jacobs I, Karlsson J & Viitasalo JT. Influence of lactate accumulation of EMG frequency spectrum during repeated concentric contractions. *Acta Physiol Scand* 1983; 119(1): 61-7.

Udo H & Yoshinaga F. Effect of a pelvic belt on abdominal pressure by various weights and bending angles. *Ind Health* 1997; 35(2): 229-34.

van Dieën, J.H. et al. Trunk extensor endurance and its relationship to electromyogram parameters. *Eur J Appl Physiol Occup Physiol* 1993; 66(5) 388-96.

van Dieën JH & Heijblom P. Reproducibility of isometric trunk extension torque, trunk extensor endurance, and related electromyographic parameters in the context of their clinical applicability. *J Orthop Res* 1996; 14(1): 139-43.

Viitasalo JT, Luhtanen P, Rahkila P & Rusko H. Electromyographic activity related to aerobic and anaerobic threshold in ergometer bicycling. *Acta Physiol Scand* 1985; 124: 287--293.

Winters JM & Woo SL-Y. Eds. (1990). *Multiple Muscle Systems. Biomechanics and Movement Organization*. Springer-Verlag.

11

EMG Analysis of a Pilates Exercise

Jefferson Fagundes Loss[1], Mônica de Oliveira Melo[2],
Débora Cantergi[1], Yumie Okuyama da Silva[1],
Artur Bonezi[1] and Aline Nogueira Haas[1]
[1]*Universidade Federal do Rio Grande do Sul*
[2]*Universidade de Caxias do Sul*
Brazil

1. Introduction

The Pilates method was originally developed by Joseph Pilates in Germany during the First World War and introduced in the United States in 1923 (Latey, 2001; Muscolino & Cipriani, 2004; Rydeard et al., 2006). The method assembles movements from gymnastics, martial arts, yoga and dance with philosophic ideas (Self et al., 1996; Latey, 2001; Rydeard et al., 2006). After the 1980's, new elements were incorporated aiming to improve both physical conditioning and rehabilitation programs. When considering physical conditioning increases in joint flexibility, muscle strength, balance and whole body conditioning were observed in Pilates' practitioners (Bertolla F, 2007; Jago et al., 2006; Segal et al., 2004). For rehabilitation, Pilates exercises have been used for joint function restoration, lumbar-pelvic stabilization, fibromyalgia control and low back pain treatment (Blum, 2002; Kolyniak et al., 2004; Donzelli et al., 2006).

In order to achieve the program goals, the health professionals can choose between mat or apparatus exercises. The apparatus, such as the reformer or the Cadillac, were designed specifically for the Pilates method. These apparatus uses springs in order to generate external load for the musculoskeletal structure. In general, each spring presents a different elastic constant and has more than one attachment possibility in the different apparatus, reflecting in the external load (Self et al., 1996; Rydeard et al., 2006). Regardless of the objectives, it is recommended that the training program uses exercises with progressive external load, according to each individual's needs. However, what have been observed is that the determination of external load in Pilates' exercises is based on subjective information, such as changing a less resistance for a higher resistance spring, without realizing how high is the difference in each situation. When this is follower, intensity is only determined based on patient's feedback and the instructor's experience (Blum, 2002), what may affect negatively the Pilates training program success.

Attentive to this situation, the Mechanics of Movement Investigation Group (*BIOMEC - Grupo de Investigação em Mecânica do Movimento*) has been using biomechanical analysis of human movement, in order to identify the resistance moments curve shape in a quantitative analysis of Pilates exercises (Silva et al., 2009; Loss et al., 2010; Melo et al., 2011). Thus, besides using load cells for measuring spring's strength (Self et al., 1996), resistance moment may be estimated in different subjects positioning and spring setups (Silva et al., 2009).

Using this kind of analysis it is possible, for example, to identify the angles where external load is maximum or internal moment is higher, what may help developing a workout with specific objectives. Although direct measurement of spring force or resistance moment analysis provides quantitative data of Pilates exercise intensity, this kind of analysis does not allow evaluating muscle activation levels during exercise.

Identifying and learning the possible changes in muscle activation arising from variations of the same exercise (such as in spring setup) can help health professionals determining, more objectively, the exercises for a Pilates training program. This way it is possible, for example, to avoid using spring adjustments or exercise positions that activate undesirable muscles during an injury recovery period, or even selecting exercises conditions that privileges the activation of specific muscle groups, according to the program's objective.

For this reason, it is believed that evaluating muscle response for imposed loads during an exercise using surface electromyography (EMG) may subsidize in an important way Pilates exercise prescription (Silva et al., 2009; Loss et al., 2010; Queiroz et al., 2010). Among several possibilities, analysis may compare different situations in the same exercise, such as changes in spring setup or in the practitioner's position. In the context that scientific studies that investigated electric activation during Pilates exercises is extremely limited, the BIOMEC group decided to analyse one of the exercises commonly used for strengthening the muscles associated to the powerhouse, performed on the Cadillac. In general this exercise may be characterized as a hip flexion-extension exercise performed in supine position with the possibility of varying subject's horizontal position (moving the subject closer or further to the apparatus edge), the spring used (the elastic constant used) and the spring's setup (the spring's vertical attachment point on the equipment, or its fixation height). Furthermore, depending of the Pilates method system followed the same exercise may be performed in different speeds. Each one of these variations may lead to different mechanical overloads on the active muscles during movement and, consequently, different patterns of muscle electrical activity (Silva et al., 2009).

Considering the importance of scientific information that may subsidize Pilates exercise prescription, this chapter will unite information from three studies on muscular activation during hip flexion-extension exercise performed in the Cadillac, including two studies already published about the use of agonist/antagonist muscle groups and trunk stabilizer muscles during the exercise. Thus, the first study aimed to compare the electrical activation of the Rectus Femoris (RF), long head of the Biceps Femoris (BF) and Semitendinosus (ST) with two spring adjustments. The second study aimed to compare the electrical activation of the Multifidus (MU) and the External Oblique (OE) adjusting spring setup and subject position. And the third study aimed to compare the electrical activation of the Multifidus (MU), the External Oblique (OE), the gluteus maximum (GM) and the Rectus Femoris (RF) performed with three different speeds.

2. General procedures

Each study sample was composed by 8 to 12 female subjects, that trained Pilates at least twice a week for a minimum of six months. The hip flexion-extension movement evaluated started at 90° of hip flexion with the subjects extending the hip until 0° of hip flexion, with two springs attached to the executioners feet and fixed to the Cadillac.

All studies collected electromyography and kinematic data. Electromyography signal was collected using a Miotool 400 (*Miotec Equipamentos Biomédicos Ltda*) equipment. Sample rate

was 2000 Hz for each muscle, and all procedures recommended by the International Society of Electrophysiology and Kinesiology were strictly followed, such as shaving, sanitizing with alcohol electrode positioning and impedance verification (accepted when lower then 10KΩ). Pairs of disposable surface electrodes were used (Kendall, Meditrace - 100; Ag/AgCl; self-adhesive 22 mm diameter, in bipolar configuration) for each muscle, following the placing location from the SENIAM project, unless otherwise informed. Electrodes were positioned over the muscle belly, parallel to the muscle fibres, separated in 2 cm from each other.
Besides the data from the hip flexion-extension exercise, signal from maximum isometric voluntary contractions (MVC) were collected in specific positions for each muscle of interest. All tests were repeated twice with 5 minutes intervals between each repetition. Electromyography signal was processed using a third order Butterworth digital filter in band pass configuration, with cut frequencies between 20 and 500 Hz. Root mean square (RMS) values from each MVC signal was calculated with a 2000 points moving-window. The highest value obtained for each muscle was used for normalization.
Kinematics used either video analysis or electronic goniometer in order to identify hip joint angle dividing the gesture in extension and flexion phases. For each set of data RMS value was calculated and normalized by the RMS value from the respective muscle MVC.

3. Study 1 – Movement agonist and antagonist muscle evaluation

Twelve subjects took part in this study. Rectos Femoris, Biceps Femoris (long head) and Semitendinosus muscles were evaluated. Rectos Femoris electrodes were positioned in the middle of a line going from anterior superior iliac spine and the patella superior part; Biceps Femoris electrodes were positioned in the middle of the line going from the ischial tuberosity and the lateral epicondyle; and Semitendinosus electrodes were positioned in the middle of the line between ischial tuberosity and medial epicondyle. Reference electrode was positioned in the right knee over the Fibula's styloideus process. Maximum isometric voluntary contraction was collected for the Rectos Femoris with the subject in supine lying position with the trunk kept still while they were instructed to try flexing the hip against manual resistance in the ankle. For Biceps Femoris and Semitendinosus subjects were in probe lying position, with the superior part of the trunk kept still in a gurney and the legs hanging with a 90° hip flexion, while they were instructed to extend the hip against manual resistance in the ankle.
The hip joint angular positions were registered during the evaluation protocol by means of an electronic goniometer (*Miotec Equipamentos Biomédicos Ltda, Porto Alegre, Brazil*). Each subject performed 2 series of 5 repetitions each of the hip flexion-extension movement using two different spring setups: i) higher position (90 cm higher than the subjects level) e ii) lower position (20 cm higher than the subjects level), as is shown in Figure 1. An interval of 1 minute was kept between positions. The spring used had been previously calibrated, and had an elastic constant of 0.013 kg/cm.
For analysis, the hip extension phase was divided in two parts: from 90° of flexion to approximately 45° of flexion and from 45° of flexion to full extension. Multiple one way ANOVA were used to verify differences in each muscle's electric activation in the following comparisons:

1. between higher and lower spring setup during the whole hip extension;
2. between higher and lower spring setup in the first half of the hip extension;
3. between higher and lower spring setup in the second half of the hip extension;
4. between first and second half of the hip extension using the higher spring setup;
5. between first and second half of the hip extension using the lower spring setup.

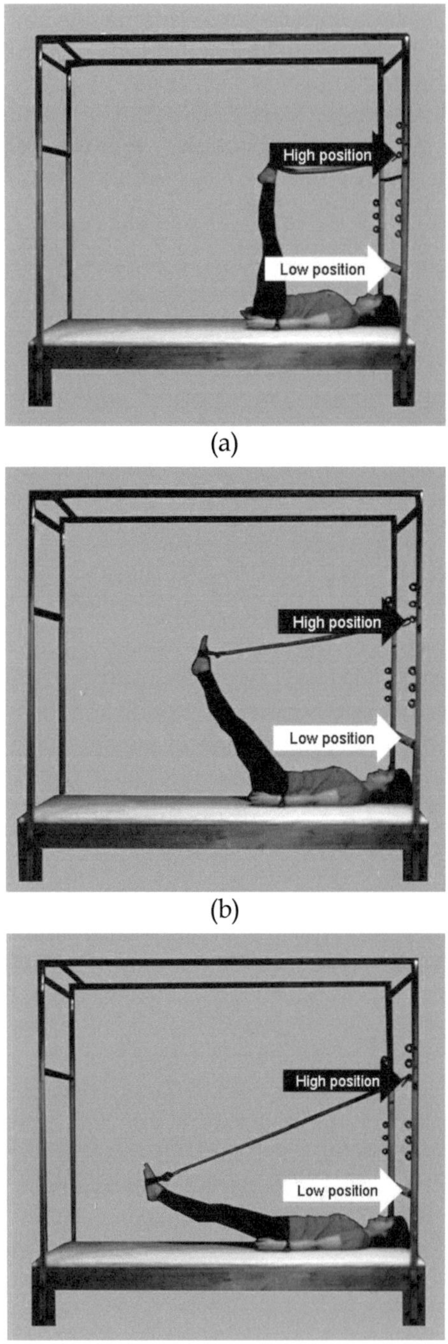

(a)

(b)

(c)

Fig. 1. Hip extension position on the Cadillac: a) near to initial position, b) intermediate position, c) near to final position. The black arrow indicates the higher spring setup and the white arrow indicates the lower spring setup. Extracted from the Brazilian Journal of Physiotherapy with permission.

Figures 2 and 3 show a typical EMG response obtained during one hip extension in only one subject. Each point in the graphic represents the RMS value of 40 consecutive points normalized by the respective muscle MVC value. It may be observed that EMG presented higher activation percentages for Biceps Femoris and Semitendinosus when compared to Rectos Femoris in the higher spring setup (Figure 2) and higher Semitendinosus values when compared to Biceps Femoris and Rectos Femoris in the lower spring setup (Figure 3). Comparing first and second halves of the hip extension subjectively in Figure 2, it may be assumed that activation is crescent and is higher during the second half, while in Figure 3 it may be assumed that Semitendinosus activation is higher than the activation of others muscles analysed, especially in the first half of the hip extension.

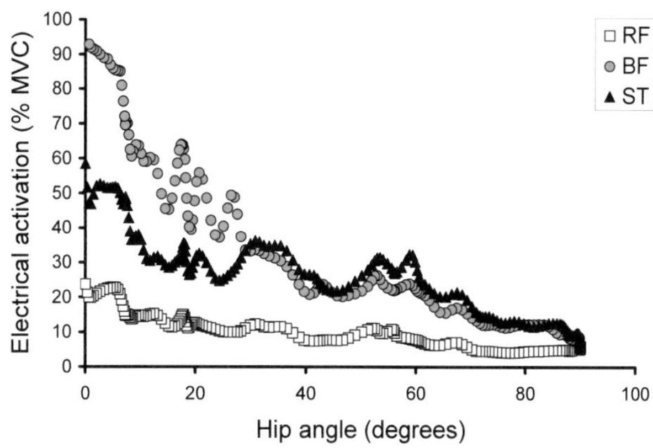

Fig. 2. Typical normalized EMG behaviour for one sample representative subject during hip extension performed on Cadillac with spring attached to the higher position.

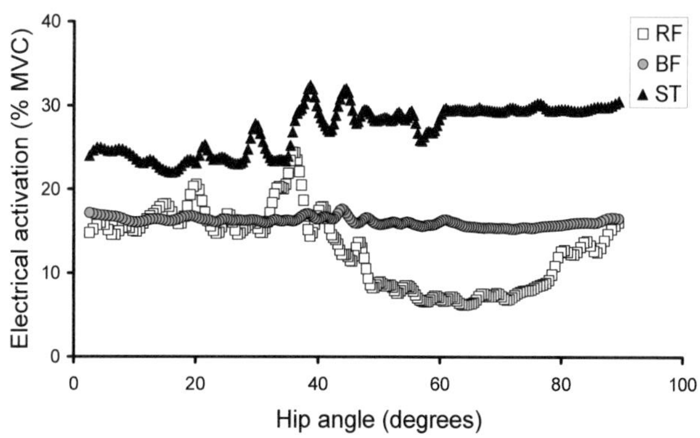

Fig. 3. Typical normalized EMG behaviour for one sample representative subject during hip extension performed on Cadillac with spring attached to the lower position.

The behaviour assumed in Figures 2 and 3 were confirmed by statistic analysis. Table 1 shows partial results of EMG divided between each half (HALF1 represents first half and HALF2 represents second half of the hip extension) of the muscles evaluated. This table show results of position comparison between positions, for the same half of the same muscle, are presented in the intermediate rows, while comparison of results between halves, for a same position of the same muscle, are presented in the last column.

Muscle	Spring setup	HALF1	HALF2	*p*
Rectos Femoris	Higher	10,8±3,8	15,2±9,4	0,038 *
	Lower	13,4±5,3	17,6±7,5	0,023 *
	p	0,015 *	0,295	
Biceps Femoris	Higher	47,5±19,4	115,1±61,7	0,003 *
	Lower	16,1±8,9	15,9±7,2	0,865
	p	0,000 *	0,000 *	
Semitendinosus	Higher	54,3±21,7	92,6±35.0	0,000 *
	Lower	28,3±15,1	20,7±4,7	0,088
	p	0,000 *	0,000 *	

Table 1. Each muscles EMG values expressed in MVC percentage, evaluated by half, separately: first half (HALF1) and second half (HALF2) of the hip extension. Intermediate lines *p* values refer to comparison between spring setup for the same half of each muscle. The last column *p* values refer to comparison between half, for the same spring setup of each muscle. * significant differences ($p<0.05$).

3.1 Practical applications

The findings in study one suggests that altering spring positions during hip extension exercise in the Cadillac as is usually prescribed in Pilates exercises, does not change only exercise intensity magnitude, but also interferes in the kineisological function that the muscles assume during exercise.

In summary, it may be observed that the agonist muscles of the hip extension movement, represented by the Bíceps Femoris and Semitendinosus muscles, were significantly more active when using the higher spring setup during the second half of the evaluated exercise. Considering that the external load in Cadillac is larger using the higher spring setup when compared to the lower spring setup (Melo et al., 2011; Silva et al., 2009), this results probably reflect the increase in motor unit recruitment due to the larger load acting on the muscle in the higher spring setup. This pattern of increased hip extensors activation was observed, mainly, in the movement's final angles; a region in which the progressive tension offered by the spring is larger than in the initial angles.

As expected, antagonist muscles in the hip extension movement, represented by Rectus Femoris muscle, presented lower values then the agonists, especially when the exercise was performed with the higher spring setup. However, co-activation values registered for Rectos Femoris show an important magnitude when compared to other studies reported in literature, even though, in this study, sample was composed by subjects with at least six months of Pilates practice. It is possible that unwanted pelvic anterior tilt occurred in extension or lowering phase due to insufficient activation of paravertebral muscles and also of trunk flexors. Because Rectos Femoris also acts on hip anterior tilt, it would justifie the activation levels observed in the present study. However, since pelvic movement was not controlled, this hypothesis could not be confirmed. Regardless, one aspect to be noted when the exercise is performed with the lower spring setup is that muscle activation pattern of the movement's agonist and antagonists that was observed is the opposite of that of the higher spring setup; in other words, as hip extension movement agonists electric activation decreases through the entire hip extension movement, antagonists

muscles present increases in electric activity values, including during the second half of the movement.
Previews studies showed (Melo et al., 2011; Silva et al., 2009) that when spring is positioned in the lower setup, inferior limb weight (thighs, lower legs and feet) may contribute more in resistance moment composition then the spring moment itself. When this occurs, an inversion in the direction of external moment happens, meaning that the moment occurring in the flexion direction and demanding from the extensor muscles may be happening in the opposite direction and demanding larger activation of the flexor muscles. This situation would explain the increase of Rectos Femoris activation, which will probably assume the function of movement agonist and contract eccentrically to keep the extension movement slow and controlled as it approached the 0° angle. Nevertheless, Biceps Femoris and Semitendinosus higher values during the movement's second half using the lower spring (as the legs approaches the horizontal) indicates that the hip extensor muscles have acted not only as co-activator, but have also helped in the pelvic neutral positions maintenance by avoiding hip anterior tilt in the attempt to keep the pelvic-lumbar region supported to the ground.
The different muscle recruitment strategies used by the central nervous system to perform hip extension movement in Pilates are a direct consequence of the external load behaviour that should *a priori* be chosen consistently by the health professional. By prescribing hip extension exercise with the higher spring setup, extensor muscles are demanded concentrically, with higher demands as the movement amplitude increases, while antagonistic muscle activation is expected to be above the levels of co-contraction due to the necessity of maintaining pelvic position. When opting for the same movement with the lower spring, hip flexor muscles may be demanded eccentrically as the movement agonists, meaning that there will be a higher contribution of passive components for the muscle force production. It is the Pilates professional that has the responsibility to choose the spring position that is more appropriate for one or another clinical objective. From this results it is considered a mistake prescribing hip flexion-extension exercise using the lower spring setup for a beginner followed by the higher spring setup as the training progresses, expecting that this change will only echoes in the intensity of the exercise, as the results presented here show that another changes will also occur influencing significantly the exercise.

4. Study 2 – Evaluation of trunk stabilizing musculature

Eight subjects took part in this study. Multifidus and External Oblique muscles were evaluated. Multifidus electrodes were positioned bilaterally in the level of the fifth lumbar vertebrae, aligned in parallel between the posterior-superior iliac spines and the first and second lumbar vertebrae interspine space. The External Oblique electrodes were positioned bilaterally in the middle of the line between the iliac crest and the most inferior point of the costal margin (same high as the third lumbar vertebrae), according to Ng (2002). Reference electrode was positioned over the seventh cervical vertebrae spinal process. Maximum isometric voluntary contractions were collected for the External Oblique with the subject positioned in a sitting position on a chair, leaning on the backrest, with the arms in the side of the body, holding himself in the chair's seat. They were instructed to flex and rotate the trunk to the left and then to the right, against a manual resistance imposed to the shoulders in the opposite direction (Arokoski et al., 1999). For Multifidus, subjects were positioned in prone lying, with tights and legs fixed, and were asked to perform trunk extension against manual resistance applied to the superior dorsal region (Arokoski et al., 1999).

The hip joint angular positions were registered by means of a webcam (25 frames/s). Each subject performed 4 series of 10 repetitions each of the hip flexion-extension movement combining two different spring setups: higher position (90 cm higher than the subjects level) and lower position (30 cm higher than the subjects level); and two different subject positions: near position (distant 10 cm from the apparatus edge) and distant position (distant 30 cm from the apparatus edge) (Figure 4) in random order. An interval of 2 minutes was kept between series. The two springs used had been previously calibrated, and had an elastic constant of 0.082 kg/cm. For standardization it was requested that subjects expire during extension and inspire during flexion.

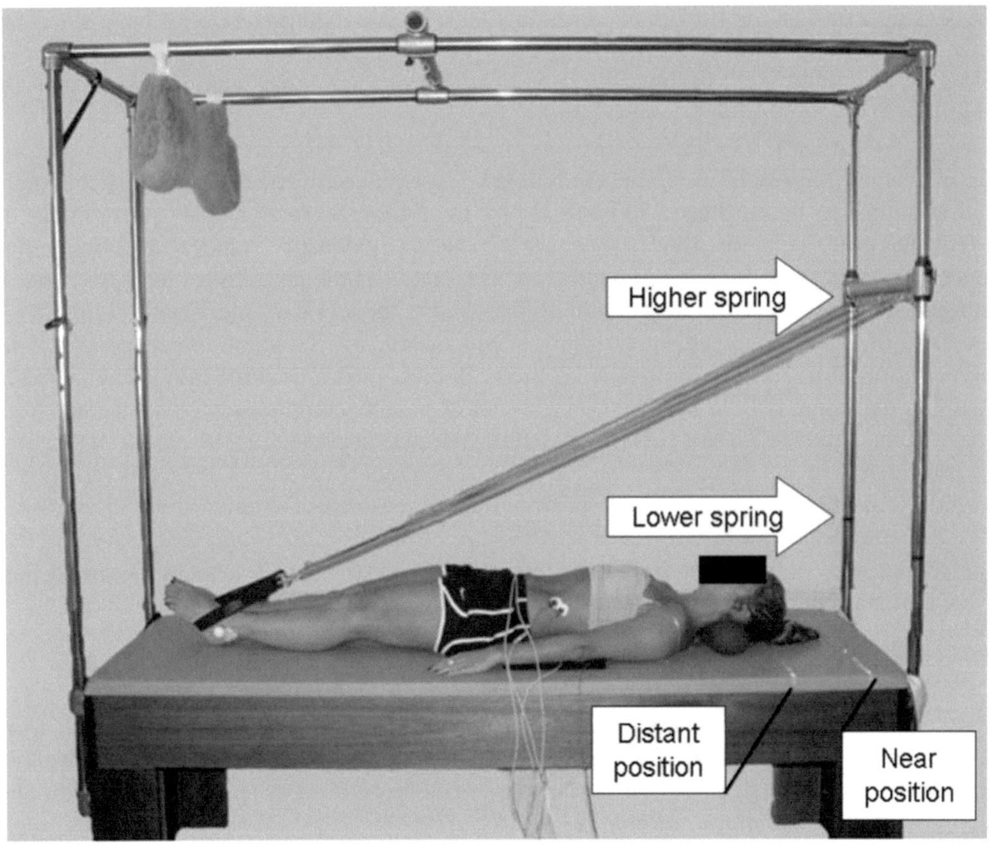

Fig. 4. Cadillac apparatus used in the study, showing different spring regulations and subjects positioning. Extracted from the Brazilian Journal of Physiotherapy with permission.

To verify electromyography differences between the distinct spring setup and subject position combinations, multiple comparisons were made using Wilcoxon test for each muscle and each phase separated. Significance level adopted for all tests was $p \leq 0.05$.

In Figures 5A and 5B is shown that during hip extension phase, right and left Multifidus presented significant differences in two situation: i) in the distant position when compared between higher and lower spring setup, and ii) in the higher spring setup, when compared between distant and near position. Figures 5C and 5D show that during the hip flexion phase significant differences occurred only in the right side of the trunk in the higher spring setup when compared distant and near positioning. Considering both phases, higher Multifidus electric activation was found in the combination higher spring setup and distant position. In figures 6A e 6B is shown that during hip extension phase significant differences occurred only in the right side of the trunk in the distant position when compared higher and lower spring setups, for the External Oblique muscle. Figures 6C and 6D show that during the hip flexion phase, right and left external oblique presented significant differences in two situation: (i) in the distant position when compared between higher and lower spring setups, and (ii) in the lower spring setup, when compared between distant and near subject positions. When both phases are considered, External Oblique electric activity was higher in the lower spring setup in the near position.

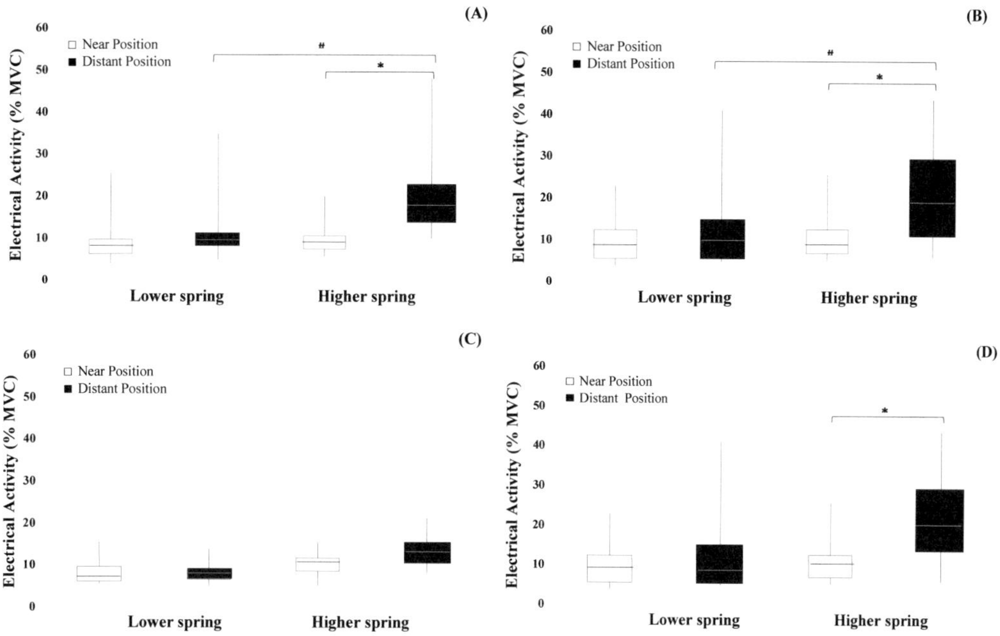

Fig. 5. Normalized electromyographyc activation maximum, minimum and median values of right and left muscle Multifidus on the evaluated spring positions and subjects positioning. (A) and (B) represent extension phase for left and right sides, respectively. (C) and (D) represent flexion phase for left and right sides, respectively. Extracted from Brazilian Journal of Physiotherapy with permission.

4.1 Practical applications

When investigating activation pattern of muscles recognized by the Pilates method as trunk stabilizers, important effects on electromyographical activation of selected muscles were found in the choice of spring setup and subjects positioning while performing hip flexion-extension exercise. Results show that during hip extension phase a 10% enhance in Multifidus activation appeared when spring setup was modified from lower to higher and subject was kept in the distant position. In the same situations, though significant difference was only found in the right side, External Oblique muscles presented an apparent decrease in the electric activation values. External Oblique are muscles responsible for maintaining the pelvic in the neutral position during hip extension performed in supine-lying (Calais-Germain & Lamotte, 2005). These results may indicate that a possible unwanted pelvic anterior tilt may have influenced the Multifidus muscles results. This hypothesis appears to be supported by previous studies that found higher Multifidus activation when pelvic posture changed from neutral to anterior tilt during the performance of a stabilizing Pilates exercise in the quadruped position (Queiroz et al., 2010).

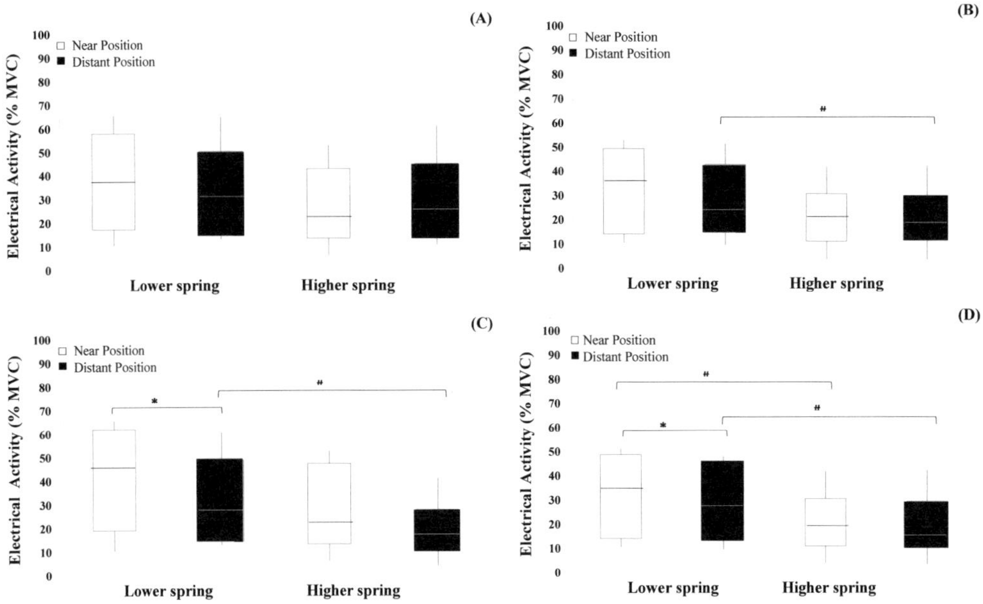

Fig. 6. Normalized electromyographical activation maximum, minimum and median values of right and left muscle external oblique on the evaluated spring positions and subjects positioning. (A) and (B) represent extension phase for left and right sides, respectively. (C) and (D) represent flexion phase for left and right sides, respectively. Extracted from Brazilian Journal of Physiotherapy with permission.

During the hip flexion phase, there was a significant increase in External Oblique activation of about 20% in the lower spring setup and distant position when compared to the higher spring setup and near position (Figure 6), probably due to a more challenging situation for keeping the pelvis in a relative neutral position and avoiding anterior tilt. The External Oblique muscle actions for maintaining the pelvis in place as the hip is flexed in a lying position was previously described by Calais-Germain and Lamotte (2005) and is consistent with global function documented by Bergmark (1989). Furthermore it should be remembered that when the spring is used in the lower position the thigh and lower leg weight may have a higher contribution in the resistance moment composition then the actual spring moment. In the mechanical point of view, in this situation the resistance moment will happen in the extension direction, even with the spring acting in the hip flexion direction. Considering this configuration of hip flexors actuation during flexion phase, there may be a higher tendency for pelvis anterior tilt with a consequent increase in lumbar lordosis (Calais-Germain & Lamotte, 2005). This idea seems to corroborate with the results in study 1, where a higher Rectus Femoris activation in the hip extension phase using the lower spring was found.

Based in the results, the hip flexion-extension exercise in the Cadillac with higher spring setup and variations in subject's position is recommended as an option of paravertrebal muscles stabilization exercise. This may be the case especially in the initial rehabilitation phase, because the electric activation levels found for Multifidos (10 to 20% of MVC) are in accordance with McGill's (2007) suggestion that an activation of 10% or less is sufficient for means of stabilization during everyday life activities. On the other side, there are studies suggesting that observed low activation levels (under 40% of MVC) for abdominal and erector spine muscles during trunk stabilization exercises, may not be enough for muscular strengthening in healthy subjects (Souza et al., 2001). Thereby, when the exercise program objective is the high performance of the trunk stabilization muscles, it is suggested that the health professional make use of other types of exercise, once activation levels obtained for Multifidos during hip flexion-extension were equal or lower than 20% of MVC.

In addition, the same hip flexion extension exercise in the Cadillac with lower spring setup and near position may be indicated as another option of exercise for trunk flexors strengthening, once the External Oblique electric activation levels obtained were similar to those found by previous studies performed outside (Mcgill & Karpowicz, 2009) and inside (Queiroz et al., 2010) the Pilates environment. Therapeutic use of hip flexion-extension exercise in the Cadillac is preferable to exercises where the abdominal actively flex the pelvis and trunk. This is because this exercises may represent a problem for individuals with disc pathologies due to the increase of intradiscal pressure (Nachemson, 1987) and lumbar spine compression (Axler & Mcgill, 1997). Nevertheless, caution is recommended when using the exercise evaluated in this study, especially for individuals with weak muscles or incapable of stabilizing pelvis and trunk against an increase in external load (Souza et al., 2001), like may be the case of elderly people.

5. Study 3 – Speed performance evaluation

Nine subjects took part in this study. External oblique, Multifidus, Rectos Femoris and Gluteus Maximum muscles were evaluated in the right side. External oblique, Multifidus, Rectos Femoris electrodes were positioned in accordance to the previous studies. Gluteus Maximums electrodes were positioned in the middle of the line between the sacral vertebrae and the greater trochanter. Reference electrode was positioned in the spine process of the seventh cervical vertebrae. Maximum isometric voluntary contraction was collected for the Gluteus maximum following the same procedure as the isquiotibialis muscles.

The hip joint angular positions were registered by means of a webcam (25 frames/s). Each subject performed 3 series of 10 repetitions each of the hip flexion-extension movement in three different speeds. First, all subjects performed the movement at self selected speed. The execution speed average was 30 degrees/s, with a very low variability. The low variability found was probably because all subjects trained at the same place and with the same instructor, having learned to perform the exercise in the same way. Then, in random order subjects performed the movement in slower speed (15 degrees/s) and in faster speed (45 degrees/s), having a digital metronome dictating the rhythm. An interval of 2 minute was kept between series. The two spring used were fixed at the higher spring setup, 90 cm high, and had been previously calibrated, having an elastic constant of 0.082 kg/cm. For standardization it was requested that subjects expire during extension and inspire during flexion.

Multiple two factors ANOVA, one for each muscle, with a Bonferroni post hoc were used to evaluate speed influence in each phase. Significance level adopted was $p < 0.05$.
For the trunk stabilizers muscle, Multifidus and External Oblique, no speed influence was found, while for Rectos Femoris and Gluteus Maximum a difference between the higher speed and the other two speeds was found, as may be seen in Figures 7 to 10. In the phase analysis, difference was only found for the External Oblique muscle, when RMS value was higher in the extension phase when compared to the flexion phase (Figure 11).

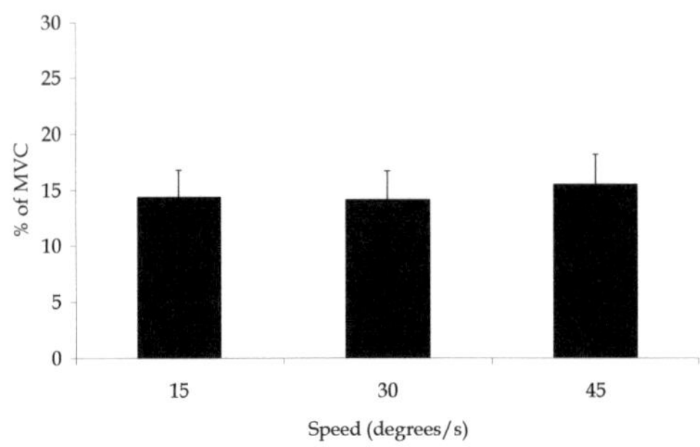

Fig. 7. External oblique muscle electric activation comparison in three angular speeds during hip flexion-extension movement in Cadillac.

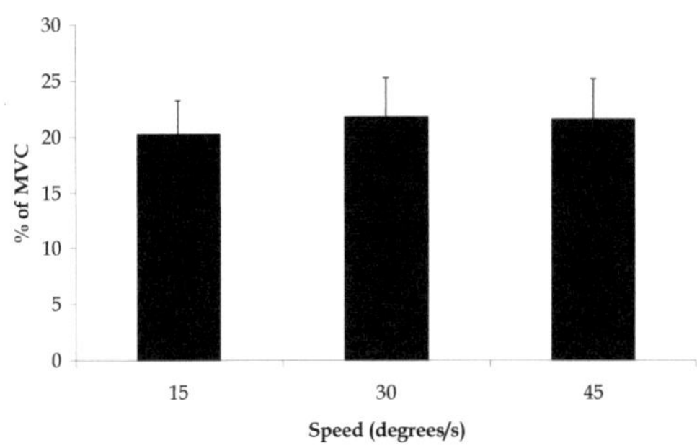

Fig. 8. Multifidus muscle electric activation comparison in three angular speeds during hip flexion-extension movement in Cadillac.

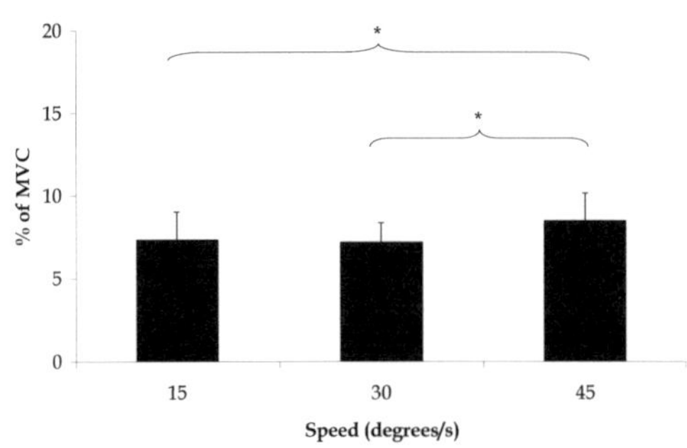

Fig. 9. Rectus Femoris muscle electric activation comparison in three angular speeds during hip flexion-extension movement in Cadillac.

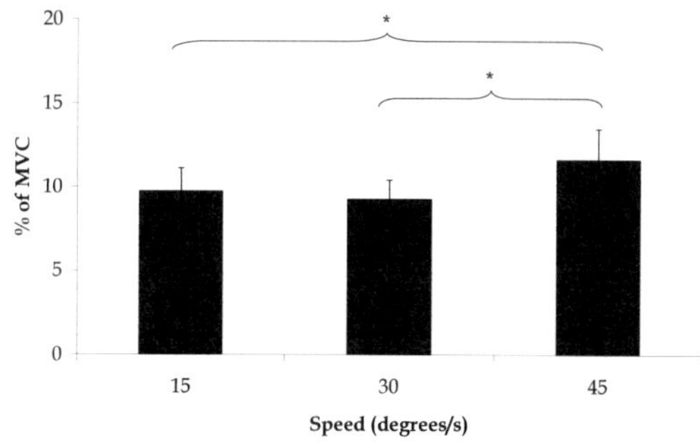

Fig. 10. Gluteus Maximum muscle electric activation comparison in three angular speeds during hip flexion-extension movement in Cadillac.

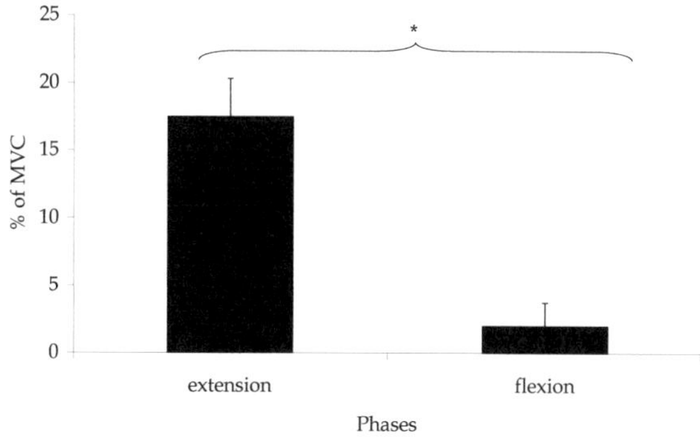

Fig. 11. External oblique muscle electric activation comparison between flexion and extension phases during hip flexion-extension movement in Cadillac.

5.1 Practical application

When verifying speed effect on the electrical activation of External Oblique, Multifidus, Rectos Femoris and Gluteus Maximum muscles during hip flexion extension movement in the Cadillac, it may be observed that only extension movement agonist and antagonist muscles were influenced by speed, showing increases in electrical activity as speed increased. Gluteus Maximum is considered by literature as the main hip extensor, having the biggest cross sectional and muscle perpendicular distance (Oatis, 2009) and Rectus Femoris (a biarticular muscle), is an important knee extensor and hip flexor (Oatis, 2009). Both muscles are fundamental in performing the analysed movement (Silva et al., 2009). Based in the force-velocity relation, that determines that in slower velocities there is a higher capability of force production (Babault et al., 2003; Hill, 1938), it is possible to speculate that using the same absolute spring load, there is a better neuromuscular efficiency in slower velocities, meaning that the muscle is capable of producing more force with a slower muscle recruitment necessity, reflecting in smaller EMG values. It may also be considered that as execution speed increases, the inertial effect is each time more significant. The inertial effect is due to the movement with variable speed of the lower limbs' mass and is part of the resistance moment. In this perspective, agonist muscles become more required to rapidly start while antagonist muscles become more required to abruptly stop faster movements.

It may also be remarked, when considering the faster speed versus the self-selected speed, that these results corroborate with those found by Hatfield et al. (Hatfield et al., 2006) that verified that execution speed exerted influence in strength training variables during squat exercise, where the self-selected speed showed better performance for the exercise. According to Purves et al (2008) when performing fast tasks and with certain time limitations, the central nervous system seems to choose speed dependent strategies, while when the individual is free to choose movement speed, the central nervous system chooses speed independent strategies (adjusting electric impulse intensity with adequate duration for complete execution of the gesture). The preferred speed used by the subject during Pilates training sections represents the necessary neural strategy to perform the hip flexion extension exercise, this being an important specific adaptation to training. Considering that execution speeds different from the self-selected may interfere in individuals muscle recruitment pattern (Germain et al., 1996; Hatfield et al., 2006; Bottaro et al., 2007), it is suggested that future studies about Pilates, also consider execution speed as a variable that may intervene significantly in the muscle electrical activity pattern.

One fundamental principle of the Pilates Method is the core musculature recruitment, having the External Oblique as a representative muscle of the anterior superficial muscle group (Bergmark, 1989) and the Multifidus a representative of the posterior deep muscle group (Rosatelli et al., 2008). Thus, another important result is that in the hip extension phase, External Oblique was significantly more active than in the hip flexion phase, regardless of execution speed. This results corroborate with anterior studies (Loss et al., 2010; Rydeard et al., 2006) and indicates that stabilizer muscles are higher influenced by pelvic positioning, that seems to vary according to the movement's phase and its association to external overload and not according to speed variation. As discussed in studies 1 and 2, it may be speculated that in the hip extension phase there is a higher external overload that increases the necessity of activation of the muscles responsible for preventing pelvis anterior tilt.

6. Conclusion

In spite of the popularity of the exercises performed on the Cadillac equipment, there is a lack of scientific research focusing on muscle electrical activity during Pilates exercise. Aiming to contribute with a step to fill the gap between science research and practical application, the present chapter presented a summary of knowledge produced by *BIOMEC* Group on EMG analysis of Pilates exercises in three studies on the hip extension movement performed on the Cadillac equipment. The first study compared the electrical activation of the Rectus Femoris, Biceps Femoris long head and Semitendinosus between two spring setups. The second study compared the electrical activation of the Multifidus and the External Oblique between two spring setup and two subjects positions. The third study compared the electrical activation of the Multifidus, the External Oblique, the Gluteus Maximum and the Rectus Femoris between three different execution speed. Together, the results of all studies showed that spring setup, subjects positioning and execution speed changes interfere in electrical activity pattern of movement agonist and antagonist muscles and muscles considered stabilizers for the Pilates methodology. In one side, the exercise performed with higher spring setup may generate larger activation levels of the hip extension movement agonists and of the Multifidus (on distant position). On the other side the exercise performed using the lower spring setup may increase the electrical activity of the hip flexors and external oblique muscles. The stabilization muscles activation pattern seems to be kept even when speed execution varies, however the same does not occur for movement agonist and antagonist muscles. In faster speeds extra motor unit recruitment appears to be necessary in front of the new motor challenge, reflecting in higher activation levels for agonist and antagonist muscles.

7. References

Arokoski, J. E., Kankaanpää, M., Valta, T., Juvonen, I., Partanen, J., Taimela, S., Lindgren, K. A. & Airaksinen, O. (1999). Archives of physical medicine and rehabilitation *Back and hip extensor muscle function during therapeutic exercises* 80(7): 842-850,

Axler, C. T. & Mcgill, S. M. (1997). Low back loads over a variety of abdominal exercises: Searching for the safest abdominal challenge *Medicine & Science in Sports & Exercise* 29(6):804-811.

Babault, N., Pousson, M., Michaut, A. & Van Hoecke, J. (2003). Effect of quadriceps femoris muscle length on neural activation during isometric and concentric contractions *Journal of Applied Physiology* 94(3):983-990.

Bergmark, A. (1989). Stability of the lumbar spine. A study in mechanical engineering *Acta Orthopaedica Scandinavica. Supplementum* 230:1-54.

Bertolla F, B. B., Leal Junior Ecp, Oltramar Jd. (2007). Effects of a training program using the Pilates method in flexibility of sub-20 indoor soccer athletes. *Revista brasileira de medicina do Esporte* 13(4): 222-226,

Blum, C. L. (2002). Chiropractic and Pilates therapy for the treatment of adult scoliosis *Journal of Manipulative and Physiological Therapeutics* 25(4),

Bottaro, M., Machado, S. M., Nogueira, W., Scales, R. & Veloso, J. (2007). Effect of high versus low-velocity resistance training on muscular fitness and functional performance in older men. *European Journal of Applied Physiology* 99(3): 257-264,

Calais-Germain, B. & Lamotte, A. (2005). *Anatomie pour le mouvement: Bases d'exercices* 2e édition. Edition DésIris.

Donzelli, S., Di Domenica, E., Cova, A. M., Galletti, R. & Giunta, N. (2006). Two different techniques in the rehabilitation treatment of low back pain: A randomized controlled trial *Eura Medicophys* 42(3): 205-210,

Germain, P., Guevel, A., Hogrel, J. & Marini, J. (1996). Incidences de la vitesse de movement el de l'angle articulaire sur des paramètres électrophysiologiques et biomécaniques lors d'un mouvement d'extension du membre inférieur *Science and Sports,* 11(39-45),

Hatfield, D. L., Kraemer, W. J., Spiering, B. A., Häkkinen, K., Volek, J. S., Shimano, T., Spreuwenberg, L. P. B., Silvestre, R., Vingren, J. L. & Fragala, M. S. (2006). The impact of velocity of movement on performance factors in resistance exercise *The Journal of Strength & Conditioning Research* 20(4):760-766.

Hill, A. V. (1938). The heat of shortening and the dynamic constants of muscle *Proceedings of the Royal Society of London. Series B, Biological Sciences* 126(843): 136-195.

Jago, R., Jonker, M. L., Missaghian, M. & Baranowski, T. (2006). Effect of 4 weeks of Pilates on the body composition of young girls *Preventive medicine* 42(3): 177-180,

Kolyniak, I., Cavalcanti, S. & Aoki, M. (2004). Avaliação isocinética da musculatura envolvida na flexão e extenção do tronco: Efeito do método Pilates *Revista brasileira de medicina do Esporte* 10(6): 487-490,

Latey, P. (2001). The Pilates method: History and philosophy *Journal of Bodywork & Movement Therapies* 5(4): 275-282,

Loss, J. F., Melo, M. D. O., Rosa, C. H., Santos, A. B. D., Torre, M. L. & Silva, Y. O. D. (2010). Electrical activity of external obliques and multifidus muscles during the hip flexion-extension exercise performed in cadillac with differents adjustment for springs and individual positions *Brasilian Journal of Physiotherapy* 14(6): 510-517,

Mcgill, S. (2007). *Low back disorders: Evidenced-based prevention and rehabilitation* Human Kinetics Publishers, Champaign.

Mcgill, S. M. & Karpowicz, A. (2009). Exercises for spine stabilization: Motion/motor patterns, stability progressions, and clinical technique *Archives of physical medicine and rehabilitation* 90(1): 118-126, 0003-9993

Melo, M. O., Gomes, L. E., Silva, Y. O., Bonezi, A. & Loss, J. F. (2011). Assessment of resistance torque and resultant muscular force during Pilates hip extension exercise and its implications to prescription and progression *Revista Brasileira de Fisioterapia* 15(1): 23-30.

Muscolino, J. E. & Cipriani, S. (2004). Pilates and the "powerhouse"—i *Journal of Bodywork & Movement Therapies* 8(1): 15-24,

Nachemson, A. (1987). Lumbar intradiscal pressure. The lumbar spine and back pain Edinburgh, Scotland, Churchill Livingstone: 191–203.

Ng, J. K., Kippers, V., Parnianpour, M. & Richardson, C. A. (2002). Emg activity normalization for trunk muscles in subjects with and without back pain. *Medicine and Science in Sports and Exercise* 34(7): 1082-1086,

Oatis, C. A. (2009). *Kinesiology: The mechanics and pathomechanics of human movement.* (2), Lippincott Williams & Wilkins, Baltimore

Purves, D., Augustine, G., Fitzpatrick, D., Hall, W., Lamantia, A., Mcnamara, J. & Williams, S. (2008). *Neuroscience,* (4), Sinauer Associates, Sunderland

Queiroz, B., Cagliari, M., Amorim, C. & Sacco, I. (2010). Muscle activation during four Pilates core stability exercises in quadruped position *Archives of physical medicine and rehabilitation* 91(1): 86-92,

Rosatelli, A. L., Ravichandiran, K. & Agur, A. M. (2008). Three-dimensional study of the musculotendinous architecture of lumbar multifidus and its functional implications. *Clinical Anatomy* 21(6): 539-546,

Rydeard, R., Leger, A. & Smith, D. (2006). Pilates-based therapeutic exercise: Effect on subjects with nonspecific chronic low back pain and functional disability: A randomized controlled trial *The Journal of orthopaedic and sports physical therapy* 36(7): 472-484,

Segal, N. A., Hein, J. & Basford, J. R. (2004). The effects of Pilates training on flexibility and body composition: An observational study *Archives of physical medicine and rehabilitation* 85(12): 1977-1981,

Self, B. P., Bagley, A. M., Triplett, T. L. & Paulos, L. E. (1996). Functional biomechanical analysis of the Pilates-based reformer during demi-plie movements *Journal of applied biomechanics* 12(3):326-337.

Silva, Y., Melo, M., Gomes, L., Bonezi, A. & Loss, J. (2009). Analysis of the external resistance and electromyographic activity of hip extension performed according to the Pilates method *Revista Brasileira de Fisioterapia* 13(1):82-88.

Souza, G. M., Baker, L. L. & Powers, C. M. (2001). Electromyographic activity of selected trunk muscles during dynamic spine stabilization exercises* 1 *Archives of physical medicine and rehabilitation* 82(11): 1551-1557.

12

Electromyography Monitoring for Complete and Incomplete Transections of the Spinal Cord in Humans Who Received a Cell Therapy Combined with LASERPONCTURE® or LASERPONCTURE® Only: Methodology, Analysis, and Results

Albert Bohbot
Laboratoire de Recherches sur le Laserponcture®
France

1. Introduction

The most difficult thing to achieve in the case of a spinal cord injury (SCI) and/or spinal trauma is to objectively assess the progress and voluntary motor recovery. The exercise becomes even more hazardous when one sets as a preliminary rule that **each SCI or spinal trauma is unique and original both in its bone and spinal anatomical location, and in its consequences on the whole body.** Starting from here, we assume that there is no standard approach but an observation process to be adapted for each special case.

For example, two SCI individuals suffering from a complete transection of the spinal cord at anatomical level T5 will show totally different clinical pictures. They may be affected, or not, by spasticity - even flaccidity for some cases with a loss of mass muscle - or neurological pain. Each case is different and should have its own approach.

Before any examination can take place, a preliminary face-to-face interview to understand the injury and its manifestations is fundamental. Every single thing should be investigated during this interview whether it concerns the motor or sensory level, as well as the bowels and bladder functions, and sexual function. The information collected should be as thorough as possible. A psychological check-up should not be discarded either as it provides the SCI individual's input regarding his/her body image and relations s/he has with others.

Electromyography monitoring is a pioneering work published in the peer-review journal Cell Transplantation and presented in various scientific meetings.

Avicenna (980-1037), a Persian philosopher and physician commonly known as **Ibn Sīnā**, was credited with the following quotation "**the sick person cannot only be encompassed through his disease**".

2. Aim

The aim of this chapter is to highlight that a voluntary muscle activity below the SCI can be measured by electromyography monitoring.

Several groups were investigated:
Group A: incomplete spinal trauma with the following subgroups:
- Laserponcture® only
- Laserponcture® combined with ensheathing stem cells
- Laserponcture® combined with ensheathing autologous stem cells
- Laserponcture® combined with autologous hematopoietic cells
- Laserponcture® combined with a therapy based on multiple autologous stem cells

Group B: complete spinal trauma (complete transection of the spinal cord) with the following subgroups:
- Laserponcture® only
- Laserponcture® combined with ensheathing stem cells
- Laserponcture® combined with ensheathing autologous stem cells
- Laserponcture® combined with autologous hematopoietic cells
- Laserponcture® combined with a therapy based on multiple autologous stem cells

The *American Spinal Injury Association Classification of Spinal Cord Injury* defines a complete or incomplete SCI in its ASIA Impairment Scale as the following:
- A = Complete: no motor or sensory function is preserved in the sacral segments S4-S5;
- B = Incomplete: sensory but not motor function is preserved below the neurological level and includes the sacral segments S4-S5;
- C = Incomplete: motor function is preserved below the neurological level, and more than half of key muscles below the neurological level have a muscle grade less than 3;
- D = Incomplete: motor function is preserved below the neurological level, and at least half of key muscles below the neurological level have a muscle grade of 3 or more;
- E = Normal: motor and sensory functions are normal.

3. Methods and material

Exclusion criteria:
- depression
- hyper spasticity

Inclusion criteria:
- complete or incomplete transection of the spinal cord treated by Laserponcture® only or Laserponcture® combined with a stem cell therapy
- cases with flaccidity post injury

Guidance and instructions for the patients were to voluntary contract the tested muscles (quadriceps, abdominal muscles, etc.) on demand. The sessions were also recorded on video.
The cases studied were selected according to the severity of the injury on MRI.
For each recording, a zeroing was performed to erase the parameters of the previous test with the aim of monitoring a change in the spasticity appearing during the examination.

Commentary

During the recordings, the following observations can be made:

a. a low curve when the individual is at rest predicts an increased response to the voluntary act during the next test

b. spasticity sometimes appears; it suggests muscle fatigue and requires to stop the test
More than 150 cases underwent the tests.

The PROCOMP5™ equipment with softwares BIOGRAPH INFINITI 5® and REHAB SUITE™ especially adapted to SCIs; the sensors MYOSCAN-PRO™ EMG (SA9401M-50) to record muscle activity, and FLEX/PRO™-SA9309M to record skin conductance were fixed on the skin. The unit of measurement is the µVolt.

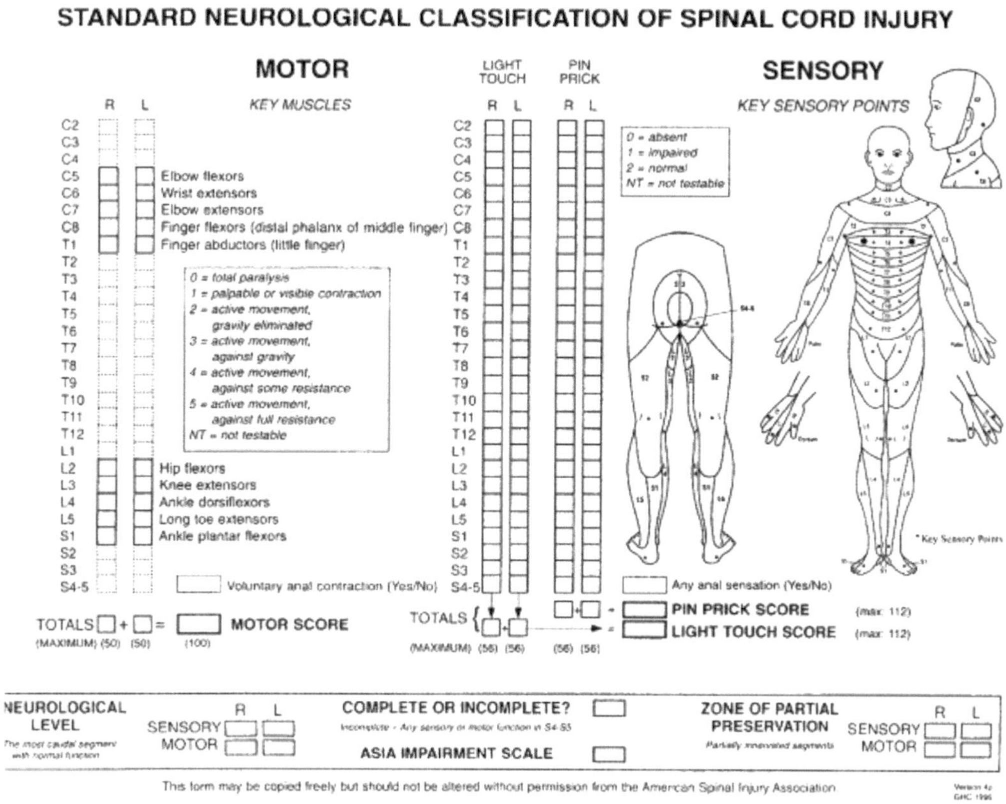

Fig. 1. Standard neurological classification of spinal cord injury.

4. Presentation of graphs and interpretation

4.1 Presentation of the graphs used

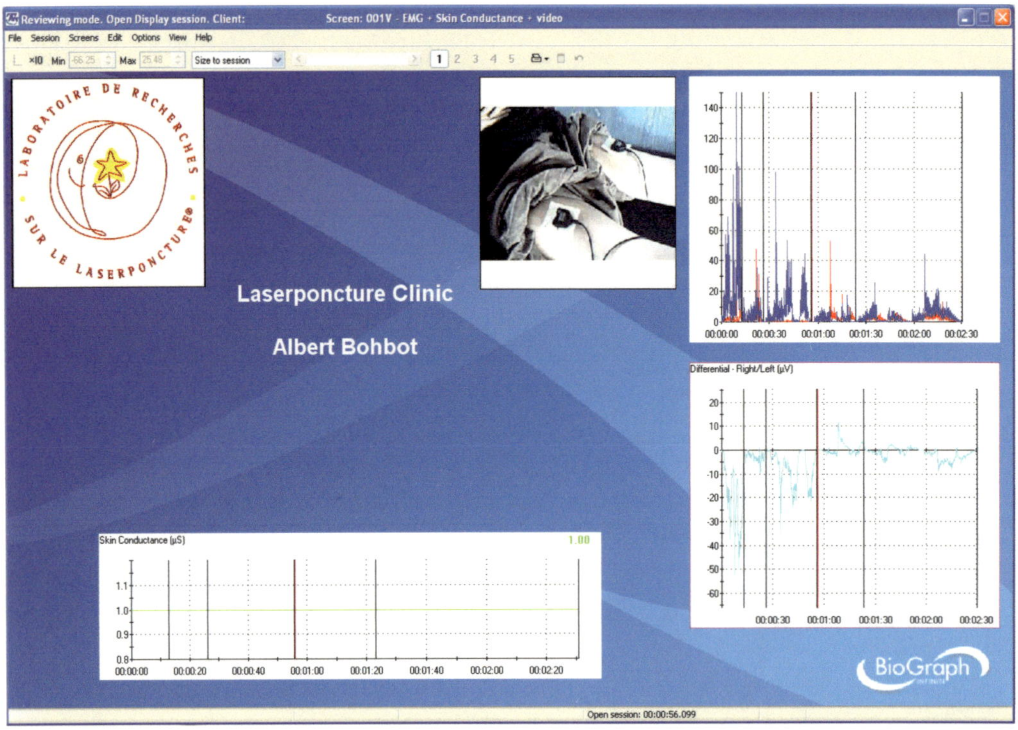

Fig. 2. Example of graphs used.
Graph A (top right): the red line represents the recorded activity of the right lower limb (RLL); the blue line represents the recorded activity of the left lower limb (LLL).
Graph B is obtained by arithmetic subtraction (bottom left): above 0: recorded activity of the RLL; below 0: recorded activity of the LLL.

4.2 Different types of activity recordings

Examples of graphs and their interpretation

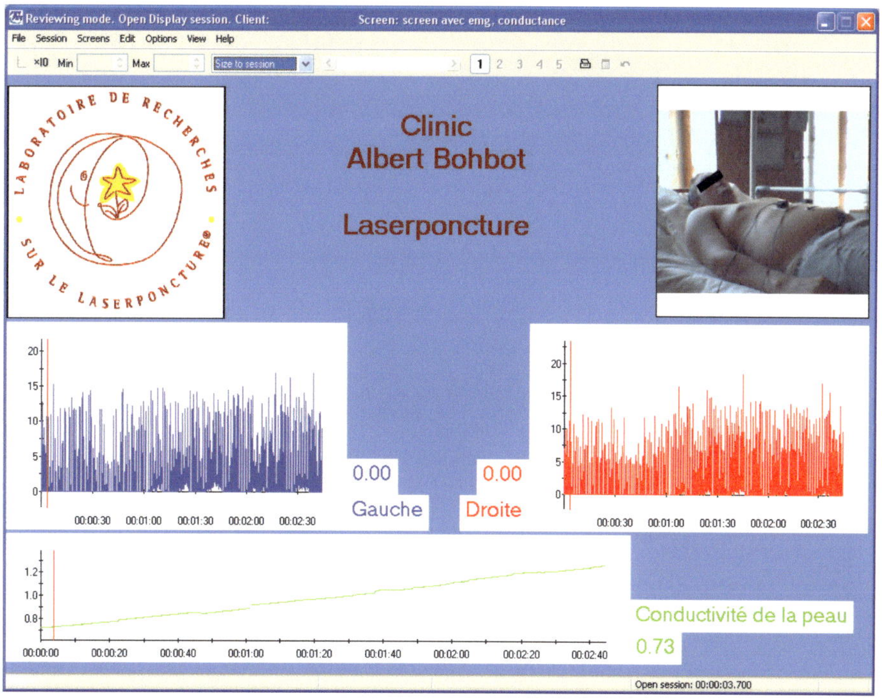

Fig. 3. Example of a muscle activity interference caused by spasticity.

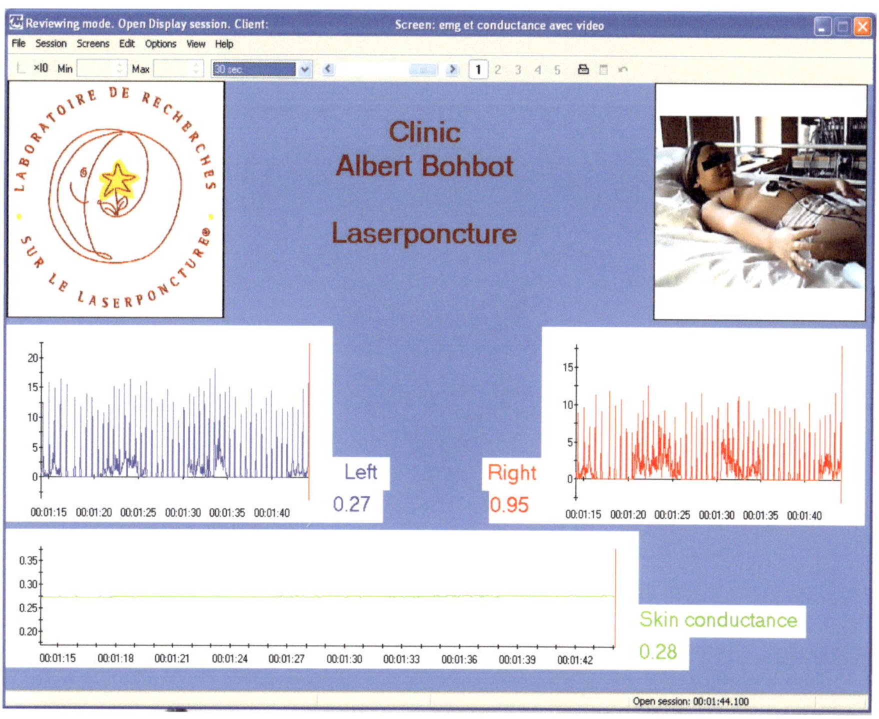

Fig. 4. Example of interference caused by the umbilical artery beatings (regular rising curve).

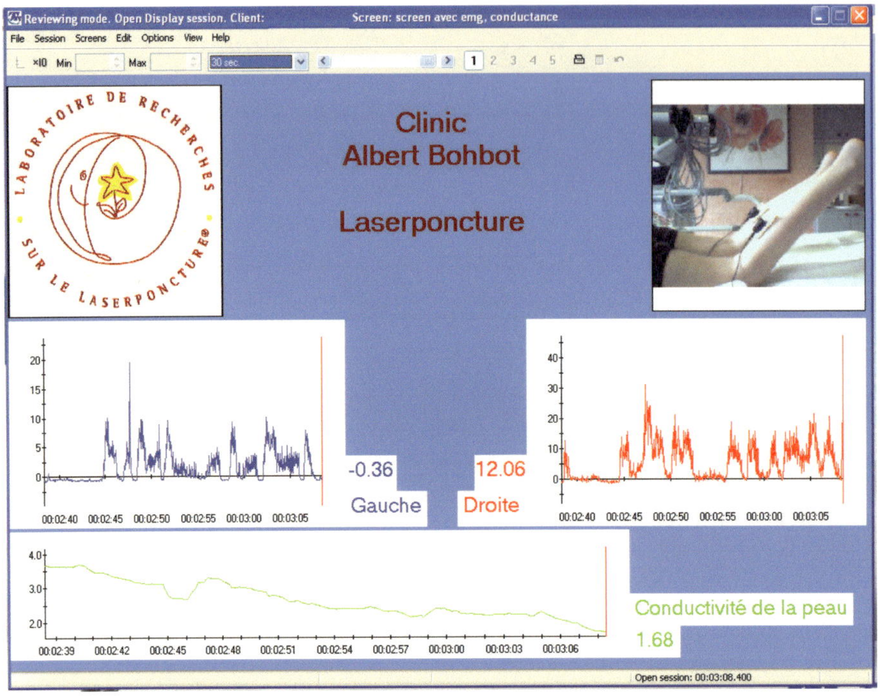

Fig. 5. Voluntary spontaneous muscle contraction (gastrocnemius muscles).

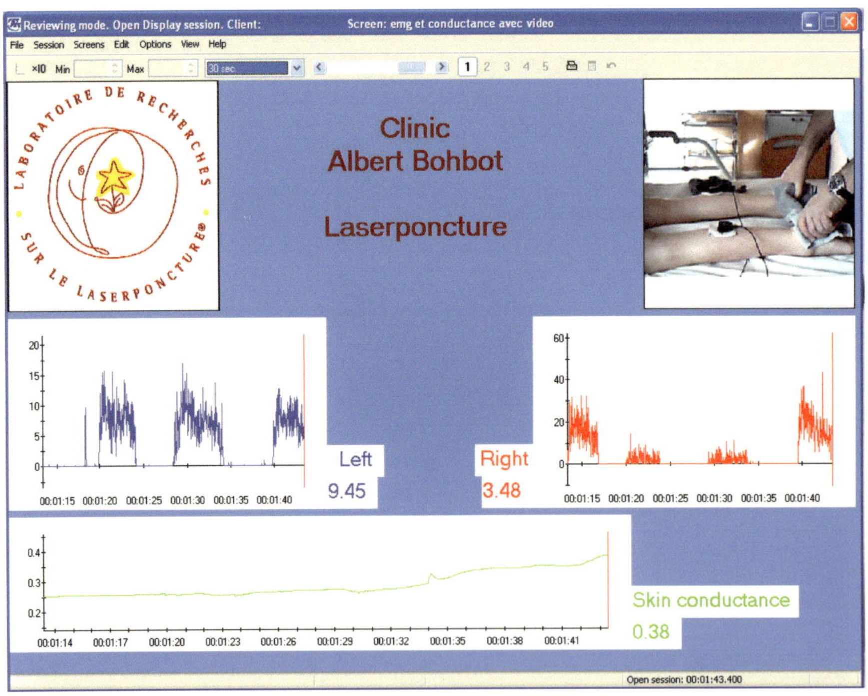

Fig. 6. Voluntary muscle contraction against resistance (gastrocnemius muscles; the operator's hand has no direct contact on the patient skin).

5. Positioning of captors

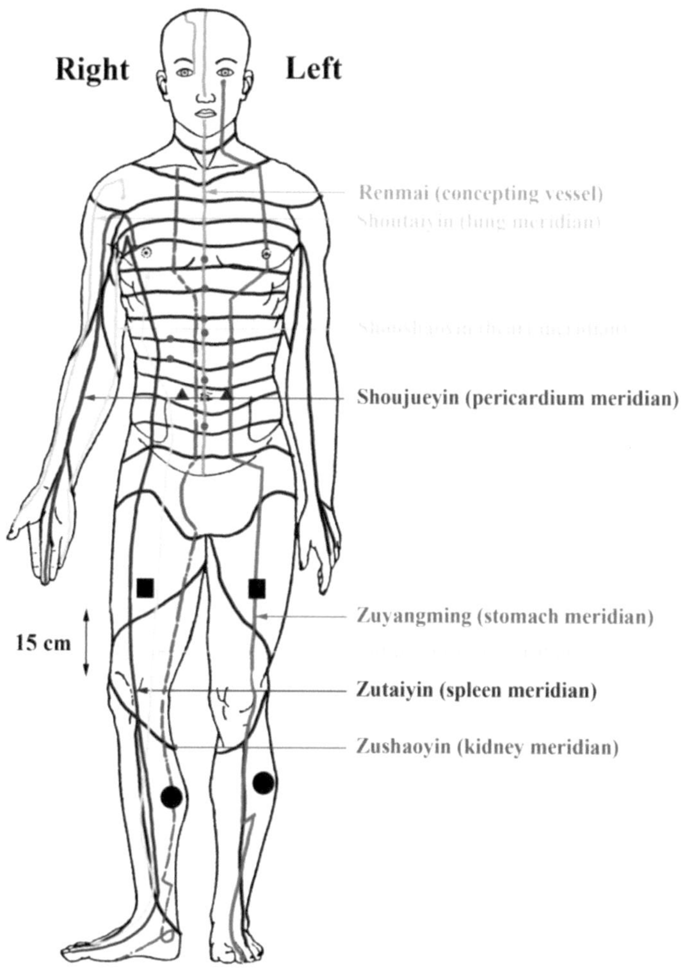

Fig. 7. Positioning of captors.

Front face
Squares: quadriceps
Triangles: abdominal muscles (upper, middle, and lower abdominal muscles)
Rounds: gastrocnemius
Other muscles can also be tested.

6. Case study

6.1 Quadriplegia with a complete SCI transection and Laserponcture® only

No MRI available for this case.

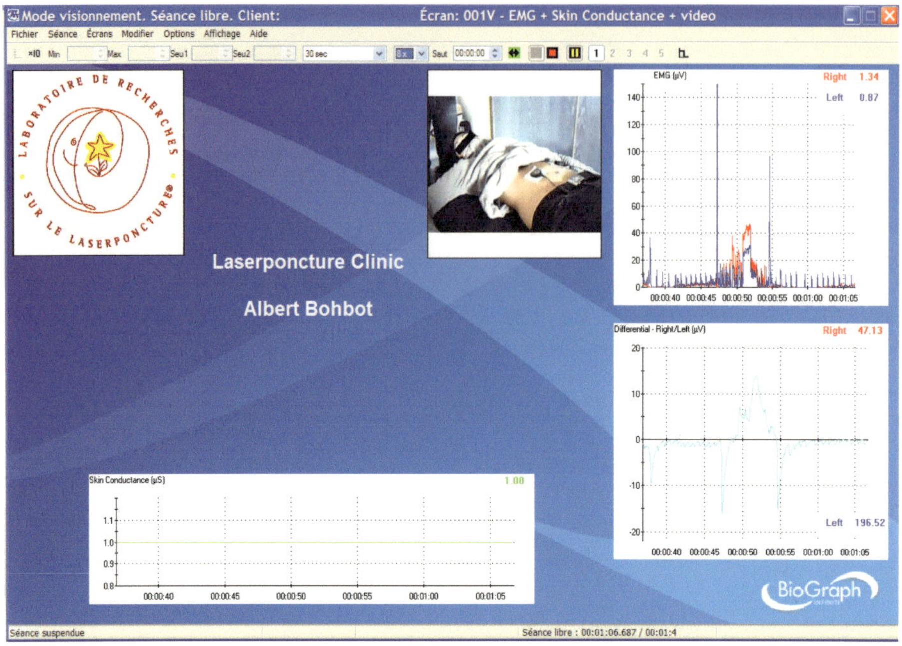

Fig. 8. Electromyography monitoring on April 1st, 2010 (upper abdominal muscles).

6.2 Quadriplegia with a complete SCI transection and Laserponcture® combined with olfactory ensheathing cells

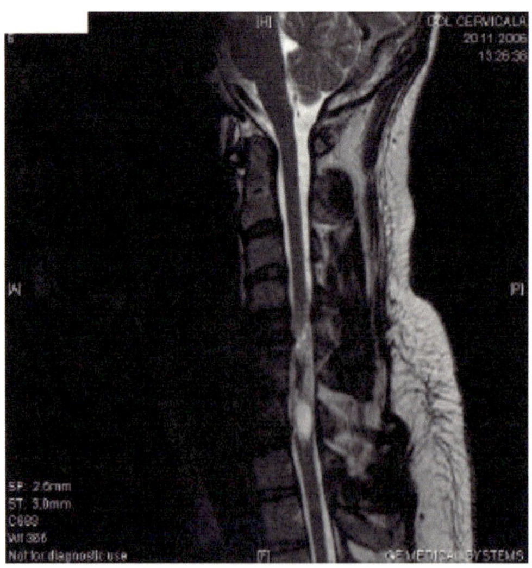

Fig. 9. MRI showing a C5-C6 complete SCI.

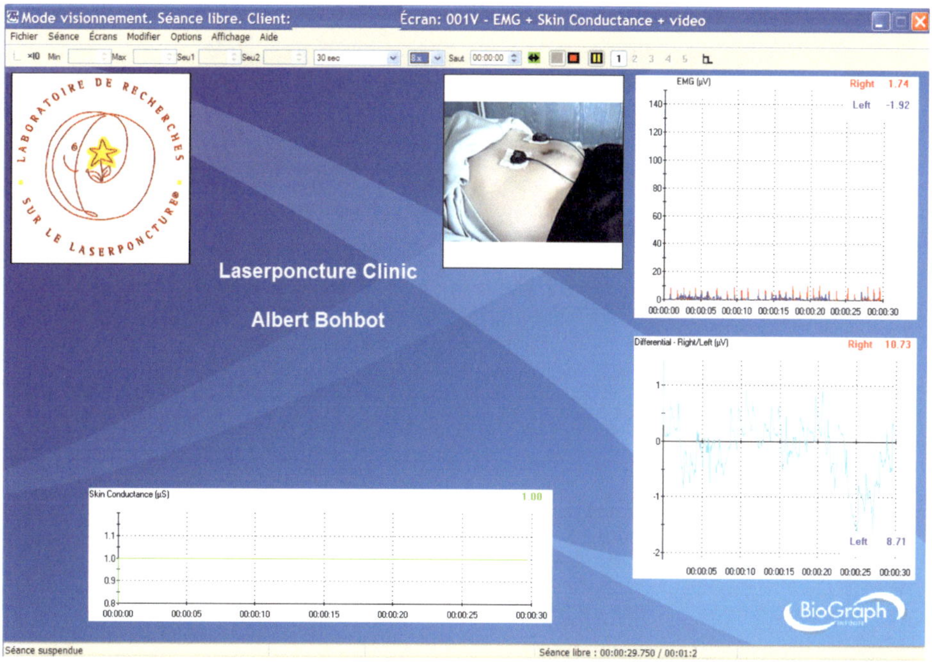

Fig. 10. Electromyography monitoring on March 17th, 2010 (upper abdominal muscles).

6.3 Quadriplegia with an incomplete SCI transection and Laserponcture® only

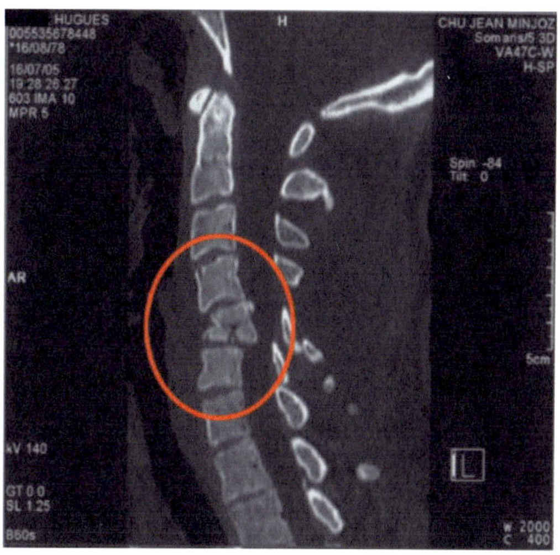

Fig. 11. MRI showing a C5-C6 incomplete SCI.

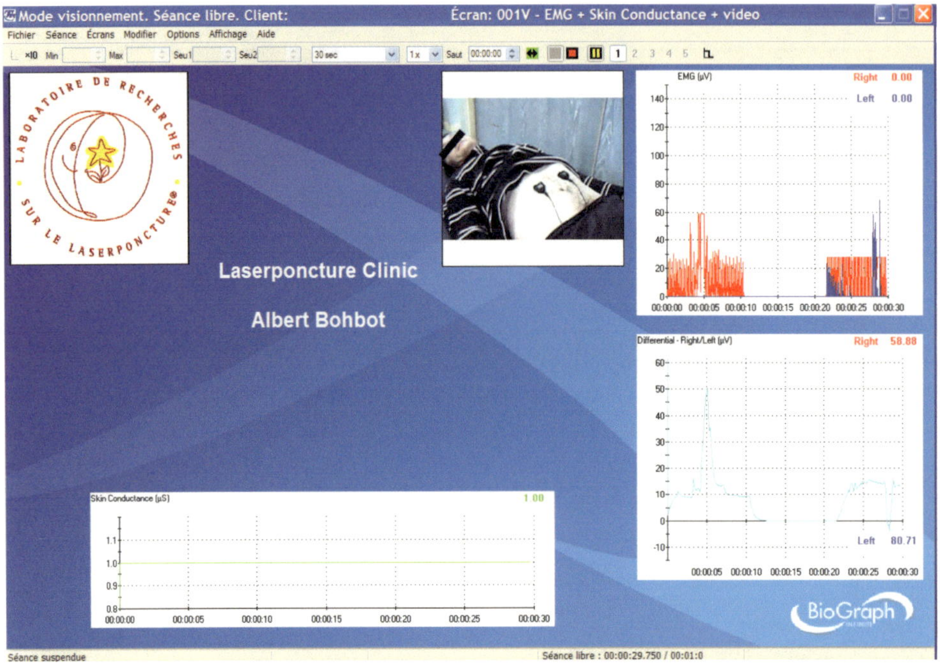

Fig. 12. Electromyography monitoring on January 12th, 2011 (upper abdominal muscles).

6.4 Quadriplegia with an incomplete SCI transection and Laserponcture® combined with cells (Nogo, Dr. Schwab's procedure)

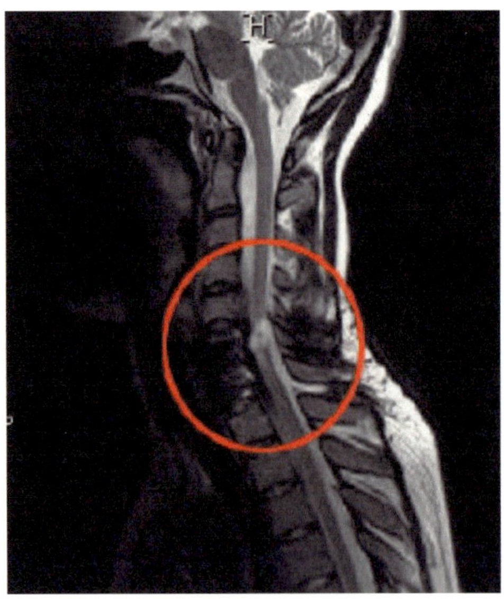

Fig. 13. MRI showing a C6-C7 incomplete SCI.

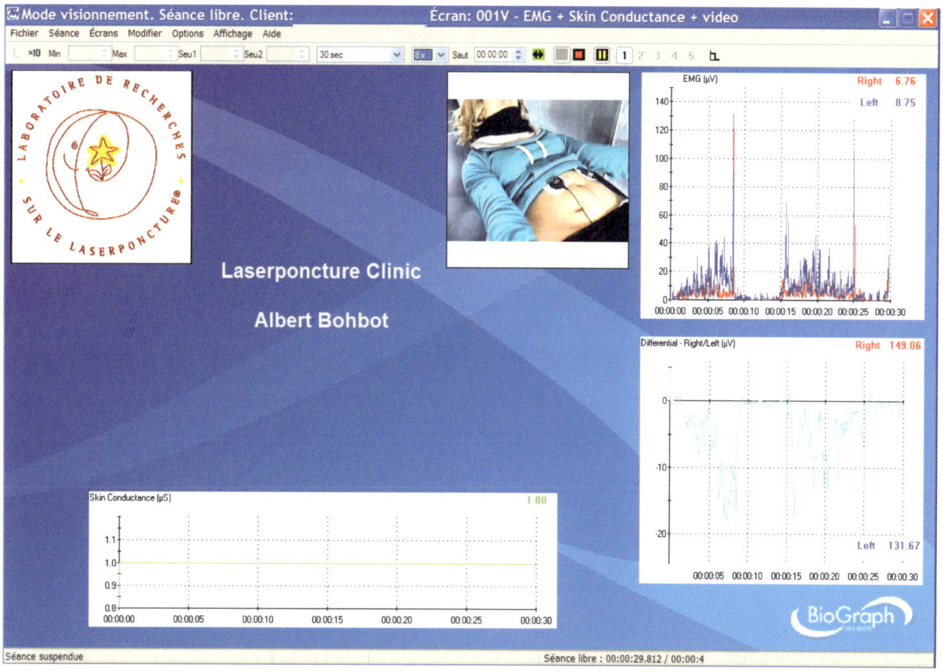

Fig. 14. Electromyography monitoring on February 28th, 2010 (upper abdominal muscles).

6.5 Paraplegia with a complete SCI transection and Laserponcture® only

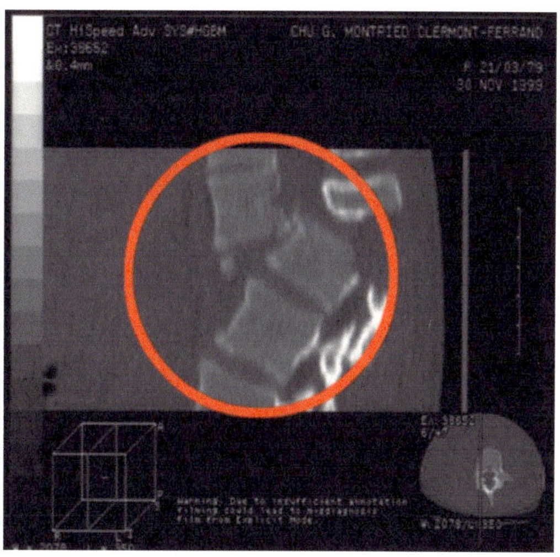

Fig. 15. MRI showing a T12-L1 complete SCI.

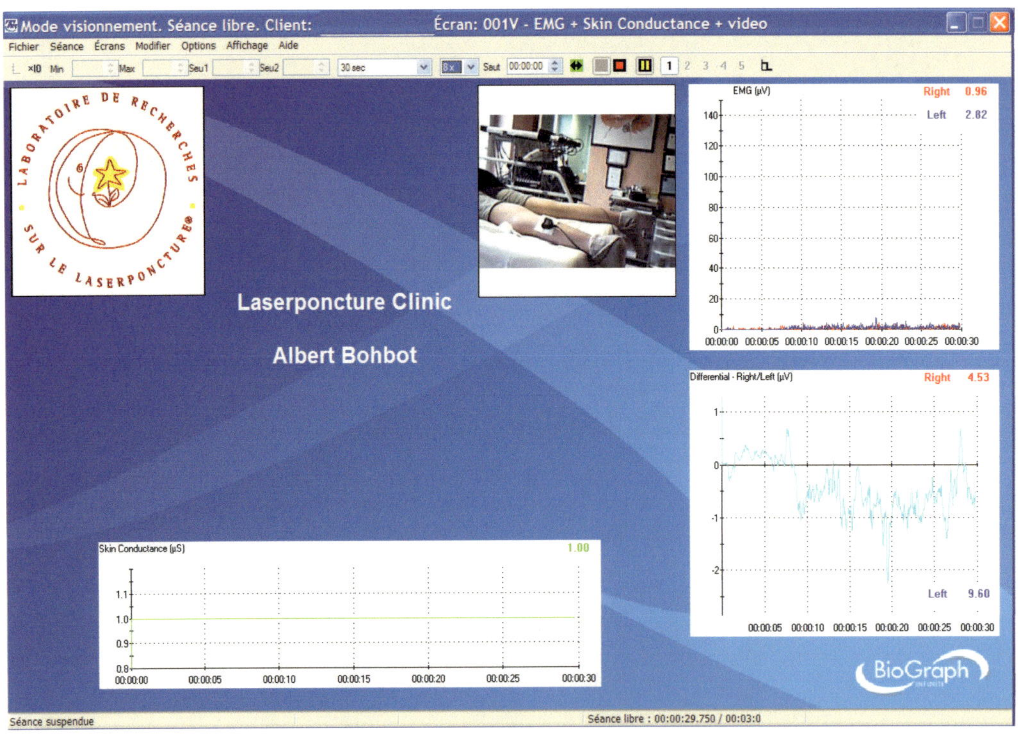

Fig. 16. Electromyography monitoring on February 9th, 2011, lateral gastrocnemius muscle.

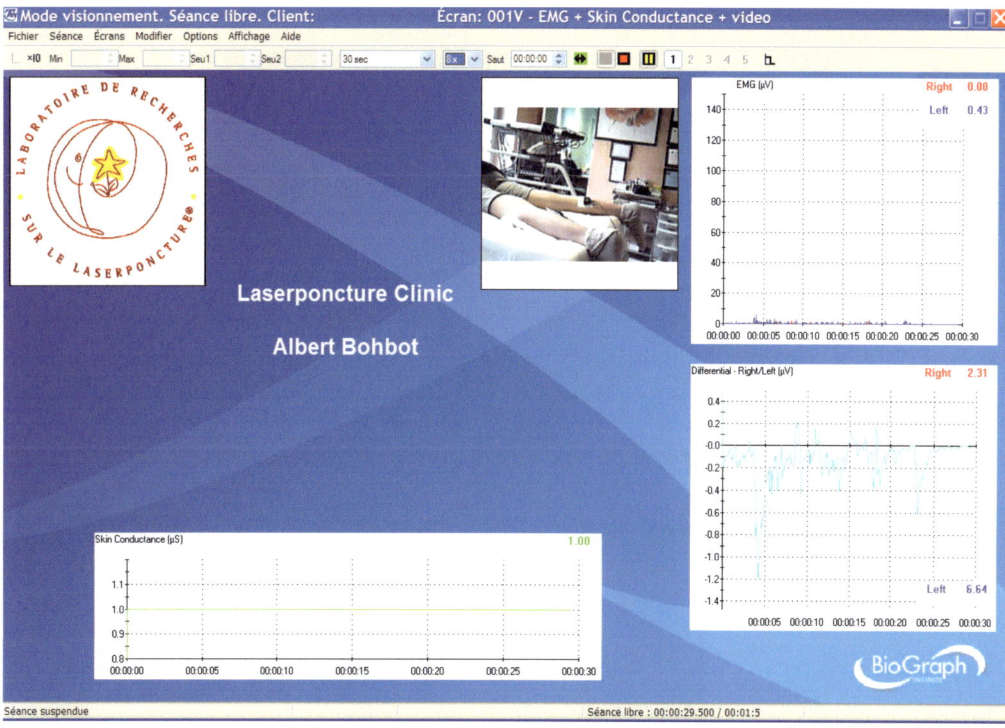

Fig. 17. Electromyography monitoring on February 9th, 2011, medial gastrocnemius muscle.

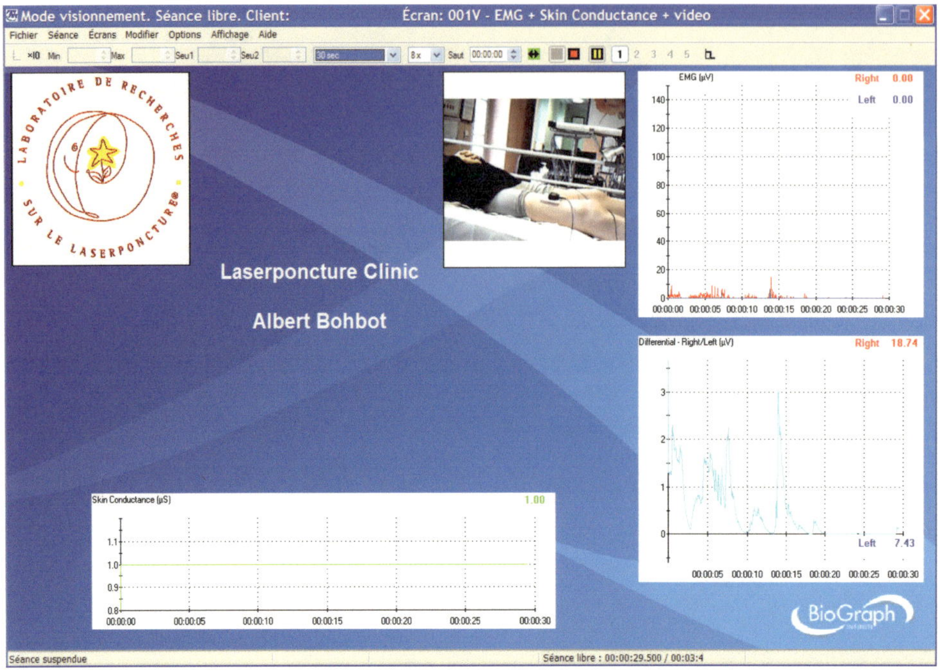

Fig. 18. Electromyography monitoring on February 9th, 2011, quadriceps.

6.6 Paraplegia with a complete SCI transection and Laserponcture® combined with olfactory ensheathing cells

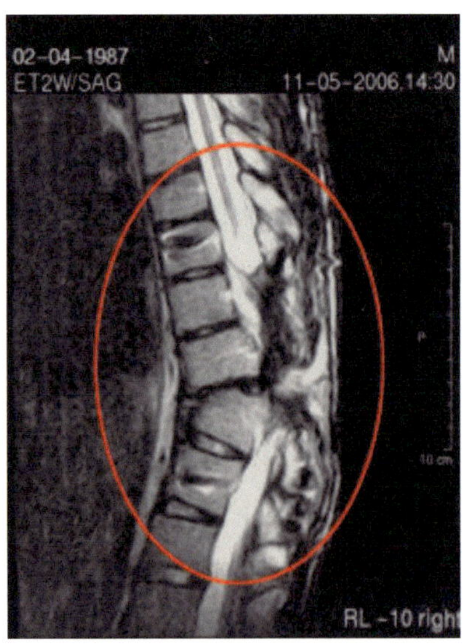

Fig. 19. MRI showing a T10 complete SCI.

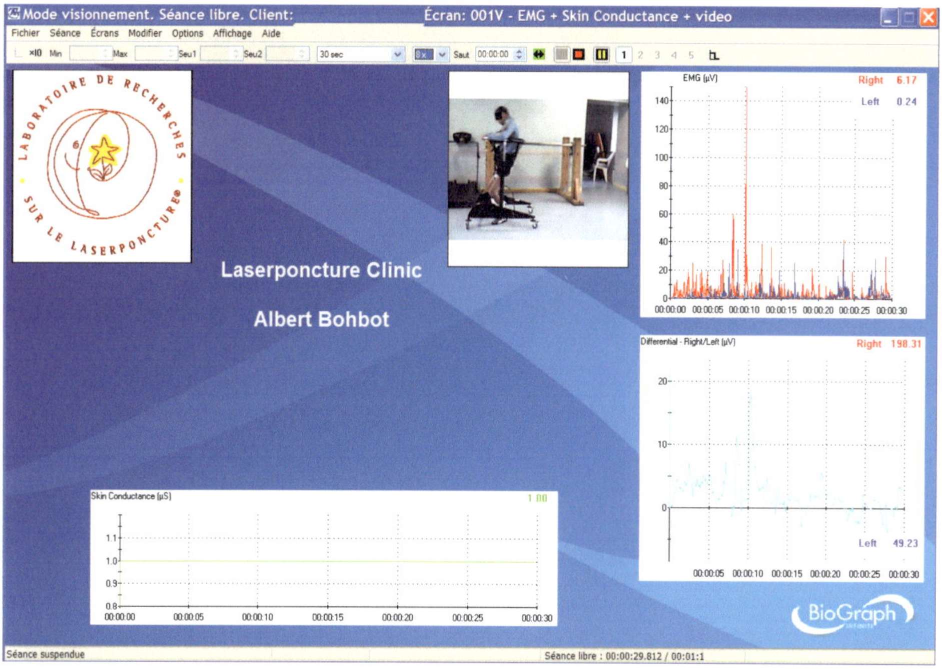

Fig. 20. Electromyography monitoring on November 22nd, 2010, quadriceps.

6.7 Paraplegia with an incomplete SCI transection and Laserponcture® only

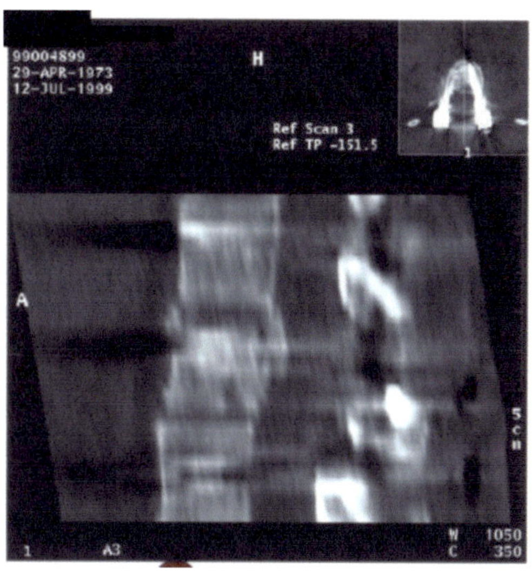

Fig. 21. MRI showing a L1 incomplete SCI.

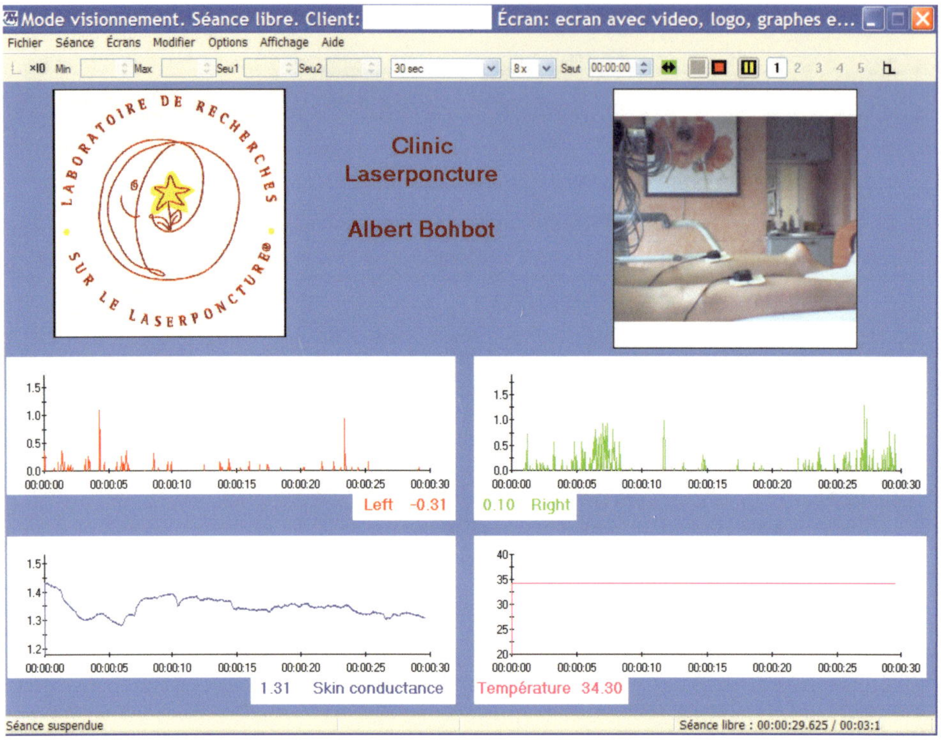

Fig. 22. Electromyography monitoring on February 26th, 2009, gastrocnemius muscles.

6.8 Paraplegia with an incomplete SCI transection and Laserponcture® combined with autologous hematopoietic cells

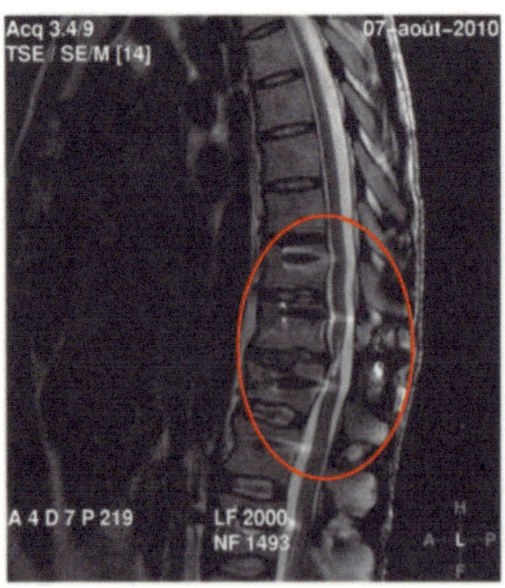

Fig. 23. MRI showing a T10-T11 incomplete SCI.

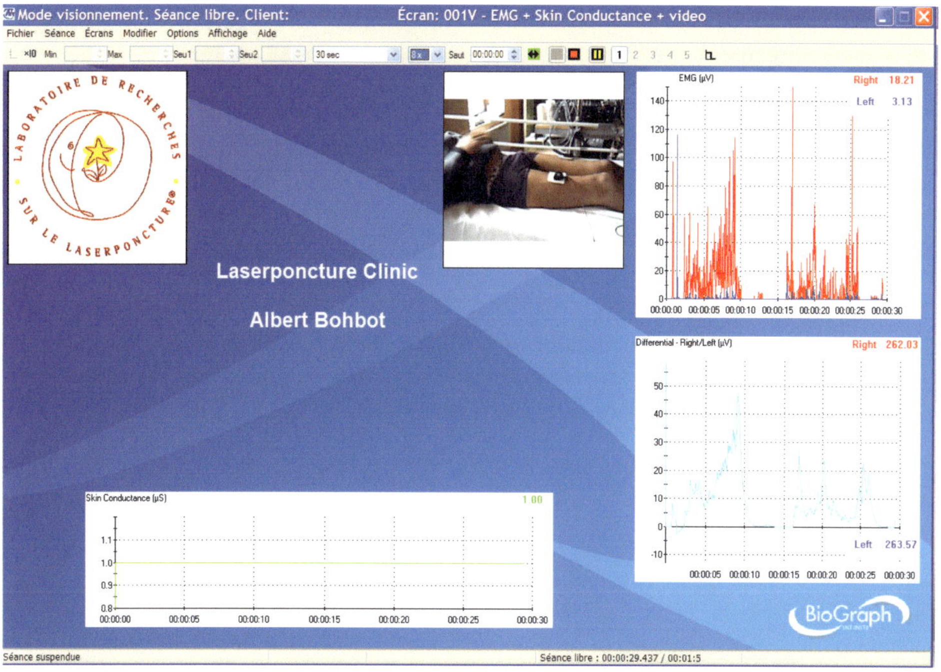

Fig. 24. Electromyography monitoring on January 26th, 2011, quadriceps.

7. Conclusion

This chapter underlines that it is important to track voluntary muscle activity below a SCI in order to possibly determine recoveries to come.

Electromyography monitoring suggests that there is muscle activity even though it may not be visible.

Despite a complete transection of the spinal cord, it also suggests that back-up networks develop to carry the brain orders through the body. It also shows that the information can be transmitted through other means, such as wavelengths, when there is a **complete anatomical transection** of the spinal axis, that is a tissue discontinuity preventing neurotransmitters to travel through synapses.

The information sent by the brain goes from an electrochemical state (neurotransmitters) to an electromagnetic state (wavelengths).

It also suggests that the brain deals with two languages of different nature, the electrochemical transmitter and the electromagnetic signal, which can relay each other.

8. Acknowledgement

Edwige Nault for her translation.

9. References

Bohbot, A. (2002). LASERPONCTURE®: an alternative for SCI. Fourth international symposium on experimental spinal cord repair and regeneration. Brescia, Italy. March 2002.

Bohbot, A. (2008). LASERPONCTURE® contribution in neural restoration. First international association of neurorestoratology annual conference. Beijing, China. May 2008.

Bohbot, A. (2008). Preliminary study on the muscle activity below the injury in complete paraplegia and quadriplegia treated by LASERPONCTURE® and monitored by electromyoscan and thermal camera. The Seventh international congress of the world association of laser therapy. Sun City, South Africa. October 2008.

Bohbot, A. (2009). OECs and LASERPONCTURE® from 2005 to today: follow-up and progress. Second international association of neurorestoratology annual conference. Beijing, China. April 2009.

Bohbot, A. Olfactory Ensheathing Glia Transplantation Combined with LASERPONCTURE® in Human Spinal Cord Injury: Results Measured by Electromyography Monitoring. *Cell Transplantation*. Vol.19, (2010), pp. 179-184.

Part 4

Sports Medicine

13

EMG Applications in Studies of Arts

Gongbing Shan and Peter Visentin
University of Lethbridge
Canada

1. Introduction

For researchers, surface electromyography (EMG) seems a seductive technology because it provides a non-invasive means to acquire in-vivo data about physiological processes that cause muscles to produce movement. It captures muscle activity during any movement of a body by measuring seizure potentials released by the muscles when they are activated. Consequently, measured potentials are typically used to fractionate a body's response process as well as get timing of neural control and coordination among muscle groups. Such analyses permit assessments of technical skills which, in turn, provide foundational information for biofeedback training and development of new pedagogical methods. Consequently, in high-skill activities such as those of the performing arts, EMG would appear to have significant relevance in terms of skill optimization and learning.

On the surface, it is apparent that arts performance shares many characteristics, including health risks, with an area where EMG research has already had a significant disciplinary impact - sports (Chesky, et al., 2002; Lehmann & Davidson, 2002; Wilson, 1986). Pedagogy and training in both sports and performance arts aim to develop physical skills efficiently while avoiding injury for participants. While EMG applications in human sports movements have been an acknowledged aid in improving sport performance for decades (e.g. the Journal of Electromyography and Kinesiology has a 21-year history in this regard), applications in arts performances are still rare. Further, a review of the literature shows that, EMG applications in the arts tend to fall into only three broad categories: skill analysis descriptions and establishment of norms, training method evaluations, biofeedback in both pedagogy and injury remediation (Kjelland, 2000).

This book chapter details selected examples where EMG technology is used in applications pertinent to arts performance. Since almost all EMG studies rely upon initial skill analysis and description in order to establish norms, research in the performance arts is often a multi-stage process. Exemplars for purposes of discussion will be drawn from instrumental and vocal performance, as well as ballet. The goals of the selected research focus on: 1) describing the activity of selected muscles, 2) identifying innate abilities or talents, 3) quantifying the efficiency and effectiveness of pedagogical methods, 4) diagnosing technical difficulties, or 5) determining loading intensity during performance and evaluating factors related to pain and injury. Given the small body of existing EMG studies in the arts, the examples below are mainly chosen to elaborate the potential and relevance of EMG research in the performing arts as well as to encourage more research in the area.

2. Representative examples

2.1 Skill analysis

In the areas of skill analysis and evaluation of training, EMG methods in music research are typically borrowed from kinesiology and sports, where they are used to quantify athletic potential and/or development, effectiveness of muscle group coordination and degree of motor control optimization (Riley & Chong, 2010). To accomplish skill analysis, researchers' choice of data processing methods and analysis techniques play an important role. Since EMG signals are dependent on individual biological make-up (e.g. skin thickness, subcutaneous layers of fat or other soft tissues, etc.) and technical factors (e.g. placement of the sensors), any raw data gathered is unavoidably non-quantitative as a measure of neural-muscular activity. For example, a sumo wrestler might generate lower measured EMG signals than a 90-pound ballerina, yet no one should be surprised at the outcome of a basho match-up between them. Thus raw data from EMG is typically processed in a number of ways. The technique of enveloping stabilizes signals for researchers and, in order to provide quasi-quantification, normalization of enveloped data is required (Kjelland, 2000; Morasky, Reynolds, & Clarke, 1981; Zinn, 1998). By expressing all measurements as a percentage of a chosen reference value (i.e. normalization), EMG provides a viable means of comparison among different subjects and trials. Commonly used references for normalization include: 1) the maximum signal level during a trial, or 2) a Maximum Voluntary Contraction (MVC) determined in a separate trial under high-load conditions.

One particularly illuminating example of music skill analysis in the existing literature looks at the singing of onsets (Shan & Visentin, 2010). "Onset" is a term used in music to describe the start of a pitch or tone. Whether singing or playing an instrument, onsets require a highly coordinated physical effort to generate sound. The articulatory nature of them is a vital component of musical expression. Thus, control of this element is important for all musicians. Since consistency and ease of effort during singing/playing can be taken as a measure of skill, analysis of this element can be equally important for researchers as an evaluative measure of skill development during training.

Figure 1 shows rectus abdominis activity of a trained mezzo-soprano singer executing onsets at three different pitch levels. Each trial consisted of ten onsets performed in two sets of five. Each set of five entailed singing a single pitch using four short vocalizations (approx. 1s. each) followed by one long vocalization (approx. 4s.). The singer was permitted to take a small breath between each of the onsets. There was about a two second break between each set of five. This same protocol was used at three different pitch frequencies - high (black), medium (dark grey) and low (light grey) covering the vocal range typical for a mezzo-soprano.

In terms of skill analysis, Figure 1 allows evaluation of training through an examination of the consistency and repeatability of the singing and the muscular activity used to accomplish the singing. Varying EMG amplitudes show that significantly different amounts of physical effort were required at different pitch levels. For low and medium pitch, although there was still a clear pattern of muscular activity, there was insignificant difference in EMG data between singing and rest with peak levels 10%-20% of the MVC. At high pitch, peak levels of EMG were above 60% of the MVC. Together these show a non-linear relationship between pitch and effort required to sing. Importantly, at the highest pitch level there was a notable difference in physical effort between the beginning of the longer sustained tone and its end. Between onsets, low EMG measurements show disciplined anticipatory preparation typical of highly skilled individuals. Such results have implications for vocal pedagogy, since perceptual awareness of physiological phenomena allows coaches to direct training.

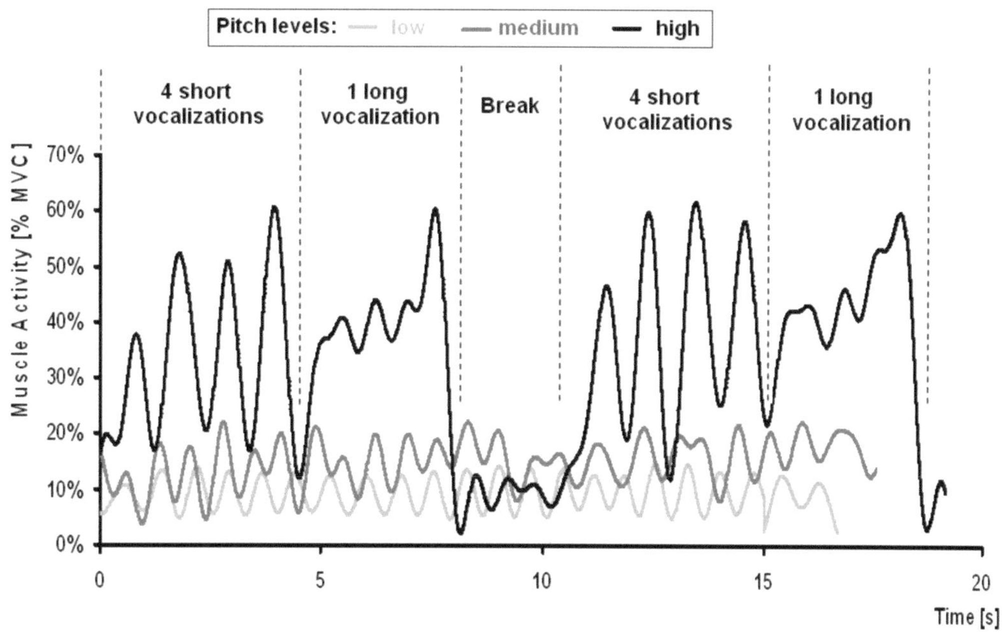

Fig. 1. Rectus abdominis activity of a trained singer at different pitch frequencies.

Evaluations of skills using EMG such as the one above can identify muscle recruitment strategies and provide information about fine motor training for music learners and professionals by showing physical adaptations resulting from training. In music, it is generally accepted among researchers and performers that that sustained levels of muscle contraction inhibit smooth motor movements and contribute to fatigue in both practicing and performing. EMG provides an excellent tool for measuring these characteristics, providing objective information that may help enhance artistic outcomes.

2.2 Pedagogical applications

A 1989 study broke new ground in the performing arts area when it used EMG to compare three different technical approaches to playing the piano (Bejjani et al., 1989). In a case study, a professional-level pianist was asked to perform three pianistic tasks using three defined postural orientations of the hand. Although it may seem to the reader somewhat artificial to have the same player adopt multiple postural orientations for the same musical passage, such adaptations are common when performing since the act of performance is by definition one of adaptation to "the moment". Rather than simply measuring a postural orientation to establish a "norm", the study validated the utility of EMG as a means to discriminate technique-related differential muscle activity. Where some muscle activity appeared to be posturally and task independent, others were clearly technique related. For the anterior deltoid, it was postulated that EMG activity during playing of arpeggios (one of the three tested tasks) was related primarily to idiosyncrasies of the performer since there was no significant difference in data among the three techniques examined. On the other hand, the flexor carpi radialis showed significant changes between techniques. Such findings have potential ramifications for pedagogy. Based on Bejjani's observations, since changes in technique do not alter the data, the deltoid muscle could effectively be neglected during training and the pedagogical focus can be directed toward those that muscles that are technique dependent. However, this conclusion might be misleading. The experiment design examined predetermined postural orientations of the hands and wrists - a three segment physics chain: hand, forearm, & upper arm - essentially eliminating the significance of the trunk. In piano performance it is more and more understood that the trunk of the body plays a vital role, an examination of which would require a minimum of a four-segment chain. It may be the case that the deltoid is vital in some other way not examined in Bejjani's work. Far from being a criticism of Bejjani's study, this underscores his assertion that there is a great need for more varied EMG studies to be undertaken in the piano performance area.

Pedagogical potential of EMG research was further underscored in 1991 in a study by Heuser and McNitt-Gray. These researchers undertook skill analyses associated with trumpet embouchure and tone production (Heuser & Mcnittgray, 1991). On the trumpet, quality of a tone's commencement is a result of careful synchronization of breath, lips and tongue. Hence from a muscular standpoint, the interaction of small and large muscles must occur in a very delicate balance. It is a fact that almost all players at one time or another can experience difficulties in achieving the effects they desire. Heuser's study examined embouchure muscles in preparation for playing both sustained and staccato (short) tones. Results indicated that EMG was an effective way to identify some aspects of tone production difficulties even for the very small muscles associated with the embouchure. In a later study, Iltis & Givens undertook similar work focussed on comparing the EMG of a horn player exhibiting embouchure distonia with that of healthy performers (Iltis & Givens, 2005). From a pedagogical standpoint such work could lead to the development of compensatory strategies for players who suffer from such vocational musculoskeletal disorders.

As in music, the use of EMG in dance can be highly varied. Its measurements can yield useful information about neuromusculoskeletal processes as well as artistic outcomes in performance. In spite of performance variability and the versatility of motor control among dancers, data has been used a means to distinguish experts from novices, track training changes and measure learning outcomes. Variability in data can illuminate temporal relationships between neural and musculoskeletal patterns with an ultimate goal of facilitating comparisons and developing normative data sets as reference points for training, performance, clinical practice, and research (Chatfield, 2003).

Studies such as the one by Chatfield (2003) show EMG to have significant pedagogical potential. For muscles that are truly technique independent, the training process can be simplified by paying more attention to other muscles. Further, idiosyncratic behaviours of a learner might be more easily observed in erratic or abnormal activity of such muscles. For muscles that are technique dependent, it is possible that either: 1) EMG patterns observed in high level professionals may be used as goals to train toward because they represent the most efficient and effective use of the body notwithstanding choice of technical approach, or 2) they can be used to evaluate the effectiveness of various training methods, and indeed develop new ones, by observing those that achieve the desired muscle activity effects most rapidly.

2.3 Vocational health and wellness applications

In addition to its pedagogical utility, EMG has important medical applications relevant to arts performance. In the arts, as in sports, preventive maintenance toward long-term personal well-being is becoming more widely understood as a foundational goal of training, even though the underlying motivations for this ethical shift may differ between the two disciplines. In many sports, it has been generally understood that injuries are a part of the "game". However, since the real cost of a multi-million dollar athlete missing a game is very high, injury avoidance can be motivated by the economics of the sports business model. In the performance arts, economic necessity is not generally the primary driver of concerns in this regard for two reasons: 1) artists generally do what they do because they love it to the degree that "self" is subjugated to the artistic goal (both from health & wellness and financial standpoints), and 2) the arts are seldom driven by a profit-oriented business model. Unfortunately, and perhaps as a consequence of the above, injury rates among performing artists are extraordinarily high but the investment in injury prevention is extremely low. Reported rates of musculoskeletal injuries in professional musicians range between 50% and 76% (Fishbein, Middlestadt, Ottati, Straus, & Ellis, 1988; Fry, 1986, 1988; Middlestadt & Fishbein, 1989; Zaza, 1998).

Fortunately, conditions are currently ripe for more arts medicine research mainly because of a dogged dedication to raising awareness by organizations such as the Performing Arts Medical Association. In its nearly 30 years of efforts, it has become an inclusive alliance of the medical, therapeutic, scientific and artistic communities that deals with vocational issues of artists ranging from musculoskeletal disorders to psychological ones. As of the year 2010, there were at least 17 specialized centers in the United States that focus on performing arts medicine, whereas a decade ago there would have been only a small handful. The rising interest is proof that there is much more to be done, both in terms of treatment and prevention. EMG has the potential to be a fundamental tool in both injury prevention and remediation research.

Some of the most effective uses of EMG in this area have been in research that brings multiple technologies to bear on a single question. Multi-modal research can provide an excellent means of better understanding factors associated with vocational injuries (Visentin, Shan, & Schultz, 2004). In a recent study of repetitive loading of the lower limb, patellar disorders, a condition common in dancers, was examined using EMG and magnetic resonance imaging MRI (Albisetti, Bartolomeo, Gabbiadini, Ventura, & Parrini, 2008). The case study involving a professional ballet dancer suffering from anterior knee pain confirmed EMG as a useful method to help diagnose and guide treatment. The research was able to demonstrate the role of particular muscles in patellar maltracking, in this case by determining a difference in onset latency of the vastus medialis obliquus and vastus lateralis of the dancer's painful knee as compared to her asymptomatic one.

Other recent research has also made efforts to enhance the significance of EMG by using multi-modal technologies. It is now well accepted that postural and behavioural practices are factors that can influence the development of musculoskeletal movement disorders. In a study investigating causal factors underlying the aetiology of repetitive stress injuries in professional violinists, EMG was used in conjunction with 3-dimensional motion analysis technology and biomechanical modeling to find relationships between posture and internal loading intensity, laying the groundwork for developing injury prevention strategies (Visentin & Shan, 2003; Visentin, et al., 2004). In these linked studies, EMG was used to determine loading patterns on the muscles and biomechanical modeling was used to confirm and further quantify the results. The left shoulder during violin playing proved to be static while right shoulder exhibited more varied behaviours ranging from quasi-static to dynamic. For the left arm, static shoulder loads were present regardless of the string being played or speed of the activity. Notably, the lowest level of the "dynamic" right shoulder was comparable to the level of the left shoulder. The maximum observed muscle intensity of the right side was four times higher than that of the left (a finding confirmed by both EMG and joint load analysis. Based on statistical studies, shoulder injury rates are comparable (51% for the right and 49% for the left) despite the differing kinematic and kinetic patterns (Fry, 1988). Through this kind of comparison the study demonstrated the significance of the type of muscle activity in terms injury causality. Looking at absolute values, the study showed that risk levels were essentially identical between static and dynamic loads even when dynamic loading was shown to be up to three or four times greater.

The implications of such research are far ranging and can influence pedagogy, learning, injury prevention and remediation. EMG can provide objective data that serves as a basis for understanding of biological and physiological process involved with arts performance. Further it can aid in evaluating and establishing pedagogical "best practices". For example, the results of the violin study above suggest the need for development of more refined teaching strategies and in a later study the same authors indeed do extrapolate from the data in developing such strategies (Visentin, Shan, & Wasiak, 2008). Discussion in this article suggested some prevention strategies might be developed to include: 1) consciously invoking movements that minimize static postures (For example, to prevent left shoulder injuries, it appears a logical strategy to change the static nature of the muscle activity), 2) transfering loads from one muscle group to another (perhaps by using subtle postural changes that alternate the motor control pattern), or 3) reconceiving the playing mechanism in a variety of different ways to minimize unnecessary muscle loading.

It must be noted that applications of EMG in the performing arts may involve changing some of the conceptual paradigms of EMG research. In the immediately preceding example, both EMG and biomechanical modeling showed violin playing to be "low-load". On average, measured EMG remained below 20% of MVC and, in fact, some muscles consistently used as little as 5%. Such conditions would be considered "safe" for most activities, but are clearly not so for the kinds of muscular (repetitive) use that is needed in the pursuit of artistic excellence in the performing arts. Such work clearly indicates that both researchers and artists need to be willing to re-examine the fundamental beliefs and understandings of their disciplines.

3. Conclusion

Even though when compared to sports and kinesiology there is a small body of EMG research investigating arts performance, the examples above illuminate the potential and relevance of EMG applications in this area. Studies based upon skill descriptions and quantification of anatomical & physiological phenomena will permit better assessments and analyses of technical skills in terms of the training process, artistic development, and the refinement of pedagogical methods - all of which provides foundational information for artists in their pursuit of a long, fulfilling and healthy career. However, artistry is typically an individualistic quest predicated on the strong vision of an outcome. This is a fact that all science-based research needs to carefully consider. As a result, research in the performance arts should be expected to involve a multi-stage process where research design is both application driven and can be viewed as relevant by the artistic community. The examples identified in this book chapter show EMG research to have significant application potential in the performing arts; it remains for researchers and artists to engage in the collaborative processes that might encourage more research in this area.

4. Acknowledgment

This work was supported by funding of CREDO program/University of Lethbridge and National Sciences and Engineering Research Council of Canada (NSERC).

5. References

Albisetti, W., Bartolomeo, O., Gabbiadini, S., Ventura, A., & Parrini, M. (2008). Surface EMG Evaluation of Patellofemoral Pain Syndrome in a Professional Ballet Dancer. Medical Problems of Performing Artists, 23(1), 29-32.

Bejjani, F., Ferrara, L., Xu, N., Tomaino, C., Pavlidis, L., Wu, J., & Dommerholt, J. (1989). Comparison of three piano techniques as an implementation of a proposed experimental design. Medical Problems of Performing Artists, 4(3), 109-103.

Chatfield, S. (2003). Variability of Electromyographic and Kinematic Measurement in Dance Medicine and Science Research. Journal of Dance Medicine & Science, 7(2), 42-48.

Fishbein, M., Middlestadt, S., Ottati, V., Straus, S., & Ellis, A. (1988). Medical problems among ICSOM musicians:overview of a national survey. Medical Problems of Performing Artists, 3(1), 1-8.

Fry, H. (1986). Overuse syndrome of the upper limb in musicians. Medical Journal of Australia, 144(4), 182-185.

Fry, H. (1988). Patterns of over-use seen in 658 affected instrumental musicians. International Journal of Music Education, 11(1), 3-16.

Heuser, F., & Mcnittgray, J. L. (1991). Emg Potentials Prior to Tone Commencement in Trumpet Players. Medical Problems of Performing Artists, 6(2), 51-56.

Iltis, P., & Givens, M. (2005). EMG Characterization of Embouchure Muscle Activity: Reliability and Application to Embouchure Dystonia. [Research]. Medical Problems of Performing Artists, 20(1), 25-34.

Kjelland, J. (2000). Application of Electromyography and Electromyographic Biofeedback in Music Performance Research: A Review of the Literature since 1985. Medical Problems of Performing Artists, 15(3), 115-118.

Middlestadt, S., & Fishbein, M. (1989). The prevelance of severe musculoskeletal problems among male and female symphony orchestra string players. Medical Problems of Performing Artists, 4(1), 41-48.

Morasky, R. L., Reynolds, C., & Clarke, G. (1981). Using biofeedback to reduce left arm extensor EMG of string players during musical performance. Biofeedback and self-regulation, 6(4), 565-572.

Riley, k., & Chong, J. (2010). Garrick Olsson on Technique: mastering the paradoxical element of control. Clavier Companion, 2(5), 12-21.

Shan, G., & Visentin, P. (2010). Arts Biomechanics - An Infant Science: Its Challenges and Future. NOVA Publishers, ISBN: 978-1-60876-809-7, New York, USA.

Shan, G., Visentin, P., & Schultz, A. (2004). Multi-dimensional Signal Analysis as a means of better understanding factors associated with repetitive use in violin performance. Medical Problems of Performing Artists, 19(3), 129-139.

Visentin, P., & Shan, G. (2003). The kinetic characteristics of the bow arm during violin performance; an examination of internal loads as a function of tempo. Medical Problems of Performing Artists, 18(3), 91-97.

Visentin, P., Shan, G., & Wasiak, E. B. (2008). Informing music teaching and learning using movement analysis technology. International Journal of Music Education, 26(1), 71-85.

Zaza, C. (1998). Playing-related musculoskeletal disorders in musicians: A systematic review of incidence & prevalence. Canadian Medical Association Journal, 158(8), 1019-25.

Zinn, M. (1998). The use of sEMG feedback for transfer of relaxation into piano technique [unpublished]. . Master, Illinois Institute of Technology, Chicago.

14

Surface Electromyography During Both Standing and Walking in *m. Ulnaris lateralis* of Diversely Trained Horses

Miss Kiara K. Salomons[1], Aziz Tnibar[2] and Adrian P. Harrison[1]

[1]IBHV, Faculty of Life Sciences, Copenhagen University
[2]Dept. of Large Animal Sciences, Medicine & Surgery, Faculty of Life Sciences, Copenhagen University
[1,2]Denmark

1. Introduction

The primary aim of any conditioning program in athletic horses is to improve performance by inducing physiological changes within the animal's body, including limb muscles and tendons (Rivero, 2007). To this end, electromyography (EMG) has been used in human studies to determine muscle fitness and general muscle strength, but it also serves as an indicator of muscle injury and/or disease (Licka et al., 2009; Heaf et al., 2010).
A good many studies have relied on needle electromyography (Tokuriki et al., 1989; Wijnberg et al., 2003a; Winjberg et al., 2003b), which in many ways is a precise technique, giving access to information about individual motor units within muscles, but this technique does not lend itself readily to muscles during periods of rapid and forceful contraction. Under such situations surface electromyography (sEMG) is preferred and in the equine, studies of primarily the back muscles have been undertaken (Licka et al., 2001; Licka et al., 2004; Peham et al. 2001), although sEMG has been used in ponies to identify forelimb muscle function (Jansen et al., 1992).
Being a rapid, painless and non-invasive method of measuring muscle activity, surface electromyography (sEMG) is potentially useful in equine athletes. For horses competing in sports events, it is essential that their limbs remain healthy and sound. Indeed, lameness and training induced injuries of the forelimb have become increasingly more common in competition horses (Kohnke, 2004; Firth, 2006), mainly as a result of a raised athletic level and increasing numbers of horses participating in competitions. It is not surprising therefore that sEMG has already begun to be used to supplement clinical findings in injured horses, and is very often explored as an informative technique when other means of clinical examination fail (Wijnberg et al., 2004).
Perhaps of greater importance, however, is the very real potential to use this technique as a measure of muscle efficiency during locomotion/exercise and in so doing, provide an insight into a horses muscle fitness and health at any given point in time, as well as enable a rider or owner to follow an individual animals response to training. sEMG reflects the force and degree of activity/coordination of a muscle during a gait cycle, revealing bursts of activity when a muscle is active (Robert et al., 1999; Butcher et al., 2009). Yet, despite this

very real potential to assist with improving and monitoring training programs, very few data exist with regard to horses, whether exercised or not.

The purpose of this study was, therefore, to validate sEMG recordings on worked and non-worked animals, and to generate reference data for further use in equine training studies. The underlying hypotheses in this study were; 1) muscle efficiency, as measured using sEMG signal analysis, is greater in worked than non-worked horses, 2) increasing age and body weight reduces muscle force and efficiency, and 3) injured horses present with a sEMG signal that is very different from that of un-injured horses.

2. Materials and methods

2.1 Animals

This study recruited 18 horses of different breed, age and training level, the later being established from FEI competition tests, as VO_{2max} could not be measured. Horses were weighed on a large animal scale where possible, whilst others were assessed using a measuring band placed around their girth (see Table 1).

Of the 18 horses, numbers 1-6 were considered to be "non-worked" (NW), and these were stabled at the Animal Hospital facility as teaching horses for veterinarians (Department of Large Animal Sciences, Medicine & Surgery, Taastrup, Faculty of Life Sciences, Copenhagen University).

Horse No.	Exercise/training level	Name	Age (years)	Body weight (kg)	Height (cm)	Body Mass (kg/m^2)
1	NW	Bella	9	558	155	248.0
2	NW	Heksehyl	6	635	160	282.2
3	NW	Nathalie	7	625	160	277.8
4	NW	Mary	7	655	155	291.1
5	NW	Ingrid	9	473	150	210.2
6	NW	Benedikte	7	550	150	244.4
7	W	Akina	6	470	164	174.7
8	W	Telle	8	592	180	182.7
9	W	Zozet	13	552	166	200.3
10	W	Madonna	20	550	167	197.2
11	W	Kento	8	498	166	180.7
12	W	Kojak	26	470	141	236.4
13	HW	Camixa	6	511	177	163.1
14	HW	Laval	13	504	170	174.4
15	HW	Akeem	14	596	171	203.8
16	HW	Gallion	16	524	165	192.5
17	HW	Lambourghini	14	478	168	169.4
18	HW	Maxi	7	448	148	204.5

Table 1. Horse data including an estimate of training/exercise level and body mass (BM). NW = non worked, W = worked to a low level, and HW = hard worked e.g. Grand-Prix standard.

Horses numbers 7-12 where measured at a private stable (Tune, Roskilde) and were fed according to their level of exercise and training, which was deemed to be "worked" (W). These horses were sent out to pasture every day and trained/exercised on a daily basis. Horses numbers 13-18 were measured at another private stable (Kokkedal), and were provided with feed appropriate to their level of work, which was assessed as being "hard worked" (HW). These were horses that were typically used for competition (primarily dressage competitions at a National level) and therefore used to travelling.

2.2 Procedures

Horses where shaved in the region of the muscle *Ulnaris lateralis* (UL) and sEMG recording electrodes were applied. A ground or reference electrode was applied to the *medial styloid process* on the tip of the radius bone. Self-sticking (Co-plus) bandaged was wrapped around the leg in the region of the electrodes in order to prevent electrodes from being dislodged.

2.2.1 sEMG measurements

This study followed the guidelines laid out in the *European Recommendations for Surface ElectroMyoGraphy* as detailed by the SENIAM project (Hermens et al., 1999). The recorded surface EMG signal was assessed as described previously in terms of signal frequency (Hz), peak-to-peak amplitude (mV), mean amplitude frequency (mVs^{-1}) and the maximum power (mV^2) using Chart analysis software (AD Instruments, Chalgrove, Oxfordshire, UK).
A double differential electrode configuration, with electrodes (N-00-S & R-00-S; Blue Sensor, Medicotest A/S, Ølstykke, Denmark) was adopted as described previously (Heaf et al., 2010; Andersen et al., 2008). sEMG recordings were taken *via* an ML 132 amplifier connected to a ML780 PowerLab/8s A/D converter (ADInstruments, Chalgrove, Oxfordshire, UK) with a further connection to a MacBook Air with Chart v. 5.5.6/s Software, Peak Parameters and Spike Histogram extensions. Input impedance was 200 MΩ differential, and a high and a low pass filter of 3 Hz and 500 Hz, respectively, were used. Sampling speed was set to 100,000 per second.
Background noise from the recording environment in which the horses were measured was checked to ensure an adequate signal was obtainable. Prior to data recording for standing and walking, the background noise was evaluated for each horse, however, none of the stable environments exhibited unduly high levels of background noise or electrical interference.
Measurements, taken during standing, were recorded for about a minute, after which the horse was walked (5-8 strides) to obtain a stable recording of ambulatory activity in the UL muscle. Horses were usually walked twice so as to obtain a more representative measurement. Leg posture was examined and noted as well as photographed. All horses except one were found to be sound and had no history of leg illnesses that we were informed of. One lame horse (no. 16) was measured on both forelimbs, since it had suffered an injury to the right forelimb at the region of the proximal phalanx. In this particular animal, the UL appeared to the naked eye to be enlarged (swollen/inflamed) in the right- *cf* the left- forelimb. In the case of horse No. 16, a recording of the superficial digital flexor tendon was made on both fore limbs in conjunction with a simultaneous recording from UL. The superficial digital flexor tendon recording was in the form of a movement artefact, representing a change in the position and thickness of the tendon relative to the fixed recording electrodes on the skin, during a period of muscle contraction.

2.3 Statistical analysis

Data are presented as mean ± SEM. Differences between means were tested for statistical significance with the use of GraphPad Instat 3 for Mac (Version 3.0b, 2003; GraphPad Inc., La Jolla, CA), with an additional test for Gaussian normal distribution. A one-way ANOVA was used to measure statistical differences between the means for all of the horse groups. Differences between means showing a *P* value >0.05 were considered non-significant.

3. Results

Ulnaris lateralis is a lateral palmar forelimb muscle connected to both the accessory carpal bone and the fourth metatarsal bone, and to the lateral humeral epicondyle. It is a muscle that is mainly comprised short fibers and is strong and stiff, with a peak isometric force of F_{max} = 5731 N, serving to stabilize the carpus during the stance phase of gait (Brown et al., 2003). In Figure 1 (see below) individual sEMG amplitudes and frequencies are presented for UL *cf* the mean of the group.

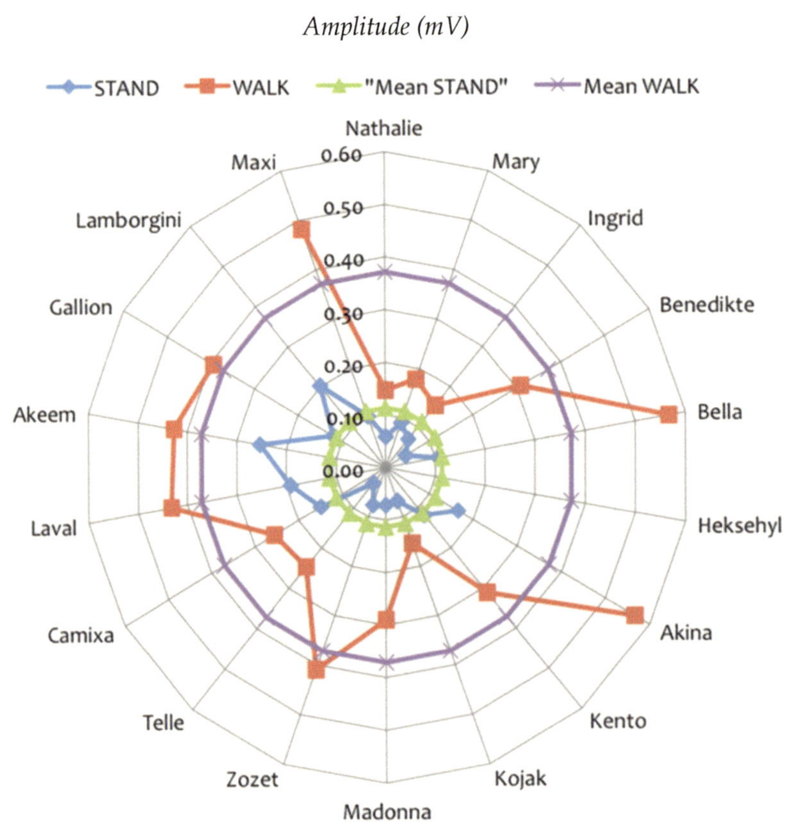

Fig. 1. (Continued)

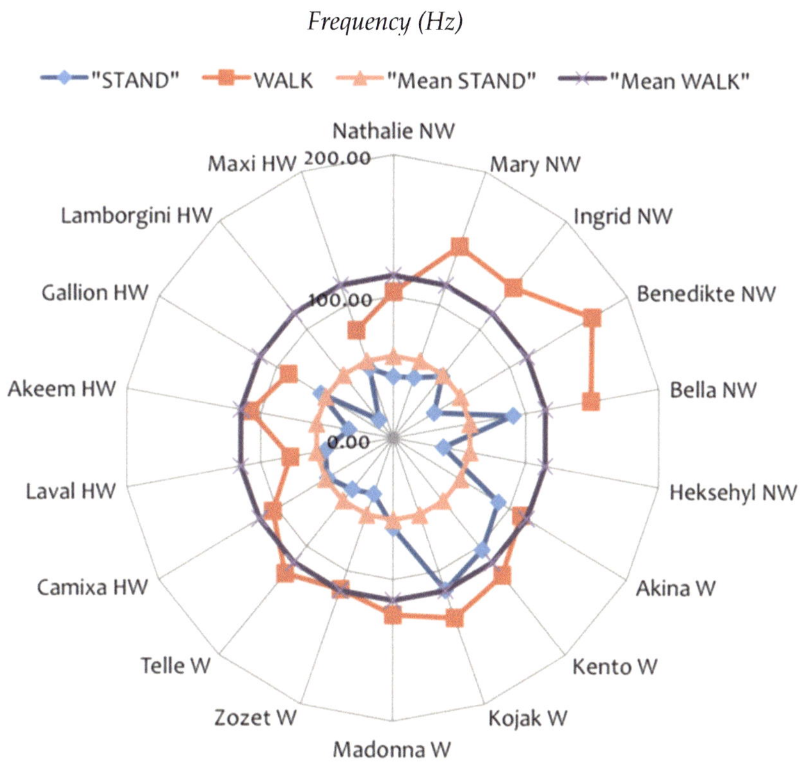

Fig. 1. A: Individual sEMG signal amplitude values for horses in this study during periods of both standing and walking compared to the mean value of the whole group. B: Individual sEMG signal frequency values for horses in this study during periods of both standing and walking compared to the mean value of the whole group. Worked (W), hard worked (HW) and non-worked (NW) horses.

3.1 sEMG amplitude data

The standing mean amplitude for the sEMG of UL was measured to be 0.17 ± 0.03 mV for HW horses, 0.09 ± 0.01 mV for W horses and just 0.07 ± 0.01 mV for the NW horses. The sEMG signal amplitude during walking was found to be more than three-fold that of the standing data with 0.50 ± 0.09 mV for HW horses, 0.33 ± 0.05 mV for W horses, and 0.27 ± 0.06 mV for NW horses (see Figure 2 below).

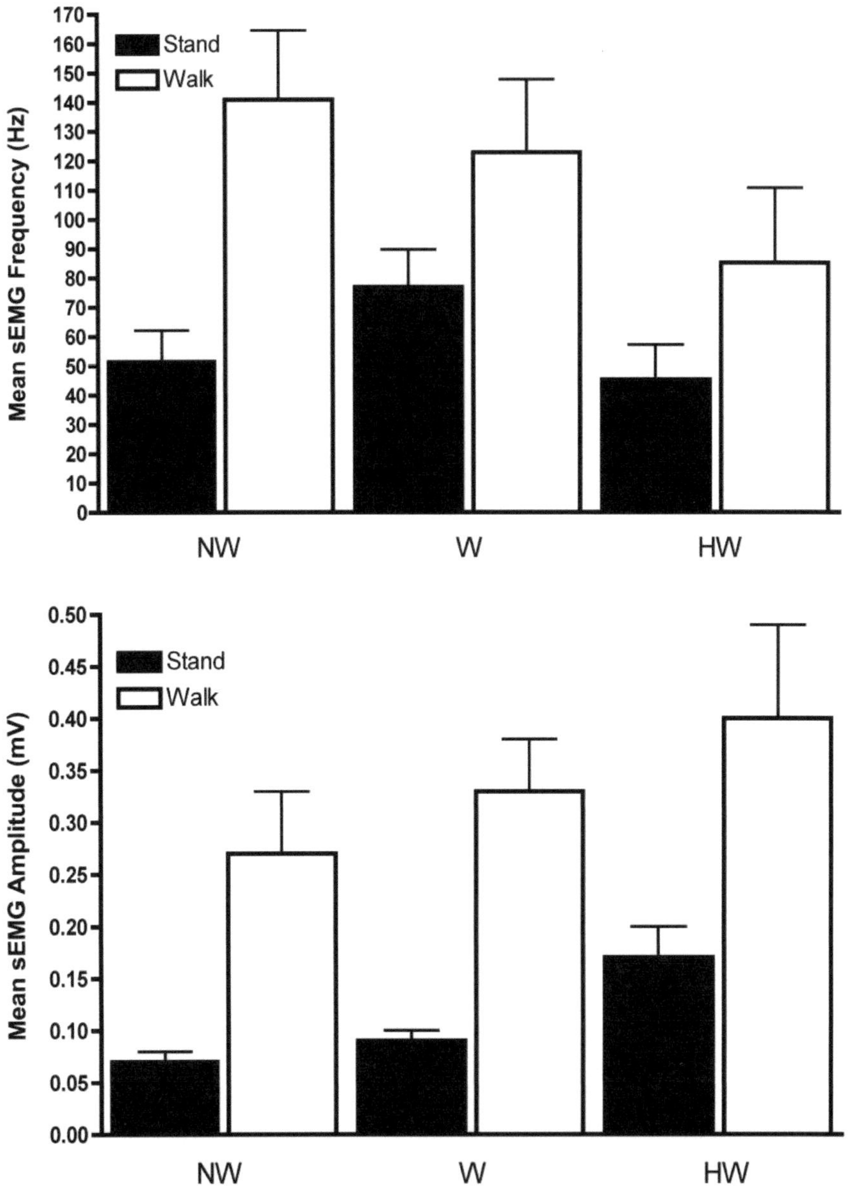

Fig. 2. Mean sEMG signal frequency (Hz) and amplitude (mV) values for *Ulnaris lateralis* during periods of standing and walking for Worked (W), hard worked (HW) and non-worked (NW) horses. Note that an increase in the level of training/exercise results in an improved degree of coordination such that the CMAP frequency falls and the amplitude rises - indicative of fast, coordinated recruitment of large MU´s.

sEMG signal amplitude varied between individual horses, and in particular among highly trained horses, which were above the mean, and where a greater individual difference between horses in terms of the degree of training/exercise was noted.

3.2 sEMG frequency data

A mean sEMG signal frequency for all the horses during standing and walking revealed values of 57.89 ± 11.83 Hz and 114.74 ± 24.78 Hz, respectively.

The mean frequency difference between standing and walking for HW horses was 39.79 Hz, whilst for W horses this was 45.69 Hz. NW horses were found to have twice the mean difference e.g. 89.43 Hz (see Figure 2). Indeed, there was a significant difference between NW and HW horses ($P<0.01$), and between W and HW horses ($P<0.05$) in terms of the sEMG signal frequency. Moreover, a positive correlation ($R^2 = 0.722$) was found between sEMG signal frequency and body weight of the W horses.

3.3 Leg posture/ lameness

A couple of horses (No.´s 2 & 16) were found to have an unusual leg posture, whilst one horse had been lame for some time. Indeed, these horses were recorded as having a very different sEMG signal from that of the healthy horses, and as a result they were excluded from most of the calculations. Horse no. 2 presented with a leg posture for the forelimbs in which it distributed its body weight to the leading edge of the hoof giving it a constant forward angle of both carpus. This resulted in a sEMG signal amplitude of 0.66 mV whereas the mean for the non-worked group was 0.07 mV during standing.

Horse no. 16 had been diagnosed lame due to right front fetlock osteoarthritis but it was still being ridden with care. Likewise, this horse was found to differ in its sEMG signal from that of the other horses in the HW group in terms of both amplitude and frequency. Furthermore, this particular horse presented with a left forelimb that performed during walking as per a normal HW horse in terms of its sEMG signal, whereas the right forelimb (injured leg) yielded a sEMG signal with a higher CMAP frequency, more typical of that for a W or NW horse; left forelimb 90 Hz & 0.39 mV *cf* right forelimb 122 Hz & 0.30 mV.

4. Discussion

This study, which endorses the sensitivity of sEMG as a non-invasive measure of muscular function in horses, confirms that muscle efficiency (short coordinated bursts), as measured using sEMG signal analysis, is greater in worked than non-worked horses. Likewise, this study has revealed that injured horses present with a sEMG signal that is very different from that of un-injured horses.

4.1 Exercise and the sEMG signal

Adaptation to physical training in both human and equine studies, has documented improvements in both neural activity patterns as well a fibre changes (Felici, 2006). In a recent study it was shown that exercise positively influences hypertrophy and neuromuscular excitability in humans and horses (Mileva et al., 2010; Wijnberg et al., 2008). Indeed, both of these authors found an increase in amplitude with exercise, a finding that is in agreement with the present study (see Figure 2). Wijnberg and colleagues (Winjberg et al., 2008) found, for the horses that they tested, an amplitude of 0.23 mV in m. vastus lateralis at rest (standing), a value that is very comparable with that of the HW horses in this study taken at rest/standing (mean amplitude of 0.17 mV in UL).

The short yet coordinated bursts of sEMG signal activity in the HW horses in the present study reflects a training induced synchronization of the individual compound muscle action potentials (CMAPs) within the UL muscle measured (Mileva et al., 2010; Wijnberg et al., 2008).

Indeed, CMAP synchronization has been cited as a means of increasing muscle strength or power (Leisson et al., 2008). To which end, the trained horses in the present study were found to have a much higher power (0.75 mVs^{-1}) than non-trained horses (0.3 mVs^{-1}).

sEMG signal frequency was also affected by training, such that HW horses had a lower frequency than NW horses ($P < 0.01$). This is not surprising in many ways, as muscle efficiency is very dependent on motor unit (MU) firing rate, with efficient muscles using a lower frequency (Hz) range when recruiting MU´s in a highly synchronized fashion, thereby producing a greater force (Winjberg et al., 2003b). Indeed the findings of the present study suggest that training/exercise induces changes in the sEMG that result in the very fast and coordinated recruitment and firing of large motor units.

This study has also found differences in the pattern of the sEMG signal over a given period of time, with respect to the level of training/exercise (see Figure 3). The horses assigned to the NW group were typically found to present with a sEMG signal in which short

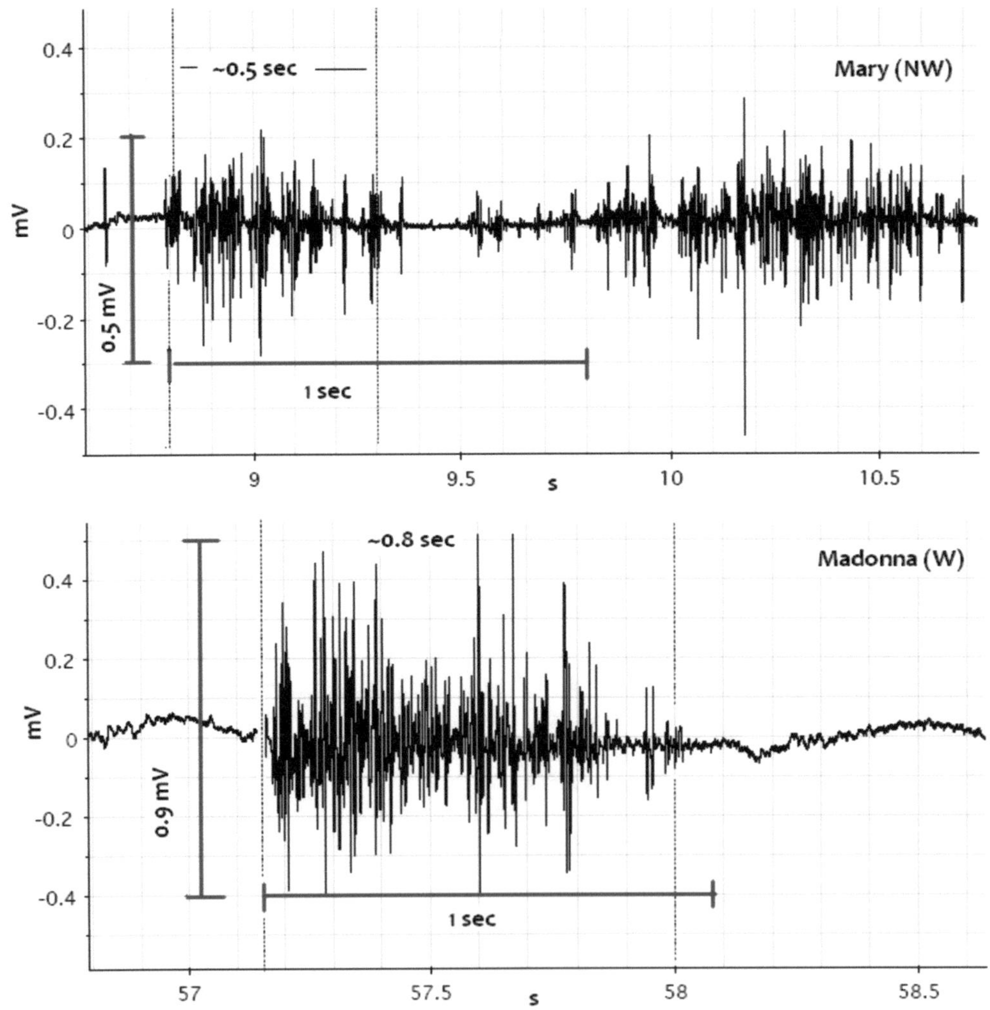

Fig. 3. (Continued)

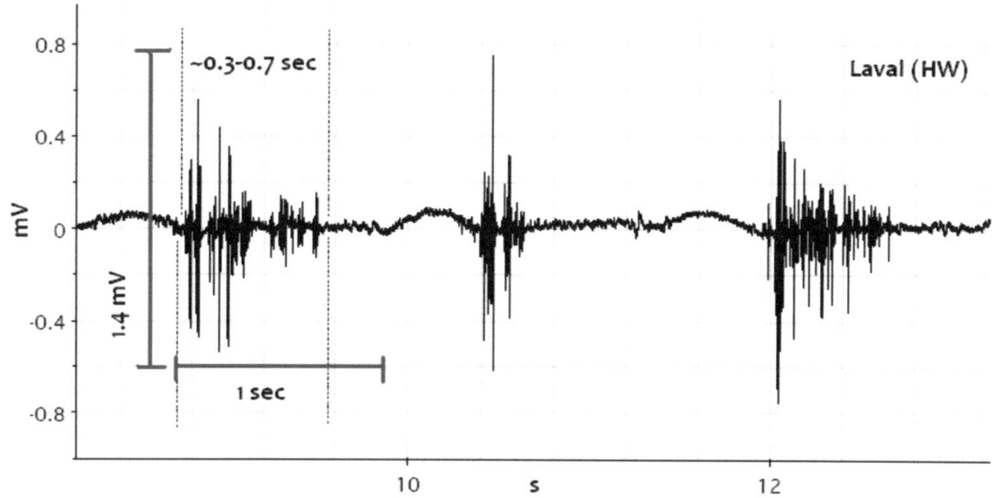

Fig. 3. Raw sEMG data for one horse in each of the three training/exercise groups; Worked (W), hard worked (HW) and non-worked (NW) horses. Data have been taken for the largest positive spike when walking. Note the difference in sEMG signal with training/exercise level of the horses - HW horses show a more controlled and immediate burst of activity *cf* the other groups where the sEMG signal is slower to reach a peak and of a longer duration. Scaling differs for mV on the Y-axis and for seconds on the X-axis between panels.

intermittent bursts of contraction were found to give rise to a constant (low-level since weak amplitude) activation of the UL muscle – something that can be considered an inefficient use of this particular muscles energy. The W horses on the other hand showed long bursts of activity of the sEMG signal followed by periods of inactivity giving rise to periods of contraction and relaxation. Finally, the HW horses typically showed a sEMG pattern comprising very short and coordinated bursts of activity with long periods of inactivity (relaxation) and a considerable signal amplitude; 1.4 mV *cf* 0.9 and 0.5 mV of the W and NW horses, respectively.

4.2 Injury and the sEMG signal

The analysis of the sEMG data collected in the present study, reveals a close similarity of values between individual horses when standing. It is really only when horses walk that differences in sEMG amplitude and frequency become more obvious.

Ulnaris lateralis has a pennation angle of 10-56°, and it is this relatively small pennation angle that gives this muscle its stiffness, contributing considerably to the stability of the carpus joint rather than producing active force as for example *Gluteus medius*. These findings along with previously published electromyography recordings indicate that *ulnaris lateralis* actively prepares for ground contact in the stance phase (Jansen et al., 1992; Brown et al., 2003). Moreover, this muscle has been found to differ between breeds, since thoroughbred horses have a greater muscle thickness than elite standard-bred horses; 70 mm *versus* 61 mm, respectively (Kearns et al., 2002).

It is of interest therefore that the sEMG signal analyses in this study have been able to determine significant changes in UL of horses presenting with signs of misuse or injury to their forelimbs. Horse no. 16 presented with a clear difference in forelimb muscle fitness, with the sEMG signal analysis of its own counterpart forelimb serving as a healthy control (see Figure 4). These findings are important for the future use of sEMG as a research tool in the assessment of muscle health. Injuries, like those of horse no. 16, in which the UL of the right forelimb had a higher firing frequency than that of the left forelimb are commensurate with its role in providing stability to the carpus joint, especially when such a joint is deficient in cartilage, and such changes can be revealed without any invasive and perhaps more damaging procedures or techniques. Indeed, if caught early enough a full and speedy recovery of this forelimb joint may very well be achievable, perhaps through the aid of orthopaedic shoes or either use of IRAP (Interleukin-1 Receptor Antagonist Protein), or PRP (Platelet Rich Plasma).

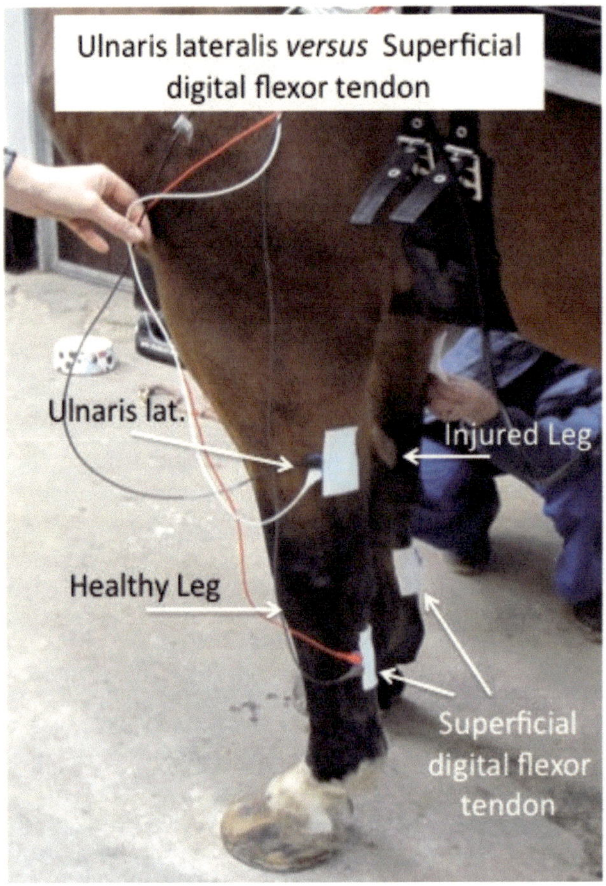

Fig. 4. Photograph of horse no. 16 showing the placement of recording electrodes on the forelimbs - both the healthy and the injured leg. Note too that electrodes were placed over the superficial digital flexor tendon on both legs, and recordings of muscle:tendon (*m. Ulnaris lateralis vs.* Superficial digital flexor) activity were taken simultaneously.

4.3 sEMG reference data

One could imagine the use of sEMG on horses suspected of having various muscle diseases in order that injuries might be caught before they become lethal, and here it is imperative that we have a clear working knowledge of normal and healthy sEMG signals for an array of diverse skeletal muscles so as to rule out any misinterpretation or misdiagnosis. To date there exists a very limited array of data concerning normal equine muscle sEMG paramaters (see Table 2). For instance, Wijnberg and colleagues (Wijnberg et al., 2004) found that myopathogenic muscles have a frequency of <150 Hz, which is far from informative, especially since all the healthy horses with normal muscle function, as defined by the present study, exhibit a frequency below 150 Hz. There is therefore clearly a great need of a reference set of data combining sEMG signal amplitude and frequency along with the horses full anatomical and medical history and work program if the true potential of this technique is to be realized.

EMG data	Muscle	Standing Frequency (Hz)	Walking Frequency (Hz)	Standing Amplitude (mV)	Walking Amplitude (mV)	Reference
Normal NW	Ulnaris lateralis	50	140	0.07	0.27	This study
Normal NW	Hind leg			<0.02		Schuurman *et al* 2003
Normal W	Ulnaris lateralis	75	120	0.09	0.33	This study
Normal HW	Ulnaris lateralis	45	85	0.17	0.5	This study
Normal HW	Hind leg				0.19-0.23	Wijnberg *et al* 2008
Joint Arthritis	Ulnaris lateralis	88	122	0.14	0.3	This study
Myopathogenic muscle	Subclavian	<150		0.28		Wijnberg *et al* 2004
Neuropathic muscle	Subclavian	>150		0.36		Wijnberg *et al* 2004
Uneven standing	Ulnaris lateralis	38		0.66		This study
Fore Head	Temporalis	19-20		0.06		Kruljc & Nemec 2006
Neck NW	Splenius			0.04-0.34		Giovangnoli *et al* 2002
Back NW	Longissimus dorsi				0.07-0.11	Licka *et al* 2009

Table 2. Comparative sEMG data for equine muscles during periods of standing and walking.

4.4 sEMG to tendon artefact

An sEMG signal can be altered/affected in many ways by what have been defined as causative, intermediate and deterministic factors (De Luca, 1997). For a more detailed explanation see the Chapter by Harrison and colleagues in this edition. The causative factors include such parameters as skin thickness and subcutaneous tissue composition and depth, blood flow etc. Thus, by placing a pair of recording electrodes over a tissue that not only moves during a period of contraction, but also changes its thickness and potentially the flow of blood supplying it, one is able to record an artefact. Just such an artefact has been recorded in this study, through the placement of two recording electrodes over the Superficial digital flexor tendon of the forelimb of horse no. 16. In the resting state (standing) the measurement obtained from the two recording electrodes remained very stable, but as the Superficial digital flexor tendon moved relative to the electrodes on the skin´s surface above the tendon (walking), an artefact was recorded - seen as a slight and transient deflection in the recorded signal (see Figure 5). In the case of horse no. 16, it was noted that the peak of this tendon artefact was significantly different in the healthy *cf.* the injured forelimb, such that the limb that had been considerably injured showed a very small time difference (δ - mSec) between the start of the sEMG signal in the *m. Ulnaris lateralis* and the peak of the tendon artefact recorded above the Superficial digital flexor tendon.

In the case of horse no. 16, the healthy left forelimb showed a greater δ compared with the injured right forelimb; 106 mSec *vs.* 49 mSec, respectively (see Figure 5). The greater the time lag between the start of the sEMG signal and the peak of the tendon artefact must be considered as indicative of a greater degree of elasticity in the muscle:tendon complex. Thus, with injury and inflammation one can expect the δ value for the muscle:tendon measurement to be reduced. Indeed, palpation of the two forelimbs gave just such an impression, and the fact that the δ for the injured forelimb was 50% that of the healthy forelimb indicates that in this forelimb very little elasticity remains in the muscle and tendon complex.

Should this condition persist, one might anticipate inflammation and damage of the tendon to bone interface and a permanent change in the tendon structure, towards one that is relatively less- to non-elastic and painful. In support of which the theory of microtrauma proposes that overuse and inflammation gives rise to joint damage e.g. tennis elbow (Roetert et al., 1995). The theory proposes that if a muscle is already at near maximum contraction, vibrations and twisting movements may be transferred directly through the muscle (muscle stiffness at this point being considerable) to the tendinous insertion, causing repeated microtrauma (Roetert et al., 1995). Clearly, there is a need for more detailed studies into muscle:tendon interactions and the incidence of tendon damage. However, studies involving rats have shown that early immobilization diminishes macrophage accumulation and leads to improved tendon-bone healing (Dagher et al., 2009), whilst untreated swollen tendons give rise to localized calcification (Ring et al., 1994).

5. Conclusion

sEMG lends itself to the detection of muscular differences in the forelimb muscle UL of diversely trained horses. Moreover, such information can be used by the owner/rider to help assist in improving and monitoring training programs. There is also a clear benefit of using this technique in the early detection of muscular/leg damage and injury. Indeed, one could envisage the use of sEMG in the assessment of diverse riding styles e.g. "low, deep and round" or "rollkur" particularly since the later has been suggested as increasing the strain on the neck and back muscles of competing horses. Clearly, more research is now needed in this area to further validate the sEMG method in terms of individual muscles, and to provide a bio-bank of data to assist in training and post injury programs.

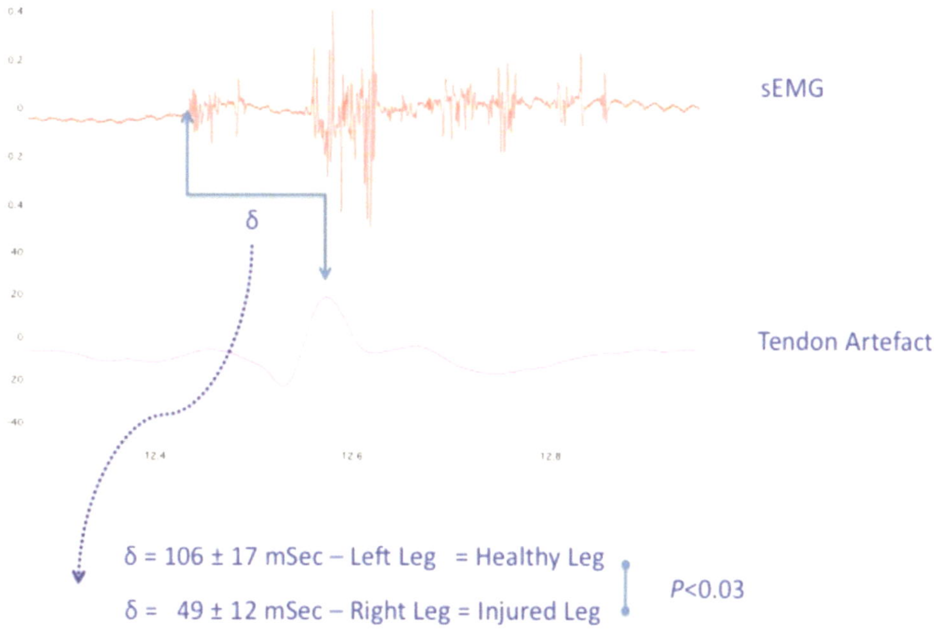

Fig. 5. The raw sEMG signal of *m. Ulnaris lateralis* in relation to the artefact signal from the Superficial digital flexor tendon. Note the significantly shorter time (δ - mSec) for the right injured leg *cf.* that for the left healthy leg. The tendon artefact represents the movement of tissue (tendon) relative to the recording electrodes during a period of muscle contraction and leg movement.

6. Acknowledgement

With thank Hanne Lander Pomykal Carlsson and Birgitte Holle for their skilled assistance during the sEMG recordings. We are most grateful to Lotte Dane, of Stald Dane, and Helene Melsen & Stine T. Jørgensen, Strandagergård, for allowing us access to their horses, their kindness and interest in this work has been a great help in terms of completing this work. We are likewise most grateful to the help and kindness shown by Susanne Nautrup Olsen at Taastrup Animal Hospital, Copenhagen University.

7. References

Andersen, N.K.; Ravn, L.S.; Guy, J.H.; Edwards, S.A. & Harrison, A.P. (2008). Postnatal changes in electromyographic signals during piglet growth, and in relation to muscle fibre types. *Livestock Science,* Vol. 115, pp. 301-312.

Brown, N.A.T.; Kawcak, C.E.; McIlwraith, C.W. & Pandy, M.G. (2003). Architectural Properties of Distal Forelimb Muscles in Horses, Equus caballus. *Journal of Morphology,* Vol. 258, pp. 106–114.

Butcher, M.T.; Hermanson, J.W.; Ducharme, N.G.; Mitchell, L.M.;Sonderholm, L.V. & Bertram, M.J.E.A. (2009). Contractile behavior of the forelimb digital flexors during steady-state locomotion in horses (Equus caballus): An initial test of muscle architectural hypotheses about in vivofunction. *Comparative Biochemistry and Physiology - Part A: Molecular & Integrative Physiology,* Vol. 152, pp. 100-114.

Dagher, E.; Hays, P.L.; Kawamura, S.; Godin, J.; Deng, X.H. & Rodeo, S.A. (2009). Immobilization modulates macrophage accumulation in tendon-bone healing. *Clinical Orthopaedics and Related Research,* Vol. 467, pp. 281-287.

De Luca, C.J. (1997). The use of surface electromyography in biomechanics. *Journal of Applied Biomechanics,* Vol. 13, pp. 135–163.

Felici, F. (2006). Neuromuscular responses to exercise investigated through surface EMG. *Journal of Electromyography and Kinesiology,* Vol. 16, pp. 578–585.

Firth, E.C. (2006). The response of bone, articular cartilage and tendon to exercise in the horse. *J. Anatomical Society of Great Britain and Ireland.* Vol. 20, pp. 513-526.

Giovagnolia, G.; Trabalza Marinuccia, M.; Bollaa A. & Borgheseb, A. (2002). Transport stress in horses: an electromyographic study on balance preservation. *Livestock Production Science,* Vol. 73, pp. 247–254.

Heaf, J.G.; Molsted, S.;, Harrison, A.P.; Eiken, P.; Prescott, L. & Eidemak, I. (2010). Vitamin D, surface electromyography and physical function in uraemic patients. *Nephron Clinical Practice,* Vol. 115, pp. c244-c250.

Hermens, H.J.; Freriks, B.; Merletti, R.; Hägg, G.G.; Stegman, D.; Blok, J.; Rau, G. & Disselhorst-Klug, C. (1999). *SENIAM 8 European Recommendations for Surface ElectroMyoGraphy*: Roessingh Research and Development, ISBN 90-75452-1.

Jansen, M.O.; van Raaij, J.A.; van den Bogert, A.J.; Riemersma, D.J.; Schamhardt, H.C. & Hartman, W. (1992). Quantitative analysis of computer-averaged electromyographic profiles of intrinsic limb muscles in ponies at the walk. *American Journal of Veterinary Research,* Vol. 53, pp. 2343-2349.

Kearns, C.F.; McKeever, K.H. & Abe, T. (2002). Overview of Horse Body Composition and Muscle Architecture: Implications for Performance. *The Veterinary Journal,*Vol. 164, pp. 224-234.

Kohnke, J.R. (2004). Bone biomechanics: a review of the influences of exercise and nutritional management on bone modeling in the growing and exercising horse. *J. Kohnke consultancy Pty Ltd, Australia,* pp. 345-353.

Kruljc, P. & Nemec, A. (2006). Electroencephalographic and Electromyographic changes during the use of Detomidine and Detomidine-Butorphanol combination in standing horses. *Acta Veterinaria Hungarica,* Vol. 54, pp. 35–42.

Leisson, K.; Jaakma, U. & Seeneb, T. (2008). Adaptation of Equine Locomotor Muscle Fiber Types to Endurance and Intensive High Speed Training. *Journal of Equine Veterinary Science,* Vol. 28, pp. 395-401.

Licka, T.; Frey, A. & Peham, C. (2009). Electromyographic activity of the longissimus dorsi muscles in horses when walking on a treadmill. *The Veterinary Journal,* Vol. 180, pp. 71–76.

Licka, T.F.; Peham, C. & Frey, A. (2004). Electromyographic activity of the longissimus dorsi muscles in horses during trotting on a treadmill. *American Journal of Veterinary Research,* Vol. 65, pp. 155-158.

Licka, T.F.; Peham, C. & Zonmann, E. (2001). Treadmill study of the range of back movement at the walk in horses without back pain. *American Journal of Veterinary Research,* Vol. 62, pp. 1173-1179.

Mileva, K.N.; Kadr, M.; Amin, N. & Bowtell, J.L. (2010). Acute effects of flexi-bar vs. Sham-bar exercise on muscle electromyography activity and performance. *Journal of Strength and Conditioning Research,* Vol. 24, pp. 737-748.

Peham, C.; Frey, A.; Licka, T. & Scheidl, M. (2001). Evaluation of the EMG activity of the long back muscle during induced back movements at stance. *Equine Veterinary Journal Supplement,* Vol. 33, pp. 165-168.

Ring, D.; Vaccaro, A.R.; Scuderi, G.; Pathria, M.N. & Garfin, S.R. (1994). Acute calcific retropharyngeal tendinitis. Clinical presentation and pathological characterization. *Journal of Bone and Joint Surgery (America),* Vol. 76, pp. 1636-1642.

Rivero, J.L. (2007). A Scientific Background for Skeletal Muscle Conditioning in Equine Practice. *Journal of Veterinary Medicine A,* Vol. 54, pp. 321–332.

Robert, C.; Valette, J.P.; Degueurce, C. & Denoix, J.M. (1999). Correlation between Surface Electromyography and Kinematics of the Hindlimb of Horses at Trot on a Treadmill. *Cells Tissues Organs,* Vol. 165, pp. 113–122.

Roetert, E.P.; Brody, H.; Dillman, C.J.; Groppel, J.L. & Schultheis, J.M. (1995). The biomechanics of tennis elbow. An integrated approach. *Clinical Sports Medicine,* Vol. 14, pp. 47-57.

Schuurman, S.O.; Kersten, W. & Weijs, W.A. (2003). The equine hind limb is actively stabilized during standing. *Journal of Anatomy,* Vol. 202, pp. 355-362.

Tokuriki, M.; Aoki, O.; Niki, Y.; Kurakawa, Y.; Hataya, M. & Kita, T. (1989). Electromyographic activity of the cubital joint muscles in horses during locomotion. *American Journal of Veterinary Research,* Vol. 50, pp. 950-957.

Wijnberg, I.D.; Back, W.; De Jong, M.; Zuidhof, M.C.; van den Belt, A.J.M. & van der Kolk, J. (2004). The role of electromyography in clinical diagnosis of neuromuscular locomotor problems in the horse. *Equine Veterinary Journal,* Vol. 36, pp. 718-722.

Wijnberg, I.D.; Franssen, H. & van der Kolk, J.H. (2003a). Influence of age of horse on results of quantitative electromyograhic needle examination of skeletal muscles in Dutch Warmblood horses. *American Journal of Veterinary Research,* Vol. 64, pp. 70-75.

Wijnberg, I.D.; van Dam, K.G.; de Graaf-Roelfsema, E.; Keizer, H.A.; van Ginneken, M.M.E.; Barneveld, A.; van Breda, E. & van der Kolk, J.H. (2008). Over-training effects on quantitative electromyography and muscle enzyme activities in standardbred horses. *Journal of Applied Physiology,* Vol. 105, pp. 1746–1753.

Wijnberg, I.D.; van der Kolk, J.H.; Franssen, H. & Breukink, H.J. (2003b). Needle electromyography in the horse compared with its principles in man: a review. *Equine Veterinary Journal,* Vol. 35, pp. 9-17.

15

Arthroscopic Treatment of Suprascapular Nerve Neuropathy

Dipit Sahu, Robert Fullick and Laurent Lafosse
Alps Surgery Institute, Clinique Generale Annecy, Annecy, France

1. Introduction

Compression of SupraScapular Nerve (SSN) was first described by Thomas in 1936 (Thomas 1936). However, Thompson and Kopell described SupraScapular Nerve (SSN) entrapment occurring at the transverse scapular notch (Thompson and Kopell 1959). Aiello et al differentiated between entrapment of this nerve at the Suprascapular notch and entrapment at the Spinoglenoid notch (Aiello, Serra et al. 1982). The incidence and prevalence of this condition has not been conclusively reported. A metanalysis by Zehetgruber showed there were 88 reports of this condition from 1959 to 2001 (Zehetgruber, Noske et al. 2002). However during the past decade there have been increasing awareness of this condition, leading to a higher reporting of SupraScapular Neuropathy. The senior author (LL) was the first to report the results of Arthroscopic SupraScapular Nerve release in 2006 in a series of 10 patients with mean follow up of 15 months (Lafosse, Tomasi et al. 2007). Reported prevalence of this entity has been reported as 7%-10%. Most of the reported incidence is in overhead athletes like volleyball player, athletic population (12-33%) (Ferretti, Cerullo et al. 1987; Witvrouw, Cools et al. 2000).

2. Anatomy and pathophysiology

Suprascapular Nerve arises from the upper trunk of Brachial Plexus with contributions from C5 and C6 nerve roots. Occasionally it also derives from C4 nerve root.

2.1 Course

The nerve initially runs posterior to the clavicle and then across the superior border of scapula and enters the Suprascapular Notch traversing under the transverse scapular ligament. The artery accompanying the nerve travels above the ligament. The transverse scapular ligament forms the roof of the notch. After exiting the suprascapular notch, the nerve runs medial to the supraglenoid tubercle and posterior glenoid rim. The nerve angles around the spine of scapula and then along with the artery runs in the spinoglenoid notch under the inferior transverse scapular ligament. This ligament has been described by different researchers (Demaio, Drez et al. 1991; Cummins, Messer et al. 2000) (Ticker, Djurasovic et al. 1998).

2.1.1 Suprascapular notch

The Suprascapular notch is a major site of SupraScapular Nerve Compression. The Suprascapular notch has been classified into 6 different types based on the morphology by

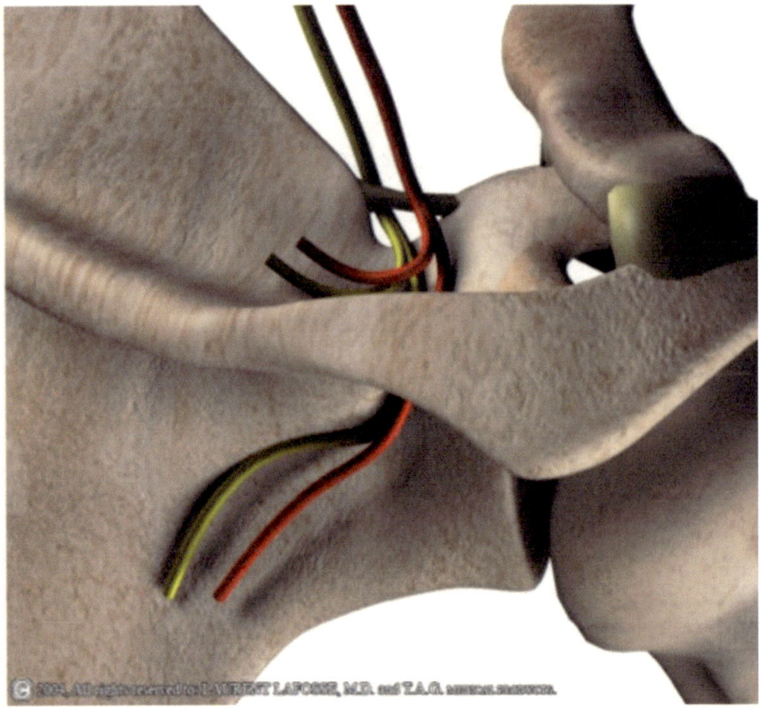

Fig. 1. 3D representation of SSN and artery and their relationships with the TSL.

Rengachary et al (Rengachary, Burr et al. 1979; Bayramoglu, Demiryurek et al. 2003). The existence of different morphologies of the notch has been corroborated by more investigators. The greatest risk of nerve entrapment is in a small scapular notch with a thick Transverse scapular ligament

2.1.2 Transverse scapular ligament

The transverse scapular ligament forms the ceiling of the Suprascapular notch. This ligament may hypertrophy and lead to stenosis within the notch. There have also been reports of calcification of the ligament which causes nerve entrapment. A sling effect mechanism of injury of Suprascapular nerve has been described in which in certain anatomical variants of the Suprascapular notch, the transverse ligament cause nerve irritation and compression during certain movement of the limb (Rengachary, Neff et al. 1979).

2.1.3 Spinoglenoid ligament

Spinoglenoid ligament, also known as inferior transverse scapular ligament is a more common site for compression of the Suprascapular Nerve. This ligament originates on the spine of the scapula and inserts on the superior margin of glenoid neck as a bilaminar structure. The spinoglenoid ligament has been classified into two types: Type I -thin band, Type 2 is a well formed ligament. The spinoglenoid ligament is dynamic because of its insertion into the posterior Glenohumeral joint capsule. In certain positions of the arm, like adduction and internal rotation, this ligament may tighten due to tensioning of the capsule and compress the nerve.

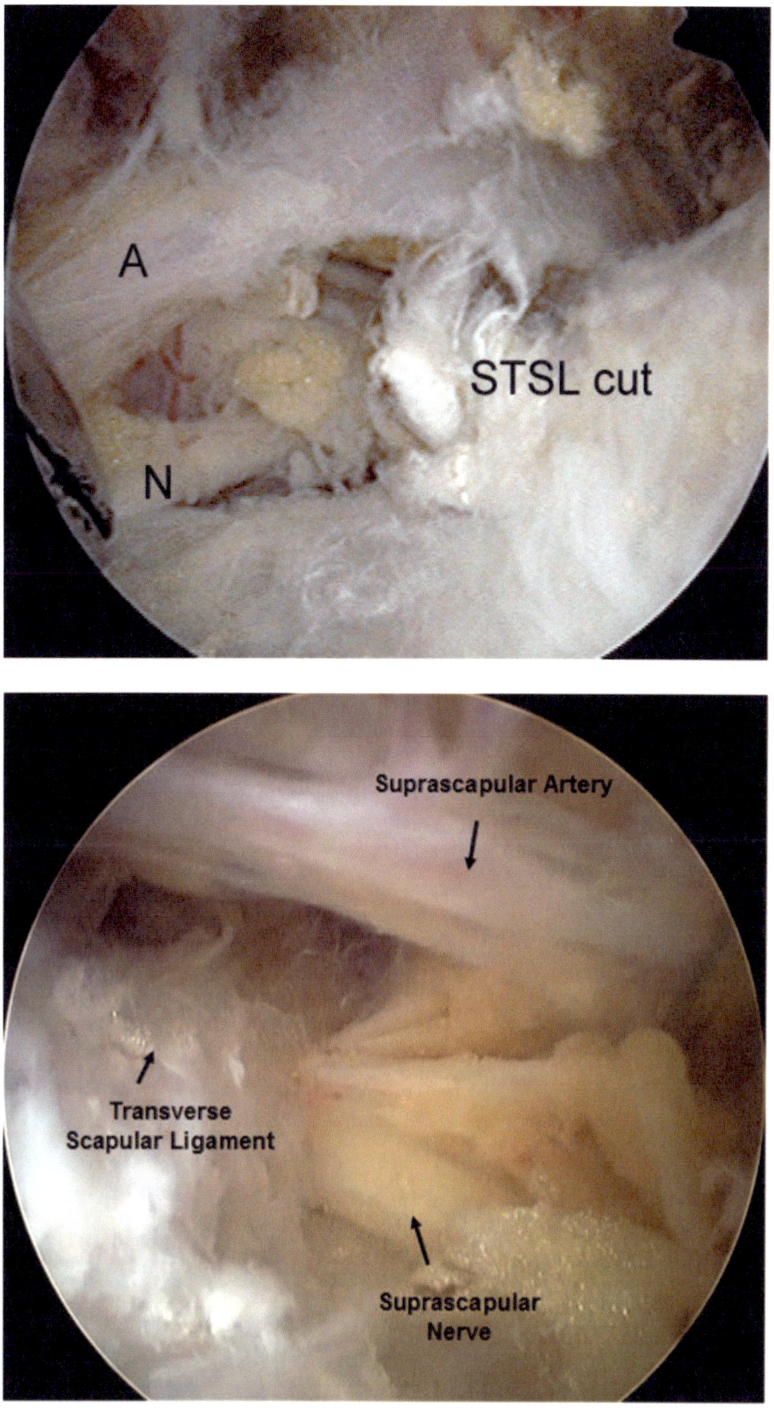

Fig. 2. Suprascapular nerve under the cut Superior transverse ligament and the artery running above.

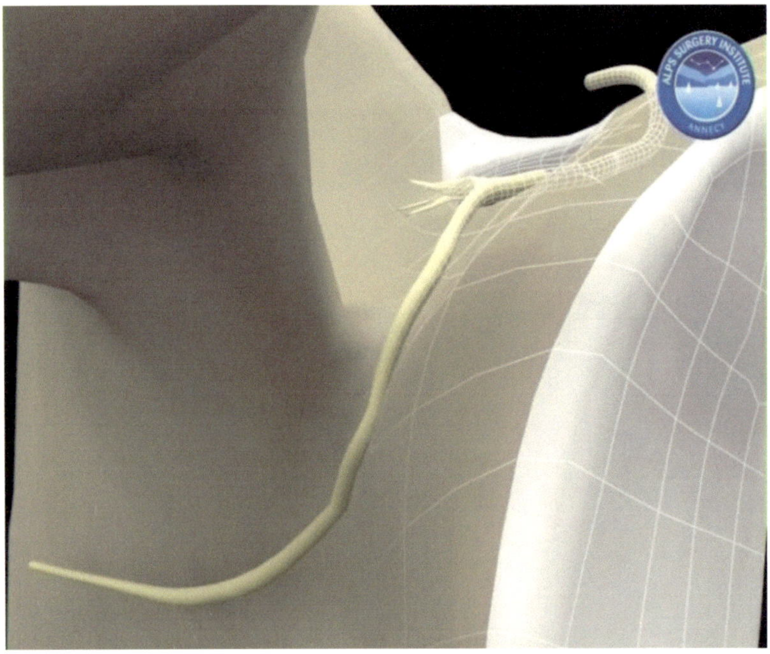

Fig. 3. 3D view of distal SSN passing around the spine of the scapula.

2.2 Distribution

The suprascapular nerve is predominantly motor nerve, but it also has nerve supply to skin and joints. Some reports by Ritchie et al and Matsumoto et al also suggest it may supply 70 % of sensations to the skin of the shoulder (Brown, James et al. 1988).

2.2.1 Muscles

The Nerve supplies two motor branches to the Supraspinatus before proceeding to the Spinoglenoid notch. After entering the Spinoglenoid Notch, the nerve supplies 2 - 4 motor branches to the Infraspinatus. Lesions of the nerve in the Suprascapular notch affect both Supraspinatus and Infraspinatus. While lesions in the Spinoglenoid notch only affect the Infraspinatus.

2.2.2 Joints

Cadaveric studies have demonstrated that Suprascapular nerve has a sensory branch to the Glenohumeral and acromioclavicular joint and coracoacromial ligament.

3. Etiology, physical examinaton and indication for arthroscopic release

3.1 Etiology

SSN compression neuropathy can primary or secondary.

3.1.1 Primary SSN neuropathy

Primary compression Neuropathy is due to repetitive trauma and microtrauma. In overhead athletes there maybe a dynamic compression by spinoglenoid ligament when shoulder is in a position of overhead throwing. There may also be compression at the suprascapular notch or spinoglenoid notch by soft tissue tumor, bone tumor, cyst secondary to capsular or labrum injury. Stenosis of the suprascapular or spinoglenoid notch, with a calcified or hypertrophied transverse scapular ligament or a spinoglenoid ligament may predispose to SSN neuropathy.

Other causes of Suprascapular nerve entrapment may include:

Compression by anterior coracoscapular ligaments

Compression by edge of hypertrophied infrascapular muscle

Compression by omohyoid muscle

Glenohumeral dislocation

Viral neuritis

Penetrating injuries to the shoulder

Posterior surgical approach to the scapula

3.1.2 Secondary SSN neuropathy

Secondary SSN neuropathy is associated with a massive rotator cuff tear. A retracted massive rotator cuff tear predisposes the nerve to traction injury at the suprascapular notch. According to Albritton et al, as the rotator muscles retract, the angle between the suprascapular nerve and its first motor branch reduces, which leads to increased tension in the nerve (Albritton, Graham et al. 2003).

Some studies have found correlation between presence of SSN neuropathy and massive retracted rotator cuff tear (Mallon, Wilson et al. 2006). Some cadaveric studies have reported that a lateral advancementof rotator cuff of more than 3 cm may increase the risk of neurovascular twisting or injury (Warner, Krushell et al. 1992). However there have been other reports of lateral advancement safe length to vary from 1 cm to 3 cm and there is no consensus as to the safe level of lateral advancement (Greiner, Golser et al. 2003).

3.2 Physical examination and electrodiagnostic tests

3.2.1 Physical examination

A thorough physical examination includes examination of the cervical spine, both shoulders to detect tenderness around posterior shoulder, muscle atrophy, strength of shoulder in external rotation.

Supraspinatus and Infraspinatus atrophy may point towards an involvement of the nerve in the Suprascapular / Spinoglenoid notch. There may be tenderness to palpation posterior to the clavicle with injury to the nerve in the Suprascapular fossa. External rotation weakness may also point towards an involvement of the Infraspinatus. Cross body adduction test which puts the spinoglenoid ligament under tension may be a good indicator of the nerve involvement in the spinoglenoid notch.

We also have described a test to detect SSN pathology. In this test, the examiner laterally rotates the patients head away from- the affected shoulder, while at the same time gently retracts the affected shoulder, resulting in an increased pain posteriorly (Figure 4).

Radiographs of the shoulder should be evaluated for the presence of callus, ossification, osseous dysplasia.

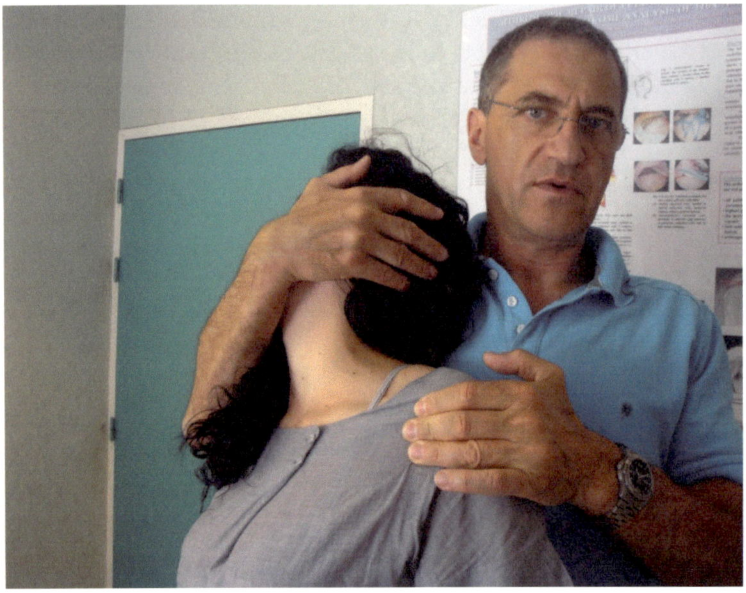

Fig. 4. Clinical test to detect Suprascapular Nerve Neuropathy.

Other imaging modalities (Ultrasound, CT scan, MRI) may give a better idea about the presence of tumor, compressing cysts, lesions in course of nerve.

3.2.2 Role of electromyography

Electromyography studies are indicated when there is an unexplained shoulder pain. However the sensitivity and specificity of Electromyography has been debated by various authors. Electromyography of a damaged nerve may show reduced amplitude of motor potentials, increased spontaneous activity, fibrillations, polyphasic activity, etc. It may show denervation of the supraspinatous or infraspinatous muscle with resultant fibrillation and sharp waves. EMG is also useful in confirming traumatic lesions of SSN.

In our study of 100 patients, we performed EMG pre operatively and at 6 months and 2 years postoperatively. A positive EMG, however, is not always the necessary criterion for diagnosing SSN neuropathy. We, believe that SSN pathology is a dynamic process and not always demonstrable on an EMG. An EMG however, may be indicated in unexplained posterior shoulder pain. EMG in retracted rotator cuff tears have shown to be abnormal suggesting Suprascapular nerve pathology.

3.3 Indications for arthroscopic release

Our Indications for Arthroscopic Release:

1. Patients with weakness of Infraspinatus/Supraspinatus with or without positive EMG
2. Patients with a thickened or ossified ligament on assessment during arthroscopic rotator cuff repair
3. Patients who present with posterior shoulder pain and a positive SSN test with or without positive EMG
4. space occupying lesion compressing SSN
5. reduction of large/massive rotator cuff tear
6. compression due to anatomical variants

4. Arthroscopic suprascapular nerve release

Technique:

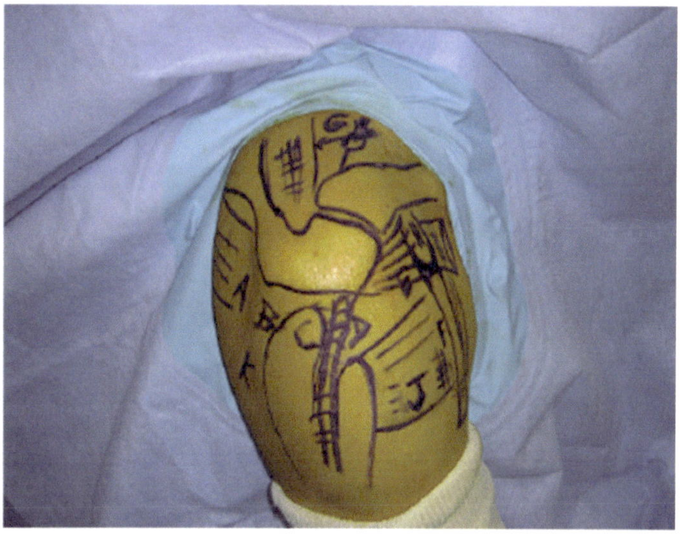

Fig. 5.

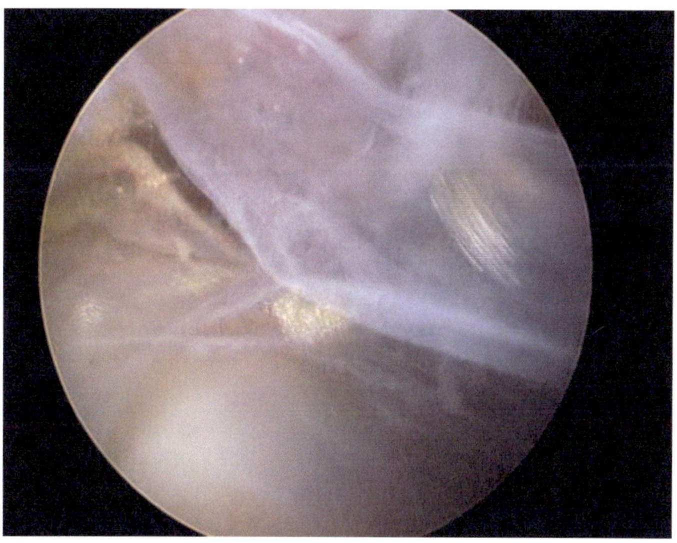

Fig. 6.

Multiple techniques exist for adequate release of the suprascapular nerve (SSN) at the suprascapular notch. In the literature, small series have shown good to excellent results using the open technique for suprascapular nerve decompression. Although no head to head comparative studies exist, it is likely that the arthroscopic technique requires less dissection and retraction, and produces less postoperative scar formation and fibrosis when compared to open surgical techniques. Subsequently, there is likely less patient morbidity and risk of recurrent nerve compression from significant scarring postoperatively.

Regardless, the surgeon should use the approach they are most familiar with to release the nerve reliably and safely. Here we present our technique as an efficient, safe, and reproducible method for arthroscopic release of the superior transverse scapular ligament (STSL) at the suprascapular notch.

Posterior visualization is achieved by inserting the arthroscope and instruments through the subacromial space to dissect medially along the anterior border of the supraspinatus muscle. Anterior visualization is accomplished through medial and inferior portals, and the notch is viewed on the medial side of the base of the coracoid process.

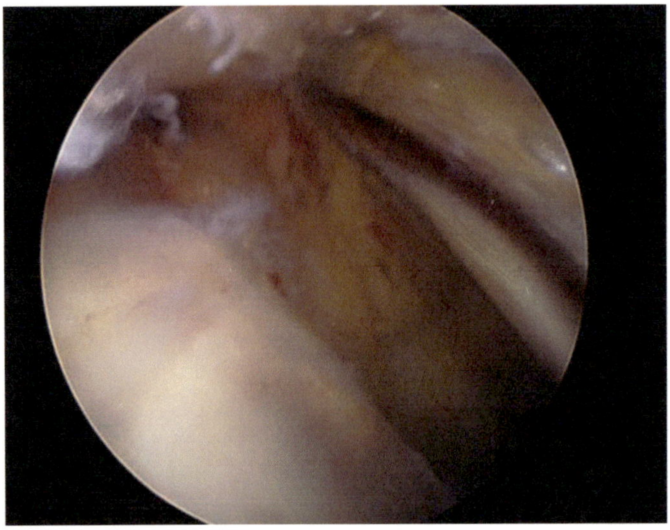

Fig. 7.

For a standard SSN release, the nerve can be easily visualized through the subacromial space as it exits the suprascapular notch posteriorly and descends into the supraspinatus fossa, beneath the muscle belly of supraspinatus. Most often, surgery to release the SSN is begun with a thorough intra-articular diagnostic arthroscopy to rule out associated shoulder pathology. After completion of the diagnostic portion of the procedure the scope may be repositioned to the subacromial space to start the bursoscopy. At this time the mid-lateral (C) portal (Figure 5) can be established in standard fashion and the initial bursectomy completed in preparation to move the camera to this portal for viewing. Commonly, a medial bursal curtain is encountered after placing the camera in the C portal, limiting medial visualization (Figure 6). At this time, is important to identify useful landmarks including the coracoacromial ligament superiorly and the anterior border of the supraspinatus tendon inferiorly. These will serve to orient the surgeon as the dissection proceeds medially. Following the identification of appropriate landmarks, a needle is used to localize the location of the anterolateral (D) working portal. This portal is usually 2 cm off the anterolateral border of the acromion and the needle is directed tangentially to the anterior border of the supraspinatus. The shaver is inserted here and the medial subacromial bursa is opened at the anterior border of the supraspinatus muscle. With the arthroscope and shaver inserted through lateral (C) and anterolateral (D) portals respectively, the anterior border of the supraspinatus muscle is used as a guide and followed medially towards the notch (Figure 7). The shaver is used to open the bursa and

remove loose connective tissue as the dissection progresses medially to the base of the coracoclavicular ligaments. The shaver blade is directed anteriorly, superiorly, and inferiorly with care taken to not damage the supraspinatus muscle. Medially, the nerve is protected from the shaver by the superior transverse scapular ligament; however, the suprascapular artery (transverse scapular artery) passes superior the ligament and is in jeopardy as the dissection is carried medially. As a result, debridement should proceed carefully once the dissection has reached the region posterior to the CC ligaments. In cases where the suprascapular artery is injured, bleeding may be stopped using a radiofrequency device. In those uncommon cases, no additional morbidity has been observed most likely due to the rich collateral circulation in the shoulder region. However, in all cases one should attempt to preserve the artery if possible.
After reaching the posteromedial aspect of the coracoid and CC ligaments, the superior (G) portal is created under direct vision, using a needle to identify the exact location of the portal. Although this portal is created under direct visualization without absolute reference to external landmarks, it is usually located 2-3cm medial to Neviaser's portal and 7cm medial to the lateral acromial border. Triangulation of the tip of the needle and view from the arthroscope is assisted if you ensure that the 30-degree scope is looking directly inferior. The needle is then introduced in line with the arthroscope, directed slightly posterior to anterior towards the ligament at the anterior border of the supraspinatus muscle. The shaver is left in position and released from the surgeon's hand. The weight of the shaver acts as a retractor to lift the trapezius muscle superiorly to improve visualization in the area. The shaver also remains immediately available if further dissection is required.

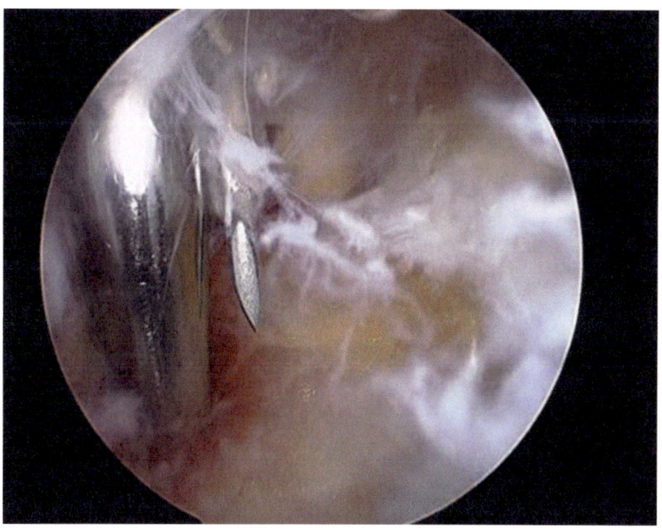

Fig. 8.

The skin is incised and a blunt trocar is then introduced through the G portal and used to dissect the remaining connective tissue above the transverse scapular ligament from the coracoclavicular ligaments posteromedially (Figures 8 & 9). The suprascapular artery and 2 accompanying veins lie on top of the ligament and are gently displaced medially with the trocar. Occasionally, an aberrant branch of the artery is found beneath the transverse ligament and is protected along with the nerve when cutting the ligament. The SSN supplies

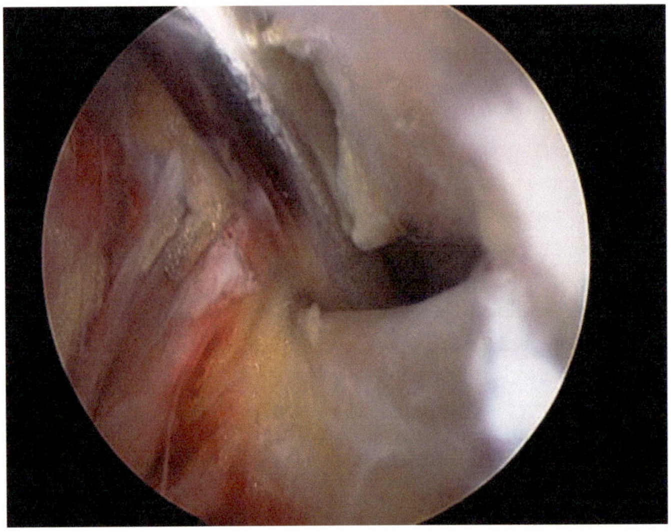

Fig. 9.

the supraspinatus muscle through very short branches that exit the notch and enter the muscle belly directly posterior the notch. Dissection with the blunt trocar is performed very gently and without excessive traction on the muscle belly to avoid avulsing the nerve branches from the supraspinatus muscle.

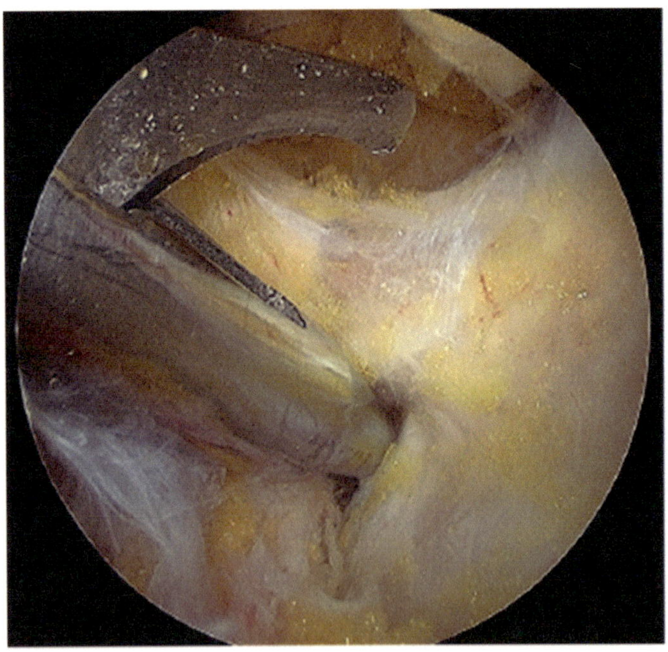

Fig. 10.

Once a clear view of the transverse ligament is obtained, the trocar is left in position, within the notch to maintain the view and protect the nerve and artery medially. The ligament can

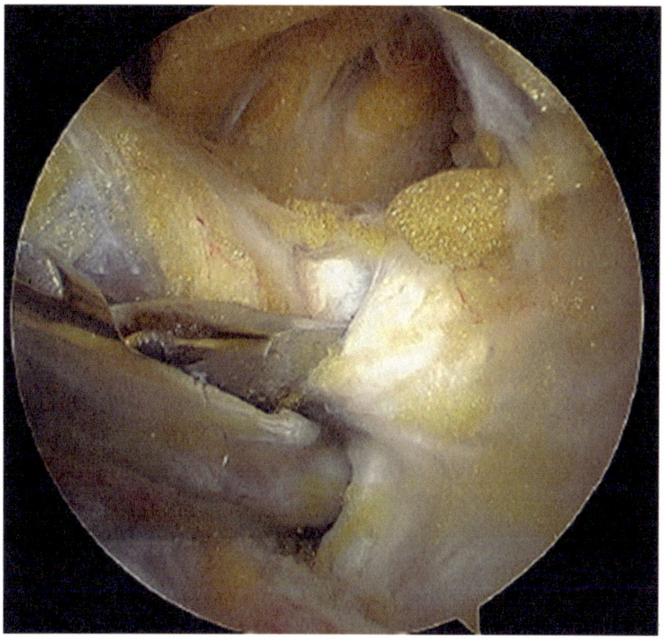

Fig. 11.

be divided with arthroscopic scissors introduced through a second stab incision adjacent to the G portal, usually 1.5 to 2cm lateral. We have developed a custom instrument that combines the blunt trocar and scissors, so that the release can be performed through one portal (Figure 10 & 11).

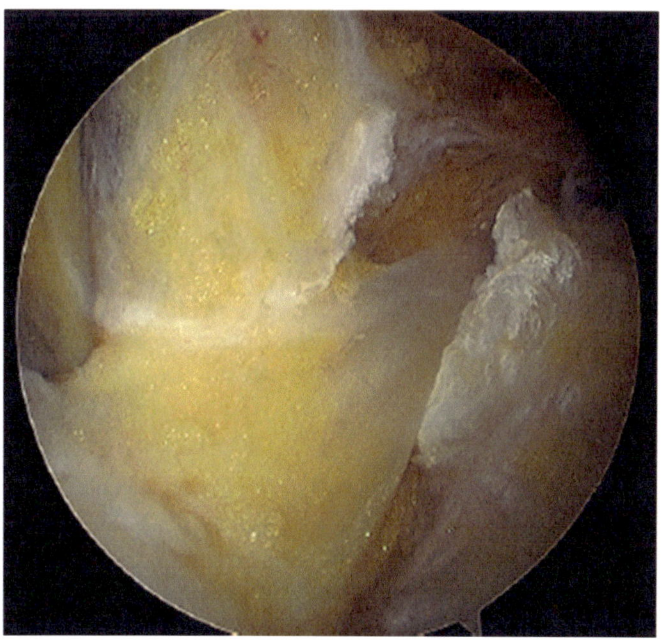

Fig. 12.

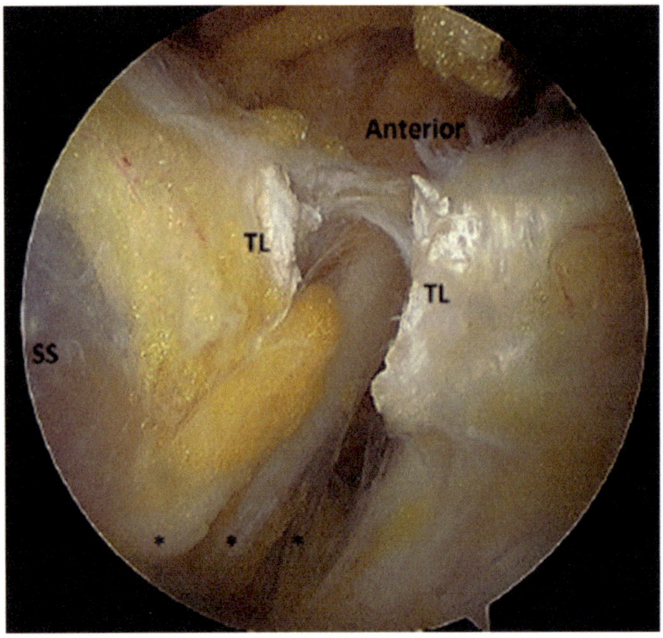

Fig. 13. Suprascapular nerve seen under the cut ligament.

In rare cases the ligament is ossified and can be removed with a combination Kerrison up-biting rongeurs, small osteotome, or small burr. In general, a notchplasty with a bur should not be performed because this creates excessive postoperative scar tissue and risks recurrent compression of the nerve. Once the ligament is removed, the nerve can be visualized in the notch (Figure 12). The delicate, short branches to the supraspinatus can be seen, separate from the major branch of the nerve, which continues to the spinoglenoid notch, under the supraspinatus muscle belly (Figure 13).

Alternatively, the nerve can be visualized through anterior portals as it enters the infraclavicular region, posterior to the brachial plexus and enters the suprascapular notch, beneath the transverse scapular ligament. To obtain this view, the arthroscope is inserted through a medial portal in line with the coracoid process and the conjoint tendon. The coracoid is viewed end-on, and the suprascapular notch, covered by the transverse scapular ligament, is found medial to the base of the process and coracoclavicular ligaments. As the nerve descends in the neck, it heads directly towards the notch, lying within loose connective tissue. Once an adequate view of the nerve entering the notch is obtained, the ligament can be divided under direct vision with arthroscopic scissors inserted through a medial portal. Care must be taken when passing instruments medially in the region of the brachial plexus and axillary artery. We only use this approach when exploring the nerve after severe trauma, to confirm its continuity more proximally.

5. Our study and results

We carried out a study on patients with symptomatic tear of the rotator cuff. The patients with a confirmed rotator cuff tear underwent a preoperative Electromyography to test the function of SSN of the index shoulder. They were tested again by EMG at 6 months and 2 years postoperatively.

There were three groups of patients. Group 1 Those who had positive EMG and underwent cuff repair only. Group 2 had positive EMG and underwent cuff repair along with SSN release. Group 3 had normal EMG and underwent cuff repair only.
We had 100 patients with average age of 58 (+/- 9.2) years. According to EMG studies, 50 pateints demonstrated normal EMG findings of SSN and 27 patients demonstrated abnormalities in EMG (23 were unclear).
Accordng to the postoperative EMG studies, 81% of patients demonstrated normal electrodiagnostic findings of SSN and 9% demonstrated abnormalities in EMG. 45 patients demonstrated the same normal level as preoperative, 22 patients were better than pre operative and 5 patients remained pathologic.
In subgroup 1, 9 patients out of group 1 postoperatively demonstrated normal EMG, 4 remained at the same pathologic level, even though SSN release had been performed, constant scores improved in all the patients.
In subgroup 2, all 11 patients post operatively demonstrated a normal EMG, despite no release of SSN being performed.
In subgroup 3, patients with a preoperative normal EMG, at the time of postoperative EMG. All showed normal EMG.

6. Discussion and overview

SSN neuropathy may have a primary etiology or may also be found in massive retracted rotator cuff. Several Authors have now identified association of SSN neuropathy with massive rotator cuff tear. Senior Author (L. L) in 2006 reported 9 of 10 patients who underwent SSN arthroscopic decompression without rotator cuff disease had excellent outcomes. 7 of these patients also had complete normalization of latency in motor fibres of SSN in EMG / NCV. The results in this study convincingly showed an improvement in Nerve conduction velocity after SSN decompression via the arthroscopic techniques (Lafosse, Tomasi et al. 2007). Costouros et al reported 6 patients with documented SSN pathology associated with massive cuff tear and found improvement in EMG function in all (Costouros, Porramatikul et al. 2007).
SSN neuropathy may be treated conservatively, but the results have been poor as shown by Callahan et al. In their series, 76% of patients required surgery eventually (Callahan, Scully et al. 1991).
Operative techniques may include open nerve release or Arthroscopic Nerve release. Open Suprascapular nerve release has been reported to give good results. In a series of 39 patients, 28 showed improvement of supraspinatus muscle strength to grade 4 (Kim, Murovic et al. 2005). However, Arthroscopic techniques of SSN release have now gained popularity due to the fact that they are less invasive, afford better visualization and require less operative time.
Arthroscopically, the SSN can be visualized and released posteriorly (Lafosse, Tomasi et al. 2007) or anteriorly (Reineck and Krishnan 2009) to the coracoclavicular ligaments.
Our unpublished data suggests EMG improves post operatively in patients undergoing massive rotator cuff repair. However, there were also 4 patients in subgroup 1 in whom the EMG stayed at the same pathologic level. In our center we do not evaluate every patient of rotator cuff tear by an EMG. We do however release the SSN in massive rotator cuff tears as we believe that a retracted rotator cuff tear does put tension on SSN and releasing the Superior transverse scapular ligament releases the tension on the nerve. Albritton et al also

proved in their study that suprascapular nerve injury may result from a retraction of a torn rotator cuff. They proved that retraction of Supraspinatus changed the course of suprascapular nerve as it passed through the notch (Albritton, Graham et al. 2003). We also assess the ligament as needed and if the ligament is found to be ossified or under tension, we go ahead and release the ligament.

In a study by Shah et al, 21 out of 24 patients who presented with deep posterior shoulder pain had EMG/NCV findings of denervation of SSN and 17 of the 24 patients showed an improvement in pain and improvement in ASES scores after SSN decompression (Shah, Butler et al.). They also concluded that there may be a subset of patients with negative electro diagnostic studies presenting with unexplained posterior shoulder pain who may respond to SSN release. Warner et al also showed that lateral reduction of rotator cuff tears of more than 3 cm during reconstruction may result in significant tension on the Supra Scapular Nerve and entrapment by the Transverse Scapular Ligament (Warner, Krushell et al. 1992).

7. Summary and our recommendation

To summarise, there are three main advantages of arthroscopic release of SSN over the traditional open technique. First it provides superior visualization of neurovascular structures and the transverse scapular ligament. The SSN is as small as 2 mm and is therefore sometimes difficult to appreciate via open exposures. The small diameter of the SSN is easily visualized with the magnification afforded by the arthroscope and permits easy release of the ligament. Secondly the arthroscopic release of the SSN is significantly less invasive and does not involve detachment of the trapezius insertion. Thirdly the operative time is considerable less and patient has significantly less pain post operatively.

We believe that by releasing the TSL, particularly in large chronically retracted tears, we improve SSN mobility both in the retracted state and for the reduction of the cuff and therefore enhancing the chances of neuromuscular recovery.

8. EMG/NCV

EMG/NCV testing and evaluation are very user dependent, and an electro physiologist skilled in evaluation of the SSN is needed for accurate interpretation of the results.

Positive EMG/NCVs are helpful; however, a negative EMG/NCV is not a contraindication to SSN release.

Similarly, our study on massive tears showed ~27% positive EMG studies. Although no significant difference in pre/post-op EMGs has been found and controversy exists regarding SSN release in the repair of large-massive cuff tears, our opinion is the procedure can be completed quickly and reproducibly without subjecting the patient to significant additional risks.

9. References

Aiello, I., G. Serra, et al. (1982). "Entrapment of the suprascapular nerve at the spinoglenoid notch." Ann Neurol 12 (3): 314-6.

Albritton, M. J., R. D. Graham, et al. (2003). "An anatomic study of the effects on the suprascapular nerve due to retraction of the supraspinatus muscle after a rotator cuff tear." J Shoulder Elbow Surg 12 (5): 497-500.

Bayramoglu, A., D. Demiryurek, et al. (2003). "Variations in anatomy at the suprascapular notch possibly causing suprascapular nerve entrapment: an anatomical study." Knee Surg Sports Traumatol Arthrosc 11 (6): 393-8.

Brown, D. E., D. C. James, et al. (1988). "Pain relief by suprascapular nerve block in gleno-humeral arthritis." Scand J Rheumatol 17 (5): 411-5.

Callahan, J. D., T. B. Scully, et al. (1991). "Suprascapular nerve entrapment. A series of 27 cases." J Neurosurg 74 (6): 893-6.

Costouros, J. G., M. Porramatikul, et al. (2007). "Reversal of suprascapular neuropathy following arthroscopic repair of massive supraspinatus and infraspinatus rotator cuff tears." Arthroscopy 23 (11): 1152-61.

Cummins, C. A., T. M. Messer, et al. (2000). "Suprascapular nerve entrapment." J Bone Joint Surg Am 82 (3): 415-24.

Demaio, M., D. Drez, Jr., et al. (1991). "The inferior transverse scapular ligament as a possible cause of entrapment neuropathy of the nerve to the infraspinatus. A brief note." J Bone Joint Surg Am 73 (7): 1061-3.

Ferretti, A., G. Cerullo, et al. (1987). "Suprascapular neuropathy in volleyball players." J Bone Joint Surg Am 69 (2): 260-3.

Greiner, A., K. Golser, et al. (2003). "The course of the suprascapular nerve in the supraspinatus fossa and its vulnerability in muscle advancement." J Shoulder Elbow Surg 12 (3): 256-9.

Kim, D. H., J. A. Murovic, et al. (2005). "Management and outcomes of 42 surgical suprascapular nerve injuries and entrapments." Neurosurgery 57 (1): 120-7; discussion 120-7.

Lafosse, L., A. Tomasi, et al. (2007). "Arthroscopic release of suprascapular nerve entrapment at the suprascapular notch: technique and preliminary results." Arthroscopy 23 (1): 34-42.

Mallon, W. J., R. J. Wilson, et al. (2006). "The association of suprascapular neuropathy with massive rotator cuff tears: a preliminary report." J Shoulder Elbow Surg 15 (4): 395-8.

Reineck, J. R. and S. G. Krishnan (2009). "Subligamentous suprascapular artery encountered during arthroscopic suprascapular nerve release: a report of three cases." J Shoulder Elbow Surg 18 (3): e1-3.

Rengachary, S. S., D. Burr, et al. (1979). "Suprascapular entrapment neuropathy: a clinical, anatomical, and comparative study. Part 2: anatomical study." Neurosurgery 5 (4): 447-51.

Rengachary, S. S., J. P. Neff, et al. (1979). "Suprascapular entrapment neuropathy: a clinical, anatomical, and comparative study. Part 1: clinical study." Neurosurgery 5 (4): 441-6.

Shah, A. A., R. B. Butler, et al. "Clinical outcomes of suprascapular nerve decompression." J Shoulder Elbow Surg.

Thomas, A. (1936)."La Paralysie du muscle sous-pineux. " Presse Med 64: 1283-4.

Thompson, W. A. and H. P. Kopell (1959). "Peripheral entrapment neuropathies of the upper extremity." N Engl J Med 260 (25): 1261-5.

Ticker, J. B., M. Djurasovic, et al. (1998). "The incidence of ganglion cysts and other variations in anatomy along the course of the suprascapular nerve." J Shoulder Elbow Surg 7 (5): 472-8.

Warner, J. P., R. J. Krushell, et al. (1992). "Anatomy and relationships of the suprascapular nerve: anatomical constraints to mobilization of the supraspinatus and infraspinatus muscles in the management of massive rotator-cuff tears." J Bone Joint Surg Am 74 (1): 36-45.

Witvrouw, E., A. Cools, et al. (2000). "Suprascapular neuropathy in volleyball players." Br J Sports Med 34 (3): 174-80.

Zehetgruber, H., H. Noske, et al. (2002). "Suprascapular nerve entrapment. A meta-analysis." Int Orthop 26 (6): 339-43.

Part 5

Gynecology/Urology

16

An Uterine Electromyographic Activity as a Measure of Labor Progression

Jerneja Vrhovec and Alenka Maček Lebar
University of Ljubljana,
Slovenia

1. Introduction

Understanding the physiology of the uterus during term and preterm parturition is essential to solving clinical problems related to gestation and labor. The uterus is a smooth muscle organ. It undergoes specific changes during gestation and is known for its unique contractility during the labor.

At the term the uterus is 10 to 20 times heavier than it is before pregnancy (from 50 g to 1000 g). This enormous expansion during pregnancy is mostly due to the increase of the size of muscle cells (hypertrophy) and less due to the proliferation of muscle cells (hyperplasia). The uterus should accommodate the growing fetus, and support the fetus through sustained muscle tone, without generating propagated contractions. This state of quiescence - the absence of the coordinated contractions - is critical to the successful outcome of pregnancy. Therefore the delicate balance should be obtained between the maintenance of tone and the resistance to propagated uterine contractions until the end of gestation and the onset of labor. At the onset of labor the uterus becomes active and at the labor's end it empties its contents through rhythmic, forceful, organized and synchronous contractions that are crucial for the successful outcome of pregnancy.

1.1 Uterine structure and activity

Functionally the pregnant human uterus can be divided into two parts: the upper part (the uterine corpus) and the lower part (the cervix). The uterine corpus is mainly composed of smooth muscle and can be divided into upper part named fundus, which is contracting and thickening during labor, and the lower part of uterus corpus named isthmus. During the labor, isthmus' main part is the junction between the fundus and the cervix; it thins and dilates around fetus (Schwalm & Dubrauszky, 1966; Chard & Grudzinskas, 1994).

The uterine corpus is composed of three layers. The uterine mucosa or endometrium is the innermost layer that lines the cavity of the uterus (inner wall). Its function is nourishing the fetus during pregnancy. The middle layer of the uterus is a smooth muscle named myometrium. The outermost layer, or serosa, is a thin fibrous layer contiguous with extrauterine connective tissue structures such as ligaments that give mechanical support to the uterus within the pelvic cavity (Devedeux et al., 1993; Chard & Grudzinskas, 1994).

The smooth muscle of myometrium is formed by three distinct anatomical layers of smooth muscle fibers organized in different ways. The outermost layer has longitudinal and circular orientation of fibers. In the middle layer of myometrium the origins of muscle fibers are tubes of horns. These muscle fibers are diagonally interlaced with each other. The innermost layer comprises muscle fibers which are mostly in a circular orientation. The distinct organization of anatomical layers of smooth muscle fibers ensures efficient contractility. While the majority of uterus corpus is composed of smooth muscle fibers, in cervix the actual count of smooth muscle fibers is from 10% - 40%. The smooth muscle fibers in cervix lay mostly in a circular orientation (Pajntar et al., 1998; Pajntar et al., 2001; Rudel & Pajntar, 1999; Word et al., 2007; Oláh, 1994). The role of the smooth muscle in cervix is namely that by contractions of muscle fibers contributes to the closing of cervical canal during pregnancy, while in the course of labor muscle fibers dilate, or through a different kind of contraction actively participate in the dilatation and retraction of the cervix. Few weeks prior to the onset of labor uterine contractions, the cervix undergoes tangible changes in consistency and length. Results from different studies using serial measurements of cervical length indicate that cervical ripening precedes myometrial contractions of labor by several weeks, suggesting that parturition in women is a process of long duration and that uterine contractions of labor are late events in the parturition progress (Word et al., 2007).

1.2 Labor and its monitoring

Labor is a physiologic process during which the products of conception (i.e. the fetus, membranes, umbilical cord and placenta) are expelled from the uterus. The onset of labor is defined as regular, painful uterine contractions resulting in progressive cervical effacement and dilatation. Labor is achieved with rhythmic uterine contractions of sufficient frequency, intensity and duration and changes in the connective tissue resulting in dilatation of the cervix (Pajntar et al., 1998).

The labor is divided into three stages that delineate milestones in a continuous process. The first stage begins with regular uterine contractions and ends with complete cervical dilatation at 10 cm. The first stage is subdivided into the latent phase and the active phase. The latent phase begins with mild, irregular uterine contractions that soften and shorten the cervix. The contractions become progressively more rhythmic and stronger. The latent phase is followed by the active phase of labor, which usually begins at about 3-4 cm of cervical dilation and is characterized by rapid cervical dilation and descent of the presenting fetal part. The first stage of labor ends with complete cervical dilation at 10 cm (Kilpatrick S.J. & Russell K.L., 1989; Albers et al., 1996). The mean frequency of contractions over the active phase of labor is four contractions in 10 min, rising to five in 10 min in the late first stage (Sabry-Rizk et al., 2000). The duration of contractions remains remarkably constant, between 70 s and 90 s. The second stage begins with complete cervical dilatation and ends with the delivery of the fetus (Chard & Grudzinskas, 1994). The third stage of labor is defined by the time period between the delivery of the fetus and the delivery of the placenta and fetal membranes.

During the labor the medical staff monitors the state of the woman and the fetus (FDA, n.d.). The monitoring of the response of the fetal heart to the uterine activity is named cardiotocography. To monitor the fetal brain activity a fetal electroencephalographic monitor is used. Ultrasonic devices can be used to determine and monitor accurately the position of the fetal head and the configuration of the cervix as well as the fetal heart rate. During the labor the blood pressure, the temperature of the patient and contractions are routinely and constantly monitored. Especially when complications occur, e.g., when labor shows poor progress, quantitative assessment of uterine contraction efficiency can guide the physician to choose a uterine contractions induction or augmentation, a Caesarean section, or other therapies. The devices for monitoring uterine contractions range in complexity from simple self-awareness of contractions to complex electronic pressure sensors. The currently used devices for monitoring uterine contractions are noninvasive tocodynamometer or 'toco' and invasive intrauterine pressure catheter. By tocodynamometers changes in abdominal contour are detected as an indirect indication of uterine contractions. The disadvantages of currently available 'tocos' are their uncomfortableness and inaccurateness (Schlembach et al., 2009). The intrauterine pressure catheters provide the best information concerning uterine contractions, but their invasiveness can increase the risk of infection and insertion requires rapture of the membranes (Maner &Garfield, 2007).

A lot of effort has been put in quantitative evaluation of uterine contractions to measure their efficiency. For example Montevideo units (MVU) was defined as a measure of uterine contraction intensity expressed as the sum of the intensity of each contraction within a 10-min period, with intensity defined as the peak pressure achieved by the contraction minus the baseline tone (Chard & Grudzinskas, 1994). Although MVU are commonly used in practice, they do not differ between labor outcomes (Cesarean section according to dystocia vs. vaginal delivery) in patients with abnormally progressing labor undergoing augmentation (Euliano et al., 2009). Another method is estimation of cumulative uterine contractions intensity defined as uterine activity units (UAU) per fixed time unit (Gibb et al., 1984; Miller et al., 1976). A correlation between UAU and MVU, was shown (Gibb et al., 1984). The method closely related to UAU is the uterine activity integral (UAI) and is defined as the integral of the intrauterine pressure above the baseline over the contraction duration (Bakker et al., 2007).

One of the simplest methods for monitoring the progress of labor is a partogram. It is a graphical representation of the head station and cervical dilatation in centimeters against the duration of labor in hours. This graph is used by labor medical staff and is based on the assumption that it facilitates early recognition of dystocia, thereby optimizing the timing of appropriate intervention, such as amniotomy, oxytocin augmentation, or, most importantly, Caesarean section (Sharf et al., 2007; Neilson et al., 2003; Windrim et al., 2007; Luria et al., 2009; Sizer et al., 2000; Basu et al., 2009). The method which could be used to help medical stuff to decide how the management of the labor should proceed is the Bishop Score. The Bishop Score (total score) is achieved by the vaginal examination and is composed of five components: fetal station, cervical dilation, cervical effacement, cervical position and cervical consistency (Bishop, 1964; Marconi et al., 2008; Newman et al., 2008).

Intrapartum assessment of uterine activity is routinely employed to guide active management of labor and delivery. The goal of such management is 2-fold: first the progress in labor resulting in vaginal delivery, and secondly the identification of unsuccessful labor that requires Caesarean delivery (Euliano et al., 2009). While the gold standard for assessing labor progress is serial cervical examinations, the risk of infection coupled with the inherent inaccuracy of the measure limits its use to the 2-3 hours intervals. Although sufficient for normal labors, in the slowly dilating patient, the inaccuracies of such judgment can complicate the diagnosis of labor arrest (Euliano et al., 2009). Only the continuous cervical dilation and fetal head station monitoring would improve the labor monitoring of this kind (Euliano et al., 2009). For now, no method is available for non-invasive monitoring and quantification of uterine contractions (Vinken et al., 2010; Euliano et al., 2006), therefore accurate measuring methods and uterine contractions understanding is a challenge for research groups for years.

1.3 Uterine electromyography

Among approaches that has been applied to improve the methods for monitoring gestation and labor changes in uterine activity, noninvasive and invasive procedures based on recording of uterine electrical signals was developed. Their aim was mainly to quantitatively evaluate the uterine activity. An outcome was the method that was called uterine electromyography (EMG) or also electrohysterography (EHG).

Uterine electromyography (uterine EMG) is a monitoring technique developed for medical diagnostics in obstetrics, like some other better known techniques, electrocardiography and electroencephalography. The technique is used for providing information about uterine activity during the pregnancy and labor. This is accomplished by measuring the action potential changes that are associated with the uterine contractions. Nowadays it is well established that uterine contractions are the results of the electrical activity propagation through the uterine muscle cells (Vinken et al., 2010). During the measurement of action potential changes the measuring electrodes are in most cases placed on the maternal abdomen. The first reports of uterine EMG studies were published in 1912 (Veit, 1912). Since 1950s uterine electromyography has been extensively investigated. The uterine electromyography was recorded either internally with endouterine electrodes, or externally with abdominal electrodes, both in animals and humans (Devedeux et al., 1993). It was assumed that abdominal electromyograms could be useful for clinical evaluations of uterine activity during pregnancy due to its noninvasive nature (Devedeux et al., 1993). For registration of the cervical EMG activity adapted spiral fetal scalp electrodes were used, which were inserted directly in cervical tissue from the vaginal side (Pajntar et al., 2001; Pajntar et al., 1998; Rudel & Pajntar, 1999). It was ascertained that the EMG signal records from the cervix reflected the actual activity of cervical smooth muscle cells. Therefore cervical EMG signal can be either independent from myometrial contractions or related to them (Rudel & Pajntar, 1999; Pajntar et al., 1998).

The abdominal uterine EMG records had poor quality comparing to uterine EMG records measured invasively. The amplitude of externally recorded bursts of spikes (from 50 to 200 μV) was about five times lower than the amplitude of the bursts obtained from the internal electrodes. The amplitude of the uterine EMG recorded from the abdominal wall can be affected by various conditions: the type and location of electrodes, the distance between them, as well as the skin impedance of the patient. Attenuation of myometrial signals occurs more for some patients and less for others, depending on a variance in subcutaneous tissues and a variance in conductivity of the skin - electrode interference. A thicker layer of the tissue between the myometrium and pickup electrodes will result in the better signal. In addition, poor conductivity due to high impedance, possibly related to salinity levels or other chemical factors on the skin surface, serves to reduce the measured uterine signal strength and to increase the background noise in the recordings of some patients. Therefore the amplitude and other connected parameters cannot be used directly to compare uterine EMG from different patients. Only the trend of variation of amplitude-based parameters can be useful in clinical applications (Jezewski et al., 2005; Maner et al., 2003).

The uterine EMG is a non-stationary signal (Terrien et al., 2008). The complete information concerning the uterine electrical activity can be obtained by recording the abdominal signal in frequency range from 0 to 5 Hz (Jezewski et al., 2005). The uterine EMG signal frequency spectrum is mainly composed of two frequency intervals, one of low frequencies between 0.1 and 1.2 Hz and the other of high frequencies between 1.2 and 4.7 Hz. They has been named fast wave low (FWL) and fast wave high (FWH) (Leman et al., 1999; Terrien et al.,

2008). Although the definition of FWL and FWH was made by observation of monkey's uterine activity, it is often used in human uterus activity analysis as well. The FWL is presumed to be related to the propagation of the electrical activity along the uterus and FWH is related to excitability of the uterus. The main frequency position of FWH may change as the gestation progresses (Terrien et al., 2010), as well as between individuals and species (Devedeux et al., 1993). The characterization of FWL and FWH may be used to detect a potential risk of preterm delivery, even in the early gestational stage (Leman et al., 1999; Terrien et al., 2008; Jezewski et al., 2005).

Most of the studies have focused on the analysis of contractility of uterus using two or four electrodes. It is generally supposed that the increase in contractility is mainly observable through an increase in frequency and/or amplitude (Terrien et al., 2009). But for investigation of propagation of electrical activity through the whole uterus the increase of system electrodes is necessary (Terrien et al., 2009).

Mainly uterine EMG signal was studied only on specific parts of the records - characteristic intermittent "bursts" of action potentials that correspond to mechanical contractions of uterus (Maul et al., 2003). The EMG segments taken during bursts of uterine activity were usually analyzed with observing amplitude distribution of the signal (Garfield & Maner, 2007; Doret et al., 2005; Jezewski et al., 2005) or calculating the power density spectrum and its modus and/or median frequency (Jezewski et al., 2005; Doret et al., 2005). Recently, approaches based on wavelet transform were used to detect a risk of preterm labor (Hassan et al., 2010).

It was demonstrated that during most of the pregnancy, uterine activity was minimal, consisting of infrequent and low amplitude electromyographic bursts. During term and preterm labor bursts of electromyographic activity were frequent and of large amplitude (Buhimschi et al., 1997). It was assumed that root mean square RMS value denotes the woman's risk for preterm delivery, independent of other possible causes (Verdenik et al., 2001). The importance of an independent activity of the smooth muscle cells in the cervix was also shown by a calculation of RMS values (Pajntar & Verdenik, 1995); namely the RMS value calculated over the intervals of cervical EMG signal is significantly greater in very unripe cervices then in riper cervices at the onset of amniotomy and oxytocin induced labors (Pajntar & Verdenik, 1995).

The shifting of the uterine EMG signal energy to higher frequencies as delivery approaches is also one of the phenomena observed in the literature (Buhimschi et al., 1997; Doret et al., 2005; Garfield et al., 2002; Maner & Garfield, 2007; Vinken et al., 2010; Maner et al., 2003). In particular, the modus frequency of the uterine EMG signal power spectral density (PSD) was commonly tested. Maner et al. reported that the modus frequency of power density spectrum increases as the measurement-to-delivery interval decreases from more than 4 days before the labor to less than 24 hours (Maner et al., 2003). It was shown that nifedipine is an effective tocolytic agent for suppressing preterm contractions with the shift of modus frequency of PSD to lower frequencies when it is expected to rise, with approaching delivery (Vinken et al., 2010). Fele-Žorž et al. showed that also the value of median frequency is higher, when the gestation is coming to the end, which may be associated with term delivery (Fele-Žorž et al., 2008).

For classifying the EMG signals recorded from patients in different state (non-laboring, in labor) the researchers used artificial neural networks, which are usually used for solving artificial intelligence problems without necessarily creating a model of a real biological system (Maner & Garfield, 2007). The bursts of uterine EMG were grouped in different groups due to the patient's state during the recording: preterm-non-laboring, term-non-laboring, term and preterm labor. The bursts were quantified by their duration, the mean value and/or standard deviation and the modus frequency of PSD. For each EMG record also the number of bursts per unit time was evaluated. According to all these measures the artificial neural networks classified the majority of bursts correctly (Maner & Garfield, 2007; Diab et al., 2009).

Oczeretko et al. showed that spontaneous uterine activity of non-pregnant uterus evaluated by inside uterus pressure measurements contains nonlinear features (Oczeretko et al. 2005). Therefore techniques that are able to characterize the dynamic behavior of underlying physiological system were applied also on uterine EMG signals. It was shown that the nonlinear synchronization measures, like the mutual correlation dimension and the cross-approximate entropy, may have a diagnostic value (Oczeretko et al. 2010). The results of synchronization between contractions were promising, especially when for evaluation the fundal and the cervical signals were used. The Sample entropy was proven to be a promising method to differ between preterm and term labors (Fele-Žorž et al. 2008). It was also shown that it would be possible to evaluate the progress of the labor with Sample entropy (Vrhovec et al. 2010; Vrhovec 2009). Sabry-Rizk et al. examined the nonlinear dynamics of the uterus EMG signals on normal and abnormal labor contractions in the first stage of the labor. An attractor structures have been calculated on abdominal EMG signals at various relaxation and contraction periods. The observed black inertness of attractors was called nucleus. Precisely, by studying its fractal behavior it was shown that the size of the nucleus increases with cervical dilatation until it takes over the entire phase-space. The weak labor contractions, typical for failure in progress in the first stage of labor, showed predominantly periodic structures with or without small-size nuclei (Sabry-Rizk et al. 2000). Maner et al. used wavelet transform on the bursts' traces and then calculated fractal dimension of the resulting transformed EMG burst-trace. They showed that this wavelet - decomposition - generated fractal dimension can successfully discern between patients who will deliver spontaneously within 24 h and those who will not; moreover, it can classify antepartum versus labor patients (Maner et al. 2006). But all nonlinear methods do not perform as expected, as it was shown with maximal Lyapunov exponent and correlation dimension (Fele-Žorž et al. 2008). Fele-Žorž et al. showed on 27 min long EMG signals segments, that there is no significant difference between preterm and term labors according to Lyapunov exponent and correlation dimension.

Researchers on the field agree that for efficient labor synchronization of uterine electrical activity is of crucial importance. Uterine EMG activity on different parts of the uterus can be observed from the abdominal surface using multi-electrode measuring systems. Jiang et al. simultaneously measured uterine EMG activity by 16 digitized channels. During the study 297 contractions were observed obtained from twenty patients who went under labor. They calculated energy on the frequency range between 0.2 and 0.45 Hz and between 0.8 and 3 Hz. The results were imaged by calculating the intermediary value of those measured by the electrodes. Visual presentation displayed the synchronization of uterine contractions (Jiang et al. 2007). It was postulated that observation of synchronization together with the classical time - frequency analysis may increase the prediction of labor (Terrien et al., 2010). Using eight channel measuring system and continuously calculating frequencies of movement patterns from normalized and filtered signals, the authors identified the center of uterine activity; Euliano et. al. (Euliano et al., 2009) followed the direction of its propagation and movement. Interestingly, the study reports that the center of uterine activity had a predominant fundal direction in women who delivered successfully. This implies that the lower uterine segment begins to relax earlier than the upper portion of the uterus in women who deliver vaginally (Euliano et al. 2009; Buhimschi 2009).

1.4 Dystocia and its recognition

Arrest in the active phase of labor or dystocia is labor abnormality refers to prolonged or slowly progressing labor. It is common in nulliparous women, as indicated by the number requiring augmentation, operative vaginal delivery, or cesarean section (Joseph et al., 2003; Kjaergaard et al., 2009). Women with a diagnosed dystocia had more often non-clear amniotic fluid, more post-partum hemorrhage, significantly increased odds of chorioamnionitis and their children were more often given low one-minute neonatal Apgar scores as compared to women delivered without a diagnosed dystocia (Kjaergaard et al., 2009; Pitkin, 2003). Although many reasons were identified such as inappropriate position or size of the fetus, congenital anomalies, cephalopelvic disproportion, abnormal uterine contractions and others (Chard & Grudzinskas, 1994), diagnosis of dystocia and optimal management recommendations are still under consideration (Shields et al., 2007).

One of the reasons for slow diagnosis of dystocia in labor progress is a lack of qualitative measurement methods for evaluating the uterus activity during labor (Euliano et al., 2009). The measurement of the uterine EMG activity provides information about myocyte electrical activity directly and investigations have indicated that it is a sensitive method having a potential in a clinical practice as a supplement tool used for monitor labor (Garfield & Maner, 2007; Doret et al., 2005; Jezewski et al., 2005). In the previous studies researchers evaluated the characteristic of the final number of burst segments, which did not describe the progress of the labor (Garfield & Maner, 2007; Doret et al., 2005; Jezewski et al., 2005). Although majority of studies are done on bursts, there are studies which showed that during labor the activity between bursts is also related to the course of labor (Pajntar et al., 1998; Verdenik et al., 2001). In this work we presented how the characteristics of uterine EMG bursts change during the last eight weeks of gestation and the evaluation of normally progressing labor as well as labor with a diagnosis of dystocia using continuously monitored uterine EMG signals. Two types of uterine EMG signal segmentation were used: successive non-overlapping segments of uterine EMG record and successive burst segments of EMG activity. By analyzing the successive non-overlapping segments of uterine EMG record we could avoid the time-consuming procedure of the bursts of EMG activity extraction. For interpretation of the uterine EMG signals Sample entropy (SampEn), the measure of time series complexity, was used.

2. Uterine EMG measurements and patients

For the purpose of the studies we used two databases. Measuring protocol that was used for recording of the "contractions" database, is described in details in Karlsson et all (Karlsson et al., 2007). The measurements were performed at the Landspitali University hospital in Iceland using a protocol approved by the relevant ethical committee. The "contraction" database was recorded by Karlsson et all (Karlsson et al., 2007) and was given to us for analysis. The subjects were seven healthy patients monitored from 32nd week of gestation to labor. The "contraction" database consists of 45 EMG signals recorded during the contractions. The EMG signals were recorded on the woman's abdominal wall by a 16-channel multi-purpose physiological signal recorder resulting in 12 bipolar EMG signals.

From each record we extract just one bipolar signal obtained with subtraction of two channels on the median vertical axis of the uterus. The signal sampling rate was 200 Hz; the recording device had a low pas filter with a cut-off frequency of 100 Hz. The EMG signals were first band-pass filtered (0.1 - 3 Hz). Each record was resampled to get as similar sampling frequency (10 Hz) as possible for the two data sets.
Measuring protocol that was used for uterine EMG recording of the "labor" database is described in details in Pajntar et all (Pajntar et al., 1998) and was approved by the National Medical Ethics Committee of Slovenia. In the study 45 patients, that have undergone their first labor at the age from 19 to 29 years, were included. After admission to the delivery room the value of Bishop Score was assessed for each patient. The values of the cervical dilatation and the fetal head station were recorded into the partogram that was carefully drawn over the whole course of the labor. During the labor, according to the protocol (Pajntar et al., 1998), quantitative information concerning uterine efficiency was provided invasively, by continuous measurement of the amniotic internal uterine pressure (IUP) with an internal uterine pressure catheter. The EMG signals were recorded on the cervix; however, in some cases an obstetrician also measured the EMG signals of the uterine corpus. Uterine EMG and IUP were measured contemporary. All signals (EMG and IUP) were sampled at 18.2 Hz, low-pass filtered at 5 Hz and saved. The "labor" database was recorded by Pajntar et all (Pajntar et al., 1998) and was given to us for analysis. We selected all labors that were, according to the partogram traces and the labor documentation, recognized as normally progressing labors or labors with a diagnosed dystocia. Therefore the database was divided into two groups: the first group consists of 15 normally progressing labors, whereas the second one consists of 13 labors with a diagnosed dystocia (Table 1). After a careful visual inspection of corresponding EMG records we rejected those records containing long or numerous noise periods. Finally, six EMG records of normally progressing labors (lasting from 1:48 to 4:18 h) and five EMG records of labors with a diagnosis of dystocia (lasting from 4:51 to 9:51 h) were included in the study.

type of labor (No.)	**Bishop score**	**length of active phase**	**weight of a newborn [g]**	**size of the head of a newborn [cm]**
normally progressing labors (15)	6 (8 2)	2h 40min (4h 15min 1h 30min)	3640 (4360 2850)	34.75 (37 33)
labors with a diagnosis of dystocia (13)	6 (9 3)	5h 18min (7h 30min 3h)	3590 (4280 3100)	35 (38 33)

Table 1. The labors were divided into two groups according to the partograms and labor documentations. The characteristics (Bischop score at the acceptation to the delivery room, length of the active phase, the weight and the size of the head of a newborn) of both labor types are listed as the median, the maximal and the minimal value in the brackets. The significant difference between the normally progressing labors and labors with a diagnosis of dystocia is present only in the length of the active phase (p=0.002). See section 3.3 for statistical details.

The uterine EMG signals were band-pass filtered using the second order Butterworth digital filter of 0.3 Hz - 3 Hz. After filtering, we decreased the sampling rate of the records by keeping every second sample. Values of SampEn were then calculated throughout the entire labor records in two ways. Firstly, each uterine EMG signal was divided into successive non-overlapping segments that lasted 8.2 min, contained 4500 samples and at least one uterine contraction. From these 4500 samples we calculated one value of SampEn. Secondly, all burst segments that correspond to successive uterine contractions were extracted from uterine EMG signal. The concurrently recorded intrauterine pressure (IUP) was used in order to ease the identification of contractions in recorded time. After identification, burst segments of the uterine EMG activity were manually extracted. All bursts segments were visually inspected and we rejected those burst segments that did not exhibit concurrent increase in IUP. The recorded uterine contractions lasted from 27.1 s to 224.3 s, therefore corresponding burst segments of the uterine EMG activity contained from 431 to 2095 samples. In this case we calculated one value of SampEn for individual burst segment.

3. Methods

Time- and frequency- domain methods have been used for evaluation of uterine EMG signals for years (see chapter 1.5), but they have not been designed to yield information on systems' inherent dynamic properties (Kuusela et al. 2002). Nonlinear time series analysis techniques can be more useful when characterizing the dynamic behavior of physiological systems (Rezek & Roberts 1998). There are many studies in which the complexity of a physiological signal was found as an important characterization of an underlying physiological process and was even proposed as a diagnostic tool (Abasolo et al. 2006; Costa et al. 2003; Costa et al. 2005; Pincus et al. 1993; Radhakrishnan & Gangadhar 1998; Radhakrishnan et al. 2000; Rezek & Roberts 1998; Richman & Moorman 2000; Xu et al. 2007; Zhang et al. 2001). In this work, both time- and frequency- domain methods, as well as nonlinear methods (measures of complexity) were used. All the analyses were made in MATLAB software (version R2010a; Inc, 2010 U.S.).

3.1 Time- and frequency- domain methods

The power spectral density (PSD), was calculated using the Welch method. Hamming window was used, which was the same length as the segment of uterine EMG signal. We evaluate median frequency of PSD and modus frequency of PSD. Additionally root mean square (RMS) was calculated.

3.2 Measures of complexity

The techniques of time series analysis measuring the complexity can be grouped: 1) information theory estimates of complexity like entropy; 2) chaos - based estimates of complexity like Lyapunov exponent; 3) Komologrov estimates like Lempel-Ziv complexity (Šliupaitė et al. 2009). In our work we concentrate on information theory estimates of complexity. In particular we focus on entropy methods especially on Sample entropy and Approximate entropy. However we also tested Lampel-Ziv complexity.

3.2.1 Approximate entropy

Approximate entropy (ApEn) was introduced as a quantification of complexity in sequences and time series data, initially motivated by applications to relatively short, noisy data sets (Rezek & Roberts, 1998; Pincus, 1991; Hornero et al., 2005). ApEn detects changes in underlying episodic behavior not reflected in a peak occurrences or amplitudes. Moreover it can be applied to finite stochastic, noisy deterministic and composite processes. Regular signals are expected to have low ApEn values (Rezek & Roberts 1998), while complex ones take on higher ApEn values. The exact algorithm is described elsewhere (Pincus, 1991).

3.2.2 Sample entropy

Richman et.al (Richman & Moorman 2000) showed that ApEn values are inconsistent due to two important expected properties. First ApEn depends on record length and is uniformly lower than expected for short records. Secondly, it lacks relative consistency. Meaning, if the value of ApEn of one data set is higher than another data set, it should remain higher for all conditions although it does not. Therefore a related complexity measure was developed as improved ApEn where self-matches are not included in calculating the probability (Richman & Moorman 2000). The exact algorithm of Sample entropy (SampEn) is described elsewhere (Richman & Moorman, 2000).

3.2.3 Lampel-Ziv complexity

Lampel-Ziv complexity (LZ) C(n) measures the generation rate of new patterns along a digital sequence (Zhang et al. 2001; Lempel & Ziv 1976). The signal has to be transformed into a sequence whose elements are only a few symbols. In the context of biomedical signal analysis, typically the discrete-time signal segment $\{x(t)\},\{ t=\{1,\ldots, N\}$ is converted into a binary sequence $P=s_1, s_2, s_3, \ldots, s_n$, where s_i is 0 if $x(i)<T_d$ otherwise it takes value 1. Usually the median is used as a threshold T_d (Radhakrishnan & Gangadhar 1998). The sequence P is scanned from left to right and the complexity counter $c(n)$ is increased by one every time a new subsequence of consecutive characters is encountered in the scanning process. After normalization, the complexity measure reflects the rate of new pattern occurrences with time. The exact algorithm is described elsewhere (Radhakrishnan & Gangadhar, 1998).

3.2.4 Uterine activity integral

Uterine activity integral (UAI) is defined as the integral of the intrauterine pressure above the baseline over the contraction duration (Bakker et al. 2007) and it represents uterine contractions intensity. The UAI are calculated from the IUP record for each successive uterine contraction. The IUP record has a specific shape; the values of IUP increase from the basal value at the beginning of uterine contraction and decrease back to the basal value at the end of uterine contraction. Usually the IUP record is first detrended to avoid possible linear trends in the signal. The UAI is then calculated as the area under the IUP curve during contraction while the basal tone is excluded from calculation.

3.3 Statistical analysis

Statistical analyses were performed by using SYSTAT software (version 11; Inc, 2004; Chicago). Descriptive data are presented as medians unless otherwise indicated. Nonparametric Friedman Two-Way Analysis was used to compare the measures between normal labors and labors with a diagnosis of dystocia, as well as to compare the measures between latent and active phase of the labors. The p value < 0.05 was accepted as significant. The values being calculated with SampEn and ApEn showed a specific trend of each labor group. Therefore we fitted polynomials to SampEn and ApEn values calculated in the first stage of labor. The fit of the polynomials was conditioned with statistic measure how successful the fit was with R-square. We required R-square 0.50 ± 0.10 or better at the lowest polynomial degree. First the polynomials were circumscribed to the values of SampEn and ApEn, which were calculated on successive non-overlapping segments of the EMG signal, since the values of SampEn and ApEn in this case were less spread out at the visual inspection. The polynomial degree was fixed. With fixed polynomial degree the polynomials were circumscribed also to the values of SampEn and ApEn, which were calculated on the burst segments of the EMG activity that correspond to successive uterine contractions. R–square of the fit of polynomial was calculated.

4. Before and during the labor evaluations using uterine EMG signal

The records of uterine EMG signals from "contraction" database were measured during the last two months of gestation. The uterine EMG signals were recorded only during uterine contractions; therefore the analyses were done on the burst segments of EMG activity. The recording of uterine EMG signals in "labor" database began at the patient's arrival to the delivery room. Therefore the EMG records have different lengths and are recorded in different phases of the labor although all EMG signals were recorded during the first stage of labor without discontinuance. As such they are not easy to compare even in the same labor group. To get an impression how the labors of normally progressing labor and labor with a diagnosed dystocia look like, we outlined a labor per group, to characterize each labor group.

4.1 End of gestation and the latent phase of the labor

We compared the bursts segments of EMG activity record in the last two months of gestation and the latent phase of the normally progressing labor. For the comparison we used the "contraction" database and 73 burst segments of the uterine EMG activity extracted from the latent phase of normally progressing labors in "labor" database.

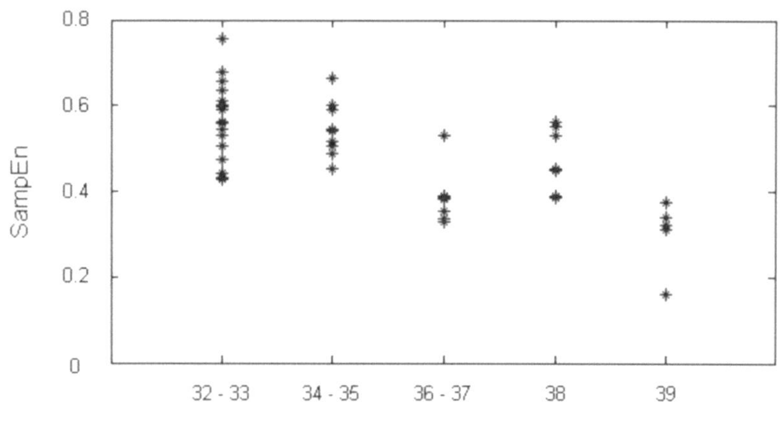

Fig. 1. The values of SampEn calculated during 32 - 33, 34 - 35, 36 - 37, 38 and 39 week of gestation.

The values of SampEn, calculated on all 45 EMG bursts obtained from 32nd to 39th weeks of gestation, are shown in Figure 1 and their basic statistics is given in Table 2. The values of SampEn calculated from EMG bursts recorded in 32nd and 33rd week of gestation were gathered in one group. They ranged from 0.43 to 0.76 (median value is 0.56). The values of SampEn calculated from EMG bursts recorded in 34th and 35th week of gestation were very similar (min 0.45, max 0.66, median 0.54) and showed no statistically significant difference from those measured in weeks 32 and 33. The values of SampEn calculated from EMG bursts recorded in 36th and 37th week of gestation ranged from 0.33 to 0.53; the median value (0.38) was significantly lower than in previous two cases. SampEn values obtained from EMG bursts in 38th week of gestation ranged from 0.39 to 0.56 with median value 0.45. The values of SampEn calculated from EMG bursts recorded in 39th week of gestation ranged from 0.16 to 0.38. The median value was 0.32. It was significantly lower than median SampEn value calculated in any other period of gestation. In the latent phase of the labor the values of SampEn increase. The values of SampEn calculated from EMG bursts record in the latent phase ranged from 0.07 to 1.03 with median value 0.71. This value is much higher then the median values obtained in any period of gestation.

Week of gestation	32-33	34-35	36-37	38	39	Latent phase
Minimal value	0.43	0.45	0.33	0.39	0.16	0.07
Maximal value	0.76	0.66	0.53	0.56	0.38	1.03
Median value	0.56	0.54	0.38	0.45	0.32	0.71

Table 2. Characteristic values of SampEn during weeks of gestation and latent phase of the labor.

The SampEn has already been presented as a promising method for analyzing the term and preterm labor. Fele-Žorž et al. (Fele-Žorž et al., 2008) used 20 min long EMG records measured before 26th week of gestation and they have shown that the values of SampEn for term labor records are higher than those for preterm labor. Moreover, due to our results the SampEn values calculated on EMG bursts significantly drop in 36th - 37th week of gestation and are even lower approaching the term; while the beginning of the labor is characterized by relatively high SampEn values.

4.2 Normally progressing labor

A typical progress of normal labor with a short latent phase is presented in Figures 2. The trace of the normally progressing labor is outlined as the partogram in the Figure 2A. The time in hours is on the abscissa; on the ordinate there are cervical dilatation (squares) and head station range (circles). The observation of the labor started at 1.8 cm cervical dilatation. The latent phase of the labor lasted for 40 minutes. In the active phase of the normal labor dilatation of cervix was progressing in the course of time and the head of the fetus was evenly drooping with no delays. The grey zone in Figures 2 marks the border between the latent and the active phase. It is marked according to partogram from 3 to 4 cm cervical dilatation.

In Figure 2B the number of contractions in 8.2 min long observation intervals (which correspond to successive non-overlapping segments of the EMG signal) in the course of time is shown. In the latent phase of the normally progressing labor only one contraction was present in 8.2 min long observation intervals. With labor progression the number of contractions in 8.2 min long intervals increased to 3 contractions at the end of the latent phase. The number of contractions was stationary around 4 contractions in 8.2 min long intervals during the active phase.

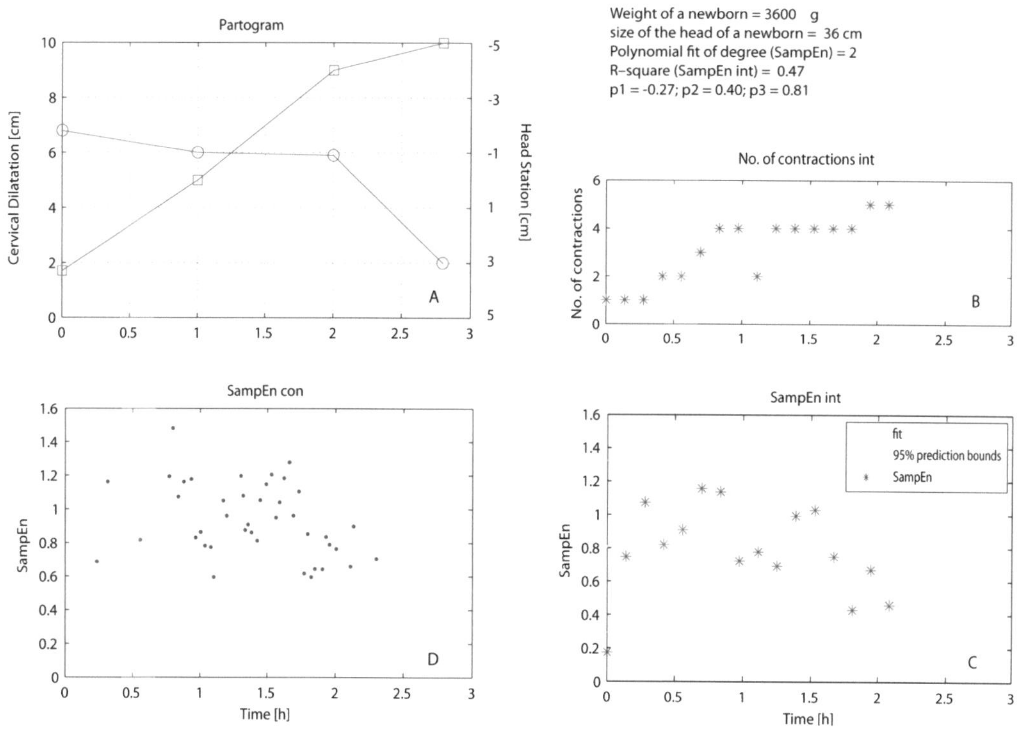

Fig. 2. The progress of normally progressing labor evaluated with different methods. A: Partogram. B: The number of contractions in 8.2 min long observation intervals. C: Values of SampEn calculated on successive non-overlapping segments of uterine EMG signal that lasted 8.2 min and polynomial fit ($p_1x^2 + p_2x + p_3$). D: Values of SampEn calculated on the burst segments of uterine EMG signal.

The trend of SampEn values calculated on successive non-overlapping segments is shown in Figure 2C. The SampEn values in the latent phase of the labor range from 0.74 to 1.15. As the active phase begins the SampEn values start to decrease. They reduce to the value 0.42 in approximately one hour when cervical dilatation already amounts 9 cm. According to all labors from our database we can conclude that at the transition from latent to active phase of the normal labor the values of SampEn start to decrease. The declining trend in values of SampEn continues with approaching the childbirth in the course of normal labor. This means that in active phase the uterine EMG activity starts to reduce its complexity, which becomes very low at the childbirth (Vrhovec, 2009; Vrhovec et al., 2010). The specific trend of SampEn values, calculated during normally progressing labors, is even more evident by the polynomial fitted to SampEn values. On the values of SampEn shown on Figure 2C the polynomial of second degree was fitted. The goodness of the fit R-square was 0.63.
The values of SampEn calculated on the burst segments of EMG activity are shown on Figure 2D start to decrease at the transition from the latent to active phase of normally progressing labor. The values of SampEn are more spread, if they are calculated on the burst segments of the uterine EMG activity, compared to the values of SampEn, calculated on successive non-overlapping segments of uterine EMG signal (Figure 2C). According to spread SampEn values calculated on the burst segments of the uterine EMG activity, we can conclude that the complexity of uterine EMG bursts differs from contraction to contraction.

The ApEn values give similar results to the SampEn values, while no specific trends were found in values of median frequency, modus frequency, RMS or LZ in the course of normally progressing labor whatever type of uterine EMG signal segmentation had been used.

4.3 Examination of the labor with a diagnosed dystocia

The trace of a labor with a diagnosed dystocia is outlined as the partogram in Figure 3A. The observation of the labor started at 1.5 cm cervical dilatation. The latent phase of the labor lasted for 2 hours. The border between the latent and the active phase is marked as the grey zone according to the partogram from 3 to 4 cm cervical dilatation. The grey zone is marked also in the rest of the parts of Figure 3. In the active phase of this labor the fetal head did not descend for two hours. Afterwards it continued the dropping trend (Figure 3A). Similar fetal head descend arrest can be noticed in the active phase of all labors in this labor group.

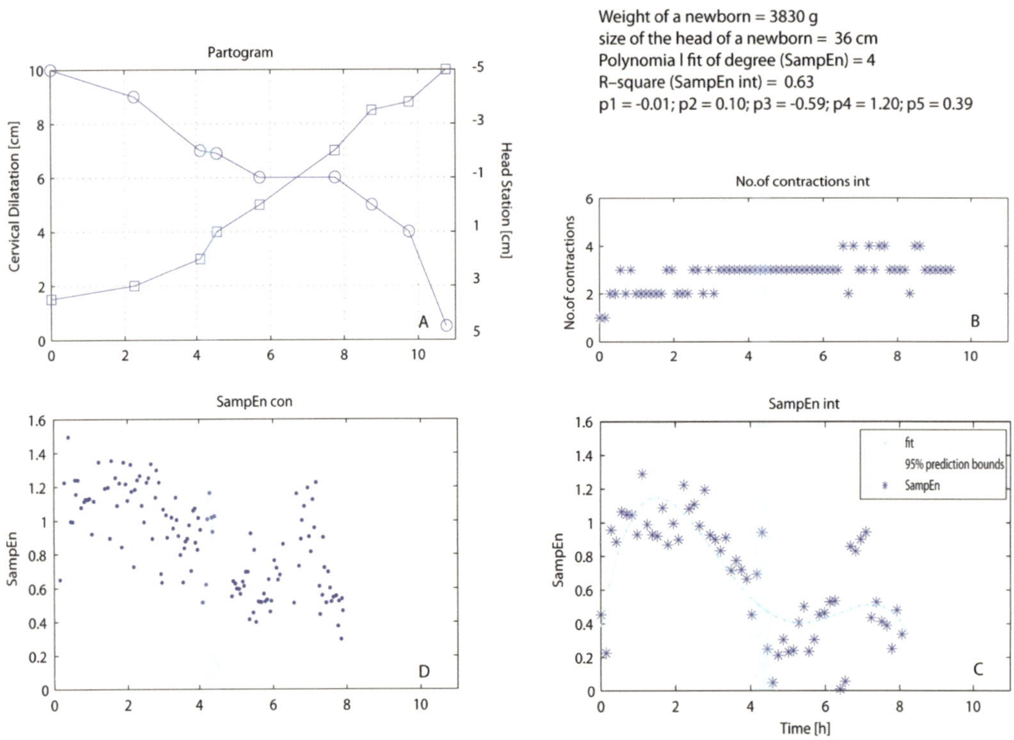

Fig. 3. The progress of normally progressing labor evaluated with different methods.
A: Partogram. B: The number of contractions in 8.2 min long observation intervals.
C: Values of SampEn calculated on successive non-overlapping segments of uterine EMG signal that lasted 8.2 min and polynomial fit ($p_1x^4 + p_2x^3 + p_3x^2 + p_4x + p_5$). D: Values of SampEn calculated on the burst segments of uterine EMG signal.

The number of contractions that were present in 8.2 min long observation intervals (which correspond to successive non-overlapping segments of the EMG signal) in the course of time is shown in Figure 3B. During the latent phase of this labor the number of contractions included in successive non-overlapping segments increased to 3. The number of contractions remained around 3 contractions in the active phase.

The values of SampEn calculated on successive non-overlapping segments of uterine EMG signal are shown in Figure 3C. The SampEn values in the latent phase of the labor range from 0.85 to 1.3. The values of SampEn start to decrease already in the latent phase, at approximately 2 cm cervical dilatation, and proceed in a decreasing trend in the active phase to the value 0.2. During the delay in the active phase the values of SampEn rise again and range from 0.2 to 0.95. As the fetal head descend proceeds, the values of SampEn drop again to the value 0.25. To confirm the specific trend of SampEn values calculated on the uterine EMG record of the labor with a diagnosed dystocia, we fitted the polynomial. On the values of SampEn that are shown on Figure 3C the polynomial of the fourth degree was fitted. The goodness of the fit R-square was 0.63.

In Figure 3D the values of SampEn calculated on the burst segments of the uterine EMG activity are shown. In the latent phase of the labor they ranged from 0.51 to 1.49. In the active phase the values of SampEn decreased to the value 0.40. During the dystocia the values of SampEn rose to the range from 0.40 to 1.20. When approaching the end of dystocia the values of SampEn dropped to the value 0.30 at the end of recorded EMG signal. The values of SampEn are more spread, if they are calculated on the burst segments of the uterine EMG activity, then if they are calculated on successive non-overlapping segments of uterine EMG signal. Also in the case of the labor with a diagnosed dystocia the values of SampEn differ from contraction to contraction, which leads to conclusion that the complexity of EMG bursts differs between contractions.

The ApEn values give similar results as the SampEn values. They start to decrease in the latent phase of the labor and keep decreasing to the value 0.23. During the dystocia the values of ApEn rise to the value 1.18. Approaching the end of the delay the values of ApEn dropped to the value 0.50. Values of median frequency, modus frequency, RMS or LZ did not show any specific trends in the course of labors with a diagnosed dystocia regardless of type of uterine EMG signal segmentation had been used.

4.4 Evaluation of labor progress

The progress of labors was evaluated by the number of contractions present in 8.2 min long observation intervals and UAI of contractions. Beside these two evaluations the values of median frequency, the values of modus frequency, the values of RMS, the values of SampEn, the values of LZ, as well as the values of ApEn were used for evaluation of the course of labor. The evaluation of the labor with the listed methods was done on the bases of two types of segmentation: successive non-overlapping segments of uterine EMG signal and the burst segments of the uterine EMG activity.

The number of contractions increased in the course of a normally progressing labor. The number of contractions had the increasing trend up to the transition between the latent phase and the active phase of the labor. The UAI of contractions did not yield any specific trend that could be noted in the course of a normally progressing labor; ordinarily UAI differed from contraction to contraction. Similarly an evaluation of the labor progress made with the values of median frequency, the values of modus frequency, the values of RMS and the values of LZ did not yield any specific trends that could be noted in the course of a normally progressing labor.

However the values of SampEn started to decrease at the transition from the latent to the active phase of the normally progressing labor. The decreasing trend of SampEn values continued with approaching the childbirth. The type of segmentation of uterine EMG signal (successive non-overlapping segments of the EMG signal and the burst segments of the uterine EMG activity) did not affect the main behavior of SampEn values in the course of a normal labor. The SampEn values were more spread when they were calculated on the burst segments of the uterine EMG activity compared to the values of SampEn, calculated on successive non-overlapping segments of uterine EMG signal. According to the spread values of SampEn, calculated on the burst segments of the uterine EMG activity during the labor, we conclude that the complexity of EMG signal differs from contraction to contraction even in the same labor phase. A specific trend of values of SampEn calculated in the course of a normally progressing labor was confirmed with polynomial fit. When we fitted the polynomials, we required R-square 0.50 ± 0.10 or better at the lowest polynomial degree. First we fitted the polynomials on the SampEn values, calculated on successive non-overlapping segments of the EMG signal, since the values were, according to visual inspection less spread out. The polynomial fit was of the first degree in the case when recorded latent phase was short. In normally progressing labors with a longer latent phase, the values were fitted with polynomial of the second degree (Table 3). The mean value of R-square was 0.52 (min: 0.47; max 0.67). If the polynomials were fitted on the values of SampEn calculated on the burst segments of the uterine EMG activity, the mean value of R-square was 0.07 (min 0.01; max 0.21). These results confirm that the values of SampEn are much more spread out when calculated on the burst segments of the uterine EMG activity.

When the normally progressing labors were evaluated with ApEn, the results were similar to those evaluated with SampEn. At the transition from the latent to the active phase of labor the values of ApEn started to decrease. The decreasing trend of ApEn values continued with approaching the childbirth in the course of a normal labor. The values of ApEn were more spread when they were calculated on the burst segments of the uterine EMG activity compared to the values of ApEn, calculated on successive non-overlapping segments of uterine EMG signal. The specific trend of values of ApEn, calculated in the course of normally progressing labor, was confirmed with polynomial fit. The polynomial fit was of the first or second degree, depending on the length of the recorded latent phase (Table 3).

In the course of labor with a diagnosed dystocia, the number of contractions increased up to the transition between the latent and the active phase of the labor, while in active phase of the labor it remained constant. The UAI of contractions did not yield any specific trend in the course of labor with a diagnosed dystocia as well as the values of median frequency, the values of modus frequency, the values of RMS and values of LZ.

The values of SampEn started to decrease with approaching the end of the latent phase or at the transition from the latent to the active phase of the labor. The decreasing trend of SampEn values continued in the active phase until, according to the partogram, the dystocia occurred. During the dystocia of the labor the values of SampEn rose. When approaching the end of the dystocia the values of SampEn dropped. The values of SampEn were, when visually inspected, more spread when for calculation the burst segments of the uterine EMG were used, although the trends were similar to the trends of SampEn values calculated on successive non-overlaping segments of the uterine EMG signal. The specific trend of SampEn values calculated in the course of labor with a diagnosed dystocia was confirmed with polynomial fit of degree. The polynomial fit was of the third degree in the case, when the record of the labor with a diagnosed dystocia had short latent phase. The labors with a diagnosed dystocia and longer recorded latent phase were fitted with polynomials of the fourth degree. The mean value of R-square was 0.51 (min 0.45; max 0.63). The successfulness of the fit on the values of SampEn calculated on the burst segments of the uterine EMG activity, using the same degree of polynomials as in previous uterine EMG

	Normally progressing labors	Labors with a diagnosed dystocia
	Active phase	
Polynomial fit of degree (SampEn)	1 or 2	4
R-square (SampEn)	0.52 (0.47 0.67)	0.51 (0.45 0.63)
Polynomial fit of degree (ApEn)	1 or 2	4
R-square (ApEn)	0.52 (0.41 0.61)	0.43 (0.38 0.57)
Values of SampEn	0.21 (0.02 1.03)* **0.71 (0.07 1.79)***	0.42 (0.01 1.40)* **0.69 (0.15 1.58)***
Values of ApEn	0.49 (0.09 1.26)* **0.77 (0.17 1.24)***	0.67 (0.12 1.46)* **0.76 (0.20 1.44)***
Median frequency value	0.36 Hz (0.18 Hz 0.75 Hz) **0.44Hz(0.18 Hz 2.06 Hz)***	0.39 Hz (0.21 Hz 1.96 Hz) **0.36 Hz(0.18 Hz 1.92 Hz)***
Modus frequency value	0.25 Hz (0.07 Hz 0.68 Hz)* **0.36 Hz(0.14 Hz 2.38 Hz)***	0.28 Hz (0.18 Hz 1.92 Hz)* **0.28 Hz (0.04 Hz 2.42 Hz)***
RMS value	80.48μV (10.84 μV 470.09μV) **70.20 μV (2.91μV 836.03μV)***	65.20 μV (7.40 μV 413.15 μV) **65.36μV (7.140 μV 386.65 μV)***
LZ value	0.6338 (0.3937 0.8360) **0.6720 (0.2699 1.4426)**	0.6621 (0.4854 0.8684) **0.6927 (0.3616 1.5127)**
	Late latent phase	
Values of SampEn	0.45 (0.04 1.16)* **0.58 (0.09 1.44)***	0.68 (0.05 1.29)* **0.87 (0.32 1.49)***
Values of ApEn	0.70 (0.17 1.31)* **0.70 (0.23 1.24)***	0.93 (0.17 1.41)* **0.89 (0.44 1.37)***
Median frequency value	0.39 Hz (0.25 Hz 1.24 Hz) **0.39 Hz (0.21 Hz 0.99Hz)**	0.39 Hz (0.21 Hz 1.31 Hz) **0.39 Hz (0.21 Hz 1.63 Hz)**
Modus frequency value	0.32 Hz (0.18 Hz 1.35 Hz) **0.32 Hz (0.04 Hz 1.31 Hz)***	0.28 Hz (0.04 Hz 1.42 Hz) **0.28 Hz (0.18 Hz 1.70 Hz)***
RMS value	54.54 μV (5.50 μV 342.32 μV) **54.35 μV (9.15 μV 318.37 μV)***	40.60 μV (9.17 μV 227.51 μV) **38.94 μV (8.52 μV 180.06 μV)***
LZ value	0.6149(0.4450 0.7281)* **0.6659 (0.3891 1.1583)***	0.6796 (0.4935 0.8765)* **0.7261 (0.3821 1.3288)***

Table 3. A comparison between normally progressing labors and labors with a diagnosed dystocia. The values listed in the table are the median, the minimal and the maximal value in the brackets. The values calculated on burst segments of the uterine EMG activity are bolded. The significant difference between labor groups is marked with *.

signal segmentation, was 0.29 (min 0.19; max 0.51). From the results of polynomial fit we can conclude that in the case of labors with a diagnosed dystocia the degree of polynomial fit was usually two degrees higher than in the case of normally progressing labors.

When the labors with a diagnosed dystocia were evaluated with ApEn, the results were similar to those evaluated with SampEn. The values of ApEn started to decrease with approaching the end of the latent phase or at the transition from the latent to the active phase of the labor. The decreasing trend of ApEn values continued in the active phase until, according to the partogram, the dystocia occurred. During the dystocia of the labor the values of ApEn rose. When approaching the end of the dystocia, the values of ApEn dropped. The values of ApEn were more spread when they were calculated on the burst segments of the uterine EMG activity. The specific trend of values of ApEn calculated in the course of the labor with a diagnosed dystocia was confirmed with polynomial fit. The polynomial fit was of the third or fourth degree (Table 3), depending on the length of the recorded latent phase. From the results we can assume that in the case of labors with a diagnosed dystocia the degree of polynomial fit is usually one or two degrees higher than in the case of normally progressing labors.

Median, maximal and minimal values of all chosen measures for labor evaluation are presented in Table 3. The values of SampEn calculated on the uterine EMG records of normally progressing labors are significantly lower than the ones calculated on the uterine EMG records of labors with a diagnosed dystocia, regardless of the used segmentation (successive non-overlapping segments of the EMG signal or burst segments of the uterine EMG activity) or the labor phase (latent or active). Significantly higher SampEn values calculated in the latent phase of the labor with a diagnosed dystocia, compared to the ones calculated on normally progressing labor records, imply SampEn potential as a diagnostic tool. Namely, high values of SampEn in the latent phase of the labor suggest the dystocia occurrence. The same significant difference between the labor's groups in the latent phase could be observed when ApEn or LZ was used as a measure for labor evaluation (Table 3).

In the latent phase of the labor with a diagnosed dystocia also significantly lower RMS values and the values of modus frequency were obtained, compared to the ones calculated on normally progressing labor records (Table 3). The differences were significant only, if the values were calculated on the burst segments of the uterine EMG activity. According to Table 3 there is no difference between the labor groups in the values of median frequency calculated in the latent phase, regardless of used segmentation. The values of median frequency showed a significant difference between a normally progressing labor and the labor with a diagnosed dystocia only in the active phase, when they were calculated on burst segments of the uterine EMG activity.

5. Discussion and conclusions

It is well known that in active phase of normal labor uterine muscles contractions, that are strong and long enough, should be present. Although lot of effort has been put in quantitative evaluation of uterine contractions to measure their efficiency (Gibb et al., 1984; Miller et al., 1976), studies have shown that various contraction-based measures (Montevideo units, uterine activity units) do not differ between labor outcomes (Euliano et al., 2009).

On the other hand obstetricians agree that a contractile pattern of the uterine muscles, that provide sufficient descending pressure gradient force, is obvious in active phase of normal labor. Therefore recognition of ineffective uterine muscles contractile patterns may be helpful in diagnosis of dystocia. Measurement of the uterine EMG activity provides information about myocyte electrical activity directly and investigations have indicated that it is a sensitive method having a potential in a clinical practice as a supplement tool used to monitor labor. Through the years researchers have studied different characteristics of the uterine EMG activity. Mostly they were based on time- and frequency- domain methods. Generally, time- and frequency- domain methods are useful and have been widely adopted in studies of the physiological signals (Rezek & Roberts, 1998), but they have not been designed to yield information on systems' inherent dynamic properties. For this purpose nonlinear time series analysis techniques can be more suitable (Richman & Moorman, 2000). Indeed, there are many studies in which the complexity of a physiological signal was found as an important characterization of an underlying physiological process and was even proposed as a diagnostic tool (Abasolo et al., 2006; Rezek & Roberts, 1998; Zhang et al., 2001). The uterine EMG is a non-stationary signal (Terrien et al., 2008); therefore we evaluated the uterine EMG signals recorded in the last two months of gestation, during normally progressing labors and during labors with a diagnosed dystocia by measures of complexity (ApEn, SampEn and LZ) as well as by time- and frequency- domain methods (median frequency, modus frequency and RMS).

The SampEn has already been presented as a promising method for distinguishing the term and preterm labor according to 20 min long EMG signals measured before 26th week of gestation (Fele-Žorž et al., 2008). They have shown that the values of SampEn for term labor records are higher than those for preterm labor. Moreover, due to our results the SampEn values calculated on EMG bursts significantly drop in 36th - 37th week of gestation and are even lower approaching the term; while the beginning of the labor is characterized by relatively high SampEn values.

Observations of normally progressing labors showed that the values of SampEn calculated on successive non-overlapping segments of the EMG signal or burst segments of the uterine EMG activity start to decrease at the transition from the latent to the active phase. The decreased trend of SampEn values continued with approaching the childbirth. Therefore we could conclude that the uterine EMG activity is regulated in the course of normally progressing labor (Vrhovec, 2009; Vrhovec et al., 2010). Observations of the labors with a diagnosed dystocia showed specific trend in SampEn values. The trend of SampEn values is similar to the trend observed in the case of normally progressing labors, until in the case of labors with a diagnosed dystocia, according to the partogram, the dystocia occurs. During the dystocia the values of SampEn rise. With approaching the end of the dystocia the values of SampEn drop again.

The values of SampEn were more spread when they were calculated on the burst segments of the uterine EMG activity compared to the values of SampEn calculated on successive non-overlapping segments of uterine EMG signal. According to the spread values of SampEn calculated on the burst segments we conclude that the complexity of EMG signals differs between contractions. Whatever type of segmentation was used to evaluate the labor (successive non-overlapping segments of the EMG signal and the burst segments of the uterine EMG activity), the trends were similar, typical for the type of labor. A specific trend of SampEn values calculated in the course of both labor groups was confirmed with polynomial fit. The polynomial fit is of the first degree in the case when normally progressing labors have a limit recorded latent phase. Normally progressing labors with a longer latent phase are fit with polynomial of the second degree. The polynomial fit is usually of the fourth degree when the labor has a diagnosed dystocia. As it could be observed in Tables 3 the same conclusions and the results can be outlined when the values were calculated with ApEn or when they were calculated with SampEn.

The correlation between EMG parameters and course of gestation shows that with duration of pregnancy the frequency of recorded electrical activity becomes lower, which is expressed as lower median frequency of uterine electrical activity (Verdenik et al., 2001). However, another study show that when the gestation is coming to an end, the higher value of median frequency occurs, which may be associated with term delivery (Fele-Žorž et al., 2008). According to our results the values of median frequency do not yield any specific trend in the course of labors. But statistical evaluation of all values of median frequency calculated on EMG segments that were recorded during both labor groups showed some differences. However, the values of the median frequency are significantly lower in labors with a diagnosed dystocia calculated on the burst segments in the active phase compared to the latent phase of the labor. The values of median frequency show a significant difference between both labor groups in the active phase, when they are calculated on burst segments of the uterine EMG activity.

Shifting of the uterine EMG signal energy to higher frequencies as delivery approaches is the phenomenon observed in the literature (Buhimschi et al., 1997; Doret et al., 2005; Garfield et al., 2002; Maner & Garfield, 2007; Vinken et al., 2010; Maner et al., 2003). In particular, the modus frequency of the uterine EMG signal power spectral density (PSD) is commonly tested. Term and preterm labors can be successfully monitored and evaluated for preparedness for labor. The modus frequency of PSD increased as the measurement-to-delivery interval decreased from more than 4 days before the labor to less than 24 hours (Maner et al., 2003). According to our results the values of modus frequency do not yield any specific trend in the course of labor. Anyway, the statistical evaluation of all values of modus frequency calculated on EMG segments that were recorded in both labor groups show some characteristics. The values of the modus frequency calculated on the burst segments are significantly higher in the active phase in the case of normally progressing labors compare to the labors with a diagnosed dystocia. However values of the modus frequency calculated on the successive non-overlapping segments are lower in the active phase in the case of normally progressing labors compare to the labors with a diagnosed dystocia.

It was shown that RMS value changes only a few days before the true labor begins (Verdenik et al., 2001). According to our results the values of RMS do not yield any specific trend in the course of both labor groups. Results of statistical evaluation show that the significantly higher RMS values are in the active phase compared to the latent phase of both observed labor groups, when for calculation burst segments of the uterine EMG activity are used. However, the significant difference is shown only in the case when the values of RMS are calculated on successive non-overlapping segments of the EMG signal and a normally progressing labor is observed. Although the RMS values have some diagnostic potential, all useful analyses can be done afterwards.

The values of LZ do not yield any specific trend in the course of normally progressing labors or labors with a diagnosed dystocia. Although the values of LZ have some diagnostic potential, all useful information can be calculated afterwards. The results of LZ between the labor groups are significantly different in the latent phase of labor regardless of the used segmentation. The median value of the LZ values is higher in the case of labors with a diagnosed dystocia regardless of the used segmentation (successive non-overlapping segments of the EMG or the burst segments of the uterine EMG activity). The values of LZ are also significantly different between the latent phase and the active phase calculated on burst segments of labors with a diagnosed dystocia. The median value of the LZ values is higher in the case of normally progressing labors calculated on the on burst segments of labors in the latent phase. According to calculated values of LZ, non of used segmentations shows any promising results.

The majority of the studies are done on bursts segments of uterine EMG. However there is one study that showed that during the labor the activity between bursts is also related to the course of labor (Pajntar et al., 1998; Verdenik et al., 2001). They proposed that the analysis of uterine EMG signals during bursts only is not as efficient as it would be if the activity between contractions is included (Pajntar et al., 1998; Verdenik et al., 2001). We use two segmentations of uterine EMG signal: segmentation on successive non-overlapping segments of the EMG signal and segmentation on the burst segments of the uterine EMG activity. From the results we can assume that segmentation on successive non-overlapping segments of the EMG signal is better in the case when the SampEn values or the ApEn values are used for characterization. However, the segmentation on the burst segments of the uterine EMG activity is a better choice in the case of values of modus frequency, values of median frequency and values of RMS.

Previous studies showed that uterine activity can be successfully monitored during pregnancy and labor using uterine EMG. Uterine EMG signals give direct assessment of uterine contractility and as such have great potential as a diagnostic or labor monitoring tool. Due to specific characteristic of uterine EMG signal during pregnancy and labor, the methods for uterine EMG signal evaluation should be carefully picked out. In this chapter we summarized the methods based on uterine EMG signals for the determination of the labor progress. The main focus was the evaluation of normally progressing labor as well as labor with a diagnosis of dystocia using continuously monitored uterine EMG signals. According to our results time series complexity measures, especially SampEn and ApEn, calculated on successive non-overlapping segments of the uterine EMG signal, are most promising for uterine EMG signals interpretation during labour.

6. References

Abasolo, D. et al. (2006). Entropy analysis of the EEG background activity in Alzheimer's disease patients. *Physiological Measurement*, Vol.27, No. 3, pp. 241-253, ISSN 0967-3334.

Albers, L.L.; Schiff, M. & Gorwoda, J.G. (1996). The length of active labor in normal pregnancies. *Obstetrics and Gynecology*, Vol.87, No.3, pp. 355-359, ISSN 1526-9523.

Bakker, P.C. et al. (2007). Uterine activity monitoring during labor. *Journal of Perinatal Medicine*, Vol.35, No.6, pp. 468-477, ISSN 0300-5577.

Basu, J.K.; Buchmann, E.J. & Basu, D. (2009). Role of a second stage partogram in predicting the outcome of normal labour. *The Australian & New Zealand Journal of Obstetrics & Gynaecology*, Vol.49, No.2, pp.158-161, ISSN 1479-828X.

Bishop, E.H. (1964). Pelvic Scoring for Elective Induction. *Obstetrics and Gynecology*, Vol.24, pp.266-268, ISSN 0029-7844.

Buhimschi, C.; Boyle, M. & Garfield, R. (1997). Electrical activity of the human uterus during pregnancy as recorded from the abdominal surface. *Obstetrics and Gynecology*, Vol.90, No.1, pp.102-111, ISSN 0029-7844.

Chard, T. & Grudzinskas, J. (1994). *The uterus*, Cambridge: Cambridge University Press, ISBN 9780521424530.

Devedeux, D. et al. (1993). Uterine Electromyography - a Critical-Review. *American Journal of Obstetrics and Gynecology*, Vol.169, No.6, pp.1636-1653, ISSN 0002-9378.

Diab, M.O.; Marque, C. & Khalil, M. (2009). An unsupervised classification method of uterine electromyography signals: classification for detection of preterm deliveries. *The Journal of Obstetrics and Gynaecology Research*, Vol.35, No.1, pp.9-19, ISSN 1341-8076.

Doret, M. et al. (2005). Uterine electromyography characteristics for early diagnosis of mifepristone-induced preterm labor. *Obstetrics and Gynecology*, Vol.105, No.4, pp.822-830, ISSN 0029-7844.

Euliano, T. et al. (2006). Prediction of intrauterine pressure waveform from transabdominal electrohysterography. *The Journal of Maternal-Fetal & Neonatal Medicine: The Official Journal of the European Association of Perinatal Medicine, the Federation of Asia and Oceania Perinatal Societies, the International Society of Perinatal Obstetricians*, Vol.19, No.12, pp.811-816, ISSN 1476-7058.

Euliano, T.Y. et al. (2009). Spatiotemporal electrohysterography patterns in normal and arrested labor. *American Journal of Obstetrics and Gynecology*, Vol.200, No.1, pp.54.e1-54.e7, ISSN 0002-9378.

FDA. (n.d.). Obstetrical and gynecological devices. *U.S. Food and Drug Administration (FDA)*, 17.12. 2010, Available from: http://www.accessdata.fda.gov/scripts/cdrh/cfdocs/cfcfr/CFRSearch.cfm?CFRPart=884

Fele-Žorž, G. et al. (2008). A comparison of various linear and non-linear signal processing techniques to separate uterine EMG records of term and pre-term delivery groups. *Medical & Biological Engineering & Computing*, Vol.46, No.9, pp.911-922, ISSN 0140-0118.

Garfield, R. & Maner, W. (2007). Physiology and electrical activity of uterine contractions. *Seminars in Cell & Developmental Biology*, Vol.18, No.3, pp.289-295, ISSN 1084-9521.

Garfield, R. et al. (2002). Uterine electromyography and light-induced fluorescence in the management of term and preterm labor. *Journal of the Society for Gynecologic Investigation*, Vol.9, No.5, pp.265-275, ISSN 1071-5576.

Gibb, D.M. et al. (1984). Characteristics of uterine activity in nulliparous labour. *British Journal of Obstetrics and Gynaecology*, Vol.91, No.3, pp.220-227, ISSN 0306-5456.

Hassan, M. et al. (2010). Interactions between Uterine EMG at Different Sites Investigated Using Wavelet Analysis: Comparison of Pregnancy and Labor Contractions. *Eurasip Journal on Advances in Signal Processing*, Vol. 2010, pp. 1-10, ISSN 1687-6172.

Hornero, R. et al. (2005). Interpretation of approximate entropy: Analysis of intracranial pressure approximate entropy during acute intracranial hypertension. *IEEE Transactions on Biomedical Engineering*, Vol.52, No.10, pp.1671-1680, ISSN 0018-9294.

Jezewski, J. et al. (2005). Quantitative analysis of contraction patterns in electrical activity signal of pregnant uterus as an alternative to mechanical approach. *Physiological Measurement*, Vol.26, No.5, pp.753-767, ISSN 0967-3334.

Joseph, K. et al. (2003). Changes in maternal characteristics and obstetric practice and recent increases in primary cesarean delivery. *Obstetrics and Gynecology*, Vol.102, No.4, pp.791-800, ISSN 0029-7844.

Karlsson, B. et al. (2007). Abdominal EHG on a 4 by 4 grid: mapping and presenting the propagation of uterine contractions. In *11th Mediterranean Conference on Medical and Biomedical Engineering and Computing 2007*. pp. 139–143, Ljubljana, Slovenia, June 26-30, 2007.

Kilpatrick S.J. & Russell K.L. (1989). Characteristics of Normal Labor. *Obstetrics and Gynecology*, Vol.74, No.1, pp.85-87.

Kjaergaard, H. et al. (2009). Incidence and outcomes of dystocia in the active phase of labor in term nulliparous women with spontaneous labor onset. *Acta Obstetricia et Gynecologica Scandinavica*, Vol.88, No.4, pp.402-407, ISSN 0001-6349.

Leman, H.; Marque, C. & Gondry, J. (1999). Use of the electrohysterogram signal for characterization of contractions during pregnancy. *IEEE Transactions on Biomedical Engineering*, Vol.46, No.10, pp.1222-1229, ISSN 0018-9294.

Luria, O. et al. (2009). Effects of the individual uterine contraction on fetal head descent and cervical dilatation during the active stage of labor. *European Journal of Obstetrics, Gynecology, and Reproductive Biology*, Vol.144 Suppl 1, pp.S101-107, ISSN 1872-7654.

Maner, W. & Garfield, R. (2007). Identification of Human Term and Preterm Labor using Artificial Neural Networks on Uterine Electromyography Data. *Annals of Biomedical Engineering*, Vol.35, pp.465-473, ISSN 0090-6964.

Maner, W. et al. (2003). Predicting term and preterm delivery with transabdominal uterine electromyography. *Obstetrics and Gynecology*, Vol.101, No.6, pp.1254-1260, ISSN 0029-7844.

Marconi, A. et al. (2008). Comparing two dinoprostone agents for cervical ripening and induction of labor: A randomized trial. *European Journal of Obstetrics Gynecology and Reproductive Biology*, Vol.138, No.2, pp.135-140, ISSN 0301-2115.

Maul, H. et al. (2003). The physiology of uterine contractions. *Clinics in Perinatology*, Vol.30, No.4, pp.665-676, ISSN 0095-5108.

Miller, F.C. et al. (1976). Quantitation of uterine activity in 100 primiparous patients. *American Journal of Obstetrics and Gynecology*, Vol.124, No.4, pp.398-405, ISSN 0002-9378.

Neilson, J.P. et al. (2003). Obstructed labour. *British Medical Bulletin*, 67, pp.191-204.

Newman, R. et al. (2008). Preterm Prediction Study: Comparison of the Cervical Score and Bishop Score for Prediction of Spontaneous Preterm Delivery. *Obstetrics and gynecology*, Vol.112, No.3, pp.508-515, ISSN 0029-7844.

Oláh, K.S. (1994). Changes in cervical electromyographic activity and their correlation with the cervical response to myometrial activity during labour. *European Journal of Obstetrics, Gynecology, and Reproductive Biology*, Vol.57, No.3, pp.157-159, ISSN 0301-2115.

Pajntar, M. (1994). The Smooth Muscles of the Cervix in Labor. *European Journal of Obstetrics Gynecology and Reproductive Biology*, Vol.55, No.1, pp.9-12, ISSN 0301-2115.

Pajntar, M. et al. (2001). Contribution of cervical smooth muscle activity to the duration of latent and active phases of labour. *British Journal of Obstetrics and Gynaecology*, Vol.108, No.5, pp.533-538, ISSN 0306-5456.

Pajntar, M. & Verdenik, I. (1995). Electromyographic activity in cervices with very low Bishop score during labor. *International Journal of Gynaecology and Obstetrics: The Official Organ of the International Federation of Gynaecology and Obstetrics*, Vol.49, No.3, pp.277-281, ISSN 0020-7292.

Pajntar, M. et al. (1998). Activity of smooth muscles in human cervix and uterus. *European Journal of Obstetrics Gynecology and Reproductive Biology*, Vol.79, No.2, pp.199-204, ISSN 0301-2115.

Pincus, S. (1991). Approximate Entropy as a Measure of System-Complexity. *Proceedings of the National Academy of Sciences of the United States Of*, Vol.88, No.6, pp.2297-2301, ISSN 0027-8424.

Pitkin, R. (2003). Commentary on Pelvic scoring for elective induction (Reprinted from Obstet Gynecol, vol 24, pg 266-8, 1964). *Obstetrics and Gynecology*, Vol.101, No.5, pp.846-846, ISSN 0029-7844.

Radhakrishnan, N. & Gangadhar, B. (1998). Estimating regularity in epileptic seizure time-series data. *Engineering in Medicine and Biology Magazine, IEEE*, Vol.17, No.3, pp.89-94, ISSN 0739-5175.

Rezek, I. & Roberts, S. (1998). Stochastic complexity measures for physiological signal analysis. *IEEE Transactions on Biomedical Engineering*, Vol.45, No.9, pp.1186-1191, ISSN 0018-9294.

Richman, J. & Moorman, J. (2000). Physiological time-series analysis using approximate entropy and sample entropy. *American Journal of Physiology-Heart and Circulatory Physiology*, Vol.278, No.6, pp.H2039-H2049, ISSN 0363-6135.

Rudel, D. & Pajntar, M. (1999). Active contractions of the cervix in the latent phase of labour. *British Journal of Obstetrics and Gynaecology*, Vol.106, No.5, pp.446-452, ISSN 0306-5456.

Sabry-Rizk, M. et al. (2000). Nonlinear dynamic tools for characterizing abdominal electromyographic signals before and during labour. *Transactions of the Institute of Measurement and Control*, Vol.22, No.3, pp.243-270, ISSN 0142-3312.

Schlembach, D. et al. (2009). Monitoring the progress of pregnancy and labor using electromyography. *European Journal of Obstetrics, Gynecology, and Reproductive Biology*, Vol.144 Suppl 1, pp.S33-39, ISSN 1872-7654.

Schwalm, H. & Dubrauszky, V. (1966). The structure of the musculature of the human uterus--muscles and connective tissue. *American Journal of Obstetrics and Gynecology*, Vol.94, No.3, pp.391-404, ISSN 0002-9378.

Sharf, Y. et al. (2007). Continuous monitoring of cervical dilatation and fetal head station during labor. *Medical Engineering & Physics*, Vol.29, No.1, pp.61-71, ISSN 1350-4533.

Shields, S. et al. (2007). Dystocia in nulliparous women. *American Family Physician*, Vol.75, No.11, pp.1671-1678, ISSN 0002-838X.

Sizer, A.R. et al. (2000). A second-stage partogram. *Obstetrics and Gynecology*, Vol.96, No.5 Pt 1, pp.678-683, ISSN 0029-7844.

Terrien, J.; Marque, C. & Germain, G. (2008). Ridge Extraction From the Time–frequency Representation (TFR) of Signals Based on an Image Processing Approach: Application to the Analysis of Uterine Electromyogram AR TFR. *Biomedical Engineering, IEEE Transactions on*, Vol.55, No.5, pp.1496-1503, ISSN 0018-9294.

Terrien, J. et al. (2009). Sources of Bias in Synchronization Measures and how to Minimize Their Effects on the Estimation of Synchronicity: Application to the Uterine Electromyogram, *Recent Advances in Biomedical Engineering*, Ganesh, R. N. pp. (73-100), InTech., ISBN 978-953-307-004-9.

Terrien, J. et al. (2010). Uterine electromyogram database and processing function interface: An open standard analysis platform for electrohysterogram signals. *Computers in Biology and Medicine*, Vol.40, No.2, pp.223-230, ISSN 0010-4825.

Veit, J. (1912). Das Electrometrogram. *Zentralbl Gynaekol*, Vol.36, pp.161.

Verdenik, I.; Pajntar, M. & Leskosek, B. (2001). Uterine electrical activity as predictor of preterm birth in women with preterm contractions. *European Journal of Obstetrics, Gynecology, and Reproductive Biology*, Vol.95, No.2, pp.149-153, ISSN 0301-2115.

Vinken, M.P.G.C. et al. (2010). Nifedipine-induced changes in the electrohysterogram of preterm contractions: feasibility in clinical practice. *Obstetrics and Gynecology International*, Vol. 2010, pp.1-8, ISSN 1687-9597.

Vrhovec, J. (2009). Evaluating the progress of the labour with sample entropy calculated from the uterine EMG activity. *Elektrotehniski vestnik - Electrotechnical Review*, Vol.76, No.4, pp.165-170.

Vrhovec, J. et al. (2010). A uterine electromyographic activity as a measure of labour progression. *Zdravniski Vestnik-Slovenian Medical Journal*, Vol.79, No.2, pp.109-116, ISSN 1318-0347.

Windrim, R. et al. (2007). A randomized controlled trial of a bedside partogram in the active management of primiparous labour. *Journal of Obstetrics and Gynaecology Canada: JOGC = Journal D'obstétrique Et Gynécologie Du Canada: JOGC*, Vol.29, No.1, pp.27-34, ISSN 1701-2163.

Word, R. et al. (2007). Dynamics of cervical remodeling during pregnancy and parturition: Mechanisms and current concepts. *Seminars in Reproductive Medicine*, Vol.25, No.1, pp.69-79, ISSN 1526-8004.

Zhang, X.; Roy, R. & Jensen, E. (2001). EEG complexity as a measure of depth of anesthesia for patients. *Biomedical Engineering, IEEE Transactions on*, Vol.48, No.12, pp.1424-1433, ISSN 0018-9294.

17

The Role of Pelvic and Perineal Muscles in Reproductive and Excretory Functions

Margarita Martínez-Gómez[1,2], Dora Luz Corona-Quintanilla[2], Yolanda Cruz-Gómez[2], René Zempoalteca[2], Jorge Rodríguez-Antolín[2] and Francisco Castelán[2]

[1]*Instituto de Investigaciones Biomédicas, Universidad Nacional Autónoma de México, Unidad Periférica Tlaxcala, Tlaxcala*

[2]*Centro Tlaxcala de Biología de la Conducta, Universidad Autónoma de Tlaxcala, Campus Rectoría, Tlaxcala*

México

1. Introduction

Excretory and reproductive functions are underlaid by autonomic- and somatic-neural control that regulates the pelvic and the perineal structures in mammals. Viscera and striated and smooth muscles are involved in complex and multiple reflexes occurring in the pelvic cavity (Komisaruk and Sansone, 2003; Pacheco et al., 1989; Thor and de Groat, 2010). In women, this region must accommodate the growing fetus during pregnancy and the passage of the newborn during childbirth (Ashton-Miller & DeLancey, 2007). For this to occur, the fetal head has to undergo a series of internal translations and rotations, aided by the maternal effort in the form of active pushing and uterine contraction (Li et al., 2010). Functions, such as urination and defecation, are also regulated by the different autonomic and somatic reflexes of the pelvic cavity.

During pregnancy and parturition, the fetal weight, translations, and rotations on pelvic structures, such as pelvic and perineal floor muscles, cause injury to the components of the pelvic reflexes (Kearney, 2006; Lanzarone & Dietz, 2008). This has been associated with visceral disorders, such as pelvic-organ prolapse and urinary and fecal incontinence (Ashton-Miller & DeLancey, 2007; Smith et al., 1989).

One of the techniques frequently used to evaluate the participation of pelvic and perineal muscles during normal and pathological functions is electromyography. The electromyographic (EMG) recordings are extremely useful to evaluate the participation of pelvic and perineal muscles during the normal and pathological functions of this female anatomy. The goal of our chapter is to review the literature of the activity of pelvic and perineal muscles and the several viscerosomatic reflexes involved in sexual response and urination in female mammals. Measurements of the pelvic- and perineal-muscle EMGs in laboratory rabbits, focusing on methods and results, and the alterations of their activity associated with dysfunctions, particularly with urinary incontinence, will be also reviewed.

1.1 Muscular reflex activity during parturition in women

Parturition is the physiological process of expelling the fetus from the uterus through uterine contractions, accompanied by cervical effacement and dilation. This process occurs in pregnant women at term and is divided into three stages; the first stage is the onset of effective uterine contractions until full dilatation of the cervix, the second stage is from full dilatation of the cervix until birth of the baby, and the third stage is from birth of the baby until delivery of the placenta.

The first stage of parturition begins with changes in the hormonal levels (and their receptors) of the mother, such as withrawal of progesterone and increasing levels of estrogen, oxytocin, prostaglandins, corticotrophin-releasing hormone, and cortisol, which starts the uterine contractions (Kamel, 2010). These contractions stimulate uterine mechanoreceptors that increase the firing rate of the hypogastric afferents and activate neurons at the thoraciclumbar level (Tong et al., 2003). Uterine stimulation also produces the uterocervical inhibitory reflex that decreases cervical pressure (Shafik, 1994).

The second stage of parturition is characterized by viscerovisceral and viscerosomatomotor reflexes occurring to support fetus expulsion, as the fetus moves downward through the birth canal and distends the perineum. Once the cervix is full dilated, the fetus-caused cervical distention activates the cervix-uterine reflex that increases uterine contraction and pressure, a positive uterine contraction feedback that leads to displacement of the fetus into the cervix (Shafik, 1994). Once the head has reached the base of the pelvis the mother experiences a strong reflexive desire to push. This represents a pushing, reflex reaction triggered by mechanoreceptors activated by cervical dilation and the downward progress of the fetal head, with the abdominal musculature as an effector. Relying on the entirely natural pushing reflex, instead of starting their pushing voluntarily at an early state, can further help mothers adopt the most effective pushing rhythm to reduce the time of fetus expulsion and postpartum fatigue (Yildirim & Beji, 2008).

Fetus expulsion requires a reduced resistance in the birth canal. Contraction of the musculature adjacent to the vagina may increase the vaginal resistance and push back on the fetal head, delaying the progress of the fetus. The pelvic floor muscle is a fanlike layering of striated muscle that encircles and supports the pelvic viscera (Lanzarone & Dietz, 2008; Li et al., 2010). It is named the *levator ani* (LA) and is made up of the pubococcygeus (Pcm), the puborectalis, and the iliococcygeus (Icm) muscles. Despite its close anatomical relation to the birth canal, there is little published work on the interaction between the pelvic floor and parturition (Lanzarone & Dietz, 2008). During this period, vaginocervical mechanoreceptors may produce an inhibitory reflex to turn off the LA motoneurons, located at the lumbar spinal-cord segments, to relax this striated musculature so that the fetus may pass through the pelvic cavity. The afferent axons may travel through the hypogastric nerve. When the fetus reaches the vagina and perineum, the birth canal mechanoreceptors activate the vaginocavernosus reflex, which then activates the ischiocavernosus and bulbospongiosus muscles. Contraction of both muscles forms a step to prevent the fetal head from sliding quickly from the cervix to the vaginal outlet and prevent tearing (Shafik, 1993).

The third stage of parturition starts once the baby has been expelled. Delivery does not end until the placenta and membranes are shed. This occurs in response to a continuous uterine contraction that produces uterine involution, which favors the detachment of the placenta. Once the placenta is completely detached from the uterine wall, a woman may feel contractions again and want to push to produce what is called birth or delivery of the placenta and membranes (Kamel, 2010).

1.2 Micturition and pelvic floor muscle activity in women

Micturition in mammals is a vital physiological process involving two coordinated events; the storage and expulsion of urine. Both events have as substrate the lower urinary tract (LUT) and are regulated by autonomic (hypogastric nerve consisting predominantly of sympathetic, and pelvic nerve, mainly parasympathetic) and somatic (represented by the pudendal and LA nerve) components triggering spinal and supraspinal reflexes to coordinate the activity between the LUT components (urinary bladder, urethra) and the striated musculature (Barber et al., 2002; Fowler et al., 2008).

The role of the striated muscles in micturition has been discussed and has been a controversial subject for several years (Bors and Blinn,1964; Lapides et al., 1957; Shafik, 2003; Yang & Huang, 2002; Thor & de Groat, 2010). To date the importance of the striated muscles to maintain normal function in both continence and urine release is recognized.

During urine storage the bladder is inactive, but the internal and external sphincter show tonic contraction (Shefchyk, 2002.) that helps to support urinary continence. This occurs when the afferents of the hypogastric nerve inhibit the bladder parasympathetic-preganglionic neurons at the 2-4 sacral spinal segments and activate the Onuf's nucleus motoneurons to contract the external urethral sphincter, causing urethral closure and preventing involuntary urine release. This process is organized by urethral reflexes known collectively as the 'guarding reflex' (Fowler et al., 2008). Whereas the contraction of the smooth muscle of the bladder neck and urethra are regulated by the hypogastric nerve (Andersson & Waldeck, 2001), other nonneural elements that contribute to the urine storage and urethral closure are vascular elements of the urethra, such as the arteriovenous plexus (Ashton-Miller & DeLancey, 2007). Through the regulation of supraspinal sites, pelvic floor muscles can also be voluntarily contracted to maintain urinary continence (Fowler et al., 2008).

During voiding, sphincter activity stops as the bladder contracts so that voiding is efficient (Yalla & Resnick, 1997). When the bladder reaches its threshold, the bladder-wall mechanoreceptors activate myelinated afferents (Aδ) and the unmyelinated or the C-fibers of the pelvic nerve. The afferents send information to the spinal cord (Fowler et al., 2008) and the ascending pathways to the brain stem, specifically to the pontine center. This integrates information from the spinal cord and brain regions, such as the hypothalamus and the cortex, acting as a micturition-reflex switch. The central pontine sends information to the 10-2 toraculumbar level to inhibit the sympathetic neurons and produce relaxation of the smooth muscle of the bladder neck and urethra, whereas at the 2-4 sacro level it inhibits the motor neurons of the pudendal and LA nerves to produce relaxation of the external urethral sphincter and pelvic floor muscles, allowing the descent of the bladder neck and the opening of the urethral lumen. At that level the parasympathetic-preganglionic neurons of the pelvic nerve are excited (Shefchyk, 2001) to trigger the detrusor contraction (Andersson & Waldeck, 2001; Morrison, 1999).

Thus, urine output requires the contraction of the detrusor muscle in coordination with the relaxation of the smooth muscle of the bladder neck, the external urethral sphincter, and pelvic floor muscles. In contrast to the pelvic muscles, activation of the abdominal and perineal-striated muscle facilitates urine expulsion during normal voiding (Shafik, 2003). Thus, the passage of urine through the urethra stimulates mechanoreceptors located in the urethral wall to produce the reflex contraction of the perineal muscles, called the urethra-corporocavernosal reflex (Shafik et al., 2008).

During the vaginal delivery, in the second stage of labor, the fetus puts pressure on the LUT and the LA, which can cause damage to these structures, nerve injury, and loss of connective tissue (Abdool et al., 2009; Branham et al., 2007; Dietz et al., 2008; South et al., 2009). The failure to recover from this trauma may lead to permanent neuromuscular, pelvic floor, and micturition disorders. These are important factors in the development of pathologies, such as pelvic-organ prolapse and fecal and urinary incontinence in parous women, which is a common medical condition.

Animal models have aid our understanding of the mechanisms underlying the pelvic visceral function and dysfunction.

2. Animal models for studying the physiology of pelvic and perineal muscles

2.1 The laboratory rat

The rat has been the animal model commonly used to study the mechanisms of urogenital function because of its maintenance cost and availability. Viscerosomatic and somatosomatic reflexes activated during mating and parturition have been well-documented in this species (Brink et al., 1980; Cueva-Rolon et al., 1996; Martínez-Gómez et al., 1992; Pacheco et al., 1989). Stimulation of mechanoreceptors located in the perineal skin and distal vagina activates pelvic floor muscles, such as the Pcm and the Icm. The Pcm and the Icm originate from the medial face of the pelvis and insert onto the proximal tail (Brink & Pfaff, 1980). Their fibers close the pelvic outlet cavity and are in close anatomical relation to the vaginal tract and rectum. The Pcm and the Icm together are part of the LA (Bremer et al., 2003). However this name may be confusing because a sexually dimorphic muscle, only present in male rats, has received the same name (Cihak et al., 1967).

Because of their anatomical position and their reflex activity, the Pcm and the Icm have been involved in sexual, reproductive, urinary, and defecator functions. In anesthetized rats the Pcm and the Icm muscles contract in response to mechanical stimulation of the perigenital skin and vagina (Martínez-Gómez et al., 1992; Pacheco et al., 1989). These reflexes may be triggered during mating by the somatosensory stimulation that the male applies during mounts and intromissions to the female perigenital skin and vaginal tract (Pfaff et al., 1977). The reflex contraction of the Pcm and the Icm may contribute to the sexual function by supporting the posture of lordosis, a typical sexual behavior assumed by female rats. This consists of arching the back, elevating the rump, and moving the tail base to expose the vaginal orifice to the male (Pfaff et al., 1977). This proposal is supported by the finding that electrical stimulation of the Pcm and the Icm in anesthetized animals causes tail movements, vaginal orifice movements, and increases the intravaginal pressure (Martínez-Gómez et al., 1992; Poortmans & Wyndaele, 1998). Increased intravaginal pressure may increase penile stimulation to achieve male ejaculation, facilitate the retention of sperm, and enhance the quality of stimulation received by the female (Martínez-Gómez et al., 1992).

From histochemical, anatomical, and electrophysiological studies, the neural elements of the genitopubococcigeus reflex described above are sensory receptors located in the perineal skin and vaginal wall, the pudendal nerve, and the viscerocutaneous branch of the pelvic nerve and are afferent pathways. The somatomotor branch of the pelvic nerve is an efferent pathway, the L6-S1 spinal cord segment is a final common pathway, and the integrator center and pubococcygeus muscle fibers are effectors (Cuevas et al., 2006; Martínez-Gómez et al., 1992; Pacheco et al., 1989).

The role of the Pcm and the Icm in the control of female reproductive or urinary functions remains unclear. Although it has been shown that cervical stimulation inhibits the activity of pelvic floor muscles, the physiological significance of this reflex it is unknown. Denervation of the Pcm and the Icm does not affect parturition (Martínez-Gómez et al., 1998). In addition, preclinical studies focused on the role of the pelvic musculature in micturition are scarce and results are conflicting. In male rats, activity of the Pcm occurs during micturition (Manzo et al., 1997). However, this result was not replicated in female rats (Jiang et al., 2010). Neither the Pcm nor the Icm discharged during voiding or during a manual increase of the bladder pressure, suggesting that the pelvic muscle activity is not necessary for voiding and does not contribute to the continence in the guardian reflex (Jiang et al., 2010). In another study, the Pcm and the Icm were activated during voiding only when the filling rate was high (0.5 mL/min) (Thor & de Groat, 2010). It is possible that these differences stem from variation in conditions, and more studies are necessary to unveil the function of the pelvic floor muscles on visceral functions.

Perineal muscles such as the bulbocavernosus, also called the bulboespongiosus (Bsm; Martínez-Gómez et al., 1997) and the ischiocavernosus (Ism), which are located outside of the pelvic bone, may also contribute to the visceral function. In women the bulbocavernosus and the Ism fibers are in close anatomical relation to the clitoris, vagina, and urethra (Shafik et al., 2008), and the contraction of these muscles may contribute to vaginal and urethral closure.

Unfortunately, studies to elucidate their role in the urogenital-tract function have not been possible in the female rat because the perineal-striated muscles are significantly involuted by adulthood. This requires further investigations into other potential laboratory animal models of pelvic and perineal physiology.

2.2 The domestic rabbit

The female rabbit is one alternative animal model known for its well-characterized and conspicuous pelvic and perineal musculature (Martínez-Gómez et al., 1997). The pelvic floor muscles, the coccygeus and the Pcm, and the perineal muscles, the Bsm and the Ism, are well-developed and accessible to manipulation and electromyographic recording. Therefore, the rabbit is an appropriate model to study the activity of pelvic and perineal muscles in relation to urogential functions.

The female rabbit is an induced ovulator and one intromission by the male accompanied by a brief series of pelvic thrusts is sufficient to ensure ejaculation, ovulation, and pregnancy (Ramírez & Lin Soufi, 1994; Soto et al., 1984). The female rabbit gives birth in a separate and well-disguised nursery burrow presumably to avoid predation but also because the umbilical cord usually ruptures in the long vagina, and the pups are expelled in rapid succession. In domestic breeds, the birth of as many as 14 pups is achieved within 10 - 15 min (Fuchs and Darwood, 1980; Hudson et al., 1995).

The reproductive tract of the female rabbit has two uterine horns with two necks attached to a long vagina, which we have regionalized as abdominal, pelvic, and perineal (Cruz et al., 2002). The pelvic vagina is covered by a prominent venous plexus and in its ventral wall is the urethral opening. The perineal vagina, the most caudal portion of the vagina, protrudes outside the pelvic cavity and ends at the urethra-vagina junction. Around this anatomical structure, also called the urogenital tract, the pelvic and perineal muscles are located (Fig. 1) and contribute to the reproductive and excretory functions (Martínez-Gómez et al., 1997; Cruz et al., 2002, 2010A, 2010B). The pelvic muscles include the *obturatorius internus*, the coccygeus, the Icm, and the Pcm. The perineal muscles include the *constrictor vestibuli*, the *constrictor vulvae*, the bulboglandularis, the Ism, and the Bsm.

Because of the anatomy of the urogenital tract, pelvic and perineal muscles could participate in the process of micturition and in those associated with reproduction. In rabbits, males and females have different ways to expell urine depending on the social context, which have been related to a role of chemical communication (Bell, 1980). To determine the role of those muscles in reproduction and micturition, our group has used electromyography and cystometrography (*see* below).

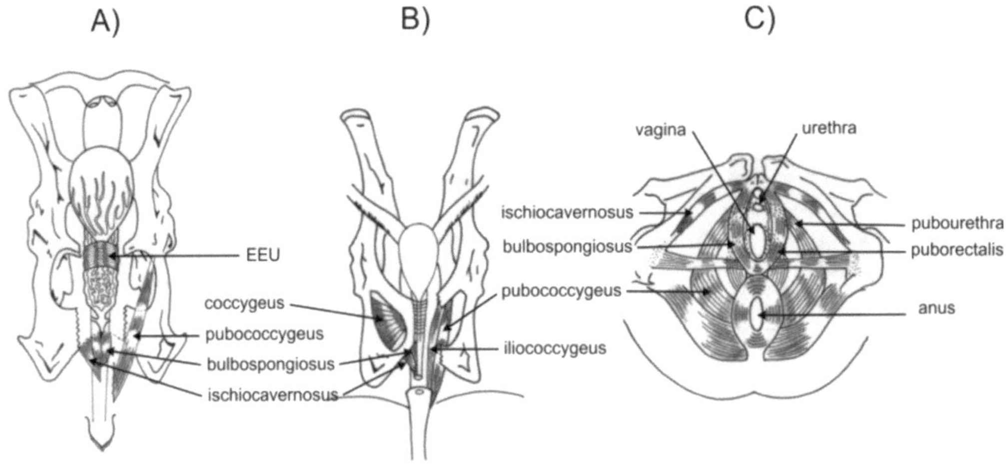

Fig. 1. Pelvic and perineal muscles in the female rabbit (A), the female rat (B) and women (C). EEU, external urethral sphincter.

3. Electromyography protocols for evaluating the role of pelvic and perineal muscles in reproduction and micturition

Electromyography methods have been widely used in research and the diagnosis of patients with neuromuscular disorders (Stalberg & Falck, 1997). The electrophysiological information is still an important part of the study of normal and abnormal nerves and muscles. In addition to morphological and histochemical methods, needle electromyography can be used to study the structure and function of the motor units (Stalberg & Falck, 1997). Electromyography has the advantage of being relatively well-tolerated, repeatable, and several muscles can be studied simultaneously. Furthermore electromyography also reflects some functional aspect of the motor units, especially those of the neuromuscular transmission.

By using electromyography in female rabbits, we have studied the activity of pelvic- and perineal-striated muscles, and some viscerosomatic reflexes, involved in the sexual response and micturition. In addition, we have evaluated how the reproductive experience affects the activity of pelvic and perineal muscles and its relationship to urodynamics.

3.1 Vaginocervical stimulation

The vaginal tract is stimulated by the intromission of the penis during mating, by the passing of the pups during parturition, and by the voiding of urine during micturition. In these processes the striated muscles associated with the vaginal tract are reflex activated, a reflex called vaginocavernosus, and this has been suggested to participate in the erection of the

clitoris and helps to prevent vaginal and perineal tearing (Shafik, 1993). In our laboratory we have evaluated the contribution of pelvic- and perineal-striated muscles to this reflex.
Stimulation of the vagina was done with a 0.5-cm diameter glass rod coated with mineral oil. This was touched to the clitoris and introduced to each level of the perineal vagina, the pelvic vagina, and the abdominal vagina, including the cervices, and then withdrawn. A possible inhibitory effect of vaginocervical stimulation on the activity of striated muscles is also analyzed. The dissection of muscles has been described elsewhere (Martínez-Gómez et al., 1997). A longitudinal incision in the skin on the right or left side of the perineum, according to the study, is made. The adipose and connective tissue, the lateral vagina, and the rectum are carefully dissected. Bipolar electrodes (0.01-mm silver wires) are inserted into the medial portion of the muscles generally, but the placement can be variable depending on the morphology and disposition of each muscle. The electrodes used for the EMG are fastened to the perigenital skin by a fine suture before inserting them into the striated muscles. The electrical activity is amplified by a preamplifier connected to a Grass PolyView Recorder 2.5 installed in a computer. Electromyographical activity is also monitored using an audio feed connected in parallel to the preamplifier.
Reflex activity in the pelvic and perineal muscles is produced by squeezing the perineal vagina between thumb and forefinger while stimulating the pelvic or abdominal vagina with the rod. In some animals, vaginal stimulation is also made after inserting a 0.7-cm diameter plastic cylinder 3-cm long into the perineal vagina, 15 min after applying a local anesthetic to the mucosa of the perineal vagina. The first method is used to prevent the rod touching the internal walls of the perineal vagina during stimulation of the pelvic or abdominal levels and the second is used to confirm that the activity of the muscles is caused by mechanoreceptors located in the walls of the perineal vagina. The activity of each muscle is recorded in each doe 2–3 min before, during, and 2–5 min after stimulation. Each stimulus is administered to the perigenital skin and at each level of the vagina at least twice, with the level and type of stimulation applied in random order. An interstimulus interval of 2-3 min is used, or if the muscle responded with afterdischarge or inhibition, an interval of 5-10 min after the after discharge or inhibition had ceased.
Another technique to measure the intravaginal pressure is the use of a balloon attached by a catheter to a pressure transducer and connected to a driver amplifier (Fig. 2). The uninflated balloon is inserted into each vaginal level and inflated via a syringe to a diameter of 2–3 cm. Then the muscles are stimulated with bipolar stainless steel electrodes using square pulses of 0.1- to 0.2-ms duration, variable voltage, and rates of 1, 5, and 10 Hz. The two distal ends of the transected nerves are bilaterally stimulated using bipolar, silver chloride electrodes connected to a stimulus isolation unit activated by a stimulator using square pulses of 0.1- to 0.2-ms duration and a variable voltage and rate.

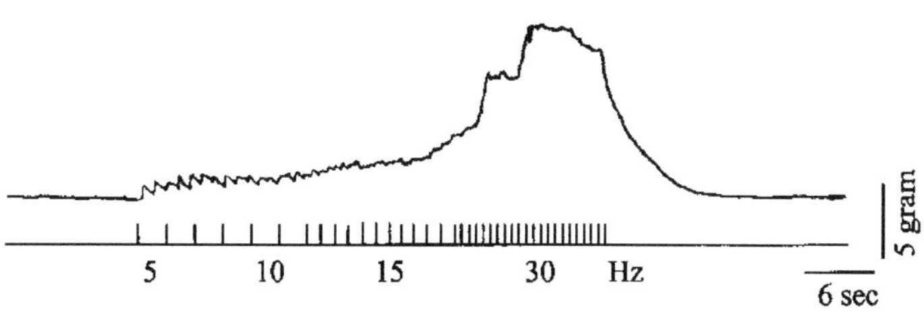

Fig. 2. Increase of the intravaginal pressure in a female rabbit during the contraction of the Bsm (Cruz et al., 2002). Physiology & Behavior by ELSEVIER INC. Reproduced with permission of Elsevier INC. in the journal format via the Copyright Clearance Center.

3.2 Simultaneous electromyography and cystometrography

Cystometry is defined as the urodynamic value that evaluates the intravesical pressure through a transducer that records the changes of pressure in the bladder during the storage and expulsion of urine. The result is a graph showing the change of bladder pressure caused by an increased volume in the bladder and these are called cystometrograms (CMGs) (McMurray et al., 2006). The recording can be made in anesthetized animals. The CMG combined with other techniques (EMG, neurectomies, or stimulation of nucleous superior centers) is used to describe the neural control of micturition, to analyze the effect of drugs and some pathologies (Pandita et al., 2000), and to evaluate the participation of pelvic- and perineal-striated muscles related to some dysfunctions.

In our work group, a CMG recordings are made using an adaptation of the previously described technique (Maggi et al. 1986). The animals are anesthetized with urethane and fixed into a dorsal supine position. The bladder is exposed through a midline incision in the abdomen and urine is expelled by applying slight manual pressure over the bladder. A 20-gauge butterfly needle is inserted into the lumen through the bladder apex to infuse warm (39 °C) saline solution (0.9% NaCl) at a constant rate of 0.8 mL per minute. The room temperature is 25 °C. Those experimental conditions were previously established at our laboratory. With polyethylene tubing (outer and inner diameter 1.6 mm and 1.2 mm) the needle is connected to a transducer to record variations in the intravesical pressure. The pressure transducer is connected to a direct current amplifier and displayed on a Grass PolyView Recorder 2.5 installed in a computer. After a 10-minute equilibration with no saline infusion, 3 reproducible bladder contractions are triggered in response to continuous saline infusion by a syringe pump.

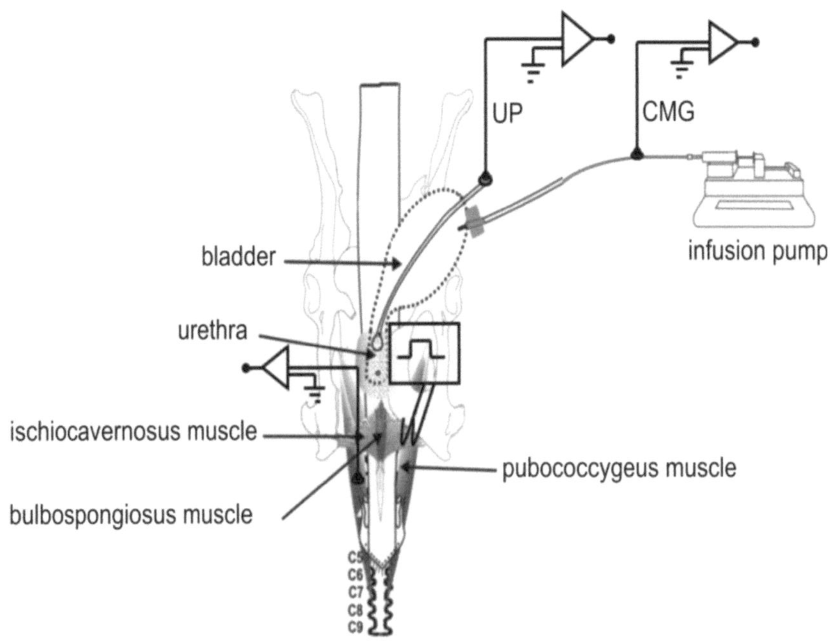

Fig. 3. Depiction showing the location of catheters used to record cystometograms (CMG) and urethral pressures (UP), and electrodes to record or stimulate pubococcygeus, ischiocavernosus, and bulspongiosus muscles in anesthetized female rabbits.

The variables analyzed to evaluate urodynamics (Fig. 4B) are 1) the volume of saline solution that triggered voiding (ThV), 2) the volume of saline expelled by the urogenital meatus during voiding (VV), 3) the volume of saline remaining inside the bladder as the result of ThV - VV (RV), 4) VE, calculated as [(VV/VV - RV) - 100], 5) the pressure that triggered the voiding phase (ThP), 6) the pressure measured from the ThP to the highest pressure observed at voiding (MP), 7) the elapsed time from the onset of ThP to the baseline pressure (VD), and 8) the elapsed time between 2 voiding phases (ICI).

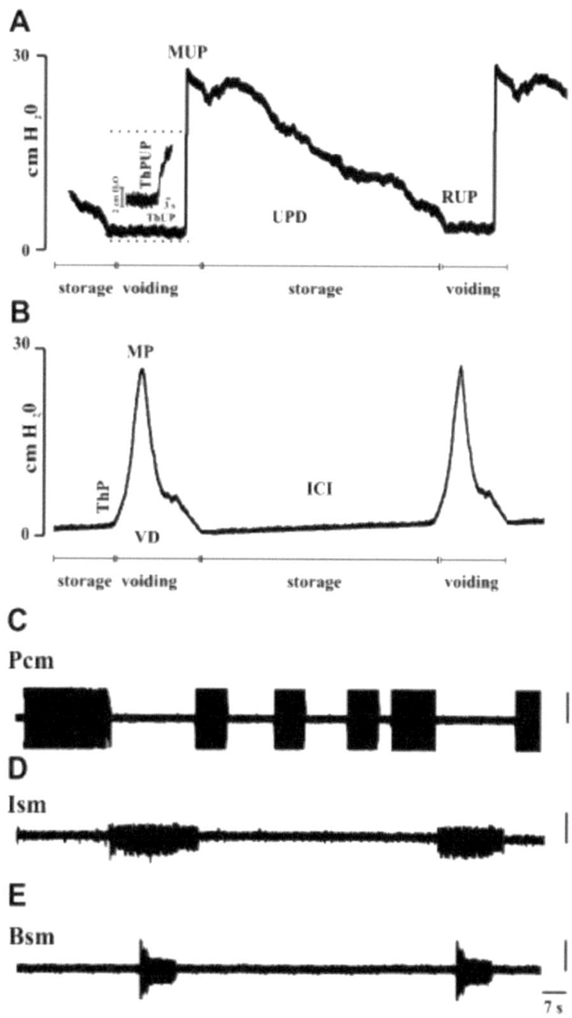

Fig. 4. Simultaneous recordings of urethral pressure (A), CMG (B), and EMG (C) of pelvic- (Pcm) and perineal- (Ism, Bsm) striated muscles during micturition caused in anesthetized female rabbits. Storage and voiding phases of the micturition are indicated. The urethral pressure is a maximum at the end of the voiding phase, preceded by the activity of the Ism and the Bsm. Thereafter, the urethral pressure decreases during the voiding phase of micturition when the activity of the Pcm occurs. s = seconds.

Electromyograms are simultaneously recorded along with the cystometograms (Fig. 3 & 4). Striated muscles (the Pcm, the Ism, or the Bsm) are dissected according to Martínez-Gómez et al. (1987) and EMG bipolar electrodes (0.01-mm silver-wires) are inserted into them. The electrical activity is amplified by a preamplifier connected to a Grass PolyView Recorder 2.5. In addition, muscle activity is monitored by using a sound unit. During the experiment, a muscle is considered to be activated or inhibited when the EMG trace is increased or decreased.

3.3 Urethral pressure

The urethral pressure (UP) is defined as the fluid pressure needed to just open a closed (collapsed) urethra (Griffiths, 1985). This definition suggests that the urethral pressure is similar to ordinary fluid pressure, i.e. it is a scalar (does not have a direction) quantity with a single value at each point along the length of the urethra. The concept of urethral pressure is only useful if the urethra collapses easily at attainable pressures to a zero cross-sectional area, as is normally the case. The use of a catheter introduces a nonzero cross-sectional area (given by the probe) and changes the natural shape of the lumen. The effect on the measured urethral pressure is small for highly distensible and collapsible tubes (Griffiths, 1985).
In our laboratory, we have established the conditions to record the urethral pressure with the EMG of pelvic and perineal muscles and the CMG, simultaneously. (Fig. 3 & 4). For this the animals are anesthetized with urethane and fixed into a dorsal supine position. For the UP recording, an adaptation of the balloon method (Lose et al., 2002) is used. A small incision is made in the bladder apex, and a balloon, mounted concentrically on a catheter (1.6-mm OD and 1.2-mm ID), is introduced into the urethra and passed though until it is exposed out of the opening of the vagina. A cotton thread (8-cm length) is tied to the balloon, which then is pulled (5 - 6 cm) inside the urethral tract. This located the balloon in the medial portion of the urethra to measure the urethral pressure. A pressure of 2-cm H_2O is required to inflate the balloon to its maximum diameter. The bladder incision is then sutured. For recording variations in the urethral pressure the catheter is connected to a transducer, which is connected to an amplifier, and the data are displayed on a Grass PolyView Recorder 2.5 installed in a computer. The urethral pressure variables analyzed are 1) the threshold urethral pressure (ThUP), defined as the pressure that triggered an abrupt rise in the urethral pressure, 2) the maximum urethral pressure (MUP), 3) the time elapsed between the ThUP and the triggering of the MUP (ThtUPD), 4) the pressure at which the UP returned to the base line (RUP), 5) the time elapsed from the ThUP to the next basal pressure (UPD), and 6) the MUP/MP ratio as an indicator of the urethral pressure required to close the urethra (UPC).

4. Reflex activity of pelvic and perineal muscles in female rabbits

4.1 Pelvic and perineal muscle activity during vaginocervical stimulation

In our laboratory, we have described the electromyographical activity of the Pcm, the Ism, and the Bsm in response to vaginal and cervical stimulation. Furthermore, mechanical stimulation, by passing a small balloon filled with saline into different regions of the vagina, differentially activated these muscles. Stimulation causes electromyographic activity of the Ism and the Bsm (Cruz et al., 2002; 2010A) and the Pcm (Cruz et al., 2010B). Such findings are similar to those described in women as the vaginocavernosus and the vaginolevator reflexes (Shafik, 1993, 1995).

In rabbits, perineal muscles such as the Bsm and the Ism are well developed, with their fibers originating at the ischiadic arch and inserting onto the ligamentum suspensorium clitoridis. Branches of the clitoral nerves innervated the BSM and the perineal nerves innervated the ISM. Bilateral electrical stimulation of these nerves caused retraction of the clitoral sheath and an increase in the intravaginal pressure at the level of the perineal vagina (Fig. 5). Though none of the muscles responded to stimulation of the perigenital skin, both were reflexively activated during mechanical stimulation of the inner walls of the perineal vagina. Prolonged cervical stimulation inhibited this reflex. Thus, in reproductive processes such as copulation and parturition, the contraction of these muscles may be produced during stimulation of the perineal vagina (Cruz et al., 2002).

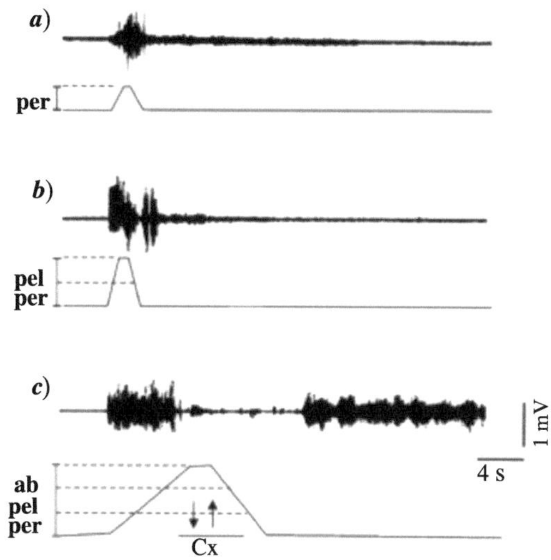

Fig. 5. Reflex EMG activity of the pubococcygeus muscle in a female rabbit in response to stimulations of the vaginal tract with a glass rod (Cruz et al., 2010b). The recording made on a polygraph before, during, and after vaginal stimulation was applied to the three levels of the vagina; a) perineal, b) pelvic, and c) abdominal. The cervix was also touched. The dotted lines shown below each EMG represent the type of stimulation. The sloping line shows when the rod was introduced, the plateau occurred when the rod reached the vaginal level (per, perineal; pel, pelvic; ab, abdominal) and the descending line shows when the rod was being withdrawn. The muscle had an afterdischarge following the removal of the glass rod.

The pelvic muscles, such as the Icm and the Pcm, are long bilateral muscles with fibers attached to the ilium bone. The muscle fibers are not attached to the pelvic viscera but they run adjacent to the vagina and rectum to be inserted into the sacral vertebrae. The iliococcygeus and pubococcygeus muscles are innervated by branches arising from S3 and S4. The reflex EMG activity was obtained during stimulation of the vaginal orifice skin and the perineal and the pelvic vagina (Fig. 6). Abdominal vaginal stimulation did not cause an EMG response. Cervical stimulation produced a temporary inhibition in the activity of both. These findings suggest that the Icm and the Pcm muscles can be activated by reflex action during reproductive processes such as mating and parturition (Cruz et al., 2010b).

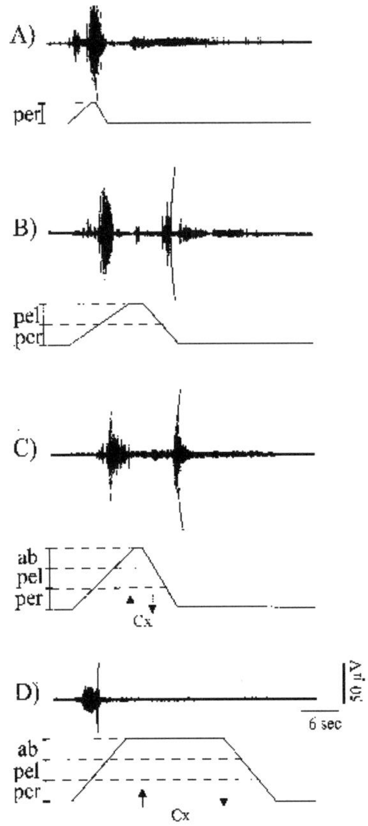

Fig. 6. Reflex EMG activity of the Bsm in a female rabbit in response to stimulation of the vaginal tract with a glass rod. Essentially, the same pattern of activation was observed in the Ism (Cruz et al., 2002). The EMGs were recorded on a polygraph before, during, and after vaginal stimulation was applied to the three levels of the vagina; (A) perineal, (B) pelvic, and (C and D) abdominal, including a brief (C) or prolonged touching of the cervix (Cx; D). The profile below each EMG shows the type of stimulation: before introducing the rod, the sloping line when the rod was introduced, the plateau when the rod reached each level of the vagina (per = perineal, pel = pelvic, ab = abdominal) and the descending line when the rod was being withdrawn. Note that except for (D), the muscle showed an afterdischarge following removal of the rod. Physiology & Behavior by ELSEVIER INC. Reproduced with permission of Elsevier INC. in the journal format via the Copyright Clearance Center.

In spite of the anatomical arrangement that the pelvic (Barber et al., 2002; Cruz et al., 2010b) and perineal muscles have in women and female rabbits (Cruz et al., 2002; Shafik et al., 2005), there are similarities of the reflex activity of those muscles. The activation of the Pcm in response to the stimulation of genital structures caused the vaginolevator reflex in women (Shafik, 1995) and female rabbits (Cruz et al., 2010b). This reflex plays a role in the sexual act that could increase the intravaginal pressure, thus increasing the stimulus received by the penis to facilitate the ejaculation (Shafik, 1995). The dysfunction of the vaginolevator reflex may result in sexual disorders (Handa et al., 2008).
Vaginal stimulation causes the reflex activity of the Bsm and the Ism (Shafik, 1993; Cruz et al., 2002; Cruz et al., 2010a), which is called the vaginocervical reflex that participates in the

erection of the clitoris (Shafik, 1993). Furthermore, the distension of the vagina by the fetal head during delivery causes the contraction of perineal muscles, which has been suggested to support the head during its descent and prevent vaginal and perineal tears (Shafik, 1993; Cruz et al., 2002; Shafik et al., 2007; Cruz et al. 2010a).

4.2 Pelvic- and perineal-muscle activities during micturition

An anatomical feature of the rabbit is that the mouth of the urethra is located in the pelvic vagina, thus forming the urogenital tract (Rodríguez-Antolín et al., 2009). Reproductive and micturition processes occur in this tract, suggesting that, as in women, pelvic and perineal muscles may be involved in the micturition process.

Micturition is a vital physiological process that involves two main phases; the continence of urine during storage in the bladder and the expelling of the urine. Because of this, in our laboratory we studied if the pelvic and perineal muscles are activated during micturition and whether the blockade of these muscles produces changes in urodynamic variables of the anesthetized rabbit (Corona-Quintanilla et al., 2009). In our study, we caused bladder emptying in young virgin rabbits by continuous infusion of saline into the bladder. During this process, the bladder pressure was measured simultaneously (CMG with the EMG of these muscles during storage and the expulsion of the saline). From our experimental observations, we established that the Pcm, the Ism, and the Bsm are active during micturition, i.e. the Pcm showed tonic activity during storage, inactivity during the voiding, and postdischarge after emptying the bladder. The Ism activity is at the end of storage and during voiding and the Bsm also showed increased EMG activity during maximum bladder pressure, corresponding to the voiding (Fig. 4B-E). In addition, another group of young virgin rabbits showed that the blockade of muscle activity by the intramuscular injection of lidocaine produces changes in the recording of the CMGs and the urodynamic variables (Corona-Quintanilla et al., 2009). The blockade of the Pcm activity, caused a significant reduction in the values of vesical efficiency and the threshold and maximum pressures. Furthermore, blocking the reflex activity of the Ism and the Bsm had a significant decrease in the vesical efficiency, intercontraction interval, and maximum pressure. With these results we concluded that pelvic and perineal muscles are differentially activated in sequence during micturition, not activated simultaneously as a unitary mass or functional unit (as seen in the literature) but as a group of structures, organized in time and space, leading us to assume the existence of a motor pattern generator in the spinal cord that generates the motion sequence for the process of micturition.

The activity of pelvic and perineal muscles during the micturition of women and female rabbits show some similarities. For example, the Pcm activity shown during the storage phase is a major component in the mechanism of urinary continence, because the electrical stimulation inhibits the bladder contraction and the urine output (Alves et al., 2011; our unpublished results). This is possible because the contraction of the Pcm during voiding is produced by the discharge of some of its afferents (from muscle spindles or tendon organs), sending information to both sacral 2 and 4 to modulate the activity of parasympathetic neurons (Manzo et al., 1997; Thor & de Groat, 2010). The Bsm and Ism activity during the voiding is mediated by a reflex called the urethrocorporocavernosal reflex. This reflex facilitates the urine voiding (Shafik et. al., 2008). Also, both women and female rabbits have been reported that during childbirth damage is produced of the pelvic floor muscles and nerves, leading to cause uncoordinated activity of pelvic and perineal muscles, modifying the micturition and producing postpartum urinary incontinence (Deindl et al., 1998; Haylen, 2009; Martínez-Gómez et al., 2011).

4.3 Pelvic and perineal muscles in virgin and multiparous rabbits

We have noted that multiparity affects pelvic and perineal muscles and this is related to the high prevalence of urinary incontinence in women with more than one vaginal delivery (DeLancey et al., 2003; Foldspang et al., 1992; Lien et al., 2004; Perucchini et al., 2002). Because of this, we studied, with the simultaneous recording of CMGs and EMGs, the Pcm, the Ism, and the Bsm. The bladder function was assessed using standard urodynamic variables. The temporal coordination of pelvic- and perineal-striated-muscle activity was changed in multiparous rabbits. The cystometrogram recordings were different from those obtained from virgin rabbits, resulting in alterations of the threshold volume, the residual volume, the voiding duration, and the maximum pressure.

Multiparity (4 consecutive vaginal deliveries) causes uncoordinated activity of pelvic and perineal muscles, and modifies urodynamics (Fig. 7; Martínez-Gómez et al., 2011). All multiparous rabbits included in that study had a pattern of muscle activity different than that of the virgin rabbits. Such a pattern involved at least one muscle in one phase of micturition. In addition, several urodynamic variables were also modified in multiparous rabbits. Those data showed that the activities of pelvic and perineal muscles are associated with the urodynamic function in rabbits. Probably the forces of the vaginal-delivery distension could injury the innervation and the morphology of those muscles, thus causing changes in their EMG activity during micturition.

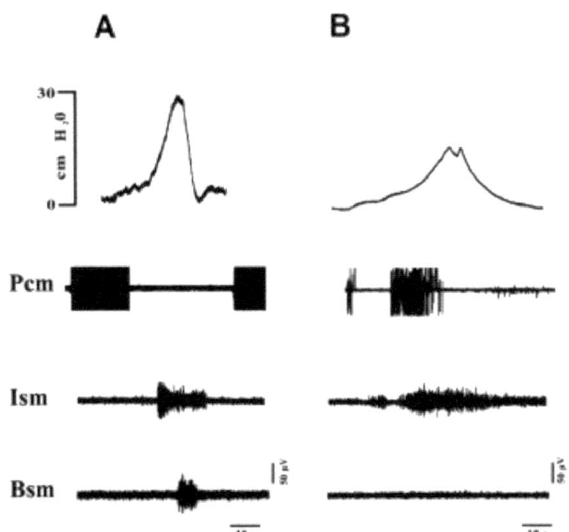

Fig. 7. Cystometrograms and EMGs of the Pcm, the Ism, and the Bsm simultaneously recorded during micturition in virgin (A) and multiparous (B) young rabbits. In virgin rabbits, temporal and coordinated activation of the Pcm, the Ism, and the Bsm occurs during the micturition phases. The cystometrogram and EMG recordings were different in multiparous rabbits and a different timing in striated-muscle activation was measured. s = seconds.

In the female rabbit, the morphology of pelvic and perineal muscles is different (Fajardo et al., 2008). The Pcm is heavier and longer than the Bsm. Though there is no difference in the number of fibers composing them, the fiber composition is different between both muscles.

By using Sudan Black stain, we have found that the Pcm is mainly composed of type I (dark) and IIa (intermediate) fibers, in contrast to that of the Bsm, which is mainly of type II (light). The morphological characteristics of those muscles are modified by multiparity. Both the Pcm and the Bsm from multiparous rabbits are lighter and longer than those of the virgin females. For each muscle, the cross-sectional fiber area of the multiparous animals was lower than that of the virgin females, without any modification about the type of fiber assessed by Sudan Black stain. Furthermore, both the Bsm and the Pcm developed lower twitch and tetanic tension force in response to electrical stimulation than the muscles of nulliparous females. In female rabbits, multiparity is associated with potentially pathological changes in the morphological and functional characteristics of these perineal and pelvic muscles, possibly as a result of stretching during parturition.

5. Conclusion

The female rabbit is an adequate model to study the physiology of pelvic and perineal muscles, and to contribute in the understanding the role of pelvic and perineal muscles in both reproductive and excretory functions. By using electromyography, our group has described the reflex activity of such muscles during the vaginal contraction and micturition. In addition, we have evaluated how the reproductive experience affects the activity of pelvic and perineal muscles, and its relationship to the urodynamics.

These findings show the importance of the participation of pelvic and perineal muscles in the reproductive and excretory processes, because in both processes the muscles are activated differentially and sequentially, not activated simultaneously as a unitary mass or functional unit. Moreover, their activity is regulated by viscerosomatic reflexes that are synchronized so that they have functions in urinary continence or fetus expulsion.

Our results in the model on the multiparity are important because they show that the uncoordinated activity of the pelvic and perineal muscles, plus other effects, such as peripheral denervation, damage to fascias, ligaments, and tissues, produced alterations in the support and dysruption in the nerve pathways of micturition. This uncoordinated activity in subsequent births can cause prolongation of the second-stage of parturition and increase the risk of urinary incontinence and pelvic organ prolapse. This knowledge will increase the accuracy of models and childbirth and may provide a better understanding about the pathologies of urinary incontinence and pelvic organ prolapse.

6. Aknowledgements

Authors thank PAPIIT-UNAM (228110, MMG), CONACYT (105882, MMG), and PROMEP-SEP (UATLAX-PTC-109, FC) for granting their research. DC was the recipient of a postdoctoral fellowship (CQDL132526) from CONACYT. Authors thank Dr. Ellis Glazier for editing this English-language text. The expert technical assistance of Laura García is also acknowledged.

7. References

Abdool, Z., Shek, K. L. & Dietz, H. P. (2009). The effect of levator avulsion on hiatal dimension and function. *American Journal of Obstetrics and Gynecology*, 201, 89–94, ISSN 0002-9378.

Alves, P.G., Nunes, F.R. & Guirro, E.C. (2011). Comparison between two different neuromuscular electrical stimulation protocols for the treatment of female stress urinary incontinence: a randomized controlled trial. *Revista Brasileira de Fisioterapia [online]*, epub ahead of print, http://www.scielo.br/scielo.php?script=sci_pdf&pid=S1413-35552011005000010&lng=es&nrm=iso&tlng=en

Andersson, E. (2001). Pharmacology of the bladder. In: *Textbook of Female Urology and Urogynaecology*, Cardozo L & Staskin D, 139-150, Isis Medical Media Ltd., ISBN 1901865053, London.

Ashton-Miller, J. A. & DeLancey, J. O. (2007). Functional anatomy of the female pelvic floor. *Annals of the New York Academy of Sciences*, 1101, 266-296, ISSN 0077-8923.

Barber, M. D., Bremer, R. E., Thor, K. B., Dolber, P. C., Kuehl, T. J. & Coates, K. W. (2002). Innervation of the female levator ani muscles. *American Journal of Obstetrics and Gynecology*, 187, 64-71, ISSN 0002-9378.

Berkley, K. J., Robbins, A & Sato, Y. (1988). Afferent fibres supplying the uterus in the rat. *Journal of Neurophysiology*, 59, 142-163, ISSN 0022-3077.

Bors, E. & Blinn, K. A. (1964). Abdominal electromyography during micturition. Proceedings Clinical Spinal Cord Injury Conference, 13, 1, 47–52.

Branham, V., Thomas, J., Jaffe, T., Crocket, M., South, M., Jamison, M & Weidner, A. (2007).Levator ani abnormality 6 weeks after delivery persists at 6 months. *American Journal of Obstetrics and Gynecology*, 197, 65-71, ISSN 0077-8923.

Bremer, R. E., Barber, M. D., Coates, K. W., Dolber, P. C. & Thor, K. B. (2003). Innervation of the levator ani and coccygeus muscles of the female rat. *The Anatomical Record. Part A, Discoveries in Molecular, Cellular, and Evolutionary Biology*, 275, 1031-1041, ISSN 1552-4884.

Brink, E. E., Modianos, D. T. & Pfaff, D. W. (1980). Ablations of lumbar epaxial musculature: effects on lordosis behavior of female rats. *Brain, Behavior and Evolution*, 17, 67-88, ISSN 0006-8977.

Brink, E. E. & Pfaff, D. W. (1980). Vertebral muscles of the back and tail of the albino rat (Rattus norvegicus albinus). *Brain, Behavior and Evolution*, 17, 1-47, ISSN 0006-8977.

Catheline, G., Touquet, B., Besson, J. & Lombard, M. (2006). Parturition in the rat: a physiological pain model. *Anesthesiology*, 104, 1257-1265, ISSN 0003-3022.

Cihak, R., Gutmann, E. & Hanzilikova, V. (1967). Morphological, physiological characteristics, development and homology of the m. levator ani of the rat. *Anatmomischer Anzeiger*, 120, 492-506, ISSN 0003-2786.

Cruz, Y., Hudson R., Pacheco, P., Lucio, R. A. & Martínez-Gómez, M. (2002). Anatomical and physiological characteristics of perineal muscles in the female rabbit. *Physiology and Behavior*, 74, 1-8, ISSN 0031-9384.

Cruz, Y., Rodríguez-Antolín, J., Nicolás, L., Martínez-Gómez, M. & Lucio, R. A. (2010a). Components of the neural circuitry of the vaginocavernosus reflex in rabbits. *Journal of Comparative Neurology*, 518, 199-210, ISSN 0021-9967.

Cruz, Y., Corona-Quintanilla, D. L., Juárez, M. & Martínez-Gómez, M. (2010b). Anatomical and physiological characteristics of pelvic muscles in the female rabbit (*Oryctoalgus cuniculus*). *Veterinaria México*, 41, 263-274, ISSN 0301-5092.

Cueva-Rolón, R., Sansone, G., Bianca, R., Gómez, L. E., Beyer, C., Whipple, B. & Komisaruk, B. R. (1996). Vagotomy blocks responses to vaginocervical stimulation after genitospinal neurectomy in rats. *Physiology & Behavior*, 60, 19-24, ISSN 0031-9384.

Cuevas, E., Camacho, M., Alvarado, M., Hudson, R. & Pacheco, P. (2006). Participation of estradiol and progesterone in the retrograde labeling of pubococcygeus motoneurons of the female rat. *Neuroscience*, 140, 1435-1442, ISSN 0306-4522.

Danuser, H. & Thor, K. B. (1996). Spinal 5-HT2 receptor-mediated facilitation of pudendal nerve reflexes in the anaesthetize cat. *British Journal of Pharmacology*, 118, 150-154, ISSN 0007-1188.

Deindl, F.M., Vodusek, D.B., Bischoff, C., Hofmann, R. & Hartung, R. (1998). Dysfunctional voiding in women: which muscles are responsible? *British Journal of Urology*, 82, 814-819, ISSN 007-1331.

DeLancey, J.O. & Kearney, R. (2003). The appearance of levator ani muscle abnormalities in magnetic resonance images after vaginal delivery. *Obstetrics & Gynecology*, 101, 46–53, ISSN 0029-7844.

Dietz, H. & Shek, C. (2008). Levator avulsion and grading ofpelvic floor muscle strength. *International Urogynecology Journal and Pelvic Floor Dysfunction*, 19, 633-636, ISSN 0937-3462.

Doi, T., Kamo, I., Imai, S., Okanishi, S., Ishimura, T., Ikeura, Y. & Natsugari H. (1999). Effects of TAK-637, a tachykin receptor antagonist, on urinary tract function in the guinea pig. *European Journal of Pharmacology*, 383, 297-303.

Fajardo, V., Pacheco, P., Hudson, R., Jiménez, I. & Martínez-Gómez, M. (2008). Differences in morphology and contractility of the bulbospongiosus and the pubococcygeus muscles in nulliparous and multiparous rabbits. *International Urogynecology Journal and Pelvic Floor Dysfunction*, 19, 843-849, ISSN 0937-3462.

Foldspang, A., Mommsen, S., Lam, G. W. & Elving, L. (1992). Parity as a correlate of adult female urinary incontinence prevalence. *Journal of Epidemiology and Community Health*, 46, 596-600, ISSN 0143-005X.

Fowler, C., Griffiths, D. & de Groat, W. C. (2008). The neural control of micturition. *Nature Reviews Neurosicence*, 9, 453-466, ISSN 1471-003X.

Fuchs, A. R. & Dawood, Y. (1980). Oxytocin release and uterine activation during parturition in rabbits. *Endocrinology*, 107, 1117-1126, ISSN 0013-7227.

Ghoniem, G. M., Shoukry, M. S. & Monga, M. (1996). Effects of anesthesia on urodynamic studies in the primate model. *The Journal of Urology*, 156, 233-236, ISSN 0022-3347.

Gintzler, A. & Komisaruk, R. (1991). Analgesia is produced by uterocervical mechanostimulation in rats: roles of afferent nerves and implications for analgesia of pregnancy and parturition. *Brain Research*, 566, 299-302, ISSN 0006-8993.

Giuliani, S., Lecci, A., Tramontana, M. & Maggi, C. A. (1998). The inhibitory effect of nociceptin on the micturition reflex in anaesthetized rats. *British Journal of Pharmacology*, 124, 1566-1572, ISSN 0007-1188.

Griffiths, D. (1985). The pressure within a collapsed tube, with special reference to urethral pressure. *Physics in Medicine Biology*, 30, 951-963, ISSN 0031-9155.

Handa, V.L., Cundiff, G., Chang, H.H. & Helzlsouer, K.J. (2008). Female sexual function and pelvic floor disorders. *Obstetrics and Gynecology*, 111, 1045-52, ISSN 0004-8666.

Harada, T., Kumazaki, T., Kigure, T., Etori, K. & Tsuchida, S. (1989). Effect of adrenergic agents on urethral compliance measurements in dog proximal urethra. *The Journal of Urology*, 142, 189-192, ISSN 0022-5347.

Haylen, B.T. (2009). Female Voiding dysfunction: prevalence and common associations. *Current Urology Reports*, 10, 421-427, ISSN 1527-2737.

Hudson, R., Müller, A. & Kennedy, G. A. (1995). Parturition in the rabbit is compromised by daytime nursing. The role of oxytocin. *Biology of Reproduction*, 53, 519-524, ISSN 0006-3363.

Jiang, H. H., Salcedo, L. B., Song, B. & Damaser, M. S. (2010). Pelvic floor muscles and the external urethral sphincter have different responses to applied bladder pressure during continence. *Urology*, 75, 1515 e1-e7, ISSN 1527-9995.

Kamel RM. (2010) The onset of human parturition. *Archives of Gynecology and Obstetrics*, 281, 975-982, ISSN 0932-0067.

Kearney, R., Miller, J. M., Ashton-Miller, J. A. & DeLancey J. O. (2006) Obstetric factors associated with levator ani mus-cle injury after vaginal birth. *Obstetrics and Gynecology*, 107, 144–149, ISSN 0029-7844.

Komisaruk, B. R. & Sansone, G. (2003). Neural pathways mediating vaginal function: the vagus nerves and spinal cord oxytocin. *Scandinavian Journal of Psychology*, 44, 241-250, ISSN 0036-5564.

Kontani, H., Nakagawa, M. & Sakai, T. (1992). Effects of adrenergic agonists on an experimental urinary incontinence model in anethetized rabbits. *Japanese Journal of Pharmacology*, 58, 339-346, ISSN 0021-5198.

Lanzarone, V. & Dietz, H. P. (2008).Three-dimensional ultrasounimagin of the levator hiatus in late pregnancy and associations with delivery outcomes. The *Australian and New Zealand Journal of Obstetrics and Gynaecology*, 47, 176–180, ISSN 0004-8666.

Lapides, J., Sweet, R. B. & Lewis, L. W. (1957). Role of striated muscle in urination. The *Journal of Urology*, 77, 247–250, ISSN 0022-5247.

Li, X., Kruger, J. A., Nash, M. P. & Nielsen P. M. F. (2010). Modeling childbirth: elucidating the mechanisms of labor. *Wiley Interdisplinary Reviews Systems Biology and Medicine*, 2, 460–470, ISSN 1939-6368.

Lien, K. C., Mooney, B., DeLancey, J. O. & Ashton-Miller, J. A. (2004). Levator ani stretch induced by simulated vaginal birth. *Obstetrics and Gynecology*, 103, 31-40, ISSN 0029-7844.

Lose, G., Griffiths, D., Hosker, G., Kulseng-Hanssen, S., Perucchini, D., Schäfer, W., Thind, P., Versi, E., Standardization Sub-Committee & International Continence Society (2002). Standardisation of urethral pressure measurement: report from the Standardisation Sub-Committee of the International Continence Society. Neurourology & Urodynamics, 21, 258-260, ISSN 0733-2467.

Maggi, C. A., Giuliani, S., Santicioli, P. & Meli, A. (1986). Analysis if factors involved in determining urinary bladder voiding cycle in urethane-anesthetized rats. *American Journal of Physiology*, 251, R250-R257, ISSN 0002-9513.

Manzo, J., Esquivel, A., Hernández, M. E., Carrillo, P., Martínez-Gómez, M. & Pacheco P. (1997). The role of pubococcygeus muscle in urinary continence in the male rat. *The Journal of Urology*, 157, 2402-2406, ISSN 0022-5347.

Martínez-Gómez, M., Chirino, R., Beyer, C., Komisaruk, B. R. & Pacheco, P. (1992). Visceral and postural reflexes evoked by genital stimulation in urethane-anesthetized female rats. *Brain Research*, 575, 279-284, ISSN 0006-8993.

Martínez-Gómez, M., Lucio, R. A., Carro, M., Pacheco, P. & Hudson, R. (1997). Striated muscles and scent glands associated with the vaginal tract of the rabbit. *The Anatomical Record*, 247, 486-495, ISSN 1932-8486.

Martínez-Gómez, M., Cruz, Y., Pacheco, P., Aguilar-Roblero, R. & Hudson, R. (1998). The sensory but not muscular pelvic nerve branch is necessary for parturition in the rat. *Physiology and Behavior*, 63, 929-932, ISSN 0031-9384.

Martínez-Gómez, M., Mendoza-Martínez, G., Corona-Quintanilla, D. L., Fajardo, V., Rodríguez-Antolín, J. & Castelán, F. (2011). Multiparity causes uncoordinated activity of pelvic- and perineal-striated muscles and urodynamic changes in rabbits. *Reproductive Sciences*, doi: 10.1177/1933719111411728, ISSN 1933-7191.

McMurray, G., Casey, J. H. & Naylor A. M. (2006). Animal models in urological disease and sexual dysfunction. *British Journal of Pharmacology*, 147, Suppl 2, S62-79, ISSN 0007-1188.

Morrison, J. (1999). The activation of the bladder wall afferent nerves. *Experimental Physiology*, 84, 131-136, ISSN 0958-0670.

Nickel, R. F. & Venker-Van Haagen, A. J. (1999). Functional anatomy and neural regulation of the lower urinary tract in female dogs: a review. *The Veterinary Quarterly*, 21, 83-85, ISSN 0165-2176.

Pacheco, P., Martínez-Gómez, M., Whipple, B., Beyer, C. & Komisaruk, B. R. (1989). Somatomotor components of the pelvic and pudendal nerves of the female rat. *Brain Research*, 490, 85-94, ISSN 0006-8993.

Pandita, R. K., Fujiwara, M., Alm, P. & Andersson, K. E. (2000). Cystometric evaluation of bladder function in non-anesthetized mice with and without bladder outlet obstruction. *The Journal of Urology*, 164, 1385-1389, ISSN 0022-5347.

Parente, M. P., Natal Jorge, R. M., Mascarenhas, T., Fernandez, A. A. & Martins, J. A. (2009). The influence of the material properties on the biomechanical behavior of thepelvic floor muscles during vaginal delivery. *Journal of Biomechanics*, 42, 1301-1306, ISSN 0021-9290.

Pfaff, D., Montgomery, M. & Lewis, C. (1977). Somatosensory determinants of lordosis in female rats: behavioral definition of the estrogen effect. *Journal of Comparative and Physiological Psychology*, 91, 134-145, ISSN 0021-9940.

Perucchini, D., DeLancey, J. O., Ashton-Miller, J. A., Peschers, U. & Kataria, T. (2002). Age effects on urethral striated muscle. I. Changes in number and diameter of striated muscle fibers in the ventral urethra. *American Journal of Obstetrics and Gynecology*, 186, 351-355, ISSN 0002-9378.

Peters, L. C., Kristal, M. B. & Komisaruk, B. R. (1987). Sensory innervationof the external and internal genitalia of the female rat. *Brain Research*, 408, 199-204. ISSN 0006-8993.

Poortmans, A. & Wyndaele, J. J. (1998). M. levator ani in the rat: does it really lift the anus? Anatomical Record, 251, 20-27, ISSN 1932-8486.

Ramírez, V. D. & Lin-Soufi, W. (1994). The neuroendocrine control of the rabbit ovarian cycle. In: The Physiology of Reproduction, 2nd ed, Knobil, E., & Neill, J. D., Raven Press, ISBN 0781700863.

Robbins, A., Sato, Y., Hotta, H. & Berkley, K. J. (1990). Response of hypogastric nerve afferent fibers to uterine distention in estrous or metestrous rats. *Neuroscience Letters*, 110, 82-85, ISSN 0304-3940.

Rodríguez-Antolín, J., Xelhuantzi, N., García-Lorenzana, M., Cuevas, E., Hudson, R. & Martínez-Gómez, M. (2009). General tissue characteristics of the lower urethral and the vaginal walls in the domestic rabbit. *International Urogynecology Journal and Pelvic Floor Dysfunction*, 20, 53-60, ISSN 0937-3462.

Shakif, A. (1993). Vaginocavernosus reflex. Description of a new reflex and its clinical significance. *Gynecologic and Obstetric Investigation*, 35, 114-117, ISSN 0378-7346.

Shafik, A. (1994). Utero-cervical inhibitory reflex. The description of a reflex and its clinical significance. *Human Reproduction (Oxford, England)*, 9, 2220-2223, ISSN 0268-1161.

Shafik, A. (1995). Vagino-levator ani reflex: description of a reflex and its role in sexual performance. *European Journal of Obstetrics, Gynecology and Reproductive Biology*, 60, 161-4, ISSN 0301-2115.

Shafik A. (2003). Straining and its role in micturition. *Urology*, 62, 199–200, ISSN 0090-4295.

Shafik, A., Ahmed, I., Shafik, A.A., El-Ghamrawy, T.A. & El-Sibai, O. (2005). Surgical anatomy of the perineal muscles and their role in perineal disorders. *Anatomical Science International*, 80, 167-171, ISSN 1447-6959.

Shafik, A., Shafik, I.A., Sibai, O.E. & Shafik, AA. (2007). The effect of external urethral sphincter contraction on the cavernosus muscles and its role in the sexual act. *International Urology and Nephrology*, 39, 541-546, ISSN 0301-1623.

Shafik, A., Shafik, A. A., El-Sibai, O. & Shafik, I. A. (2008). Effect of micturition on clitoris and cavernosus muscles: an electromyographic study. *International Urogynecology Journal and Pelvic Floor Dysfunct*, 19, 531-535, ISSN 0937-3462.

Shefchyk, S.J. (2001). Sacral spinal interneurones and the control of urinary bladder and urethral striated sphincter muscle function. *The Journal of Physiology*, 533, 57-63, ISSN 0022-3751.

Shefchyk, S. J. (2002). Spinal cord neural organization controlling the urinary bladder and striated sphincter. *Progress in Brain Research*, 137, 71–82, ISSN 0079-6123.

Silva, W. A. & Karram, M. M. (2004).Anatomy and physiology of the pelvic floor. *Minerva Ginecologica*, 56, 283-302, ISSN 0026-4784.

Smith, A. R., Hosker, G. L. & Warrell, D. W. (1989). The role of partial denervation of the pelvic floor in the aetiology of genitourinary prolapse and stress incontinence of urine. A neurophysiological study. *British Journal of Obstetrics and Gynaecology*, 96, 24-28, ISSN 0306-5456.

Soto, M. A., Reynoso, M. & Beyer, C. (1984). Sexual dimorphism in the motor mounting pattern of the New Zealand white rabbit: steroid regulation and rhythmicity of pelvic thrusting. *Hormones and Behavior*, 18, 225-234, ISSN 0018-506X.

South, M.M., Stinnet, S. S., Sanders, D. B., & Weidner, A. C. (2009). Levator ani denervation and reinnervation 6 months after childbirth. *American Journal of Obstetrics and Gynecology*, 200, 865-873, ISSN 0002-9378.

Stalberg, E. & Falck, B. (1997). The role of electromyography in neurology. *Electroencephalography and Clinical Neurology*, 103, 579-598, ISSN 0013-4694.

Tavenner, H & Green, W. W. (1958). Diagnosis of bovine pregnancy by measuring vaginal response to oxytocin. *Journal of Animal Science*, 18, 865-875, ISSN 0021-8812.

Thor, K. B. & de Groat, W. C. (2010). Neural control of the female urethral and anal rhabdosphincters and pelvic floor muscles. *American Journal of Physiology Regulatory, Integrative, and Comparative Physiology*, 299, R416-R438, ISSN 0363-6119.

Tong, C., Ma, W., Shin, S., James, R. L. & Eisenach J. C. (2003). Uterine cervical distension induces cFos expression in deep dorsal horn neurons of the rat spinal cord. *Anesthesiology*, 99, 205-211, ISSN 0003-3022.

Watanabe, T., Perkash, I. & Constantinou, C. E. (1997). Modulation of detrusor contraction strength and micturition characteristics by intrathecal baclofen in anesthetized rats. *The Journal of Urology*, 157, 2361-2365, ISSN 0022-5347.

Yalla, S. V. & Resnick, N. M. (1997). Initiation of voiding in humans: the nature and temporal relationship of urethral sphincter responses. *The Journal of Urology*, 157, 590–595, ISSN 0022-5347.

Yang, J. M. & Huang, W. C. (2002). Implications of abdominal straining in women with lower urinary tract symptoms. *Urology*, 60, 428–433, ISSN 0090-4295.

Yildirim, G. & Beji, N. K. (2008). Effects of pushing techniques in birth on mother and fetus: a randomized study. *Birth*, 35, 25-30, ISSN 0730-7659.

18

Electromyography Usefulness in Diagnosis of Functional Status of Pelvic Floor Muscles in Women with Urinary Incontinence

M.F. Lorenzo-Gomez[1], B. Padilla-Fernandez[1], F.J. Garcia-Criado[2], A. Gomez-Garcia[3], J.A. Mirón-Canelo[4], A. Geanini-Yagüez[5] and J.M. Silva-Abuin[1]

[1]*Department of Urology*
[2]*Department of Surgery*
[3]*Family and Community Medicine*
[4]*Department of Preventive and Public Health*
[5]*Department of Rehabilitation*
Hospital Universitario de Salamanca,
Spain

1. Introduction

1.1 Stress urinary incontinence

1.1.1 Definition, epidemiology and economic impact

Urinary incontinence has been defined by the International Continence Society (ICS) as the involuntary leakage of urine through the urethra, objectively demonstrable and of such magnitude that it entails a social or hygienic problem (International-Continence-Society 1977; Abrahams, Blaivas et al. 1988). It makes up a significant morbidity, affecting the social and occupational life with repercussions for the psychological, physical and sexual health of the woman (Serrano 2003).

The stress urinary incontinence is an important public health problem. In Europe it affects up to 1/3 of women over 18 years old with increasing prevalence up to 45% at 60-years-old women (Hunskaar, Lose et al. 2004).

In the last 5 years at least 12 epidemiological studies of the prevalence of urinary incontinence have been done in the United States. In 9 studies performed with women we find very different results ranging between 15% with Latin women over 65 years old (Espino, Palmer et al. 2003), 18% with Asiatic women (Huang, Thom et al. 2006), and up to 40% with non-institutionalized women (Fultz, Girts et al. 2005; Melville, Katon et al. 2005; Minassian, Stewart et al. 2008). In Spain, epidemiological studies before 2003 show a prevalence of nearly 40% in women over 65 years old, but in later studies the amount was under 35.1% in persons over 64 years, 23% in women over 18 years old, 20% in working women and 14% in women between 40 and 64 years old (Martínez-Agulló, Ruiz-Cerdá et al. 2009). Approximately 50% of women after retirement age suffer some type of incontinence, but less than half of them consult with their physicians(Viana-Zulaica 2005). Up to 91% of psychogeriatrical patients are affected, and urinary incontinence is one of the primary motivating factors for women entering a nursing

home. Therefore, success in the treatment of urinary incontinence will allow women to remain in the community with independence for a longer period of time (Bidmead 2002).
This pathology creates an important economic problem. In 1996, the cost of consumption of absorbents in Spain was more than 160 million euros, 3.2% of the total amount of the pharmaceutical allowance of the National Health System. We also must consider the economic repercussions of other direct and indirect common costs in other cost-illness studies (SNS 1996). The absorbents used to ease stress urinary incontinence represent the primary expense of this problem to the public sanitary system (Médico-Interactivo-Diario-Electrónico-de-la-Sanidad 2003).
Social and cultural conditions make it difficult to properly deal with urinary incontinence, since nowadays the specific preventive measures could eliminate up to 90% of the stress urinary incontinence cases (Serrano 2003).
With regard to the quality of life issues associated with incontinence, we have several methods to evaluate it: King´s Health Questionnaire (Kelleher, Cardozo et al. 1997) and ICIQ-SF (Espuña, Rebollo et al. 2004). The importance of these instruments lies in their capacity to explain and describe the damage that urinary incontinence does to the quality of life of the person suffering it and also his/her ability to discern between the different types of urinary incontinence.

1.1.2 Anatomy and physiology of the pelvis floor for the urine continence

In order to properly treat stress urinary incontinence and the associated pelvic floor's dysfunction, it's essential to understand the functional anatomy of the female pelvic floor and the continence's control system. The stress urine continence's control system is formed of two main elements: the urethral abutment system and the sphincteric closing system **(Castro 2002).**
The urethral abutment system consists of the bladder's wall, the endopelvic fascia, the tendinous arch of the pelvic fascia and the levator ani muscles.
The endopelvic fascia is a layer of dense fibrous connective tissue surrounding the bladder and fixing it to the levator ani muscles and the tendinous arch of pelvis fascia laterally, providing structural stability (Halban, Tandler et al. 1907). During the intraabdominal rises in pressure, the urethra puts pressures on this suburethral abutment layer. When the endopelvic fascia is changed, the urethra and the bladder's base don't have a good abutment, altering the intraabdominal pressure's transmission to the urethra.
The tendinous arch of pelvis fascia is a bilateral tensor structure located on both sides of the urethra and the vagina. It's like a cable with a chained form, like a suspension bridge that gives the necessary abutment to fix the urethra to the front vaginal wall. In the beginning it's a well-defined fibrous band, but when it approaches the pubic bone it gets wider and forms an aponeurotic structure, going dorsally to the ischial spine. This band fuses with the pelvic fascia, which joins the levator ani muscles in turn.
The levator ani muscles are the pubococcygeus muscle, the puborectalis muscle and the iliococcygeus muscle.
In comparison with other skeletal muscles in the body, the levator ani muscle has a greater connective tissue formation that is involved in the direct abutment of the pelvis organs. (Raz, Rosenblum et al. 2003). The pubococcygeus and puborectalis muscles are set out in U-form, beginning at the pubic bone on both sides of the median line, and passing after the rectum in order to form a sling. This sling is composed by type I striped muscle fibres and they are prepared to maintain a constant tone in order to close the uro-genital hiatus (Castro 2002).

The powerful levator ani aponeurosis is the most important element of the muscle-aponeurotic system which forms the abutment of the structures of the pelvis cavity. It surrounds the urethra and the bladder's neck and base, and it joins the tendinous arch of obturator internus. According to the anatomic-surgical principles postulated by Raz (Raz 1992) we find four different condensations of this fascia: the pubourethralis, the urethropelvic, the pubovesical (cervical) and the cardinal uterosacral ligaments.

Thanks to meticulous anatomic studies, the functional dynamics of the different vaginal ligament supports has become evident and the problems derived from its injury have been analyzed. DeLancey (DeLancey 1990) defines three urethral support levels dividing the vagina in three segments: *level I or of suspension, level II or of fixation and level III or of fusion.*

The sphinteric closing system consists of the striped muscle, the urethral smooth muscle and the vascular element of the submucosa layer. Each of these components equally contributes to the urethral closing pressure. The urethral most external layer is the striped sphincter muscle, which is found at an 80% of the anatomic urethra's length. It's composed of two parts: the paraurethral sphincter, in direct contact with the urethra and formed by slow contraction fibres which are able to maintain the basal tone, and the periurethral sphincter (the pubourethralis portion of levator ani) formed mostly by quick contraction fibres which can produce a voluntary compression of the urethra. When the intraabdominal pressure rises quickly, these fibres increase the urethral resistance with an active reflexive contraction.

The urethral striped sphincter is innervated by myelinic somatic fibres from level S2-S3, which run with the pudendal nerve (Castro 2002). In rest, the urethral basal tone increases with bladder's filling. When the intraabdominal pressure changes suddenly, a reflexive response of the quick spasm fibres increases the urethral closure and resistance. The reflex or voluntary contraction of the levator muscles increases the closure and the urethral resistance, improving the pelvis floor's support with a board effect and an efficient pressure's transmission to proximal urethra (Raz, Rosenblum et al. 2003).

The bladder's neck is closed in rest because of the distribution of the detrusor's smooth muscle fibres. One loop of detrusor's smooth muscle surrounds the front part of bladder's neck and can take part in its closure. The closure of the bladder's neck and proximal urethra are considered essential to maintaining continence and is more important than the external sphincter mechanism. However, it has been proven that many continent menopausal women have their bladder's neck open when coughing. It's also demonstrated that many nullipara women have their bladder's neck open in rest (Castro 2002).

Urethral length is determined by the distance between bladder's neck and the external urethral meatus. The urethral segment which receives higher pressures than the intravesical ones defines the functional length. Patients with stress urinary incontinence have a decreased functional length because of the failure of the proximal urethra.

1.1.3 Surgical treatment of stress urinary incontinence

At the present time we are experiencing a revolution in the treatment of stress urinary incontinence. Several surgical techniques have been considered. Distant seems the time when reefing sutures like those described by Nelly (1913), Stokel (1921) and Marion (1925) were suggested, until arriving at the suprapubic colposuspension described by Marshall, Marchetti and Krantz with many modifications and culminating in Burch's operation (Solà-Dalenz, Pardo-Schanz et al. 2006).

In 1995 tension-free transvaginal tape (TVT) was introduced (Ulmsten and Petros 1995). In 2001 another technique, suburethral transobturator tape (TOT) was introduced (Delorme. 2001). The main advantages were that the tape lays at a more anatomic position than in TVT, the needle doesn't cross the retropubic space, no abdominal incisions are made, there's a lower risk of vesical or intestinal injury and no cystoscopy is required (Solà-Dalenz, Pardo-Schanz et al. 2006; Delorme and Hermieu 2010).
The simplicity of these techniques and their reproducibility has dramatically increased their use, by both Urologists and Gynaecologists (Castiñeiras-Fernández 2005).

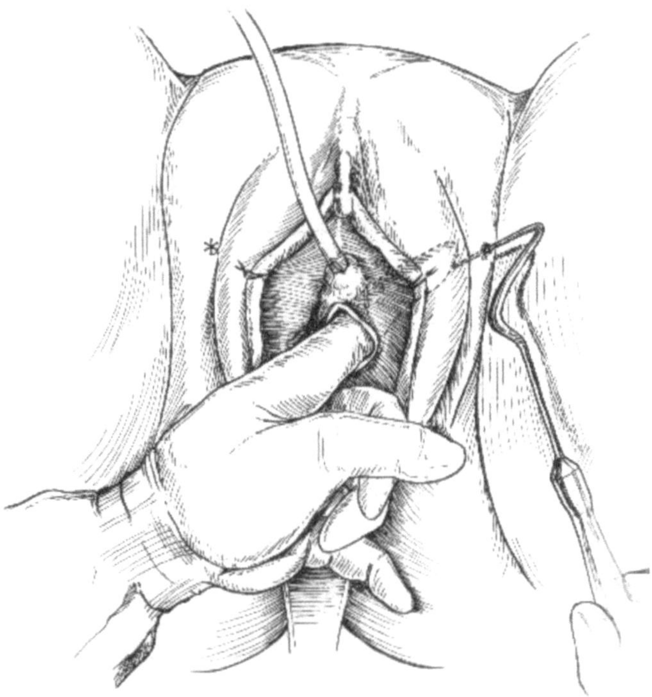

Fig. 1. Needle-passing during the TOT intervention (Castiñeiras-Fernández 2005).

When surgical treatment is indicated, the TOT procedure is chosen as the first-line election if there are no contraindications. This decision is backed up by the establishment of the TVT as a worldwide validated and demonstrated procedure for the surgical correction of the urinary incontinence. After the TVT, the transobturator treatment was accepted by the FDA. Autologous, heterologous or synthetic materials can be used.

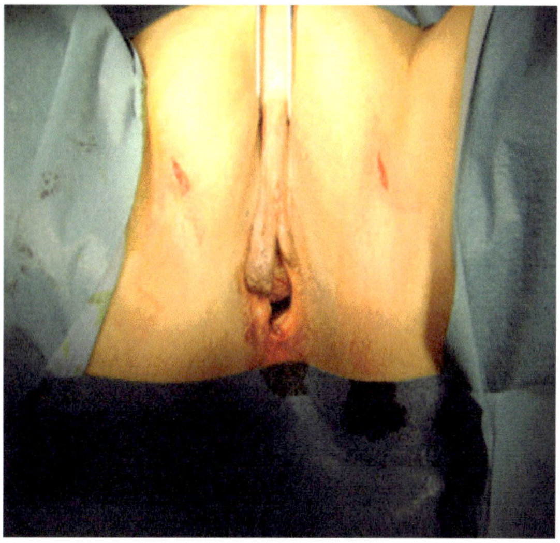

Fig. 2. Puncture sites.

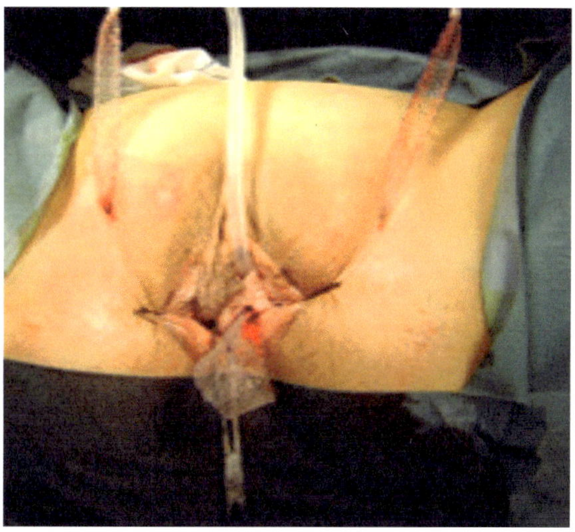

Fig. 3. Suburtehral tape already passed.

1.2 Perineal electromyography

1.2.1 Definition

The electromyography evaluates and records the electrical activity produced by skeletal muscles (Rio and Montero 2004).

The electromyography of the pelvic musculature allows us to evaluate the function of these muscles like any other striped muscle.

The use of surface electrodes is a method of registering electrical activity in a non-invasive way. There are different types of surface electrodes such as:

- Anal cylindrical electrode: two surface electrodes over Teflon which are inserted in the anal canal.

- Surface electrodes: silver discs over an adhesive surface, used on children, and stuck on the perineal skin.
- Electrodes overlaping a probe or a Foley catheter.
- Vaginal electrodes, similar to the anal cylindrical (González-Hidalgo 1998).

Biofeedback: can be employed to evaluate and/or to train the pelvic floor muscles of the patients. The procedure gives a virtual representation of a change in the measure of one of the following channels or in the combination of two of them:

- Flow channel.
- Pressure channel.
- EMG channel.

The aim of the EMG- Feedback or biofeedback with electromyography (biofeedback EMG), is to register the electrical muscular activity of the body through surface electrodes. The results are shown to the patient and to the procedure's instructor. The feedback can be visual, as in an LCD screen or auditory. For the visual feedback several representation models can be chosen. For the auditory feedback we can choose between a proportional reproduction, a reproduction depending on the threshold or an abrupt signal reproduction (only audible with headphones).

In the present study, the visual method was used for a greater resemblance to the physiotherapeutical treatment. Patients had a biofeedback session with the EMG channel, using surface electrodes: two located over the musculature and another one, neutral or ground, located at the inner face of the thigh.

Regarding the needle electromyography, some authors consider it the most precise method of exploration. A coaxial needle with an electrode at the needle's end is used. It can detect the electrical activity of a group of muscular fibres belonging to several motor units (Rio and Montero 2004).

1.2.2 Described perineal electromyography protocols

Several different methods of evaluating and/or enhancing pelvic floor function have been developed and modified.

In a strict sense, there can't be any perfect protocol for every patient affected by changes in the pelvic floor's function, since each patient begins with different parameters of muscular function.

The best method would be the most personalized one and high success rate have been indicated with the "biofeedback-therapist-guided" treatment:where the procedure's instructor stays with the patient during the whole process (Lorenzo-Gómez, Silva-Abuín et al. 2008).

The described protocols have many modalities: three 20-minutes sessions per week over a seven-week period (Amaro, Gameiro et al. 2006), twice weekly for 8 weeks (Voorham-van, Pelger et al. 2006), stimulator is activated on demand only by a sudden increase in intra-abdominal pressure (Nissenkorn, Shalev et al. 2004), 30 minutes per session, twice a week for 6 weeks (Lee and Choi 2006), 12 sessions (Rett, Simoes et al. 2007), 12 consecutive weeks (Capelini, Riccetto et al. 2006), 12 weeks training (Di-Gangi-Herms, Veit et al. 2006), six weeks, two training sessions each week (Seo, Yoon et al. 2004)

2. Aims of the chapter

If we follow the definition of urinary incontinence, i.e. that it is a problem that seriously affects the patients' life and after several unsuccessful conservative treatment attempts

(pelvic floor rehabilitation and drugs with variable efficacy), surgical treatment must be considered. The problem occurs when patients remain as incontinent as before. It is important to find a method of predicting which factors can cause a treatment's failure. Electromyographic research of the pelvic floor of each patient has been performed.
The aims of the chapter are:

1. To describe a perineal electromyography session (EMG) with surface electrodes without electro-stimulation to evaluate the functional status of the pelvic floor's muscles in patients with urinary incontinence.
2. To analyse the usefulness of the results produced in an electromyographic session as an evaluation of the pelvic floor muscles to predict a possible surgical treatment's failure.

3. Method and tools used

In 302 women planning surgical treatment via transobturator vaginal tape for urinary incontinence between April 2003 and December 2010, ages ranged between 41 and 81 years old, a monitoring session was performed to evaluate functional status of perineal muscles by means of biofeedback with superficial electrodes without electro-stimulation prior to recommending surgical treatment.
Age, time suffering urinary incontinence, perineal electromyography, secondary diagnosis (allergy; arthritis, arthrosis, depression; IDDM, NIDDM; fibromyalgia; nicotine poisoning; HTN; obesity; osteopenia; intestinal disorders; respiratory disorders), concomitant treatments (antidepressant-anxiolytic; antihypertensives), obstetric and pathological antecedents (number of eutocic, distocic childbirths, nulliparity, multiparity, previous hysterectomy, anexectomy, Cesarean, colpocele, TVT o TOT) were evaluated. ICIQ-SF questionnaire (International Consultation on Incontinence Questionnaire - Urinary Incontinence Short Form) was used to assess the outcome of treatment.
Study groups: The electromyographic values and the pathologic and non-pathologic antecedents in two groups of patients were described: Group A (n=254): operated on stress urinary incontinence through TOT with a successful result (urinary continence); and Group B (n=48): urinary incontinence through TOT with an unsuccessful result (still incontinent).
Studied variables:

- Perineal electromyography (expressed in mVol): average of the electromyographic values obtained in two stretches of the registered sequence during a 20 minutes session of pelvic floor biofeedback without electro-stimulation: first 5 and last 5 contractions of this sequence. The session took place at the urodynamics office with a Medicina y Mercado™ equipment, the patient was lying supine, with light flexing of the hips and protection of the lumbar lordosis in order to avoid fatigue. In this position the patient could see the screen of the biofeedback equipment (figures 4 and 5). The electrodes used were paediatrics pre-gelled electrodes. After explaining the anatomy and physiology of the pelvic floor, the patient was instructed to contract the perineal musculature several times and these contractions were registered, reflecting the power and the muscular tone, as well as the contraction time in accordance with the perineal electromyography. Each signal was registered continuously with a polygraph (figures 6 and 7).
- Results were produced from the answers of the Spanish validated-version of the ICIQ-SF questionnaire (International Consultation on Incontinence Questionnaire - Urinary Incontinence Short Form).

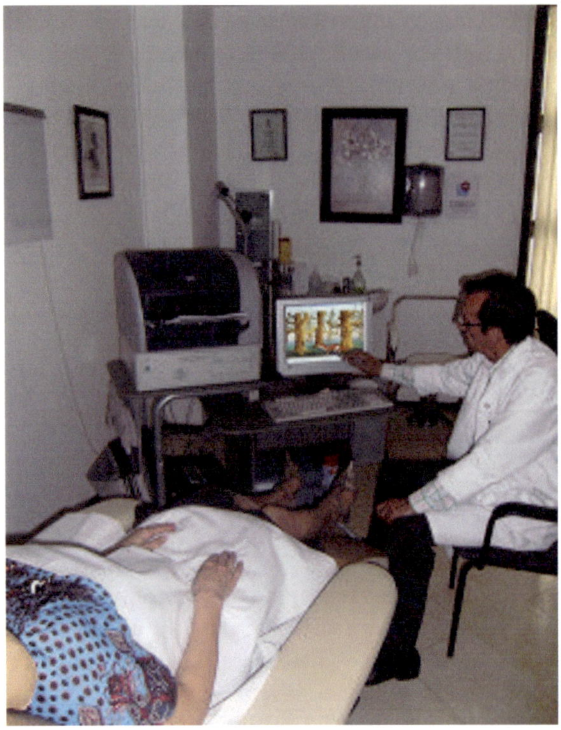

Fig. 4. BFB session.

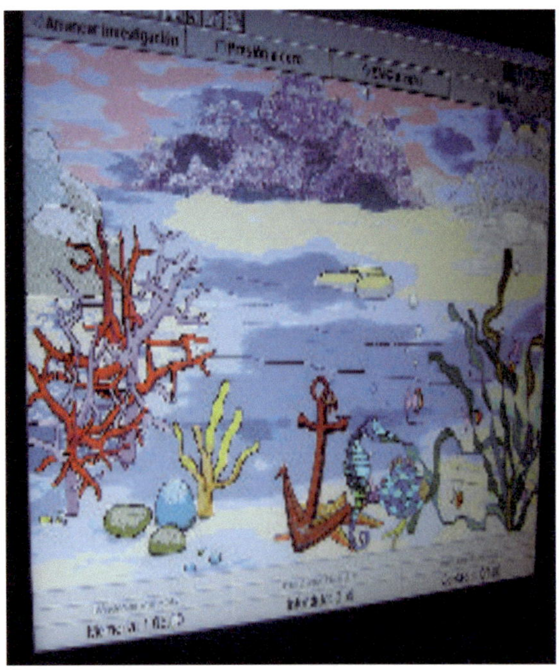

Fig. 5. Screen showing a scene for BFB.

Figures 6 and 7 show fragments of the graphics obtained from the EMG activity registry at a biofeedback session of two different patients.

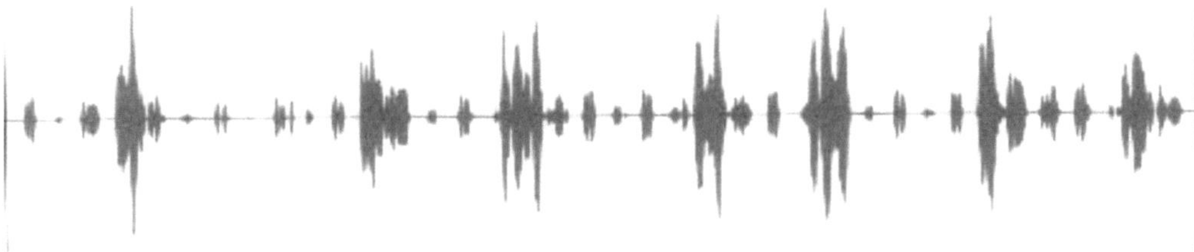

Fig. 6. EMG registry at BFB session.

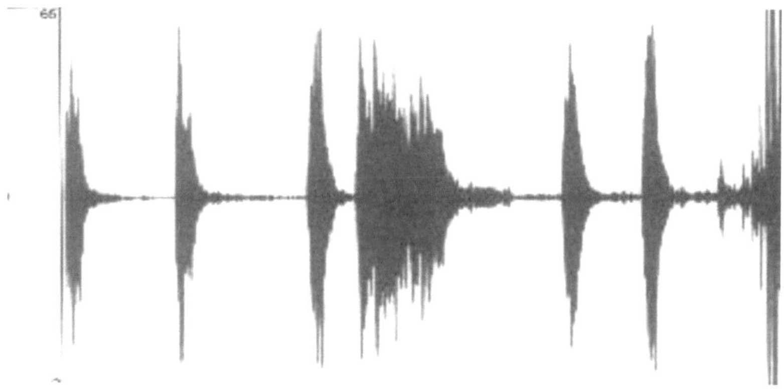

Fig. 7. EMG registry at BFB session.

All patients signed a consent form according to the specific legislation by Directive 2001/20/CE of the European Parliament and of the Council and to the performance of the Good Clinical Practise norms of the Ministry of Health and the Spanish Drugs Agency.
Qualitative and quantitative variables were analysed by NCSS-2000™ statistic program.
Descriptive and inferential studies were performed: analysis of cross tabulation, Fisher exact test, Chi-square, Student's t-test, Pearson correlation test. $p<0,05$ were accepted as statistically significant.

4. Results

4.1 A diagnostic perineal electromyography (EMG) session consists of a 20 minute session of biofeedback (BFB) of the pelvic floor (PF) with superficial electrodes without electro-stimulation, with contractions of 3-5 seconds, followed by a relaxation period of 8-10 seconds after each contraction. Perineal muscle voltage in millivolts (mV) was recorded during the contraction period, and the first five and last five intervals of the session were studied. Initial EMG average were called EMGi; and final AMG average were called EMGf.
4.2 Transobturator vaginal tape procedure was a success and achieved continence in 84% of women, while 16% continued with some grade or kind of incontinence (stress or de novo urgence).
4.2.1 Patients in Group A are younger on average (59,11 yearls old) than those in Group B (69.57 years al) in a statistically significant way (p=0.0001) (Table 1).

Age (years)	Group A	Group B
Mean	59.11	69.57
SD	11.47	9.14
SEM	1.12	49
N	254	48
Student's t-test: p<0.0001 Mean success age minus failure age= -10.45. CI 95% of this difference: from -15.51 to -5.40.		

Table 1. Age of patients with TOT being performed.

4.2.2 Patients in Group A were affected by incontinence on average for a shorter period of time (90.65 months) than those in Group B (195.17 months) (p= 0.0170) (Table 2).

Development time (months)	Group A	Group B
Mean	90.65	195.17
SD	86.61	159.06
	13.21	64.94
N	254	48
Student's t-test: p=0.0170 Development time in succeeded – time in failed= -104.52. CI 95% of this difference: from -189.49 to -19.54.		

Table 2. Development time of urinary incontinence in patients with TOT performed.

4.2.3 Development time of urinary incontinence wasn't correlated with patients' age (Table 3).

Pearson Product Moment Correlation – Ungrouped data		
Statistic	Age (years)	Development time of urinary incontinence (months)
Mean	69.57	195.17
Biased Variant	114.54545455	7278.545454
Biased Standard Deviation	10.702591020	85.31439183
Covarianza	100.8	
Correlation	0.1003590	
Determination	0.01007194	
T-Test	0.30260	
p-value (2 sided)	0.7690	
p-value (1 sided)	0.3845	
Number of observations	48	

Table 3. Relation between patients' age and development time of urinary incontinence.

4.2.4 Age can work as a confusion factor for the analysis of the researched factors, so a stratification regarding age was performed until we had two homogeneousage groups. It was possible at a range of 48-68 years old, with the distribution shown in table 4:

Range 48-68 (años)	Group A	Group B
Mean	58.27	59.38
SD	7.78	7.17
SEM	0.90	1.99
N	150	24

Table 4. Patients' distribution in two homogeneous groups regarding age.

4.2.5 Correlation between the age of the whole sample including succses and failures, N=302) and the average electromyographic values at the beginning (EMGi) and at the end (EMGf) of the session (Table 5).
A general correlation between age and EMGi (-0,067670) or EMGf (-0,100230) was not found in the women in the entire sample (N=302).
4.2.6 The correlation between age and the average electromyographic values at the beginning (EMGi-A) and at the end (EMGf-A) of the session was analysed in the group of succeses (Group A) (Table 6).

Pearson Correlations Section (Row-Wise Deletion):

	Edad	EMGi	EMGf
Age	1,000000	-0,067670	-0,100230
	0,000000	0,678223	0,538316
	40,000000	40,000000	40,000000
EMGi	-0,067670	1,000000	0,894848
	0,678223	0,000000	0,000000
	40,000000	40,000000	40,000000
EMGf	-0,100230	0,894848	1,000000
	0,538316	0,000000	0,000000
	40,000000	40,000000	40,000000

Cronbachs Alpha = 0,671004 Standardized Cronbachs Alpha = 0,489648

Table 5. Correlation between age and electromyographic values (in mVol) at the beginning (EMGi) and at the end (EMGf) of the session.

Pearson Correlations Section (Row-Wise Deletion)

	Age A	EMGi-A	EMGf-A
Age Group A	1,000000	0,043438	-0,017339
	0,000000	0,822962	0,928864
	29,000000	29,000000	29,000000
EMGi-A 0,043438	1,000000	0,904445	
	0,822962	0,000000	0,000000
	29,000000	29,000000	29,000000
EMGf-A -0,017339	0,904445	1,000000	
	0,928864	0,000000	0,000000
	29,000000	29,000000	29,000000

Cronbachs Alpha = 0,696365 Standardized Cronbachs Alpha = 0,574281

Spearman Correlations Section (Row-Wise Deletion)

	Age A	EMGi-A	EMGf-A
Age Group A	1,000000	0,005289	0,087484
	0,000000	0,566915	0,491832
	64,000000	64,000000	64,000000
EMGi-A	0,005289	1,000000	0,567339
	0,566915	0,000000	0,000001
	64,000000	64,000000	64,000000
EMGf-A	0,087484	0,567339	1,000000
	0,491832	0,000001	0,000000
	64,000000	64,000000	64,000000

Table 6.

A correlation between age and EMGi (0,043438) and EMGf (-0,017339) was not found in women who were urinary continent after surgical treatment (Group A).

4.2.7 The correlation between age and the average electromyographic values at the beginning (EMGi-B) and at the end (EMGf-B) of the BFB session was analysed in the group of failures (Group B) (Table 7):

Pearson Correlations Section (Row-Wise Deletion)

	Age B	EMGi-B	EMGf-B
Age Group B	1,000000	-0,743008	-0,263170
	0,000000	0,008792	0,434286
	11,000000	11,000000	11,000000
EMGi-B -0,743008	1,000000	0,472372	
	0,008792	0,000000	0,142340
	11,000000	11,000000	11,000000
EMGf-B -0,263170	0,472372	1,000000	
	0,434286	0,142340	0,000000
	11,000000	11,000000	11,000000

Cronbachs Alpha =- 0,621773 Standardized Cronbachs Alpha =- 0,828724

Table 7.

There was a correlation between age and EMGi (-0,743008), but not with EMGf (-0,263170) in women with continued urinary incontinence after surgical treatment (Group B).

4.2.8 No statistically significant association was found (p=0.2813) between the EMG average initial values in the successful patients (Group A; mean 18.08 mVol) and in the failed patients (Group B; mean 27 mVol) (Graphic 1):

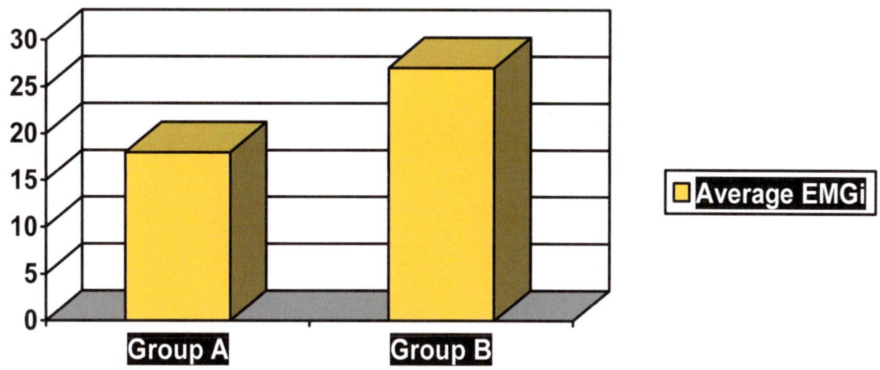

Graphic 1. Average initial EMG.

There was no statistical difference (p= 0,2813) between continent women EMGi (average 18.08mV) and incontinent women EMGi (average 27.00mV).

4.2.9 There was a statistically significant association (p=0.0406) between the final average values in success (Group A; mean 39.67 mVol) and in failure (Group B; mean 13.20 ,Vol) (Graphic 2):

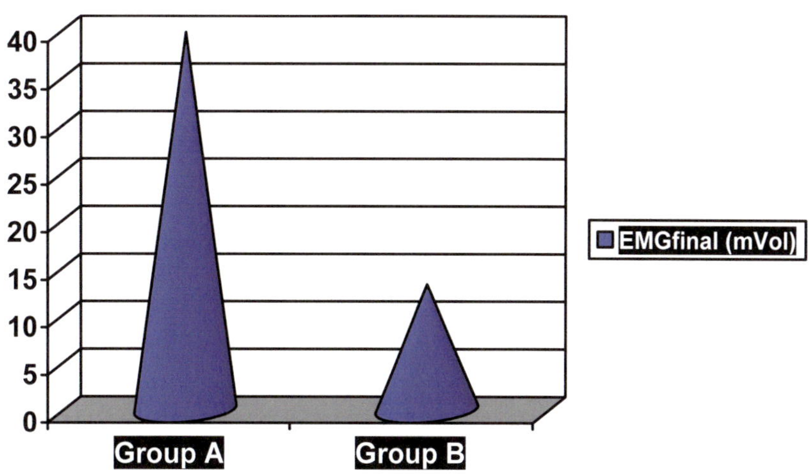

Graphic 2. Average final EMG.

4.2.10 Graphic 4 shows the distribution of the "gain" (we say difference in the graphic) between the initial EMG value and the final one in Group A age-stratified (N=150).

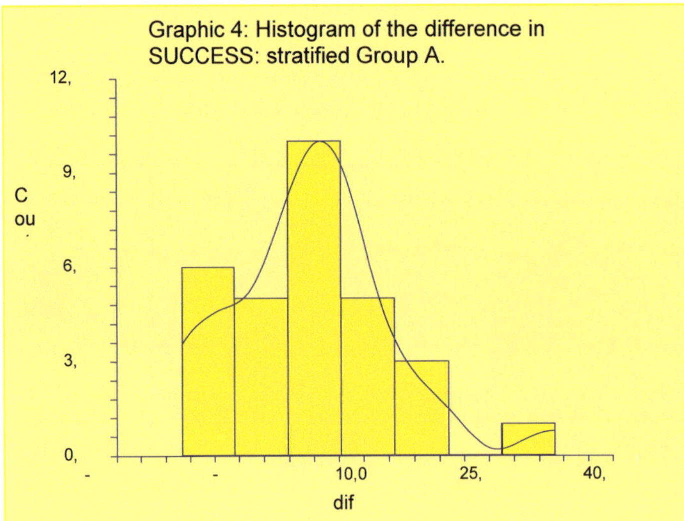

Graphic 4.

4.2.11 Graphic 5 shows the distribution of the "gain" between the initial EMG value and the final one in Group B age-stratified (N=24).

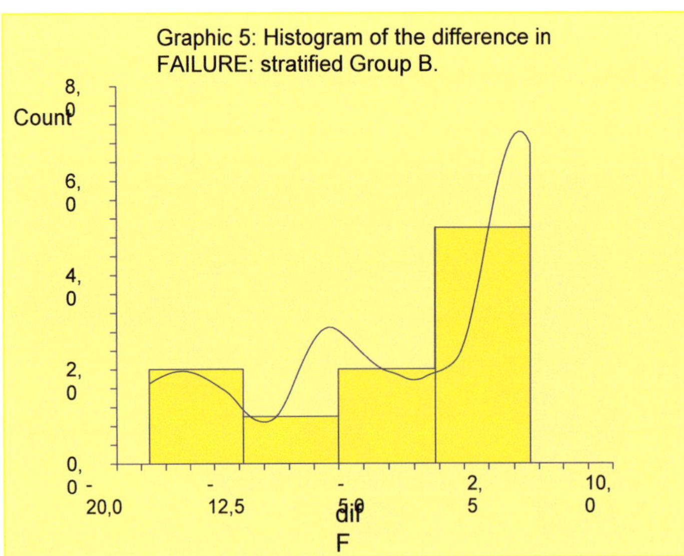

Graphic 5.

Variable	Count	Mean	Standard Deviation	Standard Error	95% LCL of Mean	95% of Mean
difE	150	4,6	9,838699	1,796292	-7,383062E-02	7,27383
difF	24	-3,7	8,472833	2,679345	8,761099	3,361099

Note: T-alpha (difE) = 2,0452, T-alpha (difF) = 2,2622

Table 8. Descriptive Statistics Section.

A statistically significant difference between the EMG gain at the BFB session in Group A and in Group B was found.

5. Discussion

5.1 Perineal electromyography

Electromyography entails the electric registry of the muscular activity. It's useful to distinguish between normal and myopathic muscle.

Some authors consider needle electromyography the most precise method of exploration. A coaxial needle with an electrode at the needle's end is used. It can detect electrical activity in a group of muscular fibres belonging to several motor units, analysing the so-called motor unit potentials.

Contact electromyography is performed locating the electrodes on the skin surface. It's a non-invasive method. Some authors criticize that the registry can be contaminated with other muscles' activity and that the amplitude of the registered activity is too low (Rio and Montero 2004).

The drawback with needle electromyography appears to be that the needle also works at the motor units of the muscle or muscular group we want to explore and at the amyelinic fibres which collect the pain caused by the prick. This painful stimulus can condition local reflexes which can affect the results of needle electromyography.

That being said after explaining the procedure and the perineal anatomy briefly to the patient surface electromyography is still completely viable. It must take place in a safe and comfortable climate, using a standarized electrode-locating method while rigorously respecting the anatomical references and understanding that the perineal electromyographic registry has proven trustworthy in the explored muscular activity.

Knowing the usefulness of surface electromyography in measuring the pelvis floor's biofeddback in incontinent women, we researched the functional status of the perineal muscles in women with genuine stress urinary incontinence who were scheduled to undergo a TOT. A 20-minute biofeedback session with surface electromyography attending to an established and rigorously observed protocol was performed; 3-5 seconds of contraction following 6-10 second of relaxation. The average electromyographic values of the first 5 and the last 5 contractions of this session were calculated. We observed a statistically significant difference in the average electromyographic values at the end of the biofeedback session; patients who remained incontinent after the surgical treatment had a lower average value, but the general average value of every contraction (the first and the last ones) was homogeneous in continent and incontinent patients. Therefore, the perineal muscular status research must be sufficiently precise to detect a possible muscular fatigue in those patients who are still incontinent after an anatomical correction. These patients with a failure of the surgical treatment could also have a defect at the muscular function of the perineum. Following this line of research, we offered many patients the convenience of rehabilitating the pelvic floor, almost 20 sessions with a therapeutic character, before considering the surgical treatment.

5.2 Stress urinary incontinence's treatment

At the present time there is a revolution in stress urinary incontinence treatment with several surgical techniques being considered, less invasive but very efficient, using synthetic materials and with few complications, which can be performed with spinal anesthesia and with only one day of admission if no complications occur.

It has been reported that six months after the surgical approach for urinary incontinence, 95% of patients felt better, but only 57% were objectively asymptomatic (Pacanowski 2002). In our sample, we have confirmed a subjective and objective improvement (totally dry) in an 84% of patients during the complete follow-up time (>6 years).

The treatment with tension free vaginal tape is, according to some authors, the first-line election in moderate to severe stress urinary incontinence (Serrano 2003). The Polypropylene tape will be covered by collagen 6 weeks after surgery, with no rejection (Serrano 2003).

The method of implantation of the tape could influence the results after correcting the incontinence. The transobturator technique seems to have less perforation risks, making unnecessary the intraoperatory vesical endoscopic exploration. This suspension type reproduces in a more physiological way the anatomic suspension of the urethra (Galmes-Belmonte and Diaz-Gómez 2004).

Urinary continence in women mainly depends on the position and the mobility of the urethra and the urethro-vesical union. The pelvis floor muscle and the endopelvic fascia are the principal elements in maintaingin the correct position and mobility of the urethra. When making an effort these muscles increase their resistance. An efficient contraction can compress the urethra onto the pubic symphysis, increasing the intraurethral pressure, with a subsequent involuntary urine leakage. The effect on urethral pressure of the voluntary contraction of the pelvis floor muscles has been reported with urodynamical studies (Espuña-Pons 2002).

Some authors have studied the knowledge that women had of their pelvis floor muscles and their ability to contract them after a theoretical explanation on how to do so. They monitored the result with vaginal touch and perineometry, and they observed that after a verbal instruction, only a 68% of 60 women studied were able to make a correct contraction. In a similar study, Bump reported that only a 41% of 47 women studied were able to contract the pelvic floor muscles after a verbal explanation made by an expert (Bump, Hurt et al. 1991). So, before beginning a pelvis floor muscle rehabilitation program it is essential to evaluate the ability that a woman has to efficiently and voluntarily contract these muscles. The evaluation methods for this objective are vaginal touch (muscular testing), perineometry and electromyography (Espuña-Pons 2002).

There is a delicate balance of physiological reflexive mechanisms that take place in each miccional cycle. Any deficiency or change of any element of this chain can follow a miccional dysfunction and alteration of the continence mechanism (Arlandis-Guzmán, Martínez-Agulló et al. 2002).

The roll of the pelvis floor musculature in this balance is essential. The pelvic floor's place in the miccional cycle is the beginning or finishing of it under a cortical control. The voluntary relaxation, cortically mediated and canalized by the pudendus nerve, is crucial in begining the drainage phase, with the subsequent reflex activation of the parasympathetic (pelvic nerve), following the detrusor's contraction, and with the sympathetic inhibition (hypogastric nerve) that relaxes the vesical neck, achieving a coordinated micturition. On the other hand, during the filling phase, the continuous contraction of the pelvic floor inhibits reflexively the detrusor's contraction, maintaining the sympathetic tone that keeps the vesical neck closed, and at the same time the periurethral muscular tone increases, which is necessary for continence during this phase, when the detrusor's stability and high urethral resistances are required (Arlandis-Guzmán, Martínez-Agulló et al. 2002).

The most complex biofeedback equipment, like the one used in this study, have three surface electrodes, two registering the activity of the pelvic floor and another registering the activity of a "control" muscular group (surface electrodes on the abdominal wall or on the inferior extremity): the information at the patient's disposal is more complex, being able to contract or relax a concrete muscular group and to observe if the exercise is being well performed or not. Not only will the inadequate performance of the exercise not reach a clinical improvement, it will aggravate the problem by strengthening antagonist musculature (Llorca-Miravet 1990). Biofeedback helps to achieve the correct performance of the exercises and is especially useful in those patients who have difficulties in locating their perineal musculature. The results reported with the vesical-sphincterian biofeedback treatment ranged from 42-80% recovery an approximately 22% improvement (Sugar and Firlit 1982; Rapariz 1994). We find an improvement rate of up to 75% in women with pelvic floor biofeedback treatment using surface electrodes, without electro-stimulation through a therapist-guided protocol (Lorenzo-Gómez, Silva-Abuín et al. 2008).

The transobturator method should remain the first-election technique for the stress urinary incontinence correction with urethral sphincter insufficiency. It is the best way to help the recovery of the functional anatomical position of the urethra and the vesical neck. But the striped external urethral sphincter and the vesical neck, composed of smooth muscle fibres, are included in a complex muscular surrounding of fine muscular bundles arranged obliquely like a lounger, which must support the column weight in bipedalism, not only of the pelvis viscera but of the whole abdomen. While seated, the direction of the tension power those perineal muscles are subjected to, changes versus a supine position. The stress-response status of the perineal musculature may require the running of a foreign material tape that is placed in order to reinforce the lounger. After the statistical correlation analysis, age was reported as the independent factor most responsible for the condition of the tone and the function of the pelvic floor muscles. Ergo the surgical treatment's result is more related to the functional status of this musculature than to concomitant illnesses or drugs which act at the vesical neck and/or the urethra.

6. Conclusion

6.1 Perineal electromyography can evaluate basal muscle tonicity and stress or exercise adaptation capacity in women planning surgical treatment by transobturator vaginal tape for urinary incontinence.

6.2 Stress and muscle fatigue due to continued exercise are more determinant of transobturator vaginal tape procedure failure that basal perineal muscle tone.

6.3 Muscle fatigue found in a perineal EMG session is associated with transobturator vaginal tape procedure failure, therefore we must offer another treatment option.

7. Concerns of the chapter

In the investigation of the excellence of surgical treatment of urinary incontinence, the perineal EMG can be included in the arsenal of tools for the evaluation of patients, as well as in the investigation of the functional status of perineum in each one of conditions or secondary diagnosis of the patients.

8. References

Abrahams, P., J. Blaivas, et al. (1988). "The standarization of terminology of lower urinary tract function." Scan J Urol Nephrol Supple: 114-5.

Amaro, J., M. Gameiro, et al. (2006). "Intravaginal electrical stimulation: a randomized, double-blind study on the treatment of mixed urinary incontinence." Acta Obstet Gynecol Scand 85(5): 619-22.

Arlandis-Guzmán, S., E. Martínez-Agulló, et al. (2002). Alternativas terapéuticas para la disfunción miccional crónica. Neuromodulación: Una nueva alternativa terapéutica para los tratornos del tracto urinario inferior. A. E. d. Urología. Madrid, ENE Ediciones: Cap 5.

Bidmead, J. (2002). "Urinary incontinence: A Gynaecologist´s Experience." Eur Urol: 21-24.

Bump, R., W. Hurt, et al. (1991). "Assessment of Kegel pelvic muscle exercise performance after brief verbal instruction." Am J Obstet Gynecol 165: 322-8.

Capelini, M., C. Riccetto, et al. (2006). "Pelvic floor exercises with biofeedback for stress urinary incontinence." Int Braz J Urol 32(4): 462-8.

Castiñeiras-Fernández, J. (2005). Anatomia funcional y quirurgica de la continencia femenina. Incontinencia urinaria de esfuerzo y reparación del suelo pélvico. J. Gonzalez and J. Angulo. Madrid, Luzán: 257-285.

Castiñeiras-Fernández, J. (2005). Técnicas de cintas sin tensión. Incontinencia de esfuerzo y reparación del suelo pélvico: Atlas de técnicas quirúrgicas. J. González and J. Angulo. Madrid, Boehringer Ingelheim: 276.

Castro, D. (2002). The pelvic floor functional anatomy. The pelvic floor functional anatomy. Pelvic Floor Reconstruction., Murcia. España, European School of Urology.

DeLancey, J. (1990). "Anatomy and physiology of the urinary continence." Clin Obstet Gynecol 33: 298.

Delorme, E. and J. Hermieu (2010). "Guidelines for the surgical treatment of female urinary stress incontinence in women using the suburethral sling." Prog Urol 20(Suppl 2): 132-142.

Delorme., E. (2001). "Transobturator urethral suspension: mini-invasive procedure in the treatment of stress urinary incontinence in women." Prog Urol 11(6): 1306-13.

Di-Gangi-Herms, A., R. Veit, et al. (2006). "Functional imaging of stress urinary incontinence." Neuroimage. 29(1): 267-75.

Espino, D., R. Palmer, et al. (2003). "Prevalence and severity of urinary incontinence in elderly Mexican-American women." J Am Geriatr Soc 51(11): 1580-1586.

Espuña, M., P. Rebollo, et al. (2004). "Validación de la versión española del ICIQ-SF. Un cuestionario para evaluar la incontinencia urinaria." Med Clin 122(8): 288-292.

Espuña-Pons, M. (2002). Criterios para la indicación de tratamiento conservador de la incontinencia urinaria de esfuerzo y tipos de tratamiento. La Opinión de los expertos. E. Glosa. Barcelona, Edit Glosa. 2: 12-14.

Fultz, N., T. Girts, et al. (2005). "Prevalence, management and impact of urinary incontinence in the workplace." Occup Med 55(7): 552-557.

Galmes-Belmonte, I. and E. Diaz-Gómez (2004). "¿Son iguales todos los sistemas empleados para corregir la incontinencia urinaria mediante mallas de libre tensión?" Actas Urológicas Españolas 28(7): 487-496.

González-Hidalgo, M. (1998). "Exploración neurológica del suelo de la pelvis." Rev Neurología 26(151): 432-438.

Halban, J., J. Tandler, et al. (1907). "Fascia endopélvia: ligamentos y envolturas." Anatomie und Atiologie der Genital prolapse beim Weibe.

Huang, A., D. Thom, et al. (2006). "Urinary incontinence and pelvic floor dysfunction in Asian-American women." Am J Obstet Gynecol 195(5): 1331-1337.

Hunskaar, S., G. Lose, et al. (2004). "The prevalence of urinary incontinence in women in four European countries." BJU International 93(3): 324-330.

International-Continence-Society (1977). "Standardization of terminology of lower urinary tract function." Urol 9: 237.

Kelleher, C., L. Cardozo, et al. (1997). "A new questionnaire to assess the quality of life of urinary incontinent women." BJOG: International Journal of Obstetrics & Gynaecology 104: 1374-1379.

Lee, I. and E. Choi (2006). "Pelvic floor muscle exercise by biofeedback and electrical stimulation to reinforce the pelvic floor muscle after normal delivery." Taehan Kanho Hakhoe Chi. 36(8): 1374-80.

Llorca-Miravet, A. (1990). Tratamiento funcional en la incontinencia urinaria. Incontinencia Urinaria: Conceptos Actuales. E. Martínez-Agulló. Valencia, Graficuatre: 629-649.

Lorenzo-Gómez, M., J. Silva-Abuín, et al. (2008). "Treatment of stress urinary incontinence with perineal biofeedback by using superficial electrodes." Actas Urol Esp 32(6): 629-36.

Martínez-Agulló, E., J. L. Ruiz-Cerdá, et al. (2009). "Prevalencia de Incontinencia Urinaria y Vejiga Hiperactiva en la población española: Resultados del Estudio EPICC." Actas Urológicas Españolas 33(2): 159-166.

Médico-Interactivo-Diario-Electrónico-de-la-Sanidad (2003). La incontinencia urinaria de urgencia podría ser abordada desde la Atención Primaria. Sección: Noticias Nacional. Meditex. Madrid, Meditex, S.L.

Melville, J., W. Katon, et al. (2005). "Urinary incontinence in US women: a population-based study." Arch Intern Med 165(5): 537-542.

Minassian, V., W. Stewart, et al. (2008). "Urinary incontinence in women: variation in prevalence estimates and risk factors." Obstet Gynecol 111(2Pt1): 324-331.

Nissenkorn, I., M. Shalev, et al. (2004). "Patient-adjusted intermittent electrostimulation for treating stress and urge urinary incontinence." BJU Int 94(1): 105-9.

Pacanowski, T. (2002). La cirugía en una sesión puede ser óptima en el suelo pélvico. Sección Cirugía General. D. Médico.com. Barcelona, Recoletos.es. 2002: http://buscador.recoletos.es/advice/pruebas/documento.jsp.

Rapariz, M. (1994). Reeducación esfinteriana en el tratamiento de la Micción no Coordinada. Departamento de Urología. Madrid, Universidad Complutense de Madrid.

Raz, S. (1992). The anatomy of pelvic support and stress incontinence. Raz S Atlas of transvaginal surgery. S. Raz. Philadelphia., Wb Saunders. 1: 1-22.

Raz, S., N. Rosenblum, et al. (2003). Cirugía reconstructiva de la vejiga. Selected topics in Urogynecology. O. E. o. A. 2003. Los Angeles, Departamento de Urología de la Universidad de California. LA. School of Medicine.

Rett, M., J. Simoes, et al. (2007). "Management of stress urinary incontinence with surface electromyography-assisted biofeedback in women of reproductive age." Phys Ther 87(2): 136-42.

Rio, C. and J. Montero (2004). "Exploración neurológica y fisiológica del suelo pelviano." Cirugía Española 76(5): 284-291.

Seo, J., H. Yoon, et al. (2004). "A randomized prospective study comparing new vaginal cone and FES-Biofeedback." Yonsei Med J 45(5): 879-84.

Serrano, C. (2003). Las mallas artificiales de polipropileno reparan fallos de suelo pélvico. Especialidades. Diariomédico.com. Madrid, Recoletos.es. 2003: http://www.diariomedico.com.

Serrano, R. (2003). El 90% de las IU de esfuerzo se evitan con medidas preventivas. Urología. D. Médico.com. Madrid, Recoletos.es. 2003: http://www.diariomedico.com/edicion/noticia/0,2458,404697,00.html.

SNS (1996). Indicadores de la prestación farmacéutica en el Sistema Nacional de Salud. Madrid, Subdirección-General-de-Coordinación Administrativa.

Solà-Dalenz, V., J. Pardo-Schanz, et al. (2006). "Cirugía minimamente invasiva de la IU femenina TVT-O. ." Actas Urológicas Españolas. 30(1): 61-66.

Sugar, E. and C. Firlit (1982). "Urodynamic biofeedback: a new therapeutic approach for childhood incontinence/infection (vesical voluntary sphincter dyssynergia)." J Urol 128: 1253.

Ulmsten, U. and P. Petros (1995). "Intravaginal slingplasty an ambulatory surgical procedure for treatment of female urinary incontinence." Scand J Urol Nephrol 29(1): 75-82.

Viana-Zulaica, C. (2005). Incontinencia urinaria en la mujer. Guías clínicas de Fisterra.com. A Coruña., Casitérides. S.L.: http://www.fisterra.com/guias2/incontinencia.asp.

Voorham-van, d.-Z., R. Pelger, et al. (2006). "Effects of magnetic stimulation in the treatment of pelvic floor dysfunction." BJU Int 97(5): 1035-8.

Part 6

Orofacial Function (Includes Dysphagia)

19

Electromyography as a Biofeedback Tool for Rehabilitating Swallowing Muscle Function

Catriona M. Steele[1], Janice W. Bennett[2], Sarah Chapman-Jay[3], Rebecca Cliffe Polacco[1], Sonja M. Molfenter[1] and Mohamed Oshalla[1]
[1]*Toronto Rehabilitation Institute, Toronto*
[2]*St. Joseph's Health Centre, Toronto*
[3]*Greater Niagara General Hospital, Niagara Falls*
Canada

1. Introduction

Dysphagia (swallowing impairment) is a common and serious problem in individuals who have suffered neurological injuries (strokes, acquired brain injury) as well as individuals with neurodegenerative conditions or head and neck cancer. The effortful swallow and Mendelsohn maneuver are two therapy techniques, recommended to address specific muscle-function related abnormalities in dysphagia due to neurological injury. The process of swallowing is a complex neuromuscular sequence, involving contributions from approximately 25 pairs of muscles in the upper aerodigestive tract. Contraction of the floor-of-mouth muscles (particularly the mylohyoid and geniohyoid) facilitates upward and forward movement of the hyoid and larynx in swallowing (Burnett et al., 2003; Pearson et al., 2010). Hyolaryngeal movement has two important functional consequences: 1) closure of the entrance to the airway; and 2) opening of the sphincter between the pharynx and the esophagus, i.e., the upper esophageal sphincter (UES), via traction forces (Cook et al., 1989). Patients with reduced hyolaryngeal excursion in swallowing are at risk for aspiration (entry of foreign material into the airway) and post-swallow residues, particularly in the pyriform sinuses, which lie just above the UES. The structures involved in swallowing are illustrated in Figure 1, which is a still shot taken from a videofluoroscopic swallowing study (VFSS) showing aspiration of material into the trachea as well as residues in the valleculae and pyriform sinuses.

Surface electromyography (sEMG) is useful for monitoring performance of the effortful swallow and Mendelsohn maneuver exercises, which are indicated as therapy techniques for patients with reduced hyolaryngeal movement in swallowing. SEMG can be used to collect and display information regarding performance of these maneuvers in treatment; such performance-contingent information can enhance motivation, compliance and task-performance. For the effortful swallow, sEMG can be used to measure the amplitude of muscle contraction used by a patient and to compare this to their regular swallowing. Amplitude targets can be used to guide a patient to work harder on this exercise, and sEMG information can be used to inform both the patient and the clinician of success in achieving these targets across the course of treatment. For the Mendelsohn maneuver, the goal is to maintain submental muscle contraction and excursion of the hyolaryngeal complex, thereby prolonging opening of the UES (Mendelsohn & McConnel, 1987); sEMG can be used to measure and display the duration of muscle contraction used in this task.

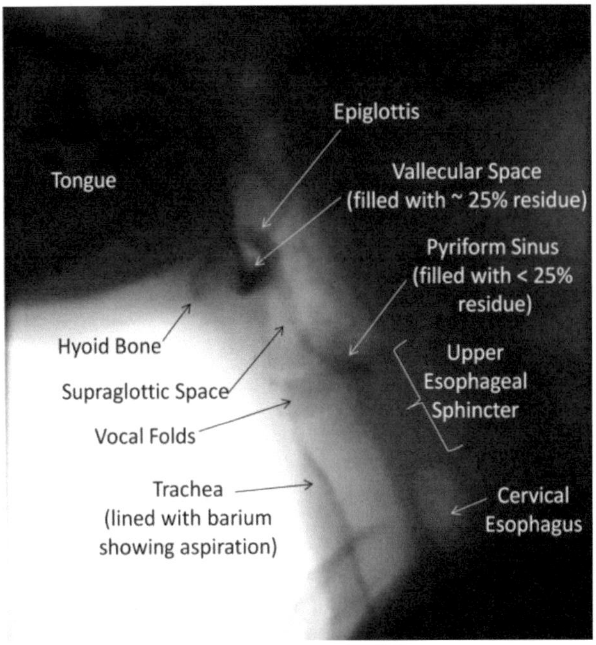

Fig. 1. A still x-ray image, taken from a videofluoroscopic swallowing study. This image shows the oropharyngeal anatomy, and includes evidence of mild residue (up to 25% of the available space) in the valleculae and pyriform sinuses. Additionally, evidence of prior aspiration is evident as a thin line of barium running down the front wall of the trachea.

In the Swallowing Rehabilitation Research Laboratory at the Toronto Rehabilitation Institute, we have developed a treatment protocol using sEMG biofeedback for patients with neurogenic dysphagia, for whom either the effortful swallow and/or the Mendelsohn maneuver are indicated. The protocol uses software that has been developed in conjunction with the Biofeedback Foundation of Europe (www.bfe.org), displaying a sEMG signal representing the composite muscle activity of the floor-of-mouth muscles (likely including the mylohyoid, geniohyoid, anterior belly digastric and genioglossus muscles). Patients who complete this protocol practice approximately 60 saliva swallows per treatment session, over 20-24 sessions, scheduled twice weekly. Tasks include amplitude target practice (for non-effortful and effortful swallows) and muscle contraction prolongation (for the Mendelsohn maneuver). Functional outcomes are measured using a standardized videofluoroscopic swallowing study (VFSS), comparing post-treatment function to baseline performance. Two videofluoroscopic measures are of particular interest: 1) the Penetration-Aspiration Scale, an 8-point ordinal scale measuring the depth of airway invasion; and 2) measures of post-swallow residue, captured using a 4-point ordinal scale reflecting the degree to which the available space in the pyriform sinuses is filled with residue (Eisenhuber et al., 2002). In this chapter, we will share sEMG and outcome data from several patients who have completed treatment using sEMG biofeedback.

2. Methods

2.1 Instrumentation

An adhesive triode electrode patch is attached under the participant's chin with the positive and negative electrodes positioned just lateral to midline, anterior to the hyoid bone (Figure 2). The reference (ground) electrode is positioned away from the muscles of interest. The electrodes are attached to an EMG device (MyoTrac Infiniti, Thought Technology, Montreal) using a sensor cable and the signal from the device is registered on a computer using specialized software (BioGraph Infiniti, Thought Technology, Montreal).

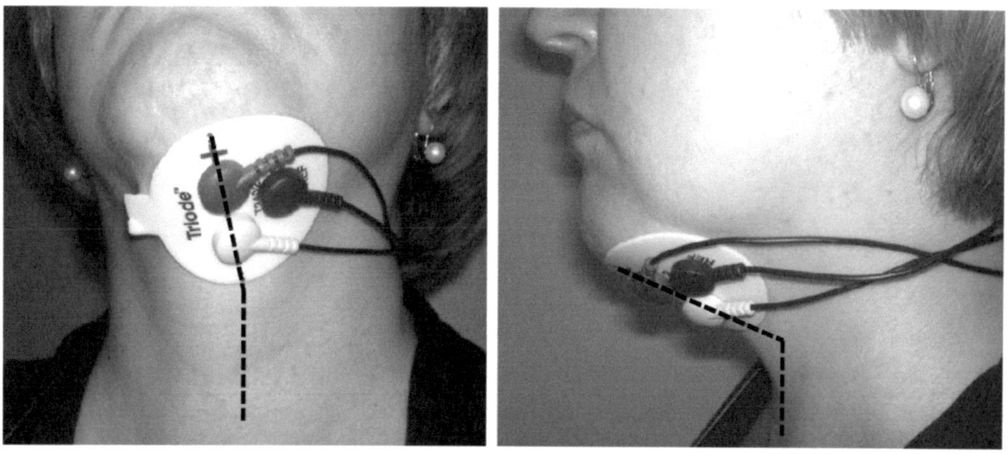

Fig. 2. Electrode attachment under the chin, just lateral to midline, with the reference electrode off to one side.

2.2 Treatment protocol

We recommend that a treatment session should include 60 swallows, practiced in 12 sets of 5 swallows. The protocol involves a progression of tasks from "regular effort saliva swallows" (RESS) to "effortful saliva swallows" (ESS) and, where indicated, "Mendelsohn Maneuver saliva swallows" (MM), as illustrated in Figure 3.

Step 1 in the protocol is a check of the submental sEMG signal to make sure that the electrodes are correctly displaying activity of the floor of mouth musculature. Once the electrodes have been positioned and connected, the clinician should ask the patient to perform some tasks that are expected to display variations in signal amplitude of the submental muscles, such as jaw opening.

Step 2 in the protocol involves a baseline measurement of sEMG amplitude during regular-effort saliva swallows. For this task, we recommend that the patient to produce one saliva swallow every 30 seconds, followed by a rest period. If the patient has extreme difficulty initiating a saliva swallow, a tiny amount of water may be taken to provide a stimulus. The 30-second cycle of resting and swallowing is repeated 5 times, allowing a measurement of the patient's average saliva swallow amplitudes for that session. All amplitude targets for other tasks in the session are then set relative to the baseline swallow measures for the session. This ensures that artifacts in sEMG amplitude due to variations in electrode placement and contact across sessions and participants do not interfere with the treatment protocol.

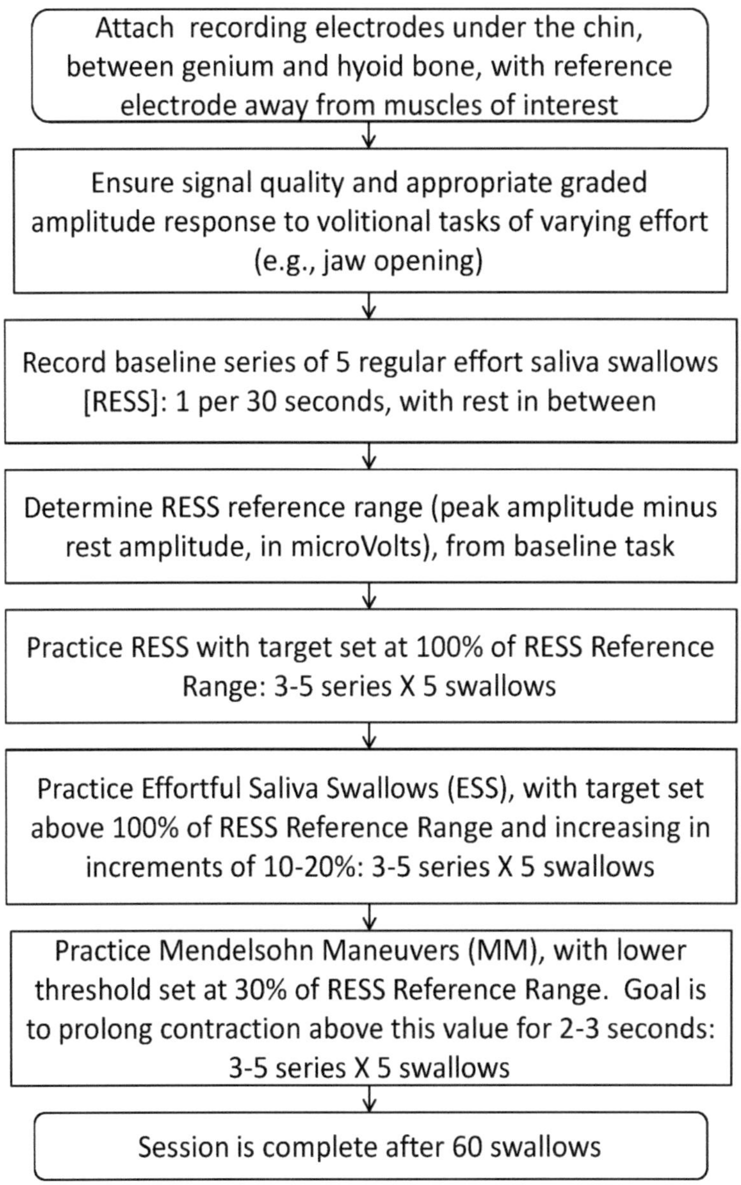

Fig. 3. Flow-chart of a typical sEMG biofeedback session for swallowing rehabilitation.

Step 3 in the treatment protocol involves further practice of RESS. The protocol proceeds in a similar manner to the previous baseline task, with alternating cycles of 20-second-long rests and 10-second intervals in which a saliva swallow should be produced. In contrast to the previous task, however, this step in the protocol involves establishing a target amplitude for the peak of each swallow. This target is set between 90% and 110% of the mean peak amplitude measured in the baseline task, and a target line appears on the screen. Success on this task is defined as a mean peak amplitude within 10% of target across a series of 5 repeated saliva swallows.

Step 4 in the treatment protocol proceeds to the practice of effortful saliva swallows (ESS). Here the goal is to contract the swallowing muscles with greater effort so that the signal amplitude reaches higher values. We begin working at 110% of the mean peak amplitude measured in the baseline reference task. Once the patient can produce swallows within 10% of this target on two successive series of 5 saliva swallows, the challenge level is increased incrementally by steps of 10%. We recommend increasing the difficulty in steps of 10%. Figure 4 displays a typical 2 ½ minute recording of submental muscle activity during practice of the ESS task.

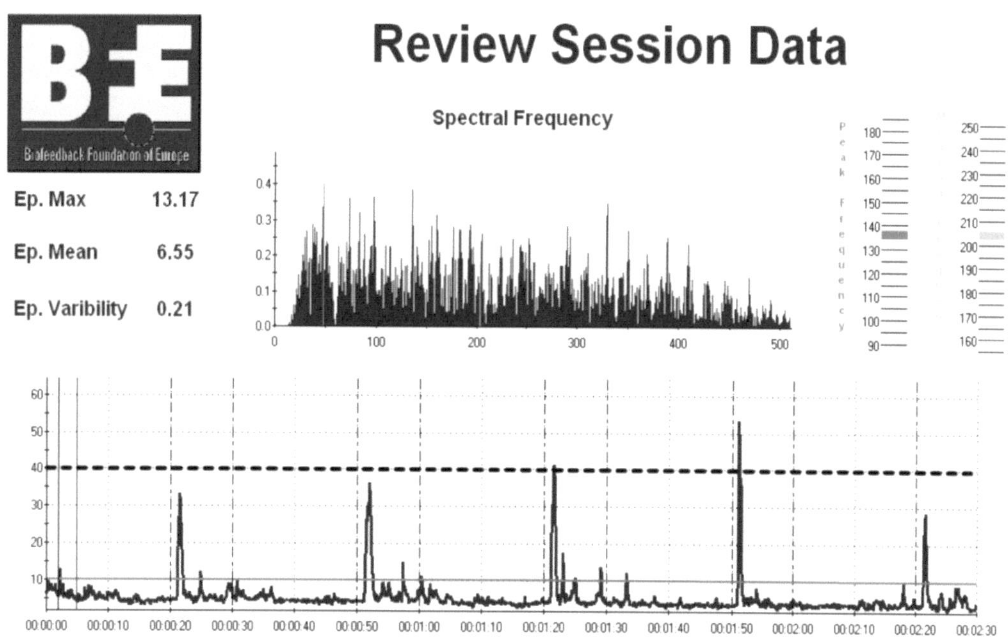

Fig. 4. A series of 5 effortful swallows is shown, one swallow per 30 seconds. The dashed black line shows an amplitude target line set at 40 microvolts. Success in reaching or surpassing this target is illustrated for the 3rd and 4th ESS of the series.

The final step in the treatment protocol is optional practice of the Mendelsohn Maneuver (MM). The goal of this task is to prolong the muscle contraction associated with swallowing. It is important that the event begins with a real swallow, leading into a sustained muscle contraction. The sEMG profile displayed on the screen is described to typically look like a straight-backed chair, where the signal first reaches a swallowing peak, then drops slightly, and is then maintained for 2-3 seconds (Figure 5). For this task, we recommend using a lower threshold of 30% of the reference amplitude range and measuring the duration of time that the patient maintains contraction above this level.

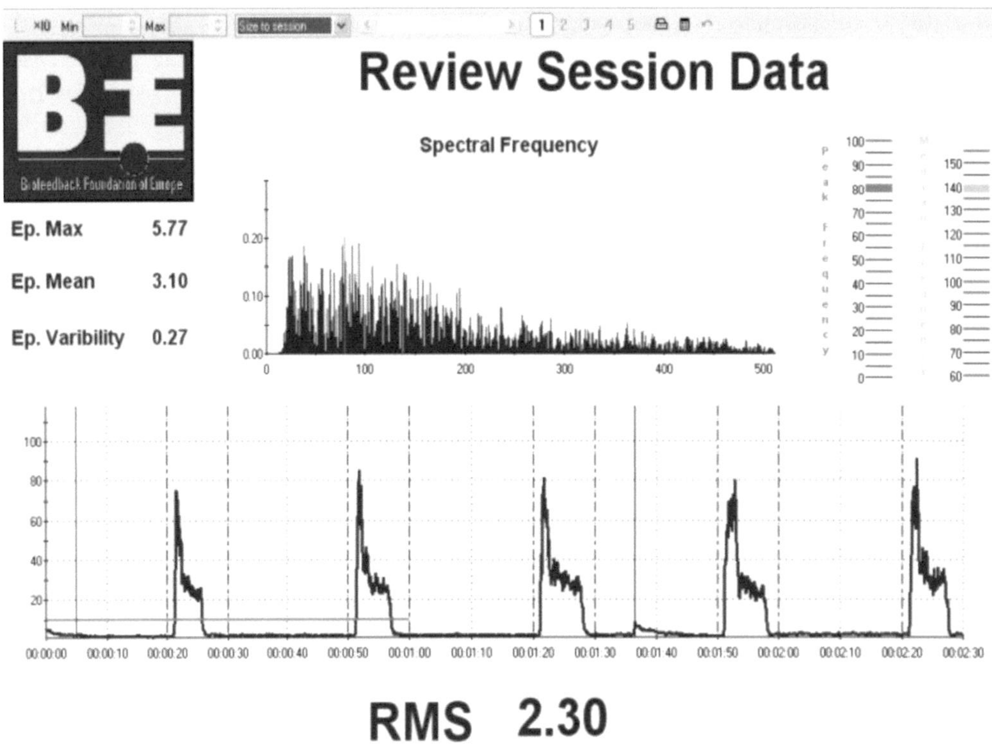

Fig. 5. A series of 5 Mendelsohn Maneuvers, displaying the characteristic straight-backed chair profile, beginning with a peak amplitude associated with a saliva swallow, and followed by prolongation of muscle contraction for 2-3 seconds, above a lower threshold set by the clinician (recommended value: 30% of regular effort saliva swallow amplitudes).

3. Case reports

Over the past three years, we have been following patients who participated in this treatment protocol at three hospitals. Patients are selected based on videofluoroscopic evidence of reduced hyolaryngeal excursion or post-swallow residues in the pyriform sinuses on a standardized VFSS examination. In a retrospective review of patients, we were able to find several cases in which fairly complete sEMG signal data were available, together with pre- and post-treatment videofluoroscopy recordings. Complete data of this nature are not always available, due to signal quality issues, or decisions by the treating clinician to retain only a portion of the data from a particular session.

In this chapter, we will use the available data to explore five questions regarding the use of sEMG biofeedback in dysphagia therapy.

1. How variable are sEMG amplitudes for the submental muscles in regular-effortsaliva swallows across repeated sessions within individual participants?
2. To what extent do effortful swallow sEMG peak amplitudes increase over time in patients with dysphagia?
3. Do videofluoroscopic measures of swallowing function improve with increases in sEMG peak amplitudes on effortful swallows?
4. To what extent does the duration of muscle contraction increase in patients who practice the Mendelsohn Maneuver?
5. Do videofluoroscopic measures of swallowing function improve with increases in the duration of muscle contraction secondary to practice of the Mendelsohn Maneuver?

3.1 How variable are sEMG amplitudes for the submental muscles in regular-effort saliva swallows across repeated sessions within individual participants?

To answer this question, we extracted sEMG data for the baseline RESS task from the first 8 available treatment sessions in 8 patients and 2 healthy, young controls (one female, one male). Signals were first visually inspected for obvious artifact, combined with a review of notes recorded by the clinician during each session; where necessary, portions of the signal containing artifact were removed using an ignore-segment function in the sEMG software. Amplitude range (peak minus rest) for the RESS baseline task is plotted by participant in Figure 6, with dashed lines showing a one standard deviation confidence interval band around the mean.

As can be seen from the varying scales on the y-axes in Figure 6, the actual value of the peak-minus-rest amplitude range (in microVolts) varied considerably across participants. The majority of participants showed maximum peak values below 100 microVolts, but this was not true for Control 2, nor for patient participants 4 and 8. Previous literature suggests that sEMG amplitudes may vary as a function of the amount of fatty tissue between the surface of the neck and the underlying muscles; this may have been one of the factors contributing to the higher amplitudes seen in these individuals. Furthermore, it can be seen that both controls and all 8 patient participants showed at least one outlier session, for which the recorded amplitude range fell outside the boundaries of a one standard deviation confidence interval. Minor variations in electrode placement and contact from session to session may contribute to such fluctuations in sEMG amplitude. The presence of fluctuating amplitudes across these data supports the need to normalize all sEMG amplitude values to a within-participant within-session reference value prior to interpretation or groupwise statistical analysis. This is a standard step in our protocol, achieved by recording a series of RESS at the beginning of the session, and subsequently transforming all other amplitude measures to a percent of the mean baseline RESS range.

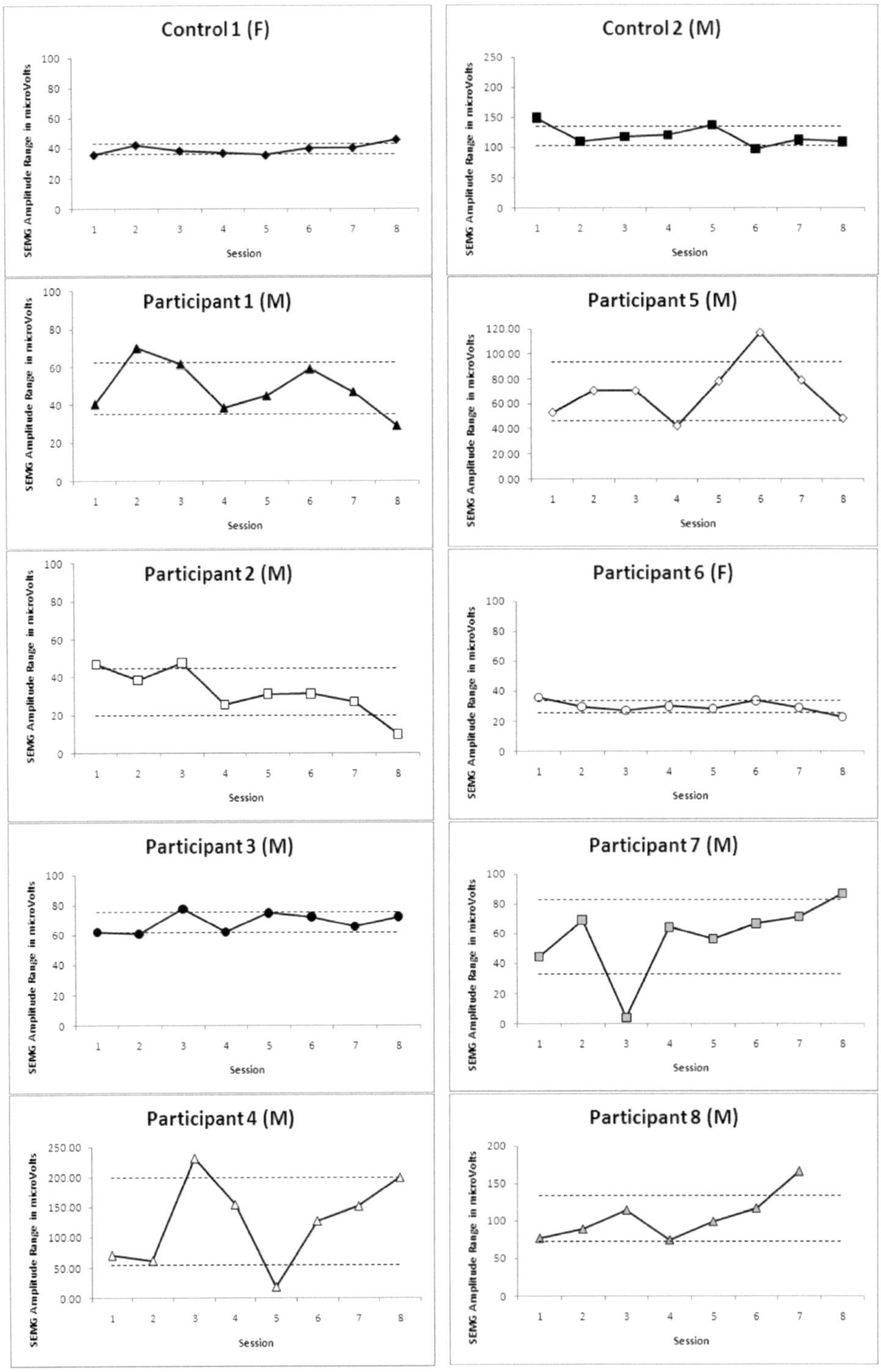

Fig. 6. Regular effort saliva swallow (RESS) amplitude range across repeated recording sessions in two healthy controls and eight patients with dysphagia.

3.2 To what extent do effortful swallow sEMG peak amplitudes increase over time in patients with dysphagia?

Six of the patient participants in this case series had available data for effortful swallows from at least 5 treatment sessions. Table 1 provides demographic information regarding these 6 participants.

Participant	Gender	Age	Primary Diagnosis
2	M	49	Acoustic neuroma; damage to adjacent cranial nerves
4	M	75	Stroke
5	M	68	Sudden onset of dysphagia with vocal fold paresis
6	F	88	Stroke
7	M	88	Stroke
8	M	69	Spinal cord injury with tetraplegia

Table 1. Demographic information regarding the cases discussed in this chapter.

For the purposes of calculating change in effortful swallow performance, all ESS amplitude data were first transformed into percentage values relative to RESS range, using the method described in section 3.1 (above). A baseline reference range for effortful swallows was then established by calculating the mean and standard deviation of all ESS values in the first two treatment sessions for each participant. As shown in Figure 7 one (grey) and two (black) standard deviation bands were plotted around the baseline mean on a control chart for each participant. Mean ESS amplitude range was then plotted for each treatment session.

Standard deviation banding methods for single subject analysis usually specify a criterion for concluding that a participant is showing change, namely the demonstration of two successive data points falling beyond a specified standard deviation boundary (Nourbakhsh & Ottenbacher, 1994). Applying a two standard deviation criterion, Figure 7 shows that participant 2 demonstrates an apparent increase in ESS values at probes 3 and 4, but this trend was not sustained and reverses at probe 5. The values seen at probe 4 are also sufficiently outlying to suggest the possibility that some sort of measurement artifact may have been affecting those data. Participants 5 and 7 both show a general trend towards increasing ESS values, but these changes fail to cross either the one or two standard deviation boundaries across more than a single session. The outlier value for probe 14 in participant 7's data is sufficiently larger than other probes to suggest an artifact effect. Participant 8 shows an overall upward trend in ESS values with the final two probes sitting at or above the two standard deviation bandwidth. Participant 6 shows very little evidence of change across treatment, remaining within the standard deviation bands. Participant 4 shows a general downward trend in ESS values across probes, but with values consistently falling within a single standard deviation band. Based on these graphs, it would appear that only participant 8 showed a convincing increase in effortful saliva swallow amplitudes, expressed as a percent of RESS range. Caution must, however, be used in accepting this interpretation, given the uneven number of data points available across participants.

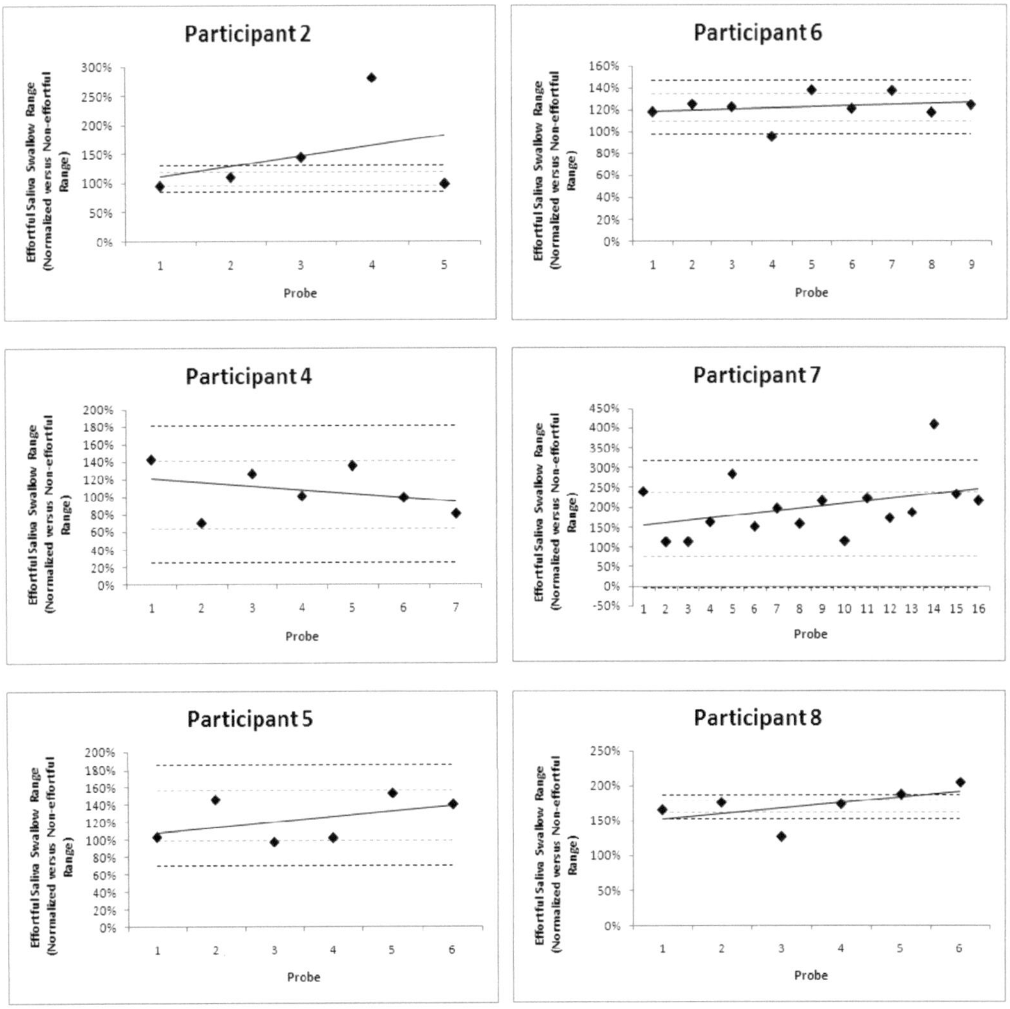

Fig. 7. Charts showing the standard deviation banding method of monitoring change in effortful saliva swallow (ESS) amplitudes, expressed as a percentage of regular effort saliva swallow (RESS) reference range, in six patients with dysphagia. Light-grey dashed horizontal lines represent a 1 standard deviation confidence interval around the patient's baseline ESS performance. Black dashed horizontal lines represent a 2 standard deviation confidence interval. Change is considered to have occurred when two consecutive data points fall outside the 2 standard deviation confidence interval boundaries.

3.3 Do videofluoroscopic measures of swallowing function improve with increases in sEMG peak amplitudes on effortful swallows?

The literature on swallowing intervention contains two impressive examples of case series, in which patients who have practiced effortful swallows and/or Mendelsohn maneuvers using sEMG biofeedback have shown dramatic functional improvement (Crary, 1995; Crary & Groher, 2000; Crary et al., 2004; Huckabee & Cannito, 1999). However, in these studies, change has been reported in terms of clinical measures of diet texture tolerance rather than using objective blinded rating of standardized videofluoroscopies. It remains unclear whether specific physiological parameters in swallowing that are logically linked to the strength or duration of suprahyoid muscle contraction change following such treatment.

Our understanding of the effortful swallow is that it should enhance bolus propulsion and clearance through the oropharynx in swallowing (Bülow et al., 1999; Bülow et al., 2001; Hind et al., 2001). Therefore, the primary videofluoroscopic parameter expected to respond to this exercise would be post-swallow residue. Other parameters that are logically related to this treatment might include the range of hyolaryngeal excursion and measures of bolus flow velocity or kinematics (Clave et al., 2006; Hind et al., 2001). In our series, pre- and post-treatment videofluoroscopy recordings were available for analysis for four of the six patients discussed previously under question 2 (participants 2, 4, 7 and 8). These recordings were spliced into clips containing the swallowing sequence for each bolus presented. The first two thin liquid and two thick liquid swallow clips were then arranged in random order and rated by two experienced speech-language pathologists, blinded to the identity of the patient participant and the timepoint of each swallow. We chose to rate post-swallow residues in the valleculae and pyriform sinuses using 4-point ordinal rating scales developed by Eisenhuber and colleagues (Eisenhuber et al., 2002). We also used the 8-point Penetration-Aspiration Scale (Rosenbek et al., 1996) to measure airway invasion, although this feature was not necessarily expected to change as a function of treatment.

Scores for post-swallow vallecular residue remained unchanged for all participants across treatment. This finding is not particularly surprising, given that vallecular residue is thought to arise primarily from weak tongue propulsion forces in swallowing, and these were not directly targeted in therapy. Pyriform sinus residues, however, were expected to respond to block practice of the effortful swallow. In this respect, participant 7 showed a marked improvement with thickened liquids, from pre-treatment values of 3 (severe) to post-treatment values of 0 (no residue). Participant 4 showed a slight improvement on this variable for thin liquids, shifting from a severe to a moderate rating. Participants 2 and 8 showed no changes in pyriform sinus residue measures, which remained in the moderate-severe range for both thin and thick liquid stimuli. The change seen in participant 7 correlates with the overall upward trend seen in this participant's effortful saliva swallow strength, as indexed by sEMG amplitude data (refer back to Figure 7). Participant 4, however, did not display a noticeable increase in effortful saliva swallow sEMG amplitudes (Figure 7), hence the apparent change in residue scores is not obviously explained by their sEMG measures. Similarly, it is important to note that participant 8, who displayed noticeable increases in effortful saliva swallowing amplitudes (Figure 7) showed no measurable change in swallowing residues, thus challenging the assumption that an association can be expected between these measures.

Penetration-Aspiration Scale scores were not seriously impaired at baseline in this subgroup of four patients. The worst baseline performance on this measure was seen in participant 7, who displayed a score of 3 (i.e., airway invasion into the supraglottic space, above the vocal folds) with thickened liquid stimuli. Participant 4 also displayed airway invasion to this level with both thin and thickened stimuli, but this was noted to clear spontaneously (score of 2). Post-treatment, all four participants showed normal scores on the Penetration-Aspiration Scale, with the exception of participant 2 who had a single episode of aspiration (entry of material into the airway below the level of the vocal folds) with a thin liquid stimulus.

3.4 To what extent does the duration of muscle contraction increase in patients who practice the Mendelsohn Maneuver?

For two of the patients in our retrospective series, the Mendelsohn Maneuver was the primary focus of treatment. As mentioned previously, this technique emphasizes prolongation of muscle contraction. The functional goal of this exercise is to enhance the degree and duration of UES opening, via biomechanical traction forces related to suprahyoid muscle contraction. In our protocol, the sEMG measures associated with performance of the Mendelsohn Maneuver include the time duration (in seconds) for which muscle contraction is maintained above a 30% lower threshold value, calculated relative to the patient's non-effortful saliva swallow sEMG amplitude range in that session. Additionally, we monitor the mean amplitude of sEMG contraction across the entire duration of the maneuver, normalized to a percentage of the patient's RESS range. It should be noted that the duration rather than a high amplitude of muscle contraction is the focus of the exercise.

Participant 1 in our series was an 82-year-old gentleman who displayed a particular impairment in UES opening, with a visible cricopharyngeal prominence suggesting failed muscle relaxation at the sphincter. The onset of his dysphagia had been sudden, and remained medically unexplained. Figure 8 shows that this patient improved in his ability to maintain muscle contraction from 0.5 to 1.23 seconds across 11 probes. Using a standard deviation banding method similar to that described previously, this patient shows convincing evidence of improvement in Mendelsohn Maneuver durations, beginning around probe 5. This contrasts with his average Mendelsohn Maneuver amplitudes, which remained fairly constant around 30% of the RESS range across treatment (Figure 9).

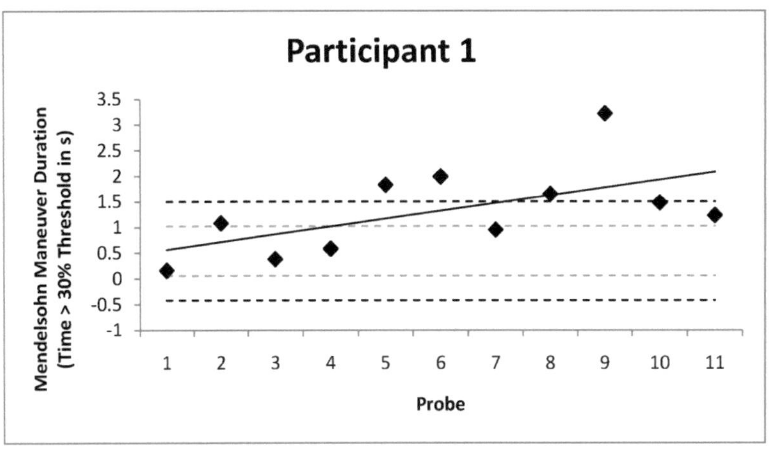

Fig. 8. Change in Mendelsohn Maneuver durations over time for participant 1. This individual showed an increase from baseline durations of 0.5 seconds to 1.23 seconds after 11 probes. The later data points approach the 2 standard deviation band confidence interval boundaries, suggesting that change has occurred.

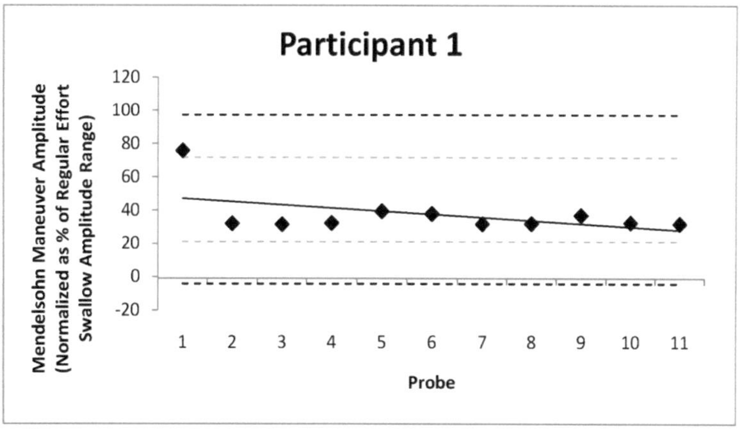

Fig. 9. Mendelsohn Maneuver amplitudes, expressed as a percentage of RESS range, plotted over time for participant 1. In contrast to the duration data shown in Figure 8, this plot shows that sEMG amplitude for this task has remained stable without evident change over 11 probes.

Participant 3 was a 55-year-old gentleman with dysphagia secondary to cervical spine surgery. He displayed a particular impairment with persistent moderate post-swallow residues, together with reduced excursion of the hyoid and larynx. Although this patient showed a slight upward trend in his Mendelsohn Maneuver duration data, he failed to show a marked change that reached or surpassed the 2 standard deviation band criterion, as illustrated in Figure 10. However, it should be noted that he started treatment with an ability to sustain the maneuver for 2 or more seconds, which is notably longer than the values seen for participant 1. His average sEMG amplitudes show a contrasting result to the

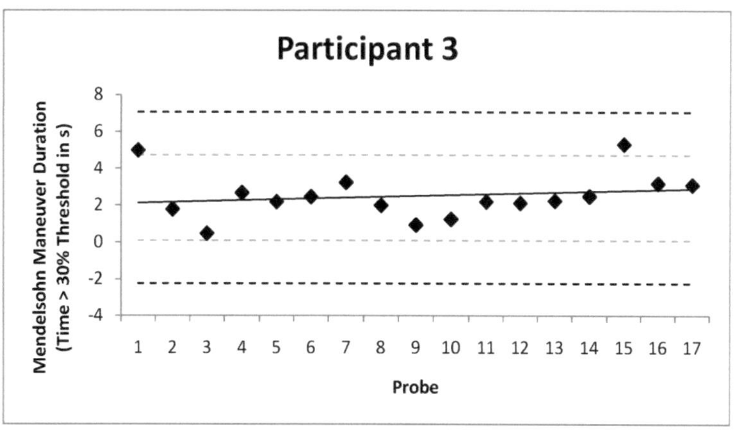

Fig. 10. Mendelsohn Maneuver durations over time for participant 3. In contrast to the data shown for participant 1 in Figure 8, this individual showed stable durations, which failed to exceed the 2 standard deviation band confidence interval boundaries, suggesting that no change occurred.

durational data, with an upward trend that surpassed the 2 standard deviation band criterion at probe 14 (Figure 11). Thus, this patient improved in his ability to sustain a strong level of muscle contraction throughout the duration of the maneuver.

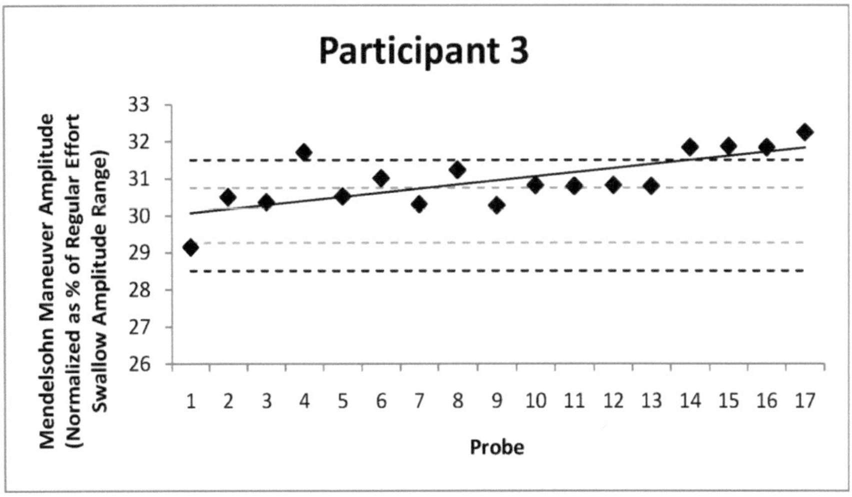

Fig. 11. Mendelsohn Maneuver amplitudes over time for participant 3, normalized to RESS range. In contrast to the durational data shown in Figure 10, an apparent increase in this measure is seen between probes 14 and 17, with data points surpassing the 2 standard deviation band confidence interval boundary.

3.5 Do videofluoroscopic measures of swallowing function improve with increases in the duration of muscle contraction secondary to practice of the Mendelsohn Maneuver?

The primary physiologic outcomes related to practice of the Mendelsohn Maneuver include upper esophageal sphincter opening width and duration, range and duration of hyoid excursion, and post-swallow pyriform sinus residues. As with the cases discussed previously, we collected pre- and post-treatment videofluoroscopies for participants 1 and 3 using a standardized protocol, and recordings were then spliced into individual swallow clips for blinded rating by expert speech-language pathologists.

From these recordings, we also extracted the following still frame images, which were used to measure UES opening width, and hyoid position and displacement in Image J software:

a. Frame of UES opening
b. Frame of maximum superior hyoid excursion
c. Frame of maximum anterior hyoid excursion
d. Frame of UES closure
e. Frame of minimum hyoid position after UES closure

All spatial measurements were performed in a coordinate system rotated into alignment with the cervical spine, using an origin positioned at the anterior inferior corner of the C4 vertebral body and normalizing all displacement and position-distance measures to the participant's height by transforming position and displacement measures to a percent of the participants C2 to C4 neck length (Steele et al., 2011). These methods correct for differences in x-ray magnification across images and control for differences in participant height. During the process of extracting these images, the timepoints of UES opening and closing were also recorded, allowing the calculation of the duration of UES opening.

Superior hyoid displacement is thought to arise primarily from contraction of the mylohyoid muscle while anterior displacement is principally achieved through geniohyoid contraction (Pearson et al., 2010). The Mendelsohn Maneuver likely engages both of these muscles; consequently, increases in hyoid excursion in both the superior and anterior direction might reasonably be anticipated as outcomes of this maneuver. Hyoid excursion in this study was measured as a percentage of the C2-C4 anatomical distance, henceforth called a "cervical unit" (CU). Current best evidence in the field suggests that vertical movements that fall below 44% and anterior movements that fall below 27% of this anatomical reference are associated with penetration-aspiration and post-swallow residues (Steele et al., 2011).

Participant 1 in our case series began treatment with substantially reduced upward movement of the hyoid (36% for thin liquids and only 22% for thick liquids); his anterior movement was not markedly impaired, falling at 46% and 51% for thin and thick liquids, respectively. Post-treatment, this patient demonstrated almost a doubling in his superior hyoid movement excursion, at 44% (thin) and 43% (thick). Anterior excursion remained stable at 44% in both planes of movement. By contrast, participant 3 began with a substantial reduction in the degree of anterior hyoid excursion at 12% and 16% for thin and thick liquids, respectively. Superior excursion was of less obvious concern, at 45% (thin) and 58% (thick). Post-treatment, anterior excursion had improved to approximately double the baseline values, at 25% (thin) and 36% (thick). Superior excursion remained fairly stable at 49% with thin liquids, but fell to 39% with thick liquids. Thus, it appears that both of these patients achieved improvements in the aspect of hyoid excursion that was most impaired following practice of the Mendelsohn Maneuver using sEMG biofeedback.

Participant 1 had average pre-treatment UES opening widths of 16% for thin liquids and 17% for thick liquids. Pre-treatment UES opening durations were 0.5 seconds for thin liquids and 0.7 seconds for thick liquids. Post-treatment his UES opening widths remained stable at 16% for thin liquids but actually decreased to 13% for thick liquids. Post-treatment UES durations increased to 0.6 seconds with thin liquids but remained stable at 0.5 seconds for thick liquids. These changes in durational and spatial measures are best appreciated in conjunction with the functional measures of interest, namely post-swallow residues. Participant 1 showed complete resolution of severe vallecular and pyriform sinus residue with thick liquids. Residues with thin liquids remained unchanged in the mild range. Thus, even though the width of UES opening decreased and durational measures remained stable for thick liquids, this patient was better able to achieve complete bolus transport from the pharynx into the esophagus post treatment.

Participant 3 had average pre-treatment UES opening widths of 19% (CUs) for thin liquids and 22% for thick liquids. Pre-treatment UES opening durations were 0.37 seconds for thin liquids and 0.33 seconds for thick liquids. Post-treatment his UES opening widths decreased to 11% for thin liquids and to 18% for thick liquids. Post-treatment UES durations decreased to 0.27 seconds for both stimuli. Participant 3 showed an improvement in vallecular residues with thick liquids from moderate to mild, and complete resolution of mild vallecular and severe pyriform sinus residues with thin liquids. Thus, like participant 1, he can be considered to have shown functional improvement related to his practice of the Mendelsohn Maneuver, with increased efficiency of pharyngo-esophageal bolus transfer represented by greater clearance despite shorter and narrower UES opening. Penetration-Aspiration Scale scores were not expected to necessarily change as a result of Mendelsohn Maneuver practice, but did improve from a level 3 to 2 with thin liquids in participant 3.

4. Discussion

These data illustrate the challenges inherent in extracting and interpreting measures of physiological change in swallowing using surface EMG signals and videofluoroscopy recordings. In this series of patients, we chose to measure penetration-aspiration and post-swallow residues as our primary functional measures, but also explored more detailed physiological change through measures of hyoid excursion and UES opening.

Several important findings can be extracted from this case series:

1. Surface EMG amplitudes should not be compared across individuals, due to fluctuations in amplitude attributable to tissue composition differences.
2. In order to track changes in sEMG amplitudes across time within an individual, care must be taken to position the recording electrodes in the same location at each session, and a data normalization procedure should be used to transform amplitudes relative to a reference task. Additionally, an adequate number of data points is needed to support single-subject monitoring for change across sessions using standard deviation banding methods.
3. Change in effortful saliva swallow performance will vary across individuals, perhaps as a function of initial strength, task load and treatment intensity.
4. Effortful saliva swallow practice appears to contribute to improvements in swallowing safety, as measured by the Penetration-Aspiration Scale (Rosenbek et al., 1996), although this interpretation should be treated with caution given that these were not compared to data from controls. Post-swallow residues appear to remain unchanged after practice of the effortful saliva swallow.
5. Change in Mendelsohn maneuver performance may vary across individuals, with change either in durational aspects or amplitude aspects of the maneuver.
6. Mendelsohn maneuver practice appears to influence hyoid excursion during swallowing, as well as swallowing efficiency, reflected by the degree of post-swallow residue achieved, despite narrower diameters and shorter durations of UES opening.

These data support the use of sEMG biofeedback to facilitate practice of the effortful swallow and Mendelsohn maneuver techniques in select patients with dysphagia, based on careful analysis of baseline videofluoroscopic swallowing studies showing evidence of the target physiological deficits. We caution that post-treatment outcome measurements require a repeat videofluoroscopic swallowing examination, to ensure that function has improved. Interpretations of swallowing function should not be made on the basis of sEMG signals alone.

5. References

Bülow, M.; Olsson, R. & Ekberg, O. (1999). Videomanometric analysis of supraglottic swallow, effortful swallow, and chin tuck in healthy volunteers. *Dysphagia,* Vol.14, No.2, pp. 67-72.

Bülow, M.; Olsson, R. & Ekberg, O. (2001). Videomanometric analysis of supraglottic swallow, effortful swallow, and chin tuck in patients with pharyngeal dysfunction. *Dysphagia,* Vol.16, No.3, pp. 190-195.

Burnett, T. A.; Mann, E. A.; Cornell, S. A. & Ludlow, C. L. (2003). Laryngeal elevation achieved by neuromuscular stimulation at rest. *Journal of Applied Physiology,* Vol.94, No.1, pp. 128-134.

Clave, P.; de Kraa, M.; Arreola, V.; Girvent, M.; Farre, R.; Palomera, E. & Serra-Prat, M. (2006). The effect of bolus viscosity on swallowing function in neurogenic dysphagia. *Alimentary Pharmacology & Therapeutics,* Vol.24, No.9, pp. 1385-1394.

Cook, I. J.; Dodds, W. J.; Dantas, R. O.; Massey, B.; Kern, M. K.; Lang, I. M.; et al. (1989). Opening mechanisms of the human upper esophageal sphincter. *American Journal of Physiology,* Vol.257, No.5, Part 1, pp. G748-759.

Crary, M. A. (1995). A direct intervention program for chronic neurogenic dysphagia secondary to brainstem stroke. *Dysphagia,* Vol.10, pp. 6-18.

Crary, M. A.; Carnaby Mann, G. D.; Groher, M. E. & Helseth, E. (2004). Functional benefits of dysphagia therapy using adjunctive sEMG biofeedback. *Dysphagia,* Vol.19, No.3, pp. 160-164.

Crary, M. A. & Groher, M. E. (2000). Basic Concepts of Surface Electromyographic Biofeedback in the treatment of Dysphagia, *American Journal of Speech-Language Pathology,* Vol.9, pp.116-125.

Eisenhuber, E.; Schima, W.; Schober, E.; Pokieser, P.; Stadler, A.; Scharitzer, M. & Oschatz, E. (2002). Videofluoroscopic assessment of patients with dysphagia: pharyngeal retention is a predictive factor for aspiration. *AJR American Journal of Roentgenology,* Vol.178, No.2, pp. 393-398.

Hind, J. A.; Nicosia, M. A.; Roecker, E. B.; Carnes, M. L. & Robbins, J. (2001). Comparison of effortful and noneffortful swallows in healthy middle- aged and older adults. *Archives of Physical Medicine and Rehabilitation,* Vol.82, No.12, pp. 1661-1665.

Huckabee, M. L. & Cannito, M. (1999). Outcomes of swallowing rehabilitation in chronic brainstem dysphagia: a retrospective evaluation. *Dysphagia,* Vol.14, pp. 93-109.

Mendelsohn, M. S. & McConnel, F. M. (1987). Function in the pharyngoesophageal segment. *Laryngoscope,* Vol.97, No.4, pp. 483-489.

Nourbakhsh, M. R. & Ottenbacher, K. J. (1994). The statistical analysis of single-subject data: a comparative examination. *Physical Therapy,* Vol.74, No.8, pp. 768-776.

Pearson, W. G., Jr.; Langmore, S. E.; & Zumwalt, A. C. (2010). Evaluating the Structural Properties of Suprahyoid Muscles and their Potential for Moving the Hyoid. *Dysphagia,* Online First, DOI 10.1007/s00455-010-9315-z.

Rosenbek, J. C.; Robbins, J. A.; Roecker, E. B.; Coyle, J. L. & Wood, J. L. (1996). A penetration-aspiration scale. *Dysphagia,* Vol.11, No.2, pp. 93-98.

Steele, C. M.; Bailey, G. L.; Chau, T.; Molfenter, S. M.; Oshalla, M.; Waito, A. A. & Zoratto, D.C.B.H. (2011). The relationship between hyoid and laryngeal displacement and swallowing impairment. *Clinical Otolaryngology*, Vol.36, pp.30-36.

20

Relating Surface Electromyograms of the Facial Muscles During Mastication to the Mechanical and Sensory Properties of Foodstuffs

E. Katherine Kemsley and Marianne Defernez
Institute of Food Research
UK

1. Introduction

Surface Electromyography (sEMG) has been widely used for studying human mastication, due to its ability to non-invasively monitor the activity of muscle groups associated with chewing (Boyar & Kilcast, 1986; Brown, 1994). It is regarded as the "gold standard" for objective measurement of simple parameters relating to chewing behaviour, such as chew rate and strength. Attempts have been made to approach a quantitative analysis of the sEMG signals, in terms of mechanical action on foods (Agrawal et al., 1998; Braxton et al., 1996; Brown et al., 1996, 1998; Horio & Kawamura, 1989; Mioche & Martin, 1998; Wilson & Brown, 1997; Yven et al., 2010). sEMG has been used to identify differences in chewing patterns between individuals, and to classify them into groups according to their chewing efficiency (Blissett et al., 2006; González et al., 2002; Lassauzay et al., 2000).

There is also interest in using sEMG data in studies of sensory texture (Duizer et al., 1996; Lee et al., 2009; Mathoniere et al., 2000; Mioche, 2004; Peng et al., 2002; Sun et al., 2001; Yven et al., 2010). Thus sEMG of the masticatory muscles provides a potential link between physical or mechanical properties of foodstuffs, and sensory evaluations, in particular of texture, made by consumers.

In this chapter we present the hardware and software needed to conduct sEMG of facial muscles during mastication, and describe the signal that is acquired, as well as options for further data treatment of this signal to obtain quantities that can be analysed by statistical means (Section 1). We highlight some of the issues that may be encountered downstream, in particular arising from the variability associated with the technique, especially between-volunteer and between-session variance (Section 2). We show that with judicious data scaling (Section 2.4), sEMG can be linked to mechanical and sensory properties of food (Section 3). Throughout, we use examples of our own data, collected during a series of related projects carried out at the Institute of Food Research in Norwich.

1.1 Collecting sEMG signals from mastication

To obtain sEMG signals from the masticatory muscles, disposable surface electrodes are attached in pairs to the surface of the skin above the masseter and temporal muscle groups, on both sides of the face (figure 1). The muscular action potentials (MUAPs) associated with chewing actions (the sum of which effectively constitutes the signal that is recorded) are small and require amplification, typically using a polygraph. The outputs from the amplifier are passed to an analogue-to-digital converter (ADC), generally operating at a sampling rate of 1kHz, and captured by a PC. The resulting signal from each electrode is a time-varying response representing each muscle group's bioelectrical activity for the duration of the chewing episode.

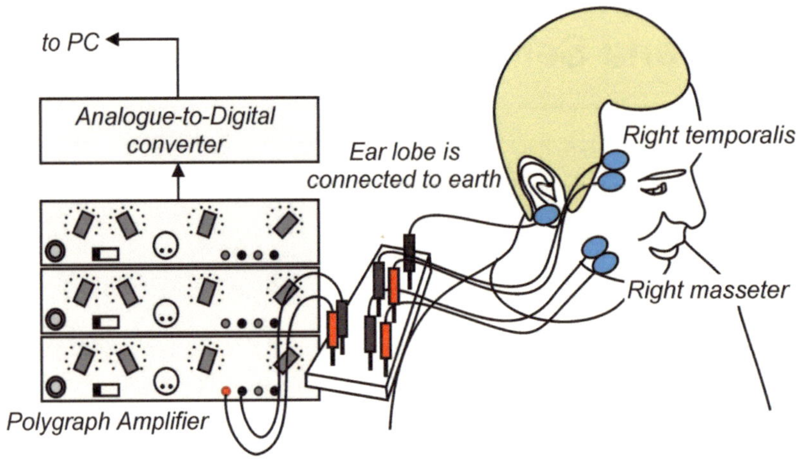

Fig. 1. Diagram showing a volunteer ready for sEMG recording of mastication. It is useful to take photographs of each volunteer once they are wired up, to assist in reducing inter-session variability.

The data presented throughout this chapter were collected using equipment as follows: bipolar disposable electrodes (Blue Sensor A-50-VS, Medicotest, Ølstykke, Denmark); a polygraph amplifier (model 7E, Grass Instrument Co., Massachusetts, USA); and an ADC interface (model 1401plus, Cambridge Electronic Design Ltd., Cambridge, UK). Data were logged by connecting the ADC to a desktop personal computer running the Spike2 data collection software package (Cambridge Electronic Design Ltd., Cambridge, UK). All subsequent signal processing was carried out in Matlab (The Mathworks, Cambridge, UK) installed with the Statistics Toolbox.

1.2 Time-domain sEMG signals – the electromyograms

Typical signals from two electrode channels (right temporalis and right masseter) obtained from a volunteer consuming one bite of apple are shown in figure 2. The main features are indicated. The first bite and subsequent chews appear as large, regularly spaced features, and these arise from the gross movements of the masticatory muscles. The end of chewing is marked by a swallow, which can be seen fairly clearly in these particular sEMG signals. However, swallow movements are not always distinctive (Hodgson et al., 2003), and we have on occasion found it useful to provide a "swallow indicator" device to be operated by the volunteer, so that the moment of swallowing is precisely located in time (Sprunt et al., 2002). Note the correspondence between the activities of the temporalis and masseter muscle groups. For normal, healthy chewing behaviour, there is involvement of both these muscle groups to similar extents. Likewise, a degree of correspondence is found between the right and left electrode channels.

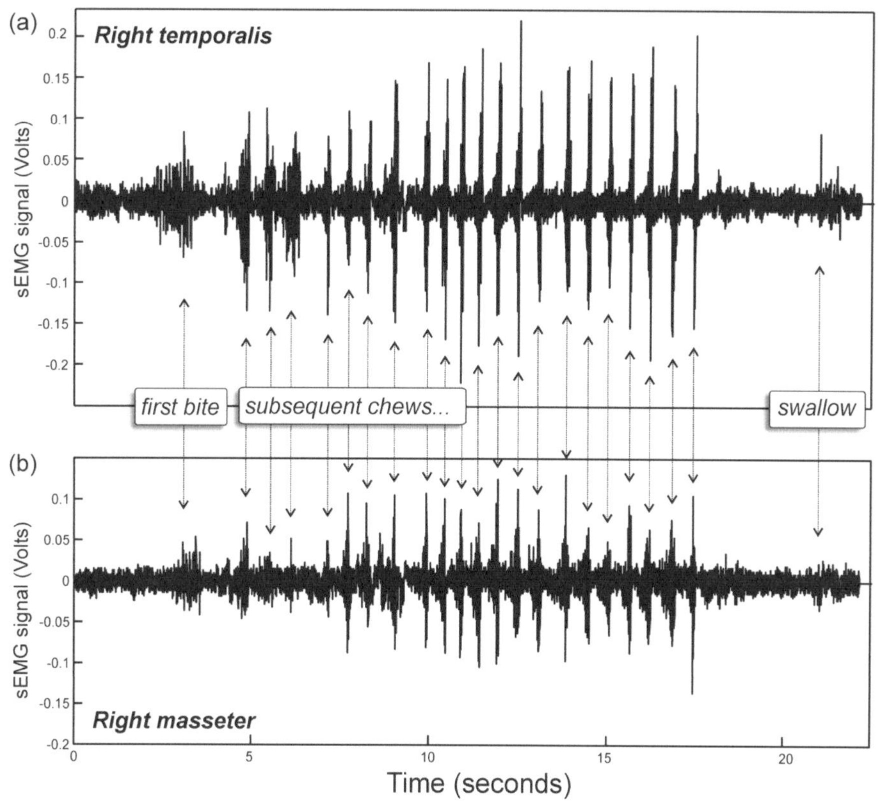

Fig. 2. Data from the right temporalis and right masseter channels from a volunteer consuming one bite of apple. The main features are marked. Note the equivalent vertical scales - in this example, the temporalis muscle group produced slightly larger signals, although there is clearly substantive involvement of both muscle groups. This is typical of normal chewing behaviour.

Depending on the food being consumed and the purpose of the study, sEMG readings may be collected over periods of up to several minutes. Consequently the amount of raw data produced can be very large. Until relatively recently, complete raw measurements have been too difficult to handle on standard desktop computers. Researchers have of necessity analysed only simplified forms of this data, such as the chew interval and rate. Figure 3 illustrates the principle by which these values are extracted from the sEMG signals. The reduction in complexity and size of the dataset is substantial: from 80,000 data points in the raw signals shown here, to a few tens of extracted values and summary statistics. Much of the literature examines how these extracted quantities relate to the properties of the food being consumed (Blisset et al., 2006; Braxton et al., 1996; Brown, 1994; Brown & Braxton, 2000; Brown et al., 1996, 1998; Duizer et al., 1996; Lee et al., 2009; Plesh et al., 1986; Tornberg et al., 1985; Veyrune & Mioche, 2000; Yven et al., 2010). However, as the power of computer processors continues to increase, so does the capacity to handle larger amounts of data, and more recently, researchers have begun to utilise the whole signal. The majority of our sEMG work has adopted this kind of approach, introduced in the following section.

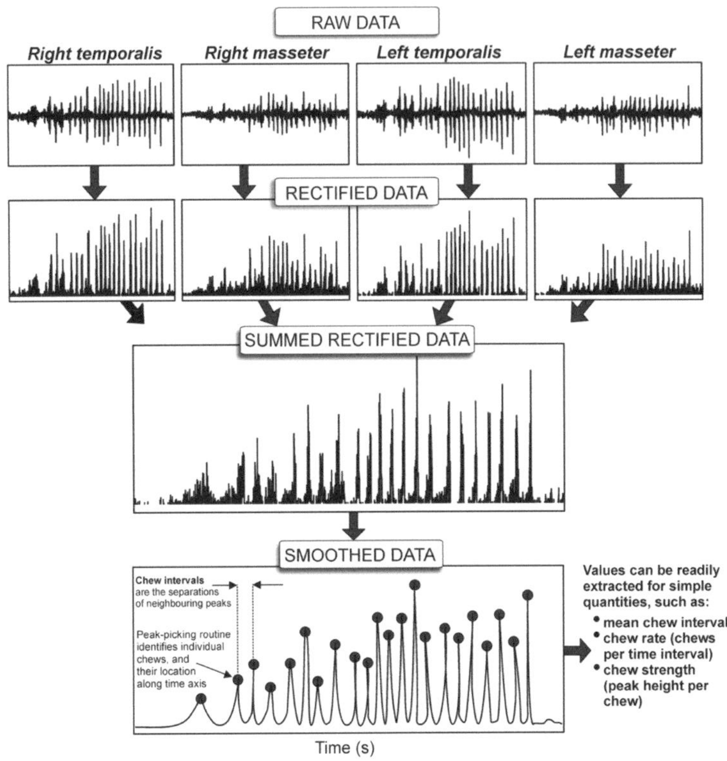

Fig. 3. Extracting parameters from the raw electromyograms.

1.3 Frequency domain signals – the power spectra

Electromyograms are collected in the time-domain, as measurements of a response as a function of time. The mathematical procedure of Fourier transformation can be used to express these readings instead as a function of frequency. The fast Fourier transform (FFT) algorithm operates on a digitized time-domain signal, sampled at a rate v, to produce a frequency-domain spectrum, in which the maximum frequency that can be detected is v/2 (a consequence of the Nyquist sampling theorem). The square of the amplitude of the Fourier-transformed signal is known as the power spectrum.

Fourier transformation has been applied to sEMG signals in the past, with the mean frequency being the most often used derived parameter as it has been found to relate to muscle fatigue (see review in Al-Mulla et al., 2011) and has also been shown to be linked to the proportions of different fiber types (Yuen et al., 1989). However there may be more subtle, frequency-specific information in the sEMG signals that can be exploited. To access this information, one needs to look separately at bands of frequencies (Schumann et al., 1994) or at the power spectrum itself (Subasi, 2006). Indeed in our own work we have investigated whether different regions of the power spectrum can be related to other data types collected during the experiment. One of the main advantages of working in the frequency domain is that registering (aligning) several electromyograms across different episodes of chewing becomes straightforward. This is because the range of the frequency scale is related solely to the ADC sampling rate. There is no need for the electromyograms to match with regard to the start or the end of recording, nor to even contain the same number of data values (a process called "zero filling" can be used to force a match between readings). All that is required is that the signals were collected at the same sampling rate.

A consequence of the inherently small electrical signals measured in sEMG is that the electromyograms, as well as the resulting power spectra, invariably contain unwanted noise arising from the electronics in the amplifier and ADC. It is useful, therefore, to improve the signal-to-noise ratio (SNR) as far as possible through signal averaging or "co-adding" of replicate measurements. Precisely what constitutes a "replicate" is an issue that needs some consideration. For example, we noted above that the electromyograms from the different electrode pairs produce highly correlated signals, and these individual signals could be co-added in the frequency-domain to improve the SNR. Another method of increasing the SNR is to co-add power spectra from successive time windows; overlapping time windows can also be used (in effect, a "moving average" smoothing process). These methods are illustrated in figure 4. The proviso is that the signal-averaging method should be consistent with the aims of the study. For instance, the window method is appropriate if there is no specific requirement to study muscle activity as a function of time; co-adding different electrode channels is appropriate if there is no desire to study the different muscle groups separately.

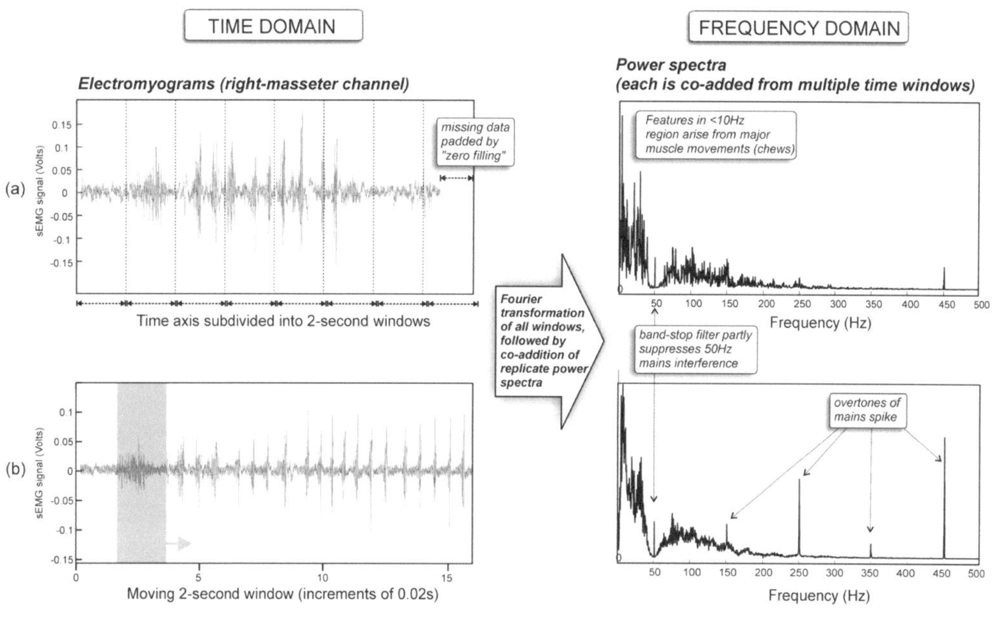

Fig. 4. Signal-averaging using windows in the time-domain. The electromyograms on the left side of the figure were collected from one electrode channel, and two different episodes of chewing. The power spectra on the right side of the figure were calculated from the electromyograms using the window method of signal-averaging. In (a), the signal was subdivided into 2-second windows (zero-filling was used to pad the last of these to give a window of the same duration). In (b), a window of 2-seconds width was "moved" along the time axis, in increments of 0.02 seconds, to effect smoothing. In both cases, all windows were Fourier transformed and the resulting spectra co-added to give a single, signal-averaged power spectrum in the frequency-domain.

Some of the main features of typical sEMG power spectra are also indicated on figure 4. The frequency scale is in Hertz, with its range determined by the ADC sampling rate. Frequency resolution is determined by the number of data points Fourier transformed (i.e., in each electromyogram window). Features arising from the main muscle movements involved in chewing can be seen in the low-frequency region ($v < 10$Hz). The broad depression centred at 50Hz arises from a band-stop filter present in the polygraph to suppress interference from the mains electricity supply. In some of the data, overtones of this $v = 50$Hz interference can be seen at $v + 2v$, $v + 4v$,... There are also some distinct features in the region 10 - 50Hz. In sEMG studies of a range of different muscle groups, these are generally attributed to synchronized activity of muscle motor units arising from rhythmic firing of the central nervous system (see for example McAuley et al., 1997, and the review of the literature included therein).

As they share a common frequency scale, power spectra can be easily collated into a matrix for processing with linear algebra techniques. This enables comparison across large collections of sEMG data, acquired for example from different volunteers, and/or from the consumption of a range of foodstuffs. This possibility is exploited extensively in different studies that will be described in the remainder of this chapter, all of which involved large collections of sEMG data from multiple volunteers. The data acquisition equipment for all studies was as described above, i.e., electromyograms were collected from four muscle groups using an ADC operating at a 1kHz sampling rate. In all cases, prior approval to conduct the study was obtained from the local ethics committee.

2. Between-volunteer differences in sEMG

2.1 A study of edible gels with characterised textural attributes

The first of the case studies comprises sEMG signals recorded from eight volunteers, who each consumed five edible gels on five separate occasions. This work formed part of a wider study on flavour release (Kemsley et al., 2002; Smith, 2004; Sprunt et al., 2002; Sprunt & Smith, 2002; Wright & Hills, 2003; Wright et al., 2003). All gels were prepared using the same nominal formulation, and then flavoured with five varying amounts of anethole. Complete details of the gel preparation and serving order can be found in Kemsley et al. (2002). Mechanical properties of the gels were determined using a TA-XT2 Texture Analyser (Stable Micro Systems, Godalming, Surrey, UK). A single-sided razor blade (length 39 mm, depth 12.5 mm, thickness 0.25 mm) was driven vertically through the gel axis at 0.05mm/sec (total travel approximately 12mm), and the work done in cutting calculated from the integrated force-distance curve.

sEMG recording was discontinued in each instance when the volunteer indicated that the gel's flavour could no longer be perceived. The minimum duration of any electromyogram was ~32 seconds. Consequently, the first 32768 ($=2^{15}$) data values in each electromyogram were passed to a fast Fourier transform algorithm and converted to power spectra, each containing 16384 data values. To improve the SNR, these were summed across the four electrode channels to give a single, signal-averaged power spectrum per chewing episode.

2.1.1 Visual examination of the data

From visual comparison of the sEMG signals from different volunteers, it was found that each volunteer exhibits highly characteristic chewing behaviour, and furthermore, this is broadly consistent between sessions. This is most evident from examination of the power spectra. In figure 5, two different representations of the frequency domain dataset are shown. On the left hand side, the complete matrix of [200 x 16384] data values is shown as a heatmap. Each row in this map represents a single power spectrum, and the data have been ordered such that the spectra from individual volunteers are grouped together (25 per volunteer: five episodes of chewing at each of five sessions). Clear blocks of data can be seen, corresponding to the 25 spectra from each individual. The right hand side of the figure shows the mean power spectra, obtained by averaging across all chewing episodes and sessions for each volunteer. Again, there are clear differences between the signals for each individual, although mean spectra alone do not convey any information about the within-volunteer variation, in contrast to the heatmap view. An expansion of the low-frequency (<10Hz) region in a selection of the power spectra is shown in figure 6, highlighting some of the volunteer-specific characteristics that persist across sessions.

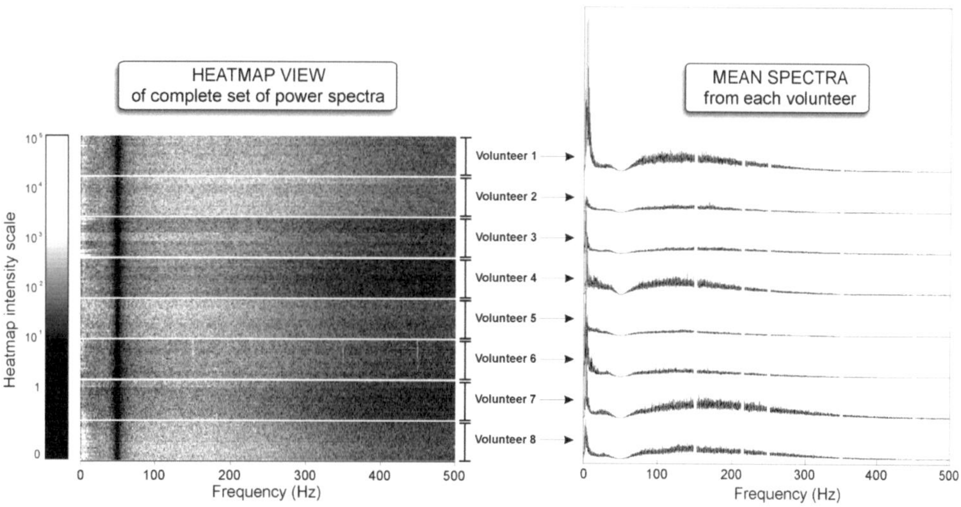

Fig. 5. Different representations of the frequency domain dataset.

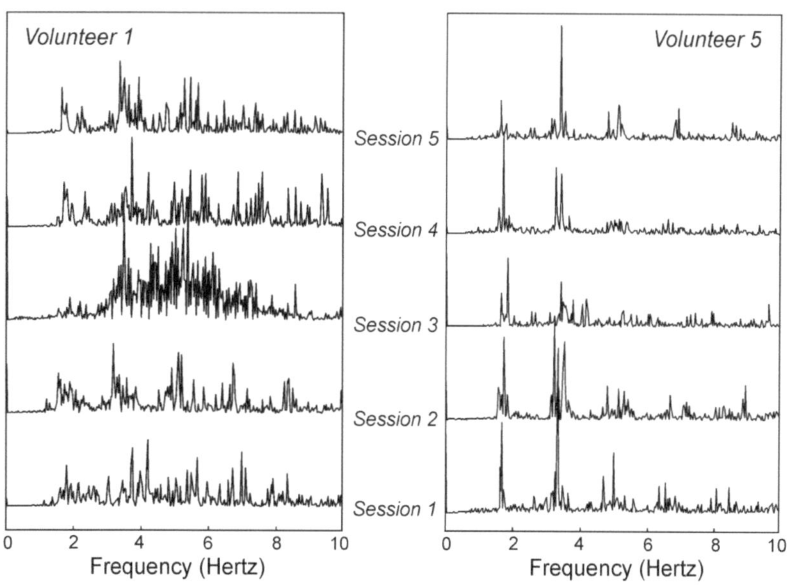

Fig. 6. An expansion of the low-frequency (<10Hz) region in a selection of the power spectra from two of the volunteers.

2.1.2 Multivariate analysis - PCA

An alternative and highly efficient means of viewing a large data matrix of this kind is to process it with a data compression technique such as principal component analysis (PCA) (Jolliffe, 1986; Krzanowshi, 1988). This method produces a transformed matrix - the PC scores - which contains most of the information that was present in the original data matrix, but in a rearranged form. Crucially, the scores matrix is much smaller in size, making it considerably easier to examine graphically. Furthermore, the scores are ranked by their variances, thus the largest (and hopefully most interesting) sources of variation are represented in the first few scores, whilst the noise component is relegated to lower scores. The PCA transformation can thus lead to an effective increase in the SNR of the systematic information of interest.

Figure 7 shows the first two PC scores obtained from the set of power spectra, using correlation-method PCA. Together, these two scores alone account for over 25% of the information content (variance) that was present in the original data set. Each point on this plot represents a power spectrum from one episode of chewing. It can be immediately seen that there is considerable clustering of the data arising from each individual. Data from volunteers 1, 2 and 6, for example, can be completely distinguished from one another, as

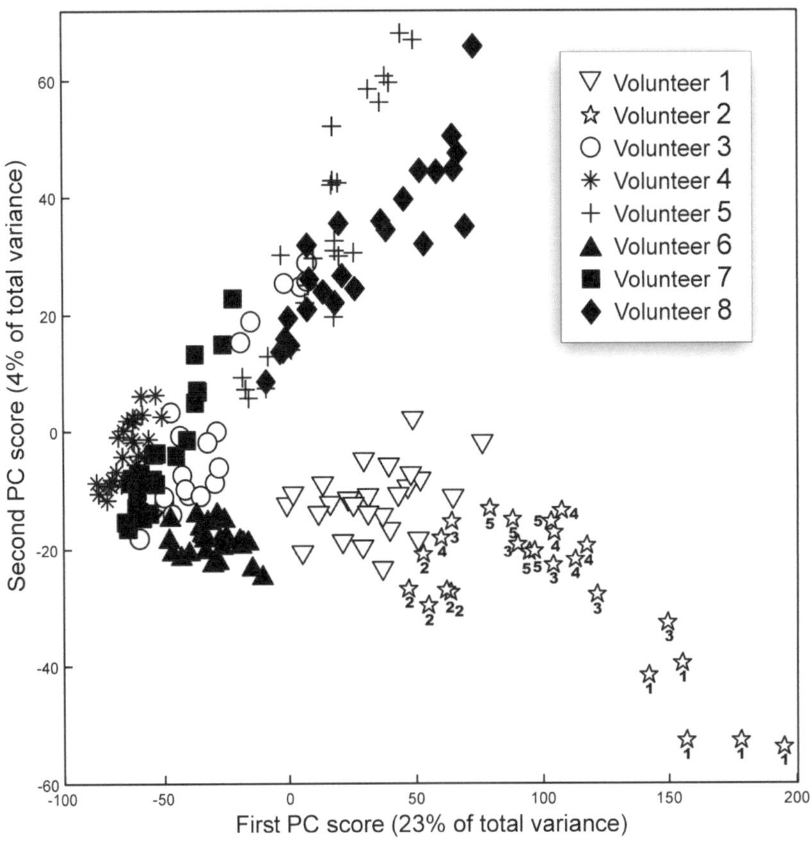

Fig. 7. PCA (correlation method) applied to sEMG power spectra from edible gels. The entire frequency range (0 – 500Hz) was used. Sessions for one volunteer (2) are marked by a number (1-5)

well as from the remaining volunteers. This is particularly remarkable considering each volunteer's data comprised measurements from five recording sessions, separated in time by periods of days. It also confirms the suggestion from qualitative examination of the spectra that volunteers can be associated with a characteristic low-frequency spectrum. Closer examination of figure 7 showed that within each volunteer's batch of signals, data from the different sessions tended to cluster together also. For clarity, this is indicated for one volunteer's readings only. Inter-session variability is likely to arise largely from irreproducibility in positioning the electrodes. This is an established source of variance in sEMG data (De Luca, 1997).

2.1.3 Discussion

The data collected in this study were also treated in the time-domain by Wright et al. (2003), who examined the distribution of the intervals between chews, and showed that a different distribution was obtained from each volunteer. Our multivariate treatment of the power spectra has further indicated that each single sEMG recording can be identified as originating from a distinct volunteer. In addition to the readily observed differences in the low-frequency region, there are characteristic differences between individuals' responses at higher spectral frequencies, as seen from the heatmap view. It is known that the shape of the frequency distribution changes in response to fatigue, with a shift in the median towards lower frequencies. This has been shown in both sEMG (see review in Al-Mulla et al., 2011) and vibromyography (VMG) studies (Herzog et al., 1994). However, volunteers will differ in the rate at which they become fatigued, and in the extent to which this is manifested in their sEMG signal. All of these findings suggested that when volunteers are asked to consume a foodstuff using their natural chewing behaviour, they do so in an individual, characteristic fashion.
Consistent differences between volunteers' sEMG characteristics could also be due to a variety of behavioural and anatomical factors. Individuals differ in terms of their efficiency in breaking down the food bolus, which is influenced by salivary flow rates and the ability to reform and move the bolus in the mouth. In addition, there is variation between individuals in their pattern of muscle activation, and hence in terms of the level of muscle recruitment and activation in the chewing sequence. This arises to some extent from the anatomy of the masticatory apparatus, as well as characteristics such as the muscle fibre-type construction (proportion of type I and II fibres), the fibre size and motor unit arrangement, the thickness of the subcutaneous layer and the electrical resistance of the skin (Westbury & Shaughnessy, 1987).

2.2 Between-volunteer differences in studies of prescribed chewing

A subsequent multi-volunteer study aimed to further explore the causes of between-volunteer variation. In particular, we sought to examine the extent to which subjectivity in sEMG signals arises from a factor potentially within the conscious control of individuals: the manner in which they chew. For this work, we dispensed with an edible stimulus (and the associated phenomena of particle breakdown and saliva stimulation). There are literature precedents for the use of model stimuli in studies of mechanical properties and sEMG responses. The use of miniature load cells was described by Mioche et al. (1993), who recorded bite forces from 25 to 124N at biting rates of 1 and 2Hz. The force-deformation behaviour of a model material, Optosil, has been compared with that of real foodstuffs by Olthoff et al. (1986). Edlund & Lamm (1980) compared sEMG signals for various foods and Optosil, and Horio & Kawamura (1989) compared sEMG signals with instrumental texture parameters for foods. There is also precedent for the use of a metronome; Plesh et al. (1987) used sEMG and a Kinesiograph to study the jaw movements of subjects chewing gum, at individuals' preferred rates, and also at rates prescribed using a metronome.

In our study, volunteers simulated chewing by elastically deforming calibrated, spring-loaded wooden pegs held between their incisors, 5mm from the end of the peg arms. The volunteers were asked to coordinate their movements with the sound produced by a metronome, which was operated at several different, predetermined rates: 30, 60, 90 and 120 bpm (beats per minute). Each of six volunteers provided duplicate measurements at the four different rates, on three separate occasions. Mechanical characterisation of the pegs was carried out by compression in a universal test machine (Stable Micro Systems Texture Analyzer, model TA-XT2). The average work done in operating the pegs was 106 mJ measured at a compression point 5mm from the ends of the peg arms.

The raw electromyograms were collected, Fourier transformed and signal-averaged in the same way as in the work on edible gels described above, although in this instance only 30 seconds of data were retained from each reading, as some volunteers indicated fatigue after this time. In all cases, the sEMG responses were greatest on the masseter-right and masseter-left channels. This is because the use of the incisor teeth involves less activity of the temporal and more of the masseter muscles, compared to the study of freestyle chewing of gels, in which more of the facial muscles tended to be involved.

2.2.1 Visual examination of the low-frequency data

The low-frequency region in a selection of the power spectra are shown in figure 8, which typify the data set as a whole. Sharp peaks can be seen in the power spectra that correspond

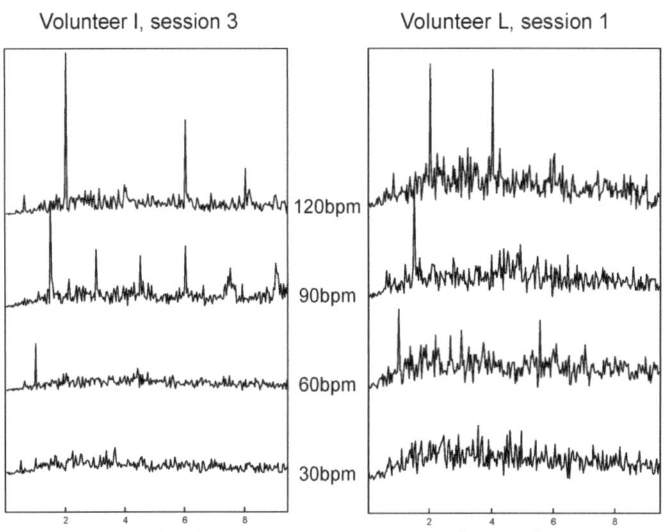

Fig. 8. Low-frequency region in spectra from prescribed chewing. For a chew rate of 120bpm, a peak is clearly seen at 2Hz, with some smaller 'overtones' at 4Hz, 6Hz,... When the chew rate is 90bpm, there are peaks at 1.5Hz with overtones at 3Hz, 4.5Hz,..., and when it is 60bpm the peaks occur at 1Hz, with overtones at 2Hz, 3Hz,... In general, volunteers found it harder to precisely coordinate their jaw movements with the lower prescribed rates. Note that no peaks are clearly seen in any volunteers' data from the chew rate of 30bpm.

directly to the prescribed chew rates. For most volunteers, this is especially clear for the chew rates of 90bpm and 120bpm. In general, volunteers appeared better able to coordinate and maintain these higher prescribed rates. These were closest to the natural chewing rhythms observed in the studies on gels (compare with figure 6).

2.2.2 Multivariate analysis: Focussing on different frequency ranges

In theory, this low frequency region is dominated by the features attributable to prescribed chewing only, and since the prescriptions were the same for all individuals in the study, it might be expected that this would reduce the degree to which their sEMG signals can be differentiated. An analysis of the chew interval data, analogous to that carried out by Wright et al. (2003) and reported in our paper (Kemsley et al., 2003) appears to indicate that this is so. From analysis of chew interval distributions, volunteers seemed to differ in their ability to precisely coordinate and maintain the prescribed chewing patterns, but individuals could not be identified by their chew interval readings alone. However, application of PCA to the power spectra, which is able to decompose different sources of systematic variation, shows that there is still some differentiation between volunteers. Figure 9(a) shows the first two PCs obtained from the low frequency (<10Hz) region, using the same method of analysis (correlation PCA) as in figure 7. The prescribed chew rates are indicated for one of the volunteer's data only, for reasons of clarity, along with a "direction" in this PC space that corresponds to variation in the chew rate as marked. It is apparent that there is still some separation of the signals by volunteer, even in this low-frequency region alone. Figure 9(b) shows the results of applying the same PCA method to the >10Hz region. The clustering according to volunteer is more marked. A further PCA analysis was applied to the whole frequency range (i.e. a direct analogue of figure 7); this showed even clearer clustering according to individual (figure 9(c)).

From examination of these figures, it would seem that variation between volunteers is an effect comparable in magnitude to the grossly different prescribed chew rates. The third and subsequent scores in all the PCA analyses (not shown) indicated some variances associated with chew rate, but smaller than those of PCs 1 and 2. This result is perhaps counter-intuitive: one might have anticipated that, when considering the dataset as a whole, by far the largest source of variance would be chew rate. This was, after all, a prescribed difference between conditions for obtaining the readings, the effects of which are clearly visible in the low-frequency region of the sEMG spectra.

Next, PCA was applied to the whole frequency range from each chew rate separately. The first two scores from the 120bpm dataset are shown in figure 10. There is now clear clustering and separation of the data from each volunteer. Similar results were obtained from analyses of the 90, 60 and 30bpm sets. This confirms that higher frequencies contain useful information for distinguishing volunteers, and moreover, the volunteer-specific nature of these higher frequencies is not removed by asking volunteers to constrain their chewing behaviour. In agreement with the gel study, our findings once more show that if sEMG signals are considered as a whole, then individual volunteers produce highly characteristic signals, which remain characteristic even when the manner in which they chew is highly controlled. In the context of examining properties of food materials, this must be regarded as an undesirable phenomenon.

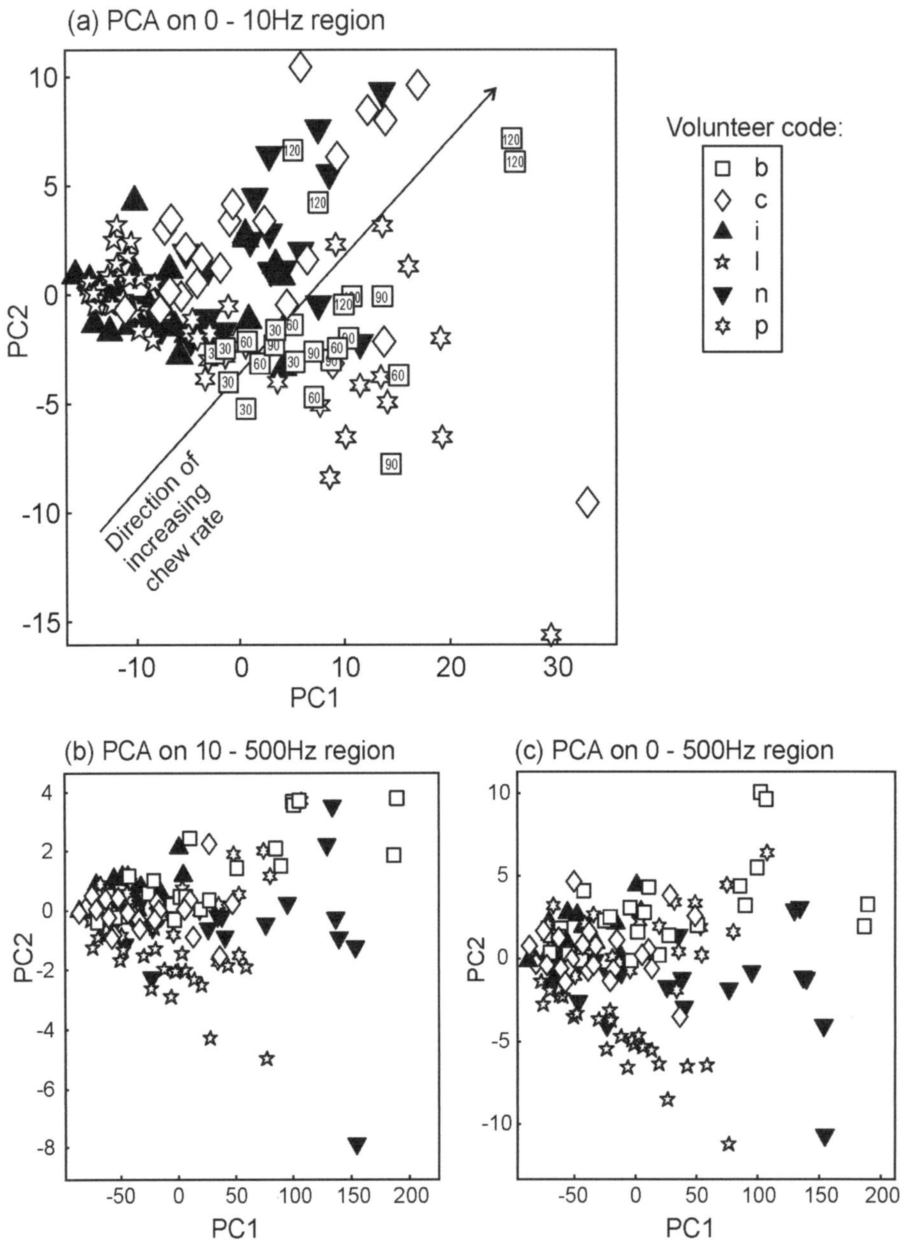

Fig. 9. PCA scores plots for different frequency ranges. In (a), one volunteer's data points are marked with the prescribed chew rate. The arrow indicates the direction in the PC space associated with the chew rate; all volunteers' data demonstrated the same directional trend. There is still noticeable grouping according to volunteer, despite the prescribed chewing behaviour. In figures (b) and (c), different regions of the power spectrum were passed to the PCA procedure; the clustering according to volunteer becomes clearer when frequencies above 10Hz are included.

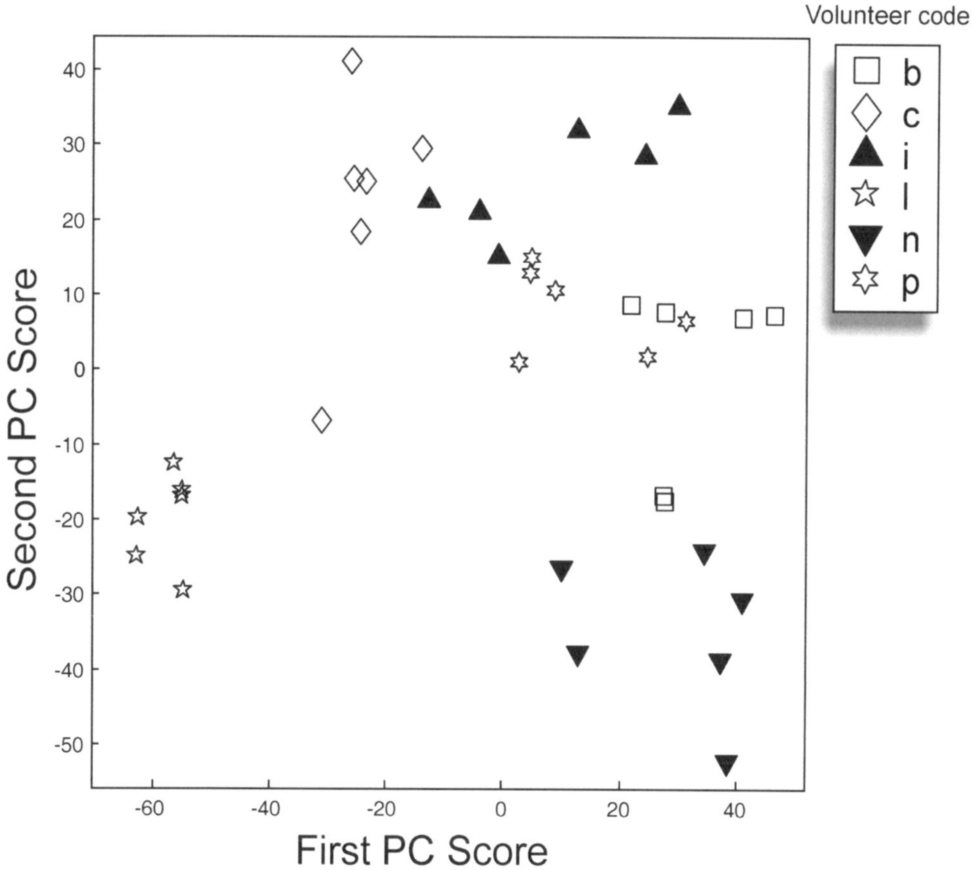

Fig. 10. PCA scores plot of first vs. second PC from the subset of data from the 120bpm chew rate only (using the whole power spectrum frequency range). Data were additionally normalized by setting the integrated spectral area to unity, before correlation-method PCA.

2.3 Summary: The extent of between-volunteer variance

These studies have clearly established that individuals exhibit highly characteristic sEMG spectra, and the relative between-volunteer and within-volunteer variances are such that individuals can be uniquely identified by their sEMG signature. Investigations using subsets of different regions of the frequency range showed that this characteristic nature is maintained even at frequencies higher than those associated with the gross muscle movement. The clustering according to volunteer was found irrespective of whether individuals use natural freestyle chewing behaviour, or were asked to chew in an artificial, highly prescribed manner.

This corroborates the findings from a number of other studies. For example, in a study involving five different foods, Horio & Kawamura (1989) found volunteers to differ in the way the food hardness affected their number of chewing strokes, and overall chewing time. Brown (1994) and Brown et al. (1998) observed significant between-volunteer variation for several temporal and amplitude parameters calculated from the time-domain signal (duration of the activity burst, period between bursts of activity, duration of the chewing period, mean voltage within activity burst, maximum voltage, and area under sEMG trace); these were recorded whilst chewing a range of different food types. Volunteers have also been classified into "chewing efficiency" groups, based on the weight loss from a stick of chewing gum, and the median particle size of almonds chewed a specified number of times (Brown & Braxton, 2000, Braxton et al., 1996); when consuming other food types (meat, biscuits), these groups exhibited different behaviours (numbers of chews, total chewing time and chew work). Similarly in a study on confectionery chews, Blisset et al. (1996) characterised groups on the basis of chewing force, chewing rate, proportion of work and total number of chews, and observed that this could influence flavour release, though this was product-dependant. Mioche & Martin (1998) observed clear differences between naïve and trained volunteers, based on their sEMG burst times, chew time, duration and work, in particular in the extent to which their behaviour was modified, comparing chewing with, and without, simultaneous sensory judgment. González et al. (2002) also found that the chewing behaviour of experts (trained subjects) was influenced by the goal of the experiment more than that of untrained subjects; in addition there were differences in chewing time, chewing work and chewing rate between experts and untrained subjects, and a larger between-session variation in untrained subjects for number of chews, chewing time, mean voltage, and chewing work.

In none of these studies was it shown, however, that volunteers exhibit consistent, individually characteristic behaviour over extended periods of time. This finding is important, because it demonstrates the inherent subjectivity of sEMG as a form of measurement. This may need to be mitigated in order to explore underlying, subtle relationships between sEMG readings and material or sensory properties of the stimulus. This is an area of work that will be examined in Section 2.4 and exploited in the remainder of this chapter. Moreover, the higher frequency components of the signal are neglected in conventional analysis of sEMG data, which processes raw signals to obtain parameters such as chew intervals, chew rate, and so on. Our findings show, however,, the high frequency region clearly contains non-trivial information, since volunteers can be distinguished by their high-frequency sEMG spectra alone.

2.4 Data scaling to remove inter-subject and inter-session variance

We return now to discuss the power spectra collected from the consumption of edible gels. Figure 7 showed clearly the between-session and between-volunteer variances. However, coding the symbols by the texture attributes of the gels revealed no conclusive clustering according to the textural properties (not shown); equally unfruitful was an exhaustive search of subsequent PC dimensions. However, this could simply be because any association with the textural properties is small and not clearly seen against the background of much larger volunteer and session effects.

A straightforward means of removing variation associated with both session and volunteer is to apply some form of scaling to the batches of signals from each volunteer and session. There are many different candidate scaling schemes. Here we use standardization, a well-known statistical technique which scales each variate (data values at each frequency in the power spectrum) so that they have mean of zero and a standard deviation of unity. When PCA is applied to the "batchwise" standardized data set, we can see from the plot of scores that variation associated with either the volunteer or session is removed (figure 11(a)). However, when we code the symbols by the different gels consumed, a new trend emerges – an association in the first PC dimension with the gel's texture as measured by work done in cutting. This is not easy to discern in the heavily populated scores plot (figure 11(b)), but much clearer when the score is plotted individually against the textural property separately (figure 12).

This amounts to strong evidence of a within-volunteer trend that associates sEMG reponse with increasing work done in cutting. We can conclude that a statistically significant association exists between the power spectra and the texture as expressed by mechanical cutting. This is an indication that quite subtle properties of foodstuffs have a discernible influence on sEMG readings; this is explored further in the subsequent section which examines data collected from a large-scale study of both the mechanical and sensory properties of apples.

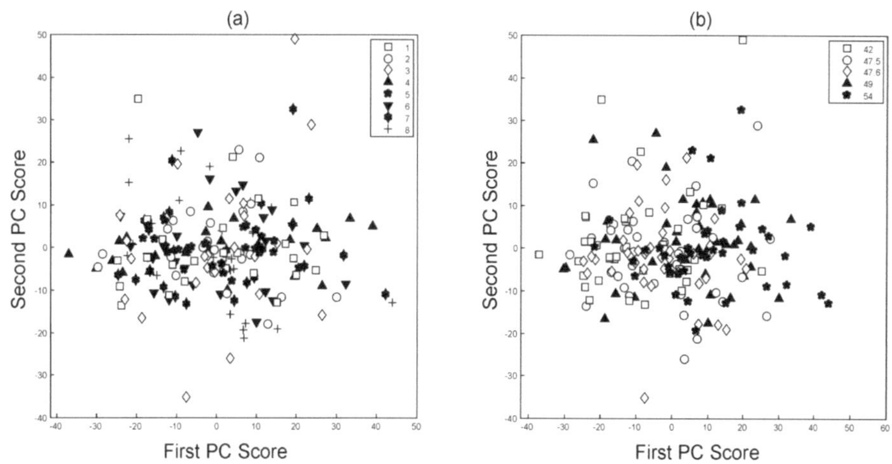

Fig. 11. PCA scores plots of "batchwise" standardized (per volunteer, per session) data set. In (a), the symbols are coded by volunteer; in (b), by edible gel. The numbers in the legend refer to the mean work done (Nmm) in cutting each of the five preparations.

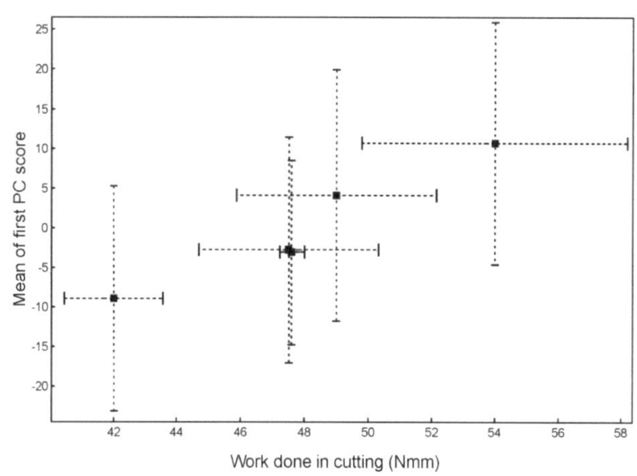

Fig. 12. Plot of gel texture (work done in cutting) versus the first PC score. Error bars represent 2 standard deviations.

3. Relating sEMG signals to mechanical and sensory texture in apples

The remainder of this chapter is concerned with textural properties of apples, in particular a single variety, Red Delicious, which is particularly vulnerable to quality deterioration during extended storage. In this work, sEMG was used to explore the link between mechanical and sensory measurements of various textural attributes.

As a term, "texture" is rather complex. The International Organisation for Standardisation defined texture in 1992 as "the mechanical, geometrical and surface attributes of a product perceptible by means of mechanical, tactile and where appropriate, visual and auditory receptors". The texture of a food, then, is perceived by humans via the sense of touch from surface responses within the mouth, deep responses by muscles and tendons, and potentially also auditory cues.

The current industry standard technique for inferring textural quality in apples is the "Magness and Taylor" test. This is conducted using a penetrometer, which comprises a metal probe that punctures a hole into the fruit, and records a value indicative of the mechanical resistance. This puncture test has been used in numerous academic studies on apple texture, where it is frequently related to sensory scores (Abbott et al., 1984; Barreiro et al., 1998; Mehinagic et al., 2003). Sensory evaluations are arguably the best reference data in this regard, as it is ultimately people who decide on the quality and acceptability of foods. Among the most common sensory terms relating to texture in apples are "*hardness*" (or "*firmness*") (Abbott et al., 1984) and "*mealiness*". These attributes are highly correlated with consumer acceptance: apples with firm texture are valued (Harker et al., 2000; Péneau et al., 2006), whereas consumers dislike mealy apples, perceiving these as soft, dry, and with poor textural quality (Daillant-Spinnler et al., 1996; Jaeger et al., 1998).

In terms of objective measurements, mealiness is the most intractable. The penetrometer, for instance, is unable to predict perceived mealiness sufficiently accurately. Brett & Waldron (1996) described the cellular changes responsible for the physical condition: the cell walls thicken and the intercellular bonds become weaker. During mastication, the cells slide apart but remain whole, so the texture is sensed as soft; and because the cell contents are not as readily released in the mouth, the fruit is perceived as dry. Mealiness develops due to ripening, senescence, temperature and humidity during storage; some cultivars (such as Red Delicious) are more prone to become mealy than others.

The work discussed in this section relates sEMG, sensory evaluations and penetrometer measurements from Red Delicious apples. The data presented here are a subset taken from a larger collection of measurements obtained from an extensive, multi-stage experiment, which is reported in Ioannides (2006) and Ioannides et al. (2007). Herein we focus on two texture-related sensory terms, hardness and mealiness, obtained by classical sensory evaluation - a single assessment by the subject representing their impression of the attribute over the entire eating period (Lee & Pangborn, 1986). Mealiness in particular is detected during chewing and not from the first bite (Lillford, 2000) and so there is a need to evaluate the whole chewing episode. Andani (2000) found that sensory mealiness was detected after 4 chews, which implied that some sensory attributes may require some manipulation of the food before the attribute can be perceived. Our wider study included a further three terms, which are outlined briefly in the methods section below, and discussed in full in the journal article (Ioannides et al., 2007).

sEMG has been used extensively to examine mastication patterns in a wide range of foods, including apples (Kohyama et al., 2005). Sakamoto et al. (1989) used sEMG to examine chewing of a range of food products with widely different textural qualities; they hypothesised that sEMG may provide an objective textural assessment tool, potentially forming a bridge between instrumental and sensory tests. Relationships have subsequently been sought between sEMG data and sensory scores: Karkazis & Kossioni (1998) compared raw carrot and peeled apple, and reported significant correlation between sensory hardness and sEMG activity in the masseter muscles.

The aim of the work presented here is to expand upon these ideas, and to explore whether sEMG can improve prediction of sensory properties compared with the use of the penetrometer alone. In the long-term this may enable sEMG to assist in assessing product quality, and crucially, obviate the need for trained panellists. Brown et al. (1994) suggested that an individuals' chewing behaviour may influence their ability to discern textural differences; this idea is also considered.

3.1 Methods

3.1.1 Samples

Red Delicious apples (Malus domestica 'Red Delicious') were obtained from a Washington State (USA) pack-house. All fruit were nominally the same size (grade 72) and same colour grade ("dark red not striped"). Mealiness can be forced onto fruit by storage at high humidity and temperature; thus, four storage regimes were devised to achieve a range of textures in the apples, detailed as follows:

Regime A: 4°C in refrigerator

Regime B: 1 week at 20°C (tray covered with polythene)

Regime C: 2 weeks at 20°C (tray covered with polythene)

Regime D: 4 weeks at 20°C (tray covered with polythene)

Preliminary work (Ioannides et al., 2006) had demonstrated that these regimes were able to induce a range of textural qualities in the fruit. Allocations of apples to each regime were made randomly. Immediately before measurements began, each apple was placed at 20°C for 12 hours, allowing it to equilibrate to room temperature.

3.1.2 Data collection

Following a number of training sessions, each of a set of thirteen panellists attended five data collection sessions, at which apple halves were consumed as follows: two halves from the same apple, three halves from different apples (5 halves in total). Each fruit was washed and cut in half before being presented cut-face down on a plate to the panellist. The presentation order was as balanced as possible with respect to the different storage regimes, to avoid order and carry-over effects. The panellist held the apple so that the skin was facing the floor, and took a natural-sized bite for each sensory attribute. Panellists took five bites per apple half, and made sensory evaluations as follows:

Bite 1: (No sensory assessment. The panellists were told to regard this as a "practice bite" only)

Bite 2: ***Hardness***, defined as the overall impression of hardness for the entire bite.

Bite 3: ***Mealiness***, defined as the extent to which the sample was dry and grainy and broke down into granular pieces during chewing.

Bite 4: ***Juiciness***, defined as the amount of juice released from the fruit into the mouth.
Bite 5: ***Skin toughness***, defined as the overall impression of how difficult it is to bite thorough and chew up the skin especially in comparison with the flesh.
These terms were chosen as they are pertinent to consumer acceptance (Daillant-Spinnler et al., 1996), and have been used in a range of other textural studies of apples (Barreiro et al., 1998; Saftner et al. 2002). The sensory assessments were made on a continuous un-structured scale, using a handle attached to a potentiometer with a nominal range of 0 - 5 volts (Sprunt et al., 2002). Extreme reference foods were used in training to enable individuals to "calibrate" their perceptions to this scale during the training and familiarization sessions, as described in Ioannides (2006). sEMG signals were recorded from all chewing episodes, using acquisition conditions as described earlier in this chapter.

3.2 Puncture test measurements

The Effegi penetrometer (Alfonsine, Italy) held in a drill stand was used to perform puncture tests on each apple. A thin slice of skin was removed and the 11 mm diameter plunger was forced into the flesh up to 8 mm; the maximum resistance reached was recorded.

3.3 Visual inspection and exploration of the sEMG data

Mean sEMG power spectra, calculated for each subject across all sessions (125 signals per subject), are shown in figure 13(a). Most striking is the very large difference in signal intensities - approximately an order of magnitude between, for instance, subjects 51 and 60. In general, features in the spectra are common to all subjects, and indeed to the data from edible gels presented earlier in this chapter. The larger number of volunteers in the present case, however, has led to an even greater range of magnitudes in response. An estimate of the total work done over each episode of chewing can be obtained by integrating the sEMG power spectra across the available frequency range (Carson et al., 2002; Kemsley et al., 2002; Peng et al., 2002; Schumann et al., 1994). The integrated values are depicted as boxplots in figure 13(b), which illustrate the range of values obtained by volunteer. The large variation in signal intensities is reflected clearly in the differences between the medians.
Figure 14(a) shows the first vs second PC scores from the complete set of power spectra. In common with previous work, the greatest source of variation in the sEMG data is due to subject, and the secondary source of variance is session. When the standardization procedure discussed earlier (section 2.4) is applied, these two sources of systematic variance are removed, and other trends in the data can be explored. One rather unexpected grouping emerges: in many of the subjects' data, there is clear clustering according to certain bite numbers, most noticeably Bite 5 (evaluation of skin toughness) and Bite 1 (the "practice" bite, with which no sensory evaluation was made). This is illustrated for one volunteer's data in figure 14(b). This indicates that an unexpectedly large amount of variance in the data is associated with the bite number, or equivalently, the sensory evaluation being undertaken. Detailed statistical analysis (one-way ANOVA, reported in full in Ioannides et al., 2009) confirmed that this was a significant effect in around half of the volunteers.
This analysis shows that the instruction given to a subject (i.e., "make no sensory evaluation", "evaluate skin toughness") can cause the subject to modify his/her chewing

behaviour such that there is a change in the sEMG signal. Perhaps the difficulty in making certain sensory evaluations caused some subjects to alter their mastication behaviour. Similarly, it seems plausible that some subjects chew differently when they are "practising" compared with when they are making sensory evaluations. Subjects were asked to use consistent habitual chewing behaviour throughout, so this modification may represent subconscious departure from the instructions. These findings provide strong quantitative evidence for an effect that has been speculated upon in the literature. Mioche & Martin (1998) showed that patterns of mastication change depending on whether or not subjects simultaneously carry out a sensory evaluation, and particularly so in trained subjects. Zimoch & Gullett (1997) suggested that different chewing behaviours may affect textural perception. Mathevon et al. (1995) proposed that subjects may alter their chewing behaviour according to their thoughts. We concur with this suggestion, and further propose that this alteration may take place subconsciously. So, the nature of the sensory evaluation must be added to the already large number of systematic factors that affect the sEMG signal. Furthermore, where the purpose of sEMG is to assist in objectively assessing texture, then this source of variability must be regarded as a confounding factor.

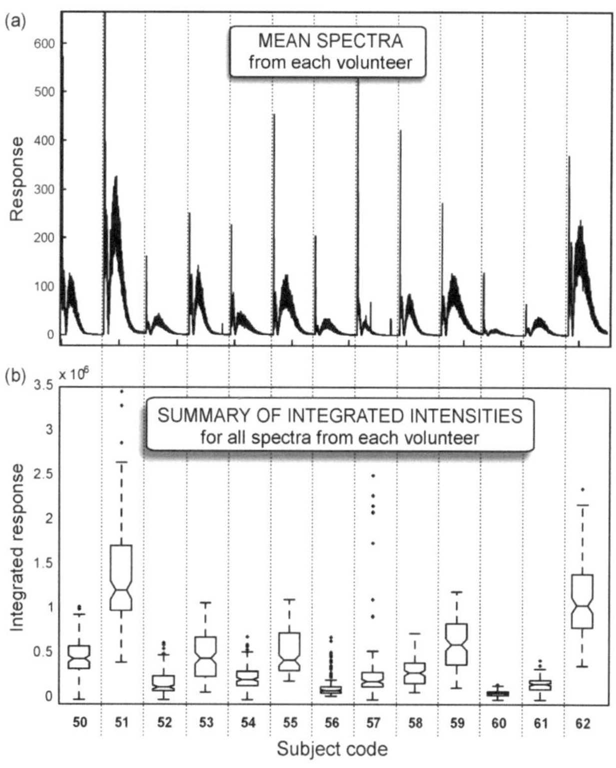

Fig. 13. (a) The mean power spectrum from each volunteer, and (b) boxplots that summarize the integrated power spectra obtained across all batches of data from each volunteer.

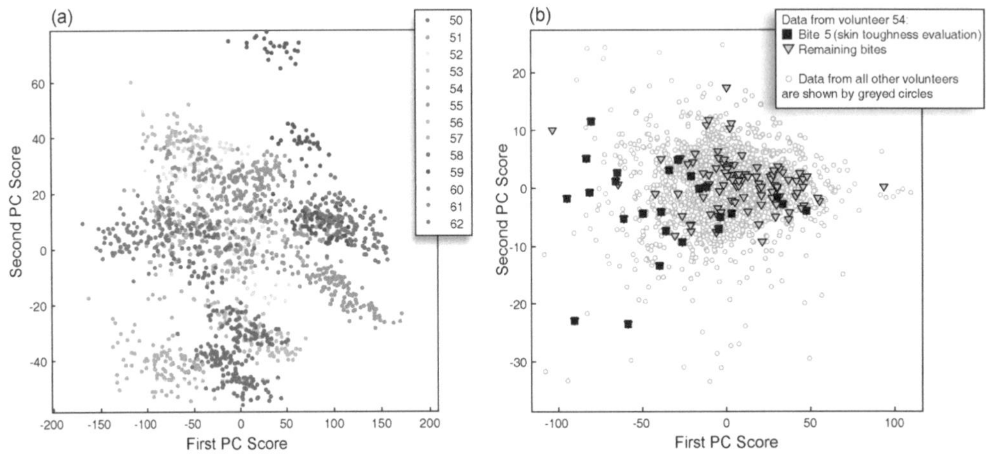

Fig. 14. (a) The first vs second PC scores (correlation method PCA, log-transformed data) from the complete set of power spectra. (b) PCA on the same original data set, but now standardized to remove volunteer and session effects. The points originating from one volunteer (54) are highlighted; data corresponding to bite 5 (= skin toughness evaluation) appears to be somewhat separated from the remaining readings.

3.4 Relationship between sEMG and puncture test data

It has been established that integrated sEMG signals are correlated with biting forces (Eves et al., 1988; Hylander & Johnson, 1989; Kemsley et al., 2003). We can hypothesize therefore that some relationship also exists between sEMG and puncture test data, since the latter involves measurement of a force exerted upon compression. However, this represents something of a challenge, given the comparatively narrow range of textural qualities encountered within a single fruit variety.

For the data set taken as a whole, we found that there is indeed a highly statistically significant relationship between the integrated sEMG intensity and the puncture test data. Furthermore, an exploration of this relationship as a function of frequency showed that the greatest correlation is obtained when the SEMG signal is integrated across higher frequencies only, and for the present dataset, specifically using parts of the spectral region greater than 15Hz. For example, figure 15(a) shows the integrated sEMG signal across the region 15 - 100Hz obtained from each apple (calculated from the standardized, co-added data) versus the puncture test data, for the entire collection of 260 apples. The R^2 value of 0.12 indicates that ~12% of the variation in the puncture test data can be explained by the sEMG data. In contrast, the frequency range below ~15Hz is the least well correlated with the puncture test data, with an R^2 of just 0.05 in comparison. The low-frequency end of the sEMG spectrum reflects gross muscle movements, whereas higher frequencies represent activation of fast and slow muscle groups (Wakeling, 2004). We surmise that it is the latter portion of the spectrum that contains information most analogous to the puncture test measurements.

This relationship was explored in more detail on a per-subject basis. It is found that there is variation in the extent to which each individual's sEMG data correlates with the penetrometer values (table 1). However, all except one of the volunteers showed a positive relationship with the penetrometer data, and for seven of these, the relationship was significant ($p<0.05$) and in some cases highly so: see for example figure 15(b).

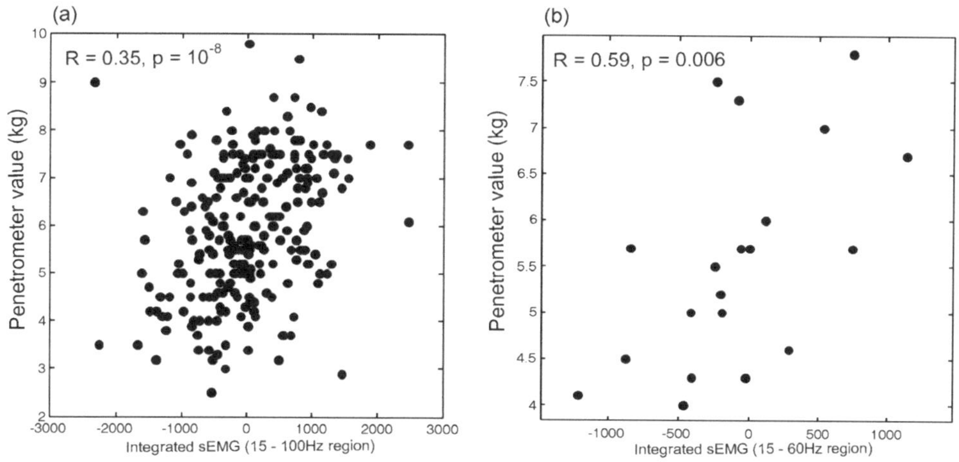

Fig. 15. Examples of the relationship between integrated sEMG data (standardized across batches of data from each volunteer and session) and the mean penetrometer values. Both the sEMG and penetrometer data were averaged to give per apple values. In (a), the relationship for the whole data set is shown (260 apples), and the sEMG integration was carried out across the 15 – 100Hz region. In (b), data from one volunteer only are used (volunteer code 59; 20 apples). Here, the sEMG integration was carried out across the 15 – 60Hz region only.

Regression of penetrometer values onto sEMG			
Volunteer code	Pearson's correlation coefficient, R	R-squared	p-value
50	0.14	0.02	0.56
51	0.63	0.39	0.00
52	0.13	0.02	0.59
53	0.41	0.17	0.07
54	0.50	0.25	0.02
55	0.64	0.41	0.00
56	-0.04	0.00	0.87
57	0.57	0.32	0.01
58	0.38	0.15	0.10
59	0.59	0.35	0.01
60	0.10	0.01	0.68
61	0.45	0.20	0.05
62	0.50	0.25	0.03

Table 1. Details of individual regressions of per apple penetrometer values onto each volunteer's sEMG data, integrated across the 15 – 60Hz region. Significant ($p<0.05$) positive relationships were found for seven of the volunteers, indicated by grey shading of the table rows.

3.5 Modelling sensory properties

The relationships between sEMG and the sensory evaluations were also explored, in particular for the properties "hardness" and "mealiness". For these two terms, we find that there are respectively clear positive and negative relationships with the sEMG data. Figure 16 shows the plots of the sensory scores for each term versus the sEMG data (figures 16(a) and (b)), and additionally the sensory scores versus the penetrometer data (figures 16 (c) and (d)). This illustrates well the similarity between sEMG and puncture tests in terms of their ability to model the sensory properties; compare the corresponding upper and lower figures in each case. Positive relationships also exist with juiciness and skin toughness (not shown), but these are much weaker, and for skin toughness, barely statistically significant. Again, a pattern of frequency dependence was found in the sEMG data: for all sensory terms, it was advantageous to integrate parts of the spectra above around 15Hz, with frequencies below this having least correlation with the sensory data. This is an important finding: it indicates that the least useful part of the sEMG power spectrum is the low-frequency region; yet it is this region that relates to the type of information that is conventionally extracted from time-domain sEMG.

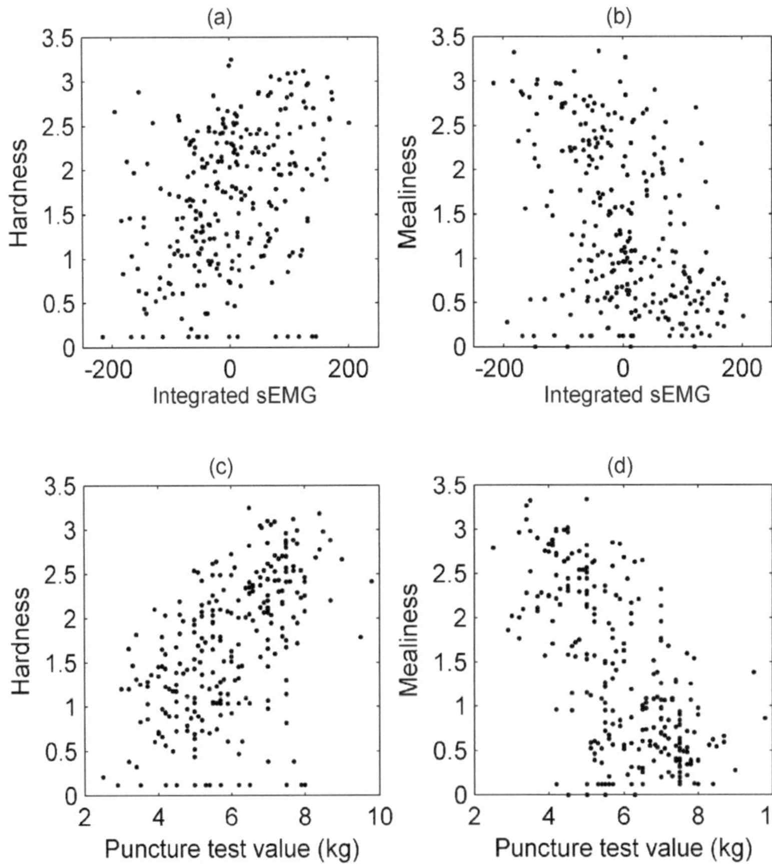

Fig. 16. Sensory hardness and mealiness versus (a) and (b) integrated sEMG signal, and (c) and (d) puncture test data. Note the qualitative similarity of plots (a) and (c), and (b) and (d).

3.6 Modelling sensory mealiness

We now focus particularly on sensory mealiness as the dependent variable of interest, since it is this property that is most challenging to measure by objective means. Sensory mealiness scores were regressed respectively onto the puncture test data, onto the sEMG data, and onto both using bivariate linear regression. All analyses were conducted on a per subject basis, and the sEMG data comprised integrated power spectra in the region 15 - 60Hz. The R^2 values are given in table 2, along with an indication of significance. There is significant ($p<0.05$) correlation of sensory mealiness with the puncture test for all subjects except one. sEMG was also found to be an effective predictor for eight out of the thirteen subjects, although the relationships (and significance levels) were generally somewhat weaker. However, this represents a substantial improvement compared with a previously reported analysis of the sEMG data (Ioannides et al., 2007) which used parameters extracted from the sEMG time domain signal, and found significant relationships for only four out of the thirteen subjects.

	Regression of sensory mealiness onto **puncture test data**		Regression of sensory mealiness onto **sEMG**		Regression of sensory mealiness onto **puncture test** and **sEMG data**	
Volunteer	Rsquared	p-value	Rsquared	p-value	Rsquared	p-value
50	0.67	0.00	0.10	0.18	0.71	0.00
51	0.61	0.00	0.49	<0.01	0.69	0.00
52	0.20	0.05	0.15	0.09	0.31	0.04
53	0.52	0.00	0.07	0.26	0.52	0.00
54	0.19	0.05	0.07	0.26	0.19	0.16
55	0.39	0.00	0.48	<0.01	0.54	0.00
56	0.52	0.00	0.00	0.92	0.52	0.00
57	0.54	0.00	0.23	0.03	0.54	0.00
58	0.43	0.00	0.27	0.02	0.51	0.00
59	0.65	0.00	0.53	<0.01	0.75	0.00
60	0.02	0.51	0.21	0.04	0.23	0.11
61	0.48	0.00	0.21	0.04	0.51	0.00
62	0.49	0.00	0.25	0.03	0.52	0.00

Table 2. Results of univariate regressions of sensory mealiness onto respectively puncture test and sEMG data, and bivariate regression onto both.

Examining now the results from the bivariate models, we see that there is better modelling of sensory mealiness in comparison with using either of the variates alone. Indeed, for the majority of subjects, the explained variance (R^2) is appreciably greater. For 10 out of the 13 subjects, ~50% of the variance in their sensory mealiness scores can be explained by the combination of sEMG and puncture test data. Furthermore, the standard deviation of the regression residuals is typically comparable in magnitude to the repeatability of the mealiness evaluations, obtained by examining the replicate blind evaluations made on the same apple halves at each session (see Ioannides et al., 2007). We conclude that the sensory mealiness has been modelled as well as could be expected, given the intrinsic error associated with the measurements involved.

4. Conclusions

The greatest obstacle preventing the use of sEMG as a routine measurement tool is that it is inherently a noisy technique. sEMG data suffers from a large amount of random noise, arising from the fact that the electrical signals generated by muscle activation are very small. This means that in practice, the SNR needs to be improved through signal-averaging by various means (for instance, co-addition of signals across replicate samples). A further considerable difficulty is that sEMG data are also affected by multiple sources of systematic noise. It is established that volunteer and recording session are major sources of unwanted variance, as demonstrated in the first sections of this chapter. We also show that an additional potential source of systematic variance is psychological in origin: changes in mastication behaviour arise from differences in the instructions given to the subject. This is strong evidence for an effect that has been speculated upon in the literature, namely that sEMG measurements are systematically affected by the nature of the sensory evaluation that the subjects are asked to make. This has clear implications for researchers engaged in sensory work.

In our analyses, we have surmounted the problems of systematic noise by using standardization of the sEMG spectra. This implicitly assumes that across each batch of data being standardized, subjects are experiencing broadly the same range of sample properties. A potential improvement to this procedure might be to ask subjects to consume standard reference materials, to establish fixed sEMG scale limits for each data subset. However, provided each session includes a sufficiently representative range of the samples under study, we have found that the within-session standardization approach is effective in allowing batches of data from different volunteers and sessions to be concatenated, increasing the power of statistical tests and the ability to explore underlying sources of information in the data.

Once the sEMG data have been appropriately treated, we find that they contain information that can be related directly to other physical properties of the foodstuffs, both mechanical and sensory. In studies of two different foodstuffs, edible gels and apples, positive and significant correlations were obtained between sEMG power spectra and mechanical measurements relating to texture. Further detailed analysis of the sEMG data in the apple study uncovered a frequency effect in the relationship between sEMG power spectra and other measurements (sensory evaluation, puncture tests) relating to texture; specifically, higher frequencies (>15Hz) proved the most useful. The work on prescribed chewing had indicated that these higher frequencies were also the least affected by major changes in gross chewing movements. In previous work on the apple data, we used parameters extracted from the time-domain sEMG signal, analogous to the low-frequency end of the power spectrum, and the number of subjects for which significant relationships were found was lower. We conclude that a fruitful approach to sEMG analysis is to use frequency-domain signals, standardized for session and subject, signal-averaged across each sample and integrated across frequency ranges above 15Hz.

5. Acknowledgement

This work was funded by the Biotechnology and Biological Sciences Research Council (BBSRC), through LINK, CASE and CSG projects. We also extend our thanks to our co-workers on these projects: A.C. Smith; J.C. Sprunt; Y. Ioannides; C.E. Raithatha; M.S. Howarth and J. Seers.

6. References

Abbott, J. A., Watada, A. E., & Massie, D. R. (1984). Sensory and instrument measurement of apple texture. *Journal of the American Society for Horticultural Science,* Vol. 109, No. 2, pp. 221-228, ISSN 0003-1062

Agrawal, K. R., Lucas, P. W., Bruce, I. C., & Prinz, J. F. (1998). Food properties that influence neuromuscular activity during human mastication. *Journal of Dental Research,* Vol. 77, No. 11, pp. 1931-1938, ISSN 0022-0345

Al-Mulla, M. R., Sepulveda, F., & Colley, M. (2011). A review of non-invasive techniques to detect and predict localised muscle fatigue. *Sensors,* Vol. 11, No. 4, pp. 3545-3594, ISSN 1424-8220

Andani, Z. (2000). *Consumer Perception of Mealiness in Apples.* PhD Thesis, University of Reading, UK

Barreiro, P., Ortiz, C., Ruiz-Altisent, M., De Smedt, V., Schotte, S., Andani, Z., Wakeling, I., & Beyts, P. K. (1998). Comparison between sensory and instrumental measurements for mealiness assessment in apples. A collaborative test. *Journal of Texture Studies,* Vol. 29, No. 5, pp. 509-525, ISSN 0022-4901

Blissett, A., Hort, J., & Taylor, A. J. (2006). Influence of chewing and swallowing behavior on volatile release in two confectionery systems. *Journal of Texture Studies,* Vol. 37, No. 5, pp. 476-496, ISSN 0022-4901

Boyar, M. M., & Kilcast, D. (1986). Electromyography as a novel method for examining food texture. *Journal of Food Science,* Vol. 51, No. 3, pp. 859-860, ISSN 0022-1147

Braxton, D., Dauchel, C., & Brown, W. E. (1996). Association between chewing efficiency and mastication patterns for meat, and influence on tenderness perception. *Food Quality and Preference,* Vol. 7, No. 3-4, pp. 217-223, ISSN 0950-3293

Brett, C. T., & Waldron, K. W. (1996). *Physiology and Biochemistry of Plant Cell Walls,* Chapman & Hall Ltd, ISBN 0-412-58060-8, London, UK

Brown, W. E. (1994). Method to investigate differences in chewing behavior in humans .1. Use of electromyography in measuring chewing. *Journal of Texture Studies,* Vol. 25, No. 1, pp. 1-16, ISSN 0022-4901

Brown, W. E., & Braxton, D. (2000). Dynamics of food breakdown during eating in relation to perceptions of texture and preference: a study on biscuits. *Food Quality and Preference,* Vol. 11, No. 4, pp. 259-267, ISSN 0950-3293

Brown, W. E., Eves, D., Ellison, M., & Braxton, D. (1998). Use of combined electromyography and kinesthesiology during mastication to chart the oral breakdown of foodstuffs: Relevance to measurement of food texture. *Journal of Texture Studies,* Vol. 29, No. 2, pp. 145-167, ISSN 0022-4901

Brown, W. E., Langley, K. R., Mioche, L., Marie, S., Gerault, S., & Braxton, D. (1996). Individuality of understanding and assessment of sensory attributes of foods, in particular, tenderness of meat. *Food Quality and Preference,* Vol. 7, No. 3-4, pp. 205-216, ISSN 0950-3293

Brown, W. E., Shearn, M., & Macfie, H. J. H. (1994). Method to investigate differences in chewing behavior in humans .2. Use of electromyography during chewing to assess chewing behavior. *Journal of Texture Studies,* Vol. 25, No. 1, pp. 17-31, ISSN 0022-4901

Carson, L., Sun, X. Z., Setser, C., & Peng, Y. K. (2002). Assessing food firmness using an electronic sensing system with a model food system. *Journal of Texture Studies,* Vol. 33, No. 5, pp. 389-399, ISSN 0022-4901

Daillant-Spinnler, B., MacFie, H. J. H., Beyts, P. K., & Hedderley, D. (1996). Relationships between perceived sensory properties and major preference directions of 12 varieties of apples from the southern hemisphere. *Food Quality and Preference,* Vol. 7, No. 2, pp. 113-126, ISSN 0950-3293

De Luca, C. J. (1997). The use of surface electromyography in biomechanics. *Journal of Applied Biomechanics,* Vol. 13, No. 2, pp. 135-163, ISSN 1065-8483

Duizer, L. M., Gullett, E. A., & Findlay, C. J. (1996). The relationship between sensory time-intensity, physiological electromyography and instrumental texture profile analysis measurements of beef tenderness. *Meat Science,* Vol. 42, No. 2, pp. 215-224, ISSN 0309-1740

Edlund, J., & Lamm, C. J. (1980). Masticatory efficiency. *Journal of Oral Rehabilitation,* Vol. 7, No. 2, pp. 123-130, ISSN 0305-182X

Eves, A. Boyar, M., & Kilcast, D. (1988). Electromyographic evaluation of the texture of confectionery products, In: *Food Acceptability,* Thomson D.M .H., pp. 459-472, Elsevier Applied Science, ISBN 1851662561, London

González, R., Sifre, S., Benedito, J., & Nogues, V. (2002). Comparison of electromyographic pattern of sensory experts and untrained subjects during chewing of Mahon cheese. *Journal of Dairy Research,* Vol. 69, No. 1, pp. 151-161, ISSN 0022-0299

Harker, F. R., Volz, R., Johnston, J., Hallett, I., & DeBelie, N. (2000). What makes fruit firm and how to keep it that way? Proceedings of Washington State University Annual Postharvest Conference

Herzog, W., Y. T. Zhang, et al. (1994). Assessment of muscular fatigue using vibromyography. *Muscle & Nerve,* Vol. 17, No. 10, pp. 1156-1161, ISSN 0148-639X

Hodgson, M., Linforth, R. S. T., & Taylor, A. J. (2003). Simultaneous real-time measurements of mastication, swallowing, nasal airflow, and aroma release. *Journal of Agricultural and Food Chemistry,* Vol. 51, No. 17, pp. 5052-5057, ISSN 0021-8561

Horio, T., & Kawamura, Y. (1989). Effect of texture of food on chewing patterns in the human subject. *Journal of Oral Rehabilitation,* Vol. 16, pp. 177-183, ISSN 0305-182X

Hylander, W. L., & K. R. Johnson (1989). The relationship between masseter force and masseter electromyogram during mastication in the monkey macaca-fascicularis. *Archives of Oral Biology,* Vol. 34, No. 9, pp. 713-722, ISSN 0003-9969

Ioannides , Y. (2006). *Textural Analysis of Red Delicious Apples.* PhD Thesis, University of East Anglia, UK

Ioannides, Y., Howarth, M. S., Raithatha, C., Defernez, M., Kemsley, E. K., & Smith, A. C. (2007). Texture analysis of Red Delicious fruit: Towards multiple measurements on individual fruit. *Food Quality and Preference,* Vol. 18, No.6, pp. 825-833, ISSN 0950-3293

Ioannides, Y., Seers, J., Defernez, M., Raithatha, C., Howarth, M. S., Smith, A., & Kemsley, E. K. (2009). Electromyography of the masticatory muscles can detect variation in the mechanical and sensory properties of apples. *Food Quality and Preference,* Vol. 20, No. 3, pp. 203-215, ISSN 0950-3293

Jaeger, S. R., Andani, Z., Wakeling, I. N., & MacFie, H. J. H. (1998). Consumer preferences for fresh and aged apples: A cross-cultural comparison. *Food Quality and Preference,* Vol. 9, No. 5, pp. 355-366, ISSN 0950-3293

Jolliffe, I.T. (1986). *Principal Component Analysis,* Springer-Verlag, ISBN 0-387-96269-7, New York, USA

Karkazis, H. C., & Kossioni, A. E. (1998). Surface EMG activity of the masseter muscle in denture wearers during chewing of hard and soft food. *Journal of Oral Rehabilitation,* Vol. 25, No. 1, pp. 8-14, ISSn 0305-182X

Kemsley, E. K., Defernez, M., Sprunt, J. C., & Smith, A. C. (2003). Electromyographic responses to prescribed mastication. *Journal of Electromyography and Kinesiology,* Vol. 13, No. 2, pp. 197-207, ISSN 1050-6411

Kemsley, E. K., Sprunt, J. C., Defernez, M., & Smith, A. C. (2002). Multivariate analysis of electromyographic (EMG) frequency spectra to characterise mastication. *Journal of Texture Studies,* Vol. 33, No. 1, pp. 15-34, ISSN 0022-4901

Kohyama, K., Nakayama, Y., Watanabe, H., & Sasaki, T. (2005). Electromyography of eating apples: Influences of cooking, cutting, and peeling. *Journal of Food Science,* Vol. 70, No. 4, pp. S257-S261, ISSN 0022-1147

Krzanowski, W.J. (1988). *Principles of Multivariate Analysis: A User's Perspective,* Oxford University Press, ISBN 0-19-852230-4, New York, USA

Lassauzay, C., Peyron, M. A., Albuisson, E., Dransfield, E., & Woda, A. (2000). Variability of the masticatory process during chewing of elastic model foods. *European Journal of Oral Sciences,* Vol. 108, No. 6, pp. 484-492, ISSN 0909-8836

Lee, W. E., & Pangborn, R. M. (1986). Time-intensity - the temporal aspects of sensory perception. *Food Technology,* Vol. 40, No. 11, pp. 71-82, ISSN 0015-6639

Lee, Y. S., Owens, C. M., & Meullenet, J. F. (2009). Tenderness perception of poultry major pectoralis muscle during mastication. *Journal of Food Science,* Vol. 74, No. 9, pp. S413-S422, ISSN 0022-1147

Lillford, P. J. (2000). The materials science of eating and food breakdown. *Mrs Bulletin, Vol. 25, No.* 12, pp. 38-43, ISSN 0883-7694

Mathevon, E., Mioche, L., Brown, W. E., & Culioli, J. (1995). Texture analysis of beef cooked at various temperatures by mechanical measurements, sensory assessments and electromyography. *Journal of Texture Studies,* Vol. 26, pp. 175-192, ISSN 0022-4901

Mathoniere, C., Mioche, L., Dransfield, E., & Culioli, J. (2000). Meat texture characterisation: Comparison of chewing patterns, sensory and mechanical measures. *Journal of Texture Studies,* Vol. 31, No. 2, pp. 183-203, ISSN 0022-4901

Mehinagic, E., Royer, G., Bertrand, D., Symoneaux, R., Laurens, F., & Jourjon, F. (2003). Relationship between sensory analysis, penetrometry and visible-NIR spectroscopy of apples belonging to different cultivars. *Food Quality and Preference,* Vol. 14, No. 5-6, pp. 473-484, ISSN 0950-3293

Mioche, L. (2004). Mastication and food texture perception: Variation with age. *Journal of Texture Studies,* Vol. 35, No. 2, pp. 145-158, ISSN 0022-4901

Mioche, L., & Martin, J. (1998). Training and sensory judgment effects on mastication as studied by electromyography. *Journal of Food Science,* Vol. 63, No. 1, pp. 1-5, ISSN 0022-1147

Mioche, L., Peyron, M. A., & Auroy, P. (1993). The use of intraoral load cells in the study of texture-perception. *Journal of Texture Studies,* Vol. 24, No. 4, pp. 361-373, ISSN 0022-4901

Olthoff, L. W., Vanderbilt, A., Deboer, A., & Bosman, F. (1986). Comparison of force-deformation characteristics of artificial and several natural foods for chewing experiments. *Journal of Texture Studies,* Vol. 17, No. 3, pp. 275-289, ISSN 0022-4901

Péneau, S., Hoehn, E., Roth, H. R., Escher, F., & Nuessli, J. (2006). Importance and consumer perception of freshness of apples. *Food Quality and Preference,* Vol. 17, No. 1-2, pp. 9-19, ISSN 0950-3293

Peng, Y. K., Sun, X. Z., Carson, L., & Setser, C. (2002). Food hardness and fracturability assessment by an electronic sensing system. *Journal of Texture Studies,* Vol. 33, No. 2, pp. 135-148, ISSN 0022-4901

Plesh, O., Bishop, B., & McCall, W. (1986). Effect of gum hardness on chewing pattern. *Experimental Neurology,* Vol. 92, pp. 502-512, ISSN 0014-4886

Plesh, O., Bishop, B., & McCall, W. (1987). Mandibular movements and jaw muscles activity while voluntarily chewing at different rates. *Experimental Neurology,* Vol. 98, No. 2, pp. 285-300., ISSN 0014-4886

Saftner, R. A., Abbott, J. A., Conway, W. S., Barden, C. L., & Vinyard, B. T. (2002). Instrumental and sensory quality characteristics of 'Gala' apples in response to prestorage heat, controlled atmosphere, and air storage. *Journal of the American Society for Horticultural Science,* Vol. 127, No. 6, pp. 1006-1012, ISSN 0003-1062

Sakamoto, H., Harada, T., Matsukubo, T., Takaesu, Y., & Tazaki, M. (1989). Electromyographic measurement of textural changes of foodstuffs during chewing. *Agricultural and Biological Chemistry,* Vol. 53, No. 9, pp. 2421-2433, ISSn 0002-1369

Schumann, N. P., Sholle, H. C., Anders, C., & Mey, E. (1994). A topographical analysis of spectral electromyographic data of the human masseter muscle under different functional conditions in healthy-subjects. *Archives of Oral Biology,* Vol. 39, No. 5, pp. 369-377, ISSN 0003-9969

Smith, A. C. (2004). Texture and mastication, In: *Texture in food: volume 2: solid foods,* Kilcast D., pp.53-81, Woodhead Publishing Ltd, 1 85573 724 8, Abington, UK

Sprunt, J. C., Raithatha, C. E., & Smith, A. C. (2002). Swallow indicator methodology as an enhancement to combined time-intensity measurement of flavour release and electromyography for monitoring mastication. *Food Quality and Preference,* Vol. 13, No. 1, pp. 47-55, ISSN 0950-3293

Sprunt, J. C., & Smith, A. C. (2002). Measurement of surface area, gel weight and saliva weight in a gelatin-based gel over the course of mastication. *International Journal of Food Sciences and Nutrition,* Vol. 53, No. 3, pp. 261-271, ISSN 0963-7486

Subasi, A., Yilmaz, M., & Ozcalik, H. R. (2006). Classification of EMG signals using wavelet neural network. *Journal of Neuroscience Methods,* Vol. 156, No 1-2, pp. 360-367, ISSN 0165-0270

Sun, X. S., Wang, F. T., Carson, L., & Setser, C. (2001). Electronic sensing system for food texture characterization. *Transactions of the Asae,* Vol. 44, No. 3, pp. 623-630, ISSN 0001-2351

Tornberg, E., Fjelkner-Modig, S., Ruderus, H., Glantz, P. O., Rnandow, K., & Stafford, D. (1985). Clinically recorded masticatory patterns as related to the sensory evaluation of meat and meat products. *Journal of Food Science,* Vol. 50, pp. 1059-1066, ISSN 0022-1147

Veyrune, J. L., & Mioche, L. (2000). Complete denture wearers: electromyography of mastication and texture perception whilst eating meat. *European Journal of Oral Sciences,* Vol. 108, No. 2, pp. 83-92, ISSN 0909-8836

Wakeling, J. M. (2004). Motor units are recruited in a task-dependent fashion during locomotion. *Journal of Experimental Biology,* Vol. 207, No. 22, pp. 3883-3890, ISSN 0022-0949

Westbury, J. R., & Shaughnessy T.G. (1987). Associations between spectral representation of the surface electromyogram and fiber type distribution and size in human masseter muscle. *Electromyography and Clinical Neurophysiology,* Vol. 27, No.6-7, pp. 427-435, ISSN 0301-150X

Wilson, C. E., & Brown, W. E. (1997). Influence of food matrix structure and oral breakdown during mastication on temporal perception of flavor. *Journal of Sensory Studies,* Vol. 12, No. 1, pp. 69-86, ISSN 0887-8250

Wright, K. M., & Hills, B. P. (2003). Modelling flavour release from a chewed bolus in the mouth: Part II. The release kinetics. *International Journal of Food Science and Technology,* Vol. 38, No. 3, pp. 361-368, ISSN 0950-5423

Wright, K. M., Sprunt, J., Smith, A. C., & Hills, B. P. (2003). Modelling flavour release from a chewed bolus in the mouth: Part I. Mastication. *International Journal of Food Science and Technology,* Vol. 38, No. 3, pp. 351-360, ISSN 0950-5423

Yuen, S. W. H., Hwang, J. C. C., & Poon, P. W. F. (1989). EMG power spectrum patterns of anterior temporal and masseter muscles in children and adults. Journal of Dental Research, Vol. 68, No. 5, pp. 800-804, ISSN ISSN 0022-0345

Yven, C., Guessasma, S., Chaunier, L., Della Valle, G., & Salles, C. (2010). The role of mechanical properties of brittle airy foods on the masticatory performance. *Journal of Food Engineering,* Vol. 101, No. 1, pp. 85-91, ISSN 0260-8774

Zimoch, J., & Gullett, E. A. (1997). Temporal aspects of perception of juiciness and tenderness of beef. *Food Quality and Preference,* Vol. 8, No. 3, pp. 203-211, ISSN 0950-3293

21

Electromyography and Facial Paralysis

Fernanda Chiarion Sassi, Paula Nunes Toledo,
Laura Davison Mangilli and Claudia Regina Furquim de Andrade
University of São Paulo
Brazil

1. Introduction

The facial motor system is responsible for functions critical to physical, social and psychological well-being (VanSwearingen & Brach, 1996). Facial nerve paralysis is a life-altering clinical condition, with functional, aesthetic and communication implications for the individuals who are afflicted (Hadlock, 2008). It differs from most other clinical conditions in that it is the end result of a very wide variety of underlying conditions; ranging from skull base trauma, congenital syndromes, skull base tumors, infectious diseases, among others, leading to a single disability (Diels, 2000; Hadlock, 2008). Several studies have presented conflicting results regarding its epidemiology. The precise annual incidence of Bell's palsy, the most common cause of unilateral facial weakness, in the Western world is probably around 20 to 25 per 100,000 people (Peitersen, 1982; Morgan & Nathwani, 1982). Bell's palsy is defined as isolated, sudden, peripheral facial paralysis of unknown etiology. However, it is generally accepted that it is a nonsuppurative, inflammatory, generative disease of the facial nerve within the stylomastoid foramen (Proctor, Corgill & Proud, 1976). The vast majority (around 80-84%) of patients will recover completely, but a few (16-20%) will remain with chronic facial paralysis or paresis (Peitersen, 1982; Morgan & Nathwani, 1982).

Although Bell's palsy may develop at any age, literature often points that it is more common among young or middle-aged adults (onset between 31-60 years) (Kukimoto et al., 1988; Gonçalves-Coelho et al., 1997; Bradbury, Simons & Sanders, 2006). The longer the recovery is delayed, the higher is the incidence of sequelae such as synkinesis and contracture (Ghali, MacQuillan & Gorbbellaar, 2001). Completeness of recovery also decreases with age with 90% complete remission up to the age of 14 compared below 40% for the over 60 age group (Peitersen, 1982). Results about distribution between genders are also conflicting. While a few authors point that the disease is equally distributed between genders (Morgan & Nathwani, 1982), others point that it is more common among females (Bradbury, Simons & Sanders, 2006; Garcia et al., 2010).

Literature indicates that head trauma is the second most frequent cause of facial paralysis (Atolini Junior et al., 2009; Pinna, Testa & Fukuda, 2004). Causes of head trauma are usually related to traffic injuries (82.5%), fall from height (7.5%), assault (5%), and gunshot (2.5%), although numbers can vary significantly from one country to the next (Pinna, Testa & Fukuda, 2004; Odebode & Ologe, 2006). Until the end of the 19th century, the treatment of facial paralysis involved non-surgical means such as ointments, medicines and electrotherapy (van de Graaf & Nicolai, 2005). With the advent and refinement of microvascular surgical techniques in the latter half of the 20th century, vascularised free muscle transfer coupled with cross-facial nerve grafts were introduced, allowing the possibility of spontaneous emotion being restored to the paralysed face became reality (Ghali, MacQuillan & Grobbelaar, 2011). The clinical or surgical treatment will depend on lesion extension.

Other causes of facial paralysis include the presence of infections, among which are the herpes group of viruses, especially herpes simplex virus and varicella-zoster virus (Morgan & Nathwani, 1992; Yeo et al., 2007), complication of acute otitis media or in the presence of cholesteatoma (Atolini Junior et al., 2009) and Schwanomas of the 7th and 8th cranial pairs (Rosenberg, 2000; Lee et al., 2007; Saito & Cheung, 2010).

Considering the anatomy and function of the facial nerve, the stylomastoid foramen marks the beginning of the facial nerve's extracranial course. The nerve becomes superficial rendering it susceptible to trauma before entering the parotid gland and dividing into two main trunks within the substance of the gland (Seikel, King & Darmright, 2010; Ghali, MacQuillan & Grobbellaar, 2010). On exiting the gland, there are between 8 and 15 branches making up the five of the facial nerve; temporal, zygomatic, buccal, marginal mandibular and cervical. Beyond the parotid gland, there is a significant arborisation and interconnection of these divisions resulting in a degree of functional overlap between branches. The facial nerve controls all the superficial facial musculature and therefore controls the appearance of the face, the ability to show expression and most of the functions about forehead, eye, cheeks and mouth (see Table 1). The main complaint in lower facial paralysis, as is the case of individuals with Bell's palsy, is the inability to smile. The most important muscles involved in smiling are zygomaticus major and levator labii superioris (Proctor, Corgill & Proud, 1976; Ghali, MacQuillan & Grobbellaar, 2010).

Muscle	Action
Corrugator supercilii	Moves eyebrow downward and medially
Procerus	Wrinkles skin of the nose
Orbicularis oculi	Closes eye
Orbicularis oris	Closes mouth
Compressor naris	Compresses nasal cartilage
Dilator naris	Dilates nostrils
Levator labii superioris	Lifts upper lip
Zygomaticus major and minor	Raise and pull upper lip laterally
Levator anguli oris	Raise corner of the mouth
Risorius	Smiling (lateral pull on the corner of the mouth)
Depressor anguli oris	Pulls down the corner of the mouth
Depressor labii inferioris	Depresses lower lip
Mentalis	Wrinkles skin of the chin
Buccinator	Compresses mouth and keeps food between teeth when chewing
Frontalis	Raises eyebrows
Platysma	Moves skin of the neck

Table 1. Action of face muscles

Given the trend of evidence-based practice (Sackett et al., 2000), it has become important to establish which facial paralysis assessment and management strategies demonstrate significant answers and benefit, either with respect to function, aesthetic appearance, ability to communicate, or a combination of these. Patients presenting with facial paralysis usually undergo subjective assessments of facial function (House & Brackmann, 1985; Berg et al., 2004), standard photographic documentation, and sometimes videographic imaging (Hadlock, 2008). As a general rule, individual practitioners have selected specific grading scales based on training, exposure and institutional experience, rather than clinical relevance to outcomes. Although these procedures may provide an accurate depiction of a patient's level of facial paresis, they do not address how this handicap may affect a patient's quality of life.

The psychological literature on the subject of facial disfigurement has consistently shown that those with facial disfigurement do experience psychological and social problems, resulting in fear of public places and impaired socialization (Tate & Tollefson, 2006; Bradbury, Simons & Sanders, 2006; Hadlock, 2008). There is evidence in the literature that individuals with facial palsy experience marked psychological and social problems. Normal face-to-face communication can be interrupted by altered or diminished facial expressions (Keillor et al., 2002). The aesthetic impact of the disfigurement caused by facial palsy is exacerbated by impaired facial movement and, therefore the individual may try to restrict expressive facial movements to minimize the disfigurement. This can be interpreted as hostile by others, provoking aggressive responses, and can increase social anxiety and avoidance. In addition the individual may become self-conscious when eating or drinking because of functional problems (Bradbury, Simons & Sanders, 2006). Symptoms can range from altered emotional well-being, decreased self-esteem, anxiety, depression, and alternative behaviors such as social isolation and addiction (Ross et al., 1991; VanSwearingen & Brach, 2003; Finn et al., 2003; Hadlock, 2008). In this sense, self-report scales are of extreme importance in order to enhance the assessment of facial neuromuscular dysfunction. Although the clinical recognition of the above mentioned problems exist, very few studies using self-reports as a form to control the outcome of treatment were found in the literature (Salles et al., 2009).

As reported in studies about disfigurement, psychological distress rather than functional impairment has been found to be the most significant predictor of social disability in patients with hemi-facial palsy (VanSwearingen, Turnbull & Mrzai, 1998). VanSwearingen and Brach (1996) have pointed that patients with facial neuromuscular dysfunction have disability associated with the disorder. The terms impairment and disability are defined within the World Health Organization's International Classification of Impairments, Disabilities, and Handicaps (Barbotte et al., 2001). Impairments refer to any physiologic or anatomic abnormalities at the organ or tissue system level, such as muscle weakness. Disabilities are person-level problems characterized by the inability to perform any of the activities considered usual for a human being, such as limitations in walking or limited ability to communicate. Wilson and Cleary (1995) suggested that the patient's emotional well-being may influence the relationship between impairment and disabilities.

To enhance the assessment of facial neuromuscular dysfunction beyond the impairment domain, VanSwearingen and Brach (1996) developed a disability assessment instrument, the Facial Disability Index (FDI). The FDI is a self-report, disease-specific instrument designed to provide the clinician with information about the disability and related social and emotional well-being of patients with facial nerve palsy. According to the authors, the FDI can be used as an initial assessment tool and as a monitoring instrument, providing the clinician with the patient's view of the outcome of the intervention in progress. The FDI is composed by two subscales: Physical Function and Social/well-being function. The Physical Function subscale involves questions related to difficulty in eating, difficulty in drinking, difficulty in speaking, excessive tearing or drying of the eye and difficulty in brushing/rinsing the teeth. The Social/well-being subscale involves questions related to feeling calm and peaceful, isolating self from people, feeling irritable toward those around, waking up early or several times at night and avoiding going out to eat, shop or participating in social activities.

Besides proposing the FDI, the authors also examined the reliability and validity of the questionnaire. The questionnaire was administered to 46 ambulatory patients with facial palsy. The results of the study indicated that the FDI subscales produced reliable scores and that the subscale of Physical Function presented a higher reliability when compared with that of Social/well-being. The authors argue that this result may be due to the fact that the facial functions assessed are largely behaviors that necessarily occur more than once a day. The authors also found a significant association of the FDI subscales with the clinical measures of facial movement and psychosocial status. Other studies have been conducted trying to correlate measures of impairment and disability using the FDI. Overall, these studies indicate a positive correlation between impairment and disability measures in patients with facial nerve paralysis (VanSwearigen et al., 1998; Coulson et al., 2004).

The most important, impeding need to improve the clinical care of the facial paralysis patient is an objective, quantitative, comprehensive evaluation of function. In this sense, surface electromyography (sEMG) can give clinicians valuable information because it provides easy access to physiological processes that cause muscle to generate force, produce movement and accomplish the countless functions which allow us to interact with the world around us (De Luca, 1997).

Studies have already been successful in reporting the outcome of neuromuscular retraining in combination with sEMG (Daniel & Guitar, 1978; Balliet et al., 1982; May et al., 1989; Ross et al., 1991; Segal et al., 1995; Brach et al., 1997; Cronin & Steenerson, 2003; VanSwearingen & Brach, 2003; Vaiman et al., 2005). Biofeedback sEMG instruments are essentially general purpose physiological monitoring devices that are designed to provide ongoing information about physiological function, such as muscle tension level (Vaiman et al., 2005). Using neuromuscular retraining in combination with sEMG is based on the plasticity of the central nervous system. The brain is capable of reorganizing using the visual and/or auditory feedback provided by sEMG (Cronin & Steenerson). Literature points that the therapeutic use of sEMG helps patients to develop selective muscle control and decreases synkinesis. No studies were found in the consulted literature related to the use of sEMG in the assessment of impairment caused by facial paralysis.

Although facial movement and muscle activity can be quantified using one of several techniques (House & Brackmann, 1985; Kayhan et al., 2000; Linstrom et al., 2000; Linstrom, 2002; Kang et al., 2002; Mehta et al., 2008) and facial disability can be quantified using self-report instruments (VanSwearingen & Brach, 1996), a relationship between objective and subjective measurements has not yet been described. The purpose of this study was to correlate electromyographic data of the anguli oris elevators to the facial disability index in long standing facial paralysis patients. We hypothesized that individuals with greater facial asymmetry (i.e. lower readings on surface electromyography) would present lower scores on the facial disability index.

2. Methods and materials

The population in this study was defined as 17 patients (mean age 42 years; age range from 35 to 60), all females, with unilateral facial nerve paralysis. All of the patients presented static and/or dynamic facial asymmetry. Patients who presented systemic or neuromuscular disease, impaired cognition and asymmetry due to craniofacial deformities were excluded from the research. A control group with 17 normal volunteers, matched for age and gender to the research group, was also included in the study. All of the selected individuals, in the research and control groups, signed an informed consent approved by the review board and ethics committee of the institution (CAPPesq HCFMUSP no 0201/08).

Inclusion criteria for the research group:

a. to present medical diagnosis of long-standing unilateral peripheral facial paralysis, i.e. with more than two years since the beginning of symptoms, with or without previous treatment by surgical methods (reconstruction or reanimation);
b. to present scores between 4 and 11 on the Clinical Score for Facial Palsy Protocol (Salles et al., 2009).

Category	N.
Acoustic neuroma	2
Bell's palsy	12
Facial nerve trauma (temporal/basilar skull fractures)	3

Table 2. Participants' distribution per diagnostic categories of facial dysfunction - Research group

Inclusion criteria for the control group:

a. to present no medical history of facial paralysis or head and neck trauma;
b. to present scores between 19 and 20 on the Clinical Score for Facial Palsy Protocol (Salles et al., 2009).

Procedure

Clinical score for facial palsy protocol

Facial symmetry was evaluated by two staff members. As already described in the literature, with this scale every voluntary movement for both sides of the face is evaluated independently, as well as the involuntary (emotional) motion. The protocol is composed by three sections: force of voluntary movement (eyebrow raise, eyelid closure, upper lip elevation - sniff, upper-lateral traction of lips, horizontal traction of lips; lip closure; lower lip depression); force of involuntary movements (eyelid closure when blinking, when speaking; when spontaneously smiling); negative findings (eyelid deformity at rest, lip deformity at rest; synkinesis/spasms). Movements were graded as absent (0), partial (1), or full (2). Negative aspects received negative scores ((0) absent, (-1) moderate, (-2) pronounced). The sum of individual scores gives a final score that ranges up to 20 points, or 100%.

Surface electromyography (sEMG) evaluation

One muscle group was examined in the study: the anguli oris elevators (zygomaticus major and minor, levator anguli oris). This muscle group was selected because it is directly involved in the action of smiling.

All EMG recordings were made using standard surface sensors (SDS500). We used the Miotool 400 (Miotec® Biomedical Equipments, Brazil) 4-channel computer-based system and disposable double electrodes (SDS 500 Ag/AgCl, contact surfaces with 10mm diameter). This EMG system has wide bandpass filter, bandwidth (RMS) 20 to 500 Hz and a 60-Hz notch filter. The system uses the Active Electrode, a compact sensor assembly that includes a miniaturized instrument preamplifier. Locating the amplifier at the electrode site allows artifacts to be canceled and the signal boosted before being transferred down the electrode cable (noise level < 5μV RMS). Each EMG record was full-wave and low-passed filtered. The computer program indicates mean, SD, minimum, maximum and range of muscle activity during each trial. Muscle activity (EMG) was quantified in microvolts (μV).
The interelectrode distance was 10mm; two sets of two bipolar pre-gelled stick-on surface electrodes were applied to the skin on each side of the face, over the anguli oris elevators to record myoelectrical activity during the production of a voluntary smile (Figure 1). This electrode arrangement had a third electrode as ground positioned on the right wrist. Electrical impedance at the sites of electrode contact was reduced because skin was scrubbed with alcohol gauze pads.

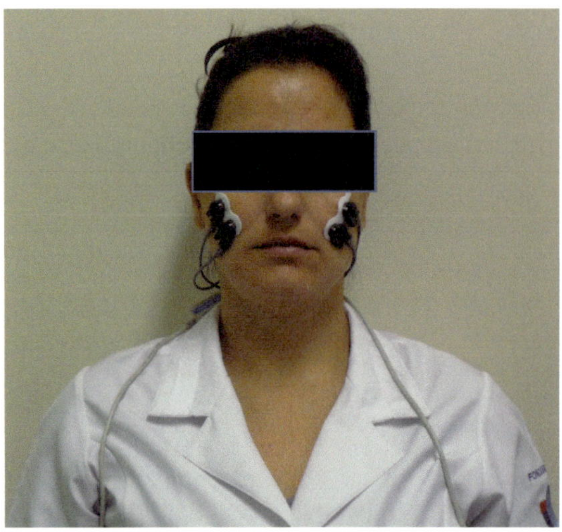

Fig. 1. Electrode placement

At first, mean electric activity of resting muscle anguli oris elevators was obtained. Following this, three tests of voluntary smiles were examined.
Step 1: Participants remained seated with their heads positioned horizontally according to the Frankfort plane. After the pairs of EMG electrodes were placed over the skin each participant was instructed to remain quiet and relaxed for the period of 1 minute. Three separate recordings of resting condition were made, with the duration of 30 seconds each.
Step 2: Each participant was asked to smile for 5 seconds and then relax for 5 seconds, three times. Participants were instructed to avoid sharp head movements. The request to begin sEMG recording was provided only when the sEMG baseline activity returned to resting levels.

sEMG data analysis

Surface EMG traces were evaluated for onset, peak and offset of activity during smiling events (Figure 2). Onset was identified as the point of upward excursion of the sEMG trace from resting baseline that led into the smiling event. Peak was the highest amplitude point of the sEMG smile trace. Offset was the point at which sEMG activity returned to baseline. Computer software calculated the mean value of the action potential during the movements (onset-peak-offset). In order to compare the results between participants, sEMG amplitude values were normalized relative to rest in order to give evidence to possible differences in symmetry.

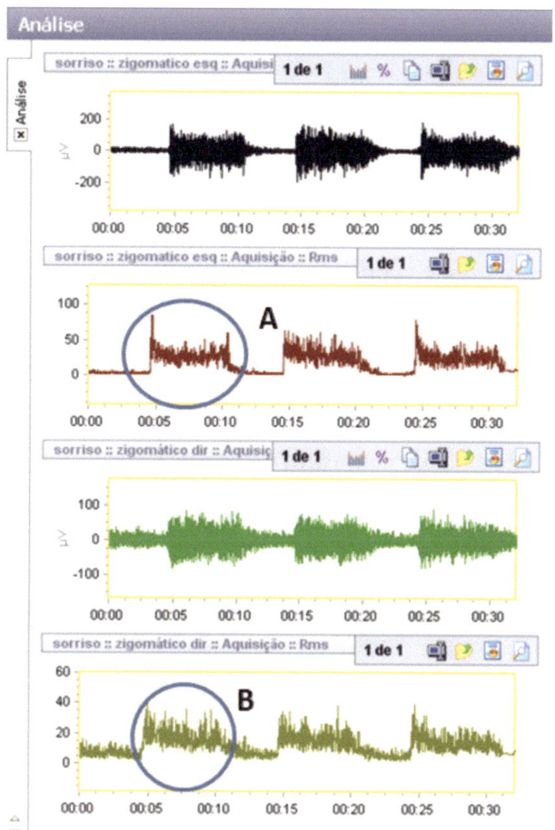

*Note: A - sEMG smile trace of the nonparalyzed side; B - sEMG smile trace of the paralyzed side

Fig. 2. sEMG smile trace

sEMG data reliability

Because subjective judgment was used for sEMG measures, interjudge reliability was estimated. To establish interjudge reliability of the measurements used in the study, a second experienced staff member, who was blinded to the original results, measured the same parameters of 30 randomly selected samples from the 204 total smiling events. Intraclass correlation coefficients were high for all comparisons (range of lower 95% confidence interval [CI] = .9788-.9965), suggesting strong consistency between examiners.

Facial Disability Index (FDI)

The FDI is a brief self-report questionnaire of physical disability and psychosocial factors related to facial neuromuscular function (VanSwearingen & Brach, 1996). It is designed to provide an account of the patient´s daily experience of living with a facial nerve disorder. It has two subscales: the Social/Well-Being Function subscale (SWBF), that contains items related to the psychological and social role aspects, and the Physical Function subscale (PF), with items that evaluate difficulties with daily activities (e.g. brushing the teeth, eating or drinking). Only participants of the research group answered the questionnaire.

Data analysis

Statistical analysis included paired-samples T- test and Spearman coefficient correlation, with a significance level of 0.05. The coefficient of asymmetry between both sides of the face during rest and muscle contraction was calculated for both groups as follows: research group – ratio Nonparalyzed side/Paralyzed side; control group - Right side/Left side.

3. Results

Surface Electromyography (sEMG) Evaluation

Differences were observed between the research and control groups. Descriptive statistics indicate that the research group presented lower electromyographic values for the resting and smiling conditions than the control group. Greater variability among the recordings was observed for the similing condition for both groups (Table 3).

Descriptive Statistics						
Group	**Condition**	**Side**	**Minimum**	**Maximum**	**Mean**	**SD**
Research	Resting	P (raw data)	2.4	7.30	4.36	1.45
		NP (raw data)	2.2	6.80	3.55	1.07
	Smiling	P (raw data)	4.7	59.70	20.41	14.13
		P (normalized data)	1.75	12.19	4.57	2.59
		NP (raw data)	15.03	183.80	61.67	46.77
		NP (normalized data)	4.42	65.64	18.39	15.37
Control	Resting	R (raw data)	2.21	17.00	6.12	3.40
		L (raw data)	2.25	9.78	5.59	2.35
	Smiling	R (raw data)	15.92	99.26	66.52	23.39
		L (raw data)	21.51	98.75	67.79	19.88
		R (normalized data)	5.84	65.10	15.70	13.57
		L (normalized data)	6.38	40.13	14.33	8.99

*Note: SD – standard deviation; NP – nonparalyzed side; P – paralyzed side; R – right side; L – left side.

Table 3. Surface electromyography descriptive statistics (μV)

When comparing both groups, participants of the research group presented a significant difference between both sides of the face for the resting (p=0.041; T=2.225) and smiling (p=0.001; T=-4.151) conditions. The coefficient of asymmetry was higher for the smiling condition (resting condition mean 1.28±0.42; smiling condition mean 11.48±8.36). On the other hand, participants of the control group did not present significant difference between the right and left sides of the face for the resting (p=0.373; T=0.917) and smiling (p=0.735; T=0.344) conditions. As observed for the research group, the control group also presented a higher coefficient of asymmetry for the smiling condition (resting condition mean 1.10±0.36; smiling condition mean 15.02±8.05).
In order to verify differences between facial asymmetry, the coefficient of asymmetry obtained for the resting and smiling conditions for both groups were compared (Figure 3). Statistical analyses indicated no differences between the groups for the resting (p=0.3; T=-1,288) and for the smiling condition (p=0.848; T=1,235).

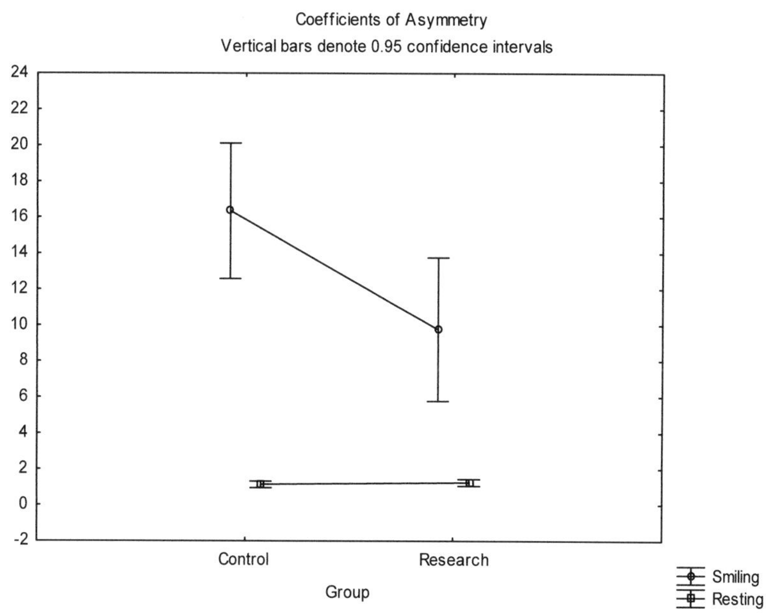

*Note: NP:P - ratio nonparalized side/paralyzed side; R:L- ratio right side/left side

Fig. 3. Coefficients of Asymmetry - Between groups comparison

Facial Disability Index (FDI)

Only participants of the research group answered the Facial Disability Index. The mean Physical Function (PF) subscale value of the FDI was of 70 (Minimum 50; Maximum 95) and of the Social/Well-Being Function (SWBF) subscale was of 68 (Minimum 40; Maximum 92).
Spearman coefficient correlation was performed in order to verify possible associations between the subscales of the FDI and between the coefficient of asymmetry (sEMG) and the subscales of the FDI. Figure 4 shows data dispersion and Table 4 and 5 shows the correlation results between the coefficient of asymmetry for resting and smiling and the FDI subscales.

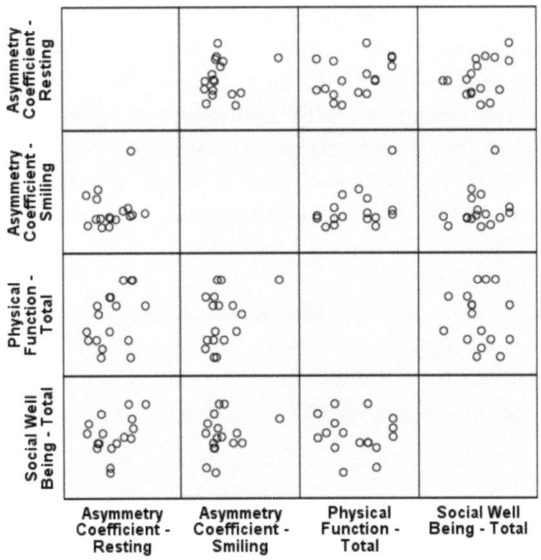

Fig. 4. Correlation between FDI subscales and sEMG - data dispersion

	Question	Correlation Coefficient	Significance
PF	1. Difficulty eating	.317	.215
	2. Difficulty drinking from a cup	.392	.119
	3. Difficulty speaking	.448	.071
	4. Excessive tearing or drying of the eye	.122	.642
	5. Difficulty brushing/rinsing teeth	.300	.242
	Total	.428	.087
SWBF	1. Feel calm and peaceful	.334	.190
	2. Isolate self from people	.269	.296
	3. Irritable toward those around you	.321	.210
	4. Wake up early, wake up several times	-.060	.819
	5. Avoid going out to eat, shop or participate in social activities	.147	.573
	Total	.324	.205

*Note: PF – Physical Function; SWBF – Social/Well being function

Table 4. Spearman correlation between Facial Asymmetry Coefficient for Resting and Scores on the FDI subscales

	Question	Correlation Coefficient	Significance
PF	1. Difficulty eating	.384	.129
	2. Difficulty drinking from a cup	-.266	.302
	3. Difficulty speaking	.133	.610
	4. Excessive tearing or drying of the eye	.344	.177
	5. Difficulty brushing/rinsing teeth	.453	.068
	Total	.333	.192
SWBF	1. Feel calm and peaceful	.571*	.017
	2. Isolate self from people	-.186	.476
	3. Irritable toward those around you	-.031	.907
	4. Wake up early, wake up several times	.286	.265
	5. Avoid going out to eat, shop or participate in social activities	.025	.924
	Total	.276	.284

*Note: PF - Physical Function; SWBF - Social/Well being function; * significant results

Table 5. Spearman correlation between Facial Asymmetry Coefficient for Smiling and Scores on the FDI subscales

Results indicate a significant correlation between the facial asymmetry coefficient for smiling and question one on the SWBF ($p=.017$). Individuals who presented greater differences in sEMG amplitude values when comparing the paralyzed and nonparalyzed sides of the face, tended to present lower scores on the question related to feeling calm and peaceful. No other significant correlations were observed.

4. Discussion

This study analyzed the correlation between electromyographic data of the anguli oris elevators (smile) to the scores obtained in a self-report questionnaire (FDI) in long standing facial paralysis patients. Our results indicated a single correlation between objective (sEMG) and self-assessment measurements; therefore our hypothesis was not confirmed. Although there was a wide variation for muscle activation among the tested individuals (sEMG), our results also indicated that individuals with facial paralysis presented significant differences between the paralyzed and nonparalyzed sides of the face, whereas healthy individuals presented no such differences. These results indicating muscle activation differences between the paralyzed and nonparalyzed side of the face have already been reported in the literature and indicate that the integrity of the facial nerve is essential for the balance and symmetry when producing facial mimetic expressions (Deleyiannis et al., 2005; Salles et al., 2009).

Facial paralysis causes both anatomical and physiological changes. Asymmetries can be caused not only by weaker muscle contractions on the paralyzed side, but also by overactivation of the nonparalyzed side (Pennock et al., 1999). A few consequences tend to appear four months after the onset, with muscle contractures and hypertrophy in association with synkinesis (Diels, 2000). A limiting factor is the viability of the facial muscles, generally because 12 months after nervous degeneration, muscles suffer atrophy very rapidly. In our study, the nonparalyzed side of the face of the research group was approximately 26% less active when compared to the muscle activation of the control group during the smiling condition (comparison for normalized data).

Management of long-standing facial paralysis has been controversial. The inability to smile effectively has been a primary motivator for surgical and nonsurgical management of the face after facial nerve palsy (Ross et al., 1991; Pennock et al., 1999; Croxson et al., 2000; Diels, 2000; VanSwearingen & Brach, 2003; Beurskens, 2004; Vaiman et al., 2005; Coulson et al., 2006; Tate & Tollefson, 2006; Salles et al., 2009). Nonsurgical management include application of botulinum toxin, phsysiotherapy techniques and muscle retraining such as mime therapy, electromyographic biofeedback and specific facial exercises. Problematically, even well-designed studies often reflect differing results, based on the inherent difficulty in precisely measuring recovery (Pinna, Testa & Fukuda, 2004; Beurskens, Heymans & Oostendorp, 2006; Hadlock, 2008; Ghali, MacQuillan & Grobbelaar, 2011). Once the field of facial nerve management reaches a consensus on quantitative facial function analysis and global results comparisons, the role of muscle retraining techniques will be clarified.

Literature has shown that the normal human face presents 6% of asymmetry during the production facial mimetic expressions (Burres, 1985). These differences were observed when combining linear measurements and integrated invasive electromyography (iEMG) and would correspond to asymmetries in anatomy, in muscle contraction caused by non-balanced forces and due to differences in measuring techniques. Our study found no such difference in muscle activation when comparing the right and left sides of the face in healthy individuals. However, the coefficient of asymmetry suggests some degree of facial asymmetry in the control group. Surface electromyography is less specific for measuring muscle activation than invasive electromyography, this will probably account for the differences in result in our study and the later. According to Castroflorio et al. (2006), methodological factors associated with the recording of sEMG may have been the cause of controversial results reported in different studies developed with muscles of the head and neck. Although no studies using sEMG for the assessment of facial paralysis where found in the literature and despite the problems with methodological difficulties inherent to use of sEMG, applications of this technological device in facial muscles seem to be promising. Moreover, technological advances in signal detection and processing have improved the quality of the information extracted from sEMG and furthered our understanding of the anatomy and physiology of the stomatognathic apparatus.

Although the literature points that FDI subscales produce reliable measurements for reporting outcomes for individuals with disorders of the facial motor system (VanSwearingen & Brach, 2003) and even to report treatment outcomes (Salles et al., 2009), our study found no correlation between these subscales and objective measurements. This fact should be carefully examined. In our study we only measured muscle activity of the anguli oris elevators (zygomaticus major and minor, levator anguli oris), mostly related to smiling. Questions on the Physical Function subscale are largely related to the functions

developed by the orbicularis oris and buccinators, the investigation of these muscles should be explored in futures studies of facial paralysis using sEMG.
The only significant correlation observed was between facial asymmetry and the question related to feeling calm and peaceful on Social/Well-being Function subscale. The literature points that facial nerve dysfunction can be a devastating handicap. Facial nerve dysfunction may be classified into two components: facial impairment which describes the anatomical abnormality, and facial disability which pertains to the functional and social deficits caused by the impairments (Saito & Cheung, 2010). Studies have shown a significant relationship of acquired facial palsy with depression, anxiety and high levels of psychological stress (Bull, 1998; VanSwearigen et al., 1998; Bradbury, Simons & Sanders, 2006).

5. Conclusion

The use of modern scientific techniques of data analysis, such as the use of sEMG, combined with self-report measurements most certainly offers great promise to clinicians and their patients. The FDI seems the capture information that goes beyond strict muscle function, i.e. the impairment rather than the function level. The combination of different measurements in randomized trials examining whether, or what type of therapy design offers optimal benefit to patients suffering from facial paralysis should be our future initiative.

6. Acknowledgements

This research was supported by grant from FAPESP (Process no. 2008/02687-5)

7. References

Atolini Junior N, Jorge Junior JJ, Gignon VF, Kitice AT, Prado LSA, Santos VGW. Facial nerve palsy: incidence of different ethiologies in a tertiary ambulatory. International Archives of Otohinolaryngology. 2009; 167-171.

Balliet R, Shinn JB, Bach-Y-Rita P. Facial paralysis rehabilitation: retraining selective muscle control. International Rehabilitation Medicine. 1982: 4:67-74.

Barbotte E, Guillemin F, Chau N, Lorhandicap group. Prevalence of impairment, disabilities, handicaps and quality of life in the general population: a review of the literature. Bulletin of the World Health Organization. 2001;79:1047-1055.

Berg T, Jonsson L, Engström M. Agreement between the Sunnybrook, House-Brackmann, and Yanagihara facial nerve grading systems in Bell's palsy. Otology & Neurotology. 2004; 25:1020-1026.

Beurskens C. Positive effects of mime therapy on sequelae of facial paralysis: stiffness, lip mobility, and social and physical aspects of facial disability. Journal of Otology & Neurotology. 2004; 24:2003.

Beurskens CHG, Heymans PG, Oostendorp RAB. Stability of benefits of mime therapy in sequelae of facial nerve paresis during a 1-year period. Otology & Neurotology. 2006; 27:1037-1042.

Brach JS, VanSwearingen JM, Lenert J, Jonhson PC. Facial neuromuscular retraining for oral synkinesis. Plastic Reconstructive Surgery. 1997; 99:1922-31.

Bradbury ET, Simons W, Sanders R. Psychological and social factors in reconstructive surgery for hemi-facial palsy. Journal of Plastic Reconstructive Aesthetic Surgery. 2006; 59:272-278.

Bull R, Rumsey N. The social psychology of facial appearance. Berlin: Springer, 1988.

Burres SA. Facial biomechanics: the standards of normal. Laryngoscope. 1985; 95(6):708-714.

Castroflorio T, Icardi K, Becchino B, Merlo E, Debernardi C, Bracco P, Farina D. Reproductibility of surface EMG variables in isometric sub-maximal contractions of jaw elevator muscles. Journal of Electromyography Kinesiology. 2006; 16:498-505.

Coulson SE, Adams RD, O'Dwyer NJ, Croxson GR. Physiotherapy rehabilitation of the smile after long-term facial nerve palsy using video self-modeling and implementation intentions. Otolaryngology - Head and Neck Surgery. 2006; 134:48-55.

Cronin GW, Steenerson RL. The effectiveness of neuromuscular facial retraining combined with electromyography in facial paralysis. Otolaryngology - Head and Neck Surgery. 2003; 128(4):534-538.

Croxson G, Quinn M, Coulson S. Temporalis muscle transfer. A further refinement. Facial Plastic Surgery. 2000; 16:351-356.

Daniel B, Guitar B. EMG feedback and recovery of facial and speech gestures following neural anastomosis. Journal of Speech and Hearing Disorders. 1978; 43:9-20.

De Luca CJ. The use of surface electromyography in biomechanics. Journal of Applied Biomechanics. 1997; 13(2):135-163.

Deleyiannis FW, Askari M, Schmidt KL, Henkelmann TC, VanSwearingen JM, Manders EK. Muscle activity in the partially paralyzed face after placement of a fascial sling: preliminary report. Annals of Plastic Surgery. 2005; 55(5):449-455.

Diels HJ. Facial paralysis: is there a role for a therapist? Facial Plastic Surgery. 2000; 16:361-364.

Finn JC, Cox SE, Earl ML. Social implications of hyperfunctional facial lines. Dermatologic Surgery. 2003; 29:450-455.

Garcia RB, Pérez SC, Suárez-Varela MM, Torella ME, Galofre JD. Sequelae of peripheral facial palsy. Acta Otorrinolaringológica Española. 2010; 61:89-93.

Ghali S, MacQuillan A, Gobbelaar AO. Reanimation of the middle and lower face in facial paralysis: review of the literature and personal approach. Journal of Plastic, Reconstructive and Aesthetic Surgery. 2011; 64:423-431.

Gonçalves-Coelho TD, Pinheiro CN, Ferraz EV, Alonson-Nieto JL. Clusters of Bell's palsy. Arquivos de Neuropsiquiatria. 1997; 55:722-727.

Hadlock T. Facial paralysis: research and future directions. Facial Plastic Surgery. 2008; 24(2): 260-266.

House JW, Brackmann DE. Facial Nerve grading system. Otolaryngology - Head and Neck Surgery. 1985; 93(2):146-147.

Kang TS, Vrabec JT, Giddings N, Terris DJ. Facial Nerve Grading Systems (1985–2002): Beyond the House-Brackmann Scale. Otology & Neurotology. 2002; .23(5):767-771.

Kayhan FT, Zurakowski D, Rauch SD. Toronto facial grading system: interobserver reliability. Otolaryngol Head and Neck Surgery. 2000; 122(2):212-215.

Keillor JM, Barrett AM, Crucian GP, Kortenkamp S, Helman KM. Emotional experience and perception in the absence of facial feedback. Journal of the International Neuropsychology Society. 2002; 8:130-135.

Kukimoto N, Ikeda M, Yamada K, Tanaka M, Tsurumachi M, Tomita H. Viral infections in acute peripheral facial paralysis. Nationwide analysis centering on CF. Acta Otolaryngology [Suppl] (Stokh). 1988; 97:3-4

Lee J, Fung K, Lownie SP, Parnes LS. Assessing impairment and disability of facial paralysis in patients with vestibular schwannoma. Archives of Otolaryngology Head and Neck Surgery. 2007; 133:56-70.

Linstrom CJ, Silverman CA, Susman WM. Facial –motion analysis with a video and computer system: a preliminary report. American Journal of Otology. 2000; 21(1):123-9.

Linstrom CJ. Objective facial motion analysis in patients with facial nerve dysfunction. Laryngoscope. 2002; 112: 1129-1147.

May M, Croxson G, Klein S. Bell's palsy. Management of using EMG rehabilitation, botulinum toxin and surgery. American Journal of Otolaryngology. 1989; 10:220-229.

Mehta RP, Zhang S, Hadlock TA. Novel 3-D video for quantification of facial movement. Otolaryngology - Head and Neck Surgery. 2008; 138(4): 468-472.

Odebode TO, Ologe FE. Facial nerve palsy after head injury: case incidence, causes, clinical profile and outcome. The Journal of Trauma. 2006; 61:388-391.

Peitersen E. The natural history of Bell's palsy. American Journal of Otolaryngology. 1982; 4:107.

Pennock JD, Peter C, Manders EK, VanSwearingen JM. Relationship between muscle activity of the frontalis and the associated brow displacement. Plastic & Reconstructive Surgery. 1999; 104(6):1789-1797.

Pinna BR, Testa JRG, Fukuda Y. Traumatic facial paralysis's study: clinical and surgical review. Revista Brasileira de Otorrinolaringologia. 2004; 70:479-482.

Proctor B, Corgill DA, Proud G. The pathology of Bell's palsy. Transactions of the American Academy of Ophtalmology and Otolaryngology. 1976;82:ORL 70-80.

Morgan M, Nathwani D. Facial Palsy and Infection: The Unfolding Story. Clinical Infectious Diseases. 1992;14:263-71.

Rosenberg SI. Natural history of acoustic neuromas. Laryngoscope. 2000; 110:497-508.

Ross B, NNedzelski JM, McLean JA. Efficacy of feedback training in long-standing facial nerve paresis. Laryngoscope. 1991; 101:744-750.

Sackett D, Strauss, SE, Richardson WS, Rosemberg W, Haynes RB. Evidence-based medicine: how to practice and teach EMB. Edinburgh:Churchill Livingstone, 2nd ed, 2000. P.436.

Saito DM, Cheung SW. A comparison of facial nerve disability between patients with Bell's palsy and vestibular shwannoma. Journal of Clinical Neuroscience. 2010; 17:1122-1125.

Salles AG, Toledo AN, Ferreira MC. Botulinum toxin injection in long-standing facial paralysis patients: improvement of facial symmetry observed up to 6 months. Aesthetic Plastic Surgery. 2009; 33:582-590.

Segal B, Zompa I, Danys I, Black M, Shapiro M, Melmed C, Arthurs B. Symmetry and synkinesis during rehabilitation of unilateral facial paralysis. Journal of Otolaryngology. 1995; 24:143-148.

Seikel JA, King DW, Darmright DG. Anatomy & Physiology for Speech, Language and Hearing. 4th ed,. Delmar Cengage Learning: New York, 2010.

Tate JR, Tollefson TT. Advances in facial reanimation. Current Opinion on Otolaryngology Head and Neck Surgery. 2006; 14:242-248.

Vaiman M, Shlamkovich N, Kessler A, Eviatar E, Segal S. Biofeedback training of nasal muscles using internal and external surface electromyography of the nose. American Journal of Otolaryngology. 2005; 26:302-307.

Van de Graaf RC, Nicolai JP. Bell's palsy before Bell: Cornelis Stalpart van der Wiel's observation of Bell's palsy in 1683. Otology Neurotology. 2005; 26:1235-1238.

VanSwearingen JM, Brach JS. The facial disability index: reliability and validity of a disability assessment instrument for disorders of the facial neuromuscular system. Physical Therapy. 1996; 76:1288-1300.

VanSwearingen JM, Cohn JF, Turnbull J, Mrzai T, Johnson P. Psychological distress: linking impairment with disability in facial neuromotor disorders. Otolaryngology Head and Neck Surgery. 1998; 118:790-796.

VanSwearingen JM, Brach JS. Changes in facial movement and synkinesis with facial neuromuscular reeducation. Plastic Reconstructive Surgery. 2003; 111:2370-2375.

Wilson JB, Cleary PD. Linking clinical variables with health-related quality of life. JAMA. 1995; 273:59-65.

Yeo SW, Lee DH, Jun BC, Chang KH, Park YS. Analysis of prognostic factors in Bell's palsy and Ramsay Hunt syndrome. Auris Nasus Larynx. 2007; 34:159-164.

22

Movement-Related Cortical Potentials Associated with Oral and Facial Functions in Humans

Nakajima Ichiro, Oka Schunichi,
Ohba Hiroiku and Yoshida Masafumi
*Nihon University School of Dentistry,
Japan*

1. Introduction

It is possible to record the electrical activities of the human brain by placing electrodes on the surface of the scalp. Event-related potentials (ERPs) are the cortical potentials associated with higher brain functions of perception, cognition and movement in humans. They are regarded as manifestations of brain activities that occur in preparation for, or in response to, discrete events (internal or external factors). ERPs can be considered to be one of the useful indicators for understanding information processing of the human brain, as well as other measurement techniques for brain activity, such as positron emission tomography (PET), functional magnetic resonance imaging (fMRI), magnetoencephalography (MEG).
Movement-related cortical potentials (MRCPs) and contingent negative variations (CNVs) are classified into ERPs that are related to the preparation, execution, and evaluation of motor responses. There have been many research reports on the diagnosis of patients with neurological motor diseases based on the recording of these potentials. Presently, the recording of these potentials is the most established method in cognitive and behavioral sciences among noninvasive human brain imaging methods.
In recent years, there has been a growing need for the accurate diagnosis and treatment of patients with dysphagia. For the development of research on dysphagia, it is necessary to clarify the nervous system of mastication and swallowing in the maxillofacial regions. However, there have been fewer reports on maxillofacial movements than on other body movements (i.e., hand, finger, and foot movements). To clarify how motor preparation processes of the brain are affected by the features of jaw muscle activities of maxillofacial regions, we have investigated the scalp distribution and waveform components of MRCPs and CNVs in relation to oral and facial functions in humans. We demonstrated that MRCPs and CNVs necessarily occur in humans during oral and facial motor tasks, reflecting the features of cognitive and motor functions of the neural system. In this chapter, therefore, we review the findings of previous studies and discuss the importance of establishing neurological research of oral and facial motor disorders based on these ERPs.
The contents of this chapter are as follows.

1. Mastication and swallowing.
2. Pain research using somatosensory evoked potentials.
3. MRCPs associated with jaw movements in humans.
4. CNVs associated with swallowing in humans.
5. Wavelet transform analysis for ERPs associated with jaw motor function.
6. Frequency changes of jaw muscle activity during reaction to a warning signal.

Furthermore, in this chapter, we discuss their implications in both future research and practice.

2. Mastication and swallowing

Mastication and swallowing are two tightly integrated components of food intake behavior. Jaw muscle activity is a basic parameter related to both chewing and swallowing. Both movements are controlled by complicated neural mechanisms involving the central pattern generator (CPG) in the brainstem as compared with mechanisms for other body movements. It is noteworthy that the motor cortices have an important role in the fine control and coordination of these oral and facial functions.

2.1 Mastication

Mastication is the action of breaking down food, in preparation for deglutition. This action involves a complex highly organized neuromuscular and digestive activities that, in normal individuals, integrate the various components of the masticatory system, such as the teeth and their investing structures, the muscles, the temporomandibular joints, the lips, the cheeks, the palate, the tongue, and the salivary glands. The aim of chewing is to crush, triturate, and mix food with saliva, so that food can be transported by deglutition down the digestive canal. The masticatory muscle is not only an agonist of an actual jaw movement but also a sensory organ involved in sensing the mandible position through stretch receptors (Morimoto et al., 1983). An overview of the neural system of mastication is shown in Fig. 1. Figure 1A shows examples of recordings of jaw muscle EMG activity during mastication. The masseter muscle (jaw-closing muscle) and digastric muscle (jaw- opening muscle) are alternately activated and produce rhythmical jaw movements during mastication. Figure 1 B shows a schema of the neural mechanism of mastication. Mastication is controlled by a rhythmical contraction of bilateral jaw-closing and jaw-opening muscle groups under the control of CPG in the brainstem (Lund & Kolta, 2006). From the results of animal studies, it has been found that the fundamental pattern of mastication—rhythmic opening and closing of the jaws—and the associated repetitive movements of the tongue, cheeks, and lips can be generated by a brainstem CPG in the absence of sensory feedback. On the other hand, oral sensation information from the peripheral sensory receptors (periodontal membrane, oral mucous membrane, and masticatory muscles) is also inputted in the central nervous system to control jaw movements intricately. On the other hand, the activity of most neurons in the masticatory cortex is higher during ingestion than during mastication, suggesting a major role of these neurons in setting the parameters of the first bite. In many species, including the cat, rabbit, and monkey, repetitive electrical stimulation of a certain area in the cerebral cortex induces coordinated rhythmic movement of the jaw and tongue (Nakamura & Katakura, 1995).

Recent studies by fMRI and PET in humans have revealed that several regions of the brain are activated during mastication, including the primary somatosensory cortex (SI),

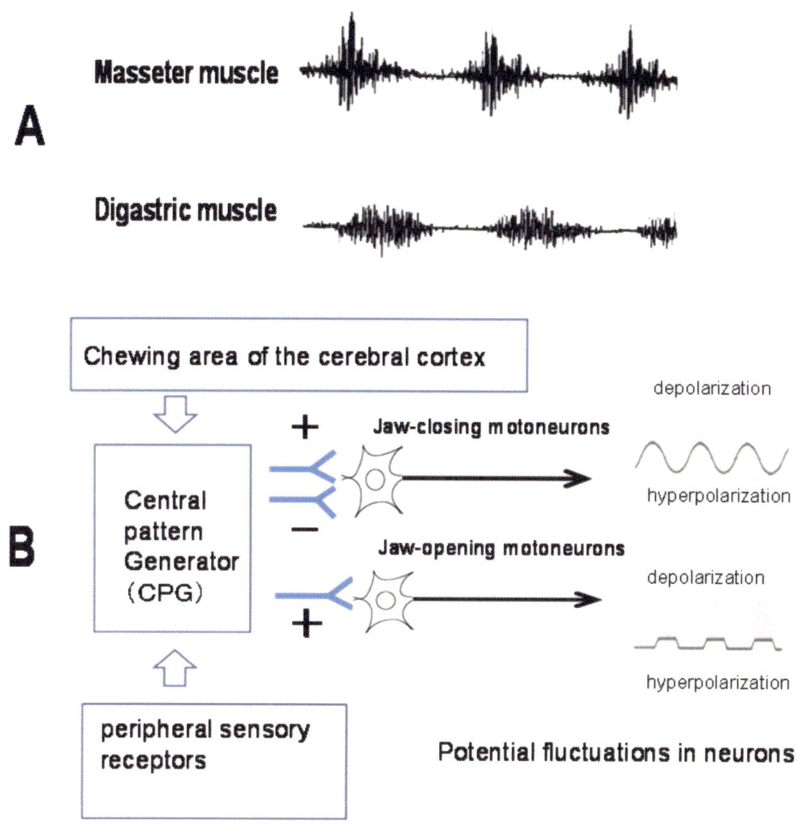

Fig. 1. Neural system of mastication. (Modified from Inoue T, 2008)
A: Masticatory muscle activities during chewing; B: Generation of masticatory rhythm in the brainstem. Efferent/afferent impulses are indicated by arrows.

primary motor cortex (MI), supplementary motor area (SMA), premotor area (PM), prefrontal cortex (PFC), insula, posterior parietal cortex (PPC), thalamus, striatum, and cerebellum (Momose et al., 1997; Onozuka et al., 2002). However, it is still unclarified how CPG in the brainstem is controlled by the cerebral cortex in humans.

2.2 Swallowing

Swallowing consists of three phases, the oral, pharyngeal, and esophageal phases. In swallowing, many orofacial muscles are activated during jaw-closing movements. Figure 2 shows an example of EMG recording during the swallowing of water in a human subject. It has been presumed that in volitional swallowing, cortical control is dominant in the oral phase, whereas the swallowing reflex arising from the brainstems is dominant in the later phases.

From the results of animal studies, it has been found that the sequential and rhythmic patterns of swallowing are formed and organized by CPG. CPG can be subdivided into three systems (Andre´, 2001):

- The afferent system corresponding to the central and peripheral inputs to the center

- The efferent system corresponding to the outputs from the center, consisting of various motoneuron pools involved in swallowing
- The organizing system located in the medulla oblongata, corresponding to the interneuronal network that programs the motor pattern

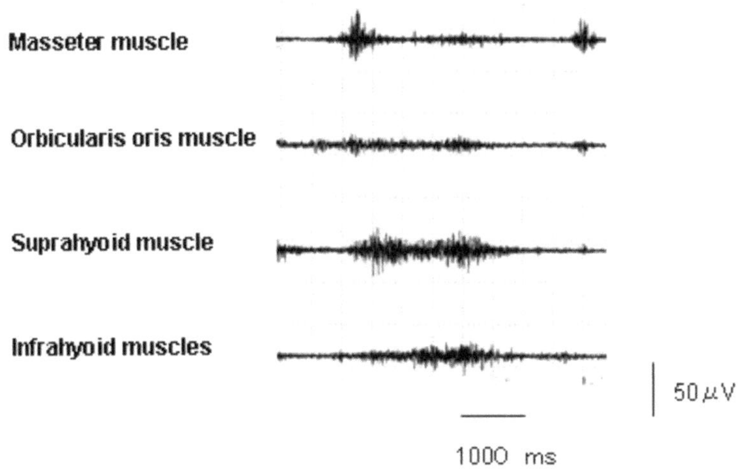

Fig. 2. Example of EMG recording of swallowing.

Recent neuroimaging studies using various techniques, such as PET, f-MRI, and MEG, have revealed that swallowing activates multiple cerebral regions including the face area of the primary sensorimotor cortex, premotor cortex, insular cortex, frontal operculum, anterior cingulate cortex, and other cerebral regions (Dziewas et al., 2003; Hamdy et al., 1999; Hamdy et al., 2000; Kern et al., 2001;Watanabe et al., 2004; Toogood et al., 2005). In particular, f-MRI research revealed that multiple cerebral regions are recruited during swallowing, most notably the anterior cingulate cortex, pericentral cortex, insula, and premotor cortex, with different degrees of symmetry between hemispheres. These findings are consistent with those of previous PET activation studies of swallowing, that showed a similar recruitment pattern, thereby demonstrating strong and relatively direct connections from the regions of the motor and premotor cortices to the muscles of the pharynx and esophagus.
However, the limitations of these techniques are as follows. f-MRI cannot distinguish among cortical activities before, during, and after swallowing, given that changes in f-MRI signal intensity signal reflect the average cortical activity throughout all phases of swallowing. Although MEG is often considered a complementary technique with a higher temporal resolution, it also has some limitations because magnetic fields generated deep within brain tissues decay rapidly over distance and are less likely to be detected at the surface than electrical fields. Thus, the correspondence between the phases of swallowing and various cortical activities has not been elucidated completely.

3. Maxillofacial pain research using somatosensory evoked potentials (SEPs)

Pain, an intimately personal phenomenon, is difficult to assess. There are many studies of oral pain sensation in humans. In this section, we introduce some studies of SEPs in oral sensation and pain sensation.

3.1 Overview of SEPs

Evoked potentials are electrical signals generated by the nervous system in response to sensory stimuli. Auditory, visual, and somatosensory stimuli are used commonly in clinical evoked potential studies. SEPs consist of a series of waves that reflect the sequential activation of neural structures along the somatosensory pathways. Although SEPs can be elicited by mechanical stimulation, clinical studies use electrical stimulation of peripheral nerves, which induces larger and more robust responses.

3.2 Pain research using SEPs

To measure pain, it is important that subjective and objective methods should be performed simultaneously. Pain-related evoked potentials are commonly used in studies in which pain-related brain activities in humans are objectively evaluated. N150 and P250 are the two major components constantly recorded in pain-related evoked potentials. Using this late evoked potential, we have conducted a few studies as follows.

Commercially prepared local anesthetic solutions usually contain a vasoconstrictor agent in dental treatment. First, therefore, we evaluated the effects of different types and concentrations of the vasoconstrictors on local anesthesia. Twelve young healthy volunteers from 18 to 24 years old participated in this study. To estimate subjective pain intensity, the visual analogue scale (VAS) was used. To estimate objective pain intensity, the late component of SEPs recorded from the vertex was analyzed. On the basis of Oono's method (Oono et al., 2008), a monopolar electrode was fixed to the surface of the upper central incisors and single electrical square pulses were administrated at 1 Hz. In this study, stimuli inducing bearable pain sensation (VAS = 5 -7) were administered. After baseline VAS score and SEP were determined, one of the local anesthetics was injected, and then postinjection VAS score and SEP were determined 22 times. The local anesthetics tested in this study were as follows: 2% lidocaine with 1/80,000 adrenaline (EL-8), 2% lidocaine with 1/200,000 adrenaline (EL-20), 2% lidocaine with 1/300,000 adrenaline (EL-30), 2% lidocaine (L), and 3% propitocaine with 0.03 IU felypressin (FP). Each local anesthetic (0.5 ml) was injected into the gingiva.

Five minutes after the injection of each local anesthetic, all the subjects felt numbness throughout their mouth. There were no distinguishable SEP components and their mean VAS score markedly decreased to zero. After the injection of a local anesthetic, the time of the reappearance of SEPs agreed with the time of increase in VAS score from zero. The following shows the duration of the effect of each local anesthetic as determined from VAS score and SEPs. EL-20 showed the same duration of its anesthetic effect as EL-8, but EL-30, and FP showed shorter durations than EL-20. These findings suggest that SEP assessment serves as a useful method for the study of dental analgesic and anesthetic agents in humans.

Second, we examined SEPs in subjects inhaling graded concentrations of nitrous oxide (N_2O) in oxygen (O_2) (Oka et al., 2007). In dental practice, a nitrous oxide inhalation sedation technique is usually used for the patients, to reduce their pain and anxiety. In this study, we used various mixture concentrations of N_2O in O_2 (0%, 10%, 30% and 50%), and measured and analyzed SEP and VAS scores in responses to painful electrical fingertip stimulation using the standard method first introduced by Bromm and Chen at high and low intensities in 15 volunteers (Bromm & Chen, 1995). Mixed effect model statistical analyses revealed that SEP and VAS score decreased significantly with increasing mixture concentration (Fig. 3)

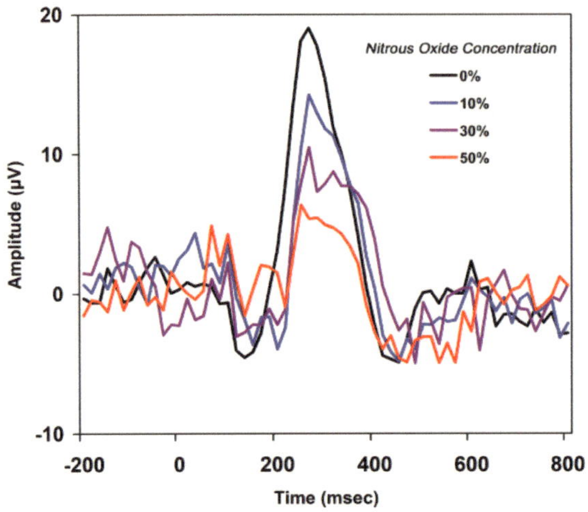

Fig. 3. Relationship between SEP amplitude and N_2O concentration.

Clinical observations suggest that the perceived intensity of a painful event increases as the unpredictability of its occurrence increases. Therefore, third, we examined the effect of varying stimulus predictability on SEP and pain report (PR) and fear report (FR) scores in 25 healthy volunteers experiencing repeated noxious fingertip shocks (Oka et al., 2010). Each volunteer was exposed to high and low stimulus intensities administered in four stimulus patterns defined by the stimulus sequence (SEQ) and interstimulus interval (ISI) as follows: A) serial stimulus intensity SEQ with a fixed ISI; B) serial stimulus intensity SEQ with varying ISI; C) random stimulus intensity SEQ with fixed ISI; and D) random stimulus intensity SEQ with varying ISI. Results revealed that a lower stimulus predictability led to higher PR and FR scores, and a greater SEP amplitude. These results would conform with the hypothesis that a low stimulus predictability is associated with high PR and FR scores, and a larger SEP amplitude.

The amplitudes of N150 and P250 components are considered to reflect the intensity of perceived pain (Kakigi et al., 2000), and reflect the activities of operculoinsular and cingular cortices, respectively (Iannetti, et al., 1990; Tarkka & Treede, 1993). Numerous investigators have used SEP extensively to study both pain and fear. Recent studies have shown that both the N 150 and P250 peaks are related, at least for some types of stimulus, to the orienting response (Dowman, 2004; Dowman et al., 2007). Nociceptive processing intrinsically involves attentional factors (Bushnell et al., 1985). Pain-related SEP may indicate, in part, attention to a threatening stimulus (Yamasaki, et al., 2000). Some investigators have found that N 150 base-to-peak amplitude-amplitude is related to attentional processing (Gratton et al., 1990; Miltner & Weiss, 1998). Others have reported that pain-related P250 is sensitive to attention (Lorenz & Garcia, 2003).

These findings indicate that SEP appears to be a useful indicator in studies of the analgesic effect and in psychological studies.

4. MRCPs and CNVs

Recently, noninvasive techniques for human brain mapping during movement have been developed in the fields of clinical neurophysiology. In general, these brain mapping techniques are mainly classified into two types on the basis of their parameters measured, that is, electrophysiological and hemodynamic responses (Shibasaki, 2008). The former type includes EEG and MEG, and the latter type includes PET and fMRI. The former type has a higher temporal resolution than the latter type. In contrast, the former has a lower spatial resolution than the latter. On the other hand, EEG has been commonly used for many years because of it being a simple analytical technique in addition to its excellent temporal resolution. Thus, various cortical potentials reflecting higher central nervous system functions in humans (cognitive, motor, and sensory functions) can be obtained by averaging EEG data. Today, clinical EEG analysis is well developed for the diagnosis of brain functions in patients with neurological motor diseases. Cortical potentials obtained by EEG that are related to motor responses can be classified into MRCPs and CNVs.

4.1 Overview of MRCPs

MRCP is a slow negative potential in an electroencephalographic recording that occurs about 2 s before voluntary movement production in humans (Kornhuber & Deecke, 1964). MRCP is obtained by averaging EEG data before the onset of voluntary movement. This potential reflects the cortical processes involved in movement planning and movement preparation. In general, MRCP consists of two main components, Bereitschaftspotential and negative slope (Shibasaki et al., 1980; Ikeda et al., 1992). A schema of MRCP waveform is shown in Fig.4. Ikeda et al. (1992) have determined the cortical source of MRCPs by the direct recording of cortical potentials through chronically implanted subdural electrodes in patients with epilepsy as part of presurgical evaluation.

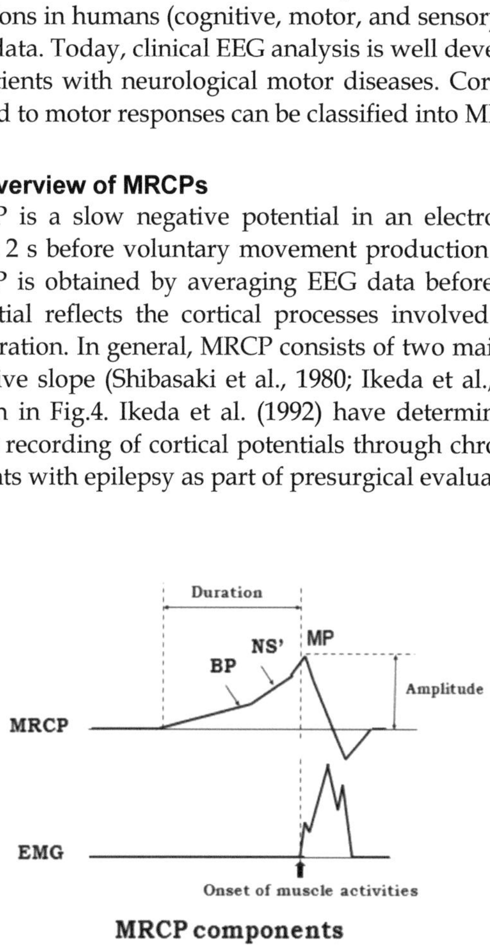

(1) Bereitschaftspotential (BP): BP is a gradually increasing, bilaterally widespread surface negativity with the maximum over the midline vertex region regardless of the site of movement, beginning about 1-1.5 s before the movement onset.

(2)Negative slope (NS'):NS' is a much steeper slope starting about 400 ms before the movement onset, and is characterized by a more localized negativity over the central and vertex regions contralateral to the movement.

(3)Motor potential (MP): MP is well localized to a small area of the contralateral central scalp, corresponding to the movement site, and occurs immediately before the movement onset.

Fig. 4. Schema of MRCP waveform.

From extensive studies, it is the current consensus that BP starts first in the SMA including pre-SMA and SMA itself, and then shortly thereafter in the lateral premotor cortices bilaterally. About 400 ms prior to the movement onset, NS′ starts in M1 and the premotor cortex mainly contralaterally. In general, MRCPs recorded from Cz over the human scalp are considered to reflect SMA activity.

MRCPs are also generated from subcortical structures. Sasaki et al. (1981) reported that in monkeys trained to perform spontaneous hand movements, MRCPs recorded before the initiation of movement disappear following cerebellum resection. Ikeda et al. (1994) reported that in cerebellar infarction patients performing an upper-limb movement task, no MRCP was recorded.

4.2 Features of MRCPs associated with jaw movements

Unilateral limb movements on the unilateral side are controlled mainly from the contralateral hemisphere. Recently, it has been clarified that there are differences in the features of the waveform components of MRCPs between the limb and jaw motor tasks.

Figure 5 shows a typical example of grand averaged waveforms of MRCPs associated with jaw-closing movements in eight subjects. Negative potentials appeared bilaterally and symmetrically approximately 1.5 s before the onset of jaw-closing muscle EMG activity.

The amplitudes of the cortical potentials preceding jaw closing can be classified into two components: BP, the cortical negative potential that initially develops slowly 1.0-1.5 s before the onset of EMG activity; and NS', the gradient of BP that rapidly develops 100-200 ms before the onset of EMG activity. These components are consistent with those of MRCPs associated with limb movements. After the movement onset, it was difficult to identify motor potential, because cortical potentials were mixed with jaw muscle EMGs. It is concluded that the supplementary motor area is necessarily activated preceding the onset of jaw movements as well as limb movements. However, MRCPs associated with jaw biting movements are different from those associated with limb movement, with respect to the NS' component. Previously, we compared the distribution of MRCPs on both sides of the scalp preceding jaw biting movements in 10 healthy subjects (Nakajima et al. 1991).

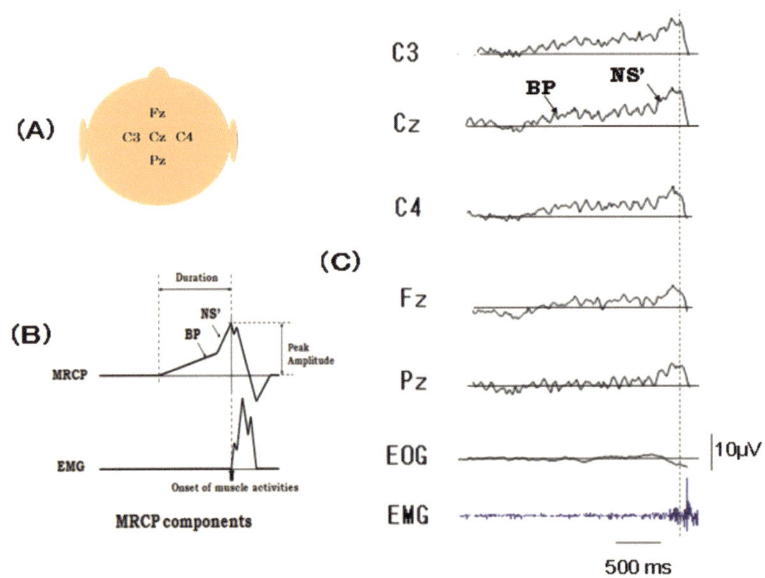

Fig. 5. Grand averaged waveforms of MRCPs associated with jaw-closing motor task in eight subjects. (A): Recording sites of EEGs. (B): MRCP components. (C): MRCP waveforms recorded at five electrodes.

In this study, a subject made a biting movement as instructed, with a 0.5-cm thick gauze pad held between the upper and lower molars on the right or left side, permitting ample biting motion. Figure 6 shows examples of the three traces of MRCPs from five regions of the scalp obtained on different days with a 1-week interval in the same subject.

BPs were recorded from the midline-central, central, and temporal areas of the scalp in accordance with the international 10–20 system, preceding self-paced biting on one side. The cortical negative potentials began 1.0-1.5 s before the EMG activity onset of the masseter muscle. All of these negative potentials could be considered to be BPs, and the additional NS' appeared 70-80 ms before the EMG activity onset of the masseter muscle. BPs were detected from all the recorded regions of the scalp, whereas NS's were observed only from the bilateral temporal areas. In contrast, NS's were more frequently detected on the side contralateral to the wrist movement in this subject. This is consistent with previous reports. There was a difference in the localization of the MRCP components between unilateral biting and wrist movements.

In this study, the amplitudes of BPs and NSs were largest in the temporal areas that were ipsilateral to the side of biting movement in all subjects.

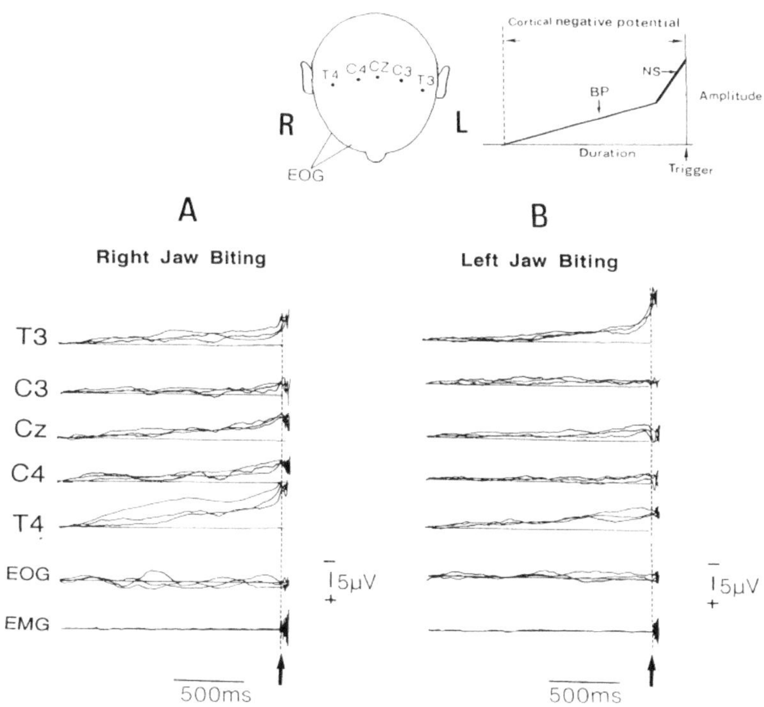

Fig. 6. Examples of cortical potentials preceding unilateral biting on either the right or left side. (From Nakajima et al. 1991)

This difference in localization indicated that impulses from the biting area of the human cerebral cortex descending to the masseter muscle on the ipsilateral side are more powerful than those on the side contralateral to the biting.

Yoshida et al. (2000) compared the MRCPs accompanying various mandibular movements to study the motor control mechanism underlying these movements. The cortical maps of BP/NS' (BP and NS' combined), immediately prior to mouth opening and closing, showed a symmetrical distribution, whereas those for the lateral movements tended to predominate over the hemisphere ipsilateral to the direction of the movement. They found that BP/NS' amplitudes at the onset of movement differed significantly or tended to differ between mouth opening, mouth closing, and lateral movements. There is a significant difference in the relationship between MRCP components and the agonist muscle activities during the jaw and limb movements.

The above-mentioned findings indicate that the lateral movements of the mandible may be controlled mainly from the ipsilateral hemisphere. This control might be explained in terms of the complicated coordination of the bilateral muscles in the maxillofacial areas in humans.

However, the amplitude of a component's peak identified at one electrode location can radically change and sometimes even cross the zero baseline and switch polarity as a function of the position of the reference electrode. That is, MRCP amplitudes do not represent absolute values of electrical brain activities because of the position of the reference electrode and the use of a limited montage (Desmedt et al., 1990; Michel et al., 2004). Therefore, it is necessary to validate the results obtained by other research methods.

Figure 7 shows examples of averaged fMR images of the human cortex during the jaw-biting motor task on the right side (habitual biting side) in six subjects.

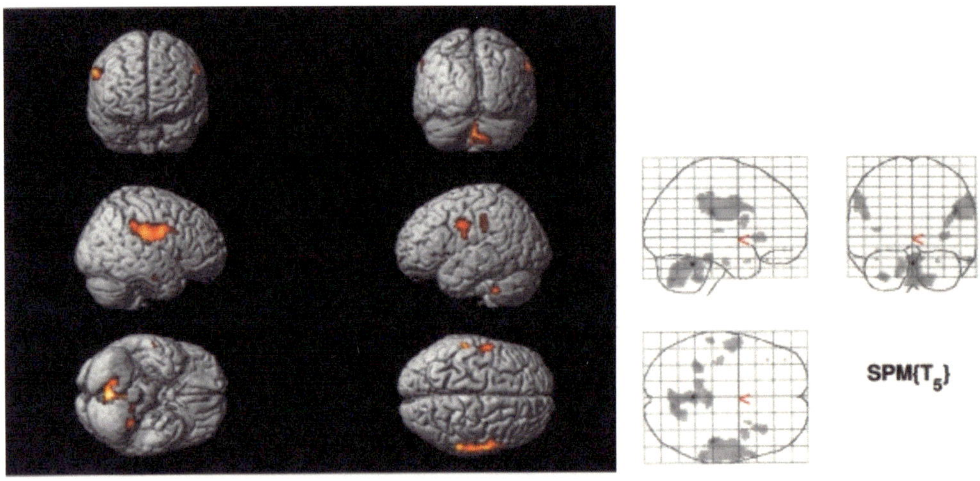

Fig. 7. fMRI recording during unilateral jaw-biting motor task in six subjects.

MRI (Toshiba VISART-EX 1.5T) was carried out in this study. Functional MR images were obtained using a superconducting MRI scanner at 1.5 tesla. To enhance blood oxygenation level (BOLD) contrast, images were taken in a T2-weighted echo-planar imaging (EPI) sequence. The imaging conditions were as follows: field of view (FOV), 240 mm; repetition time (TR)/echo time (TE), 4000/45 ms; flip angle, 90 deg; and slice thickness, 8.0 mm. The transverse thickness, 8.0 mm. EPI conditions were as follows. The entire brain was dissected into 18 slices (8 mm/slice for the longitudinal axis of the body; slice thickness, 8 mm). The EPI resolution (voxel) was $2.5 \times 2.5 \times 8$ mm^3. T1-weighted autopsy images were also taken at the same position and using the same number of slices. The image resolution was $1 \times 1 \times 8$ mm^3. The data obtained from all the subjects were analyzed by the t-test using Statistical Parametric Mapping, SPM99. Areas showing activation with a statistical significance of $p<0.01$ were considered to be "activated" and extracted for the standard brain. In this study, the subjects were instructed to strongly bite on a 3-cm-thick plastic block held between the upper and lower molars on the right side, for 30 s.

As seen in Fig. 7, the sensorimotor areas were strongly activated on the side ipsilateral to the side of biting movement. It is possible to confirm the activation of the sensorimotor area corresponding to the jaw biting movements, on the basis of the changes in cerebral blood flow. This suggests the possibility that unilateral jaw biting movements may activate mainly the motor cortex on the ipsilateral hemisphere. However, because of the limitations of temporal resolution, fMRI cannot distinguish among cortical activities before, during, and after biting, given that changes in f-MRI signal intensity reflect the average cortical activity throughout all phases of unilateral jaw biting. On the basis of the results of these experiments, we studied the projection of the afferent inputs from the receptors of the periodontal ligament in humans, as a factor that activates the human cortex.

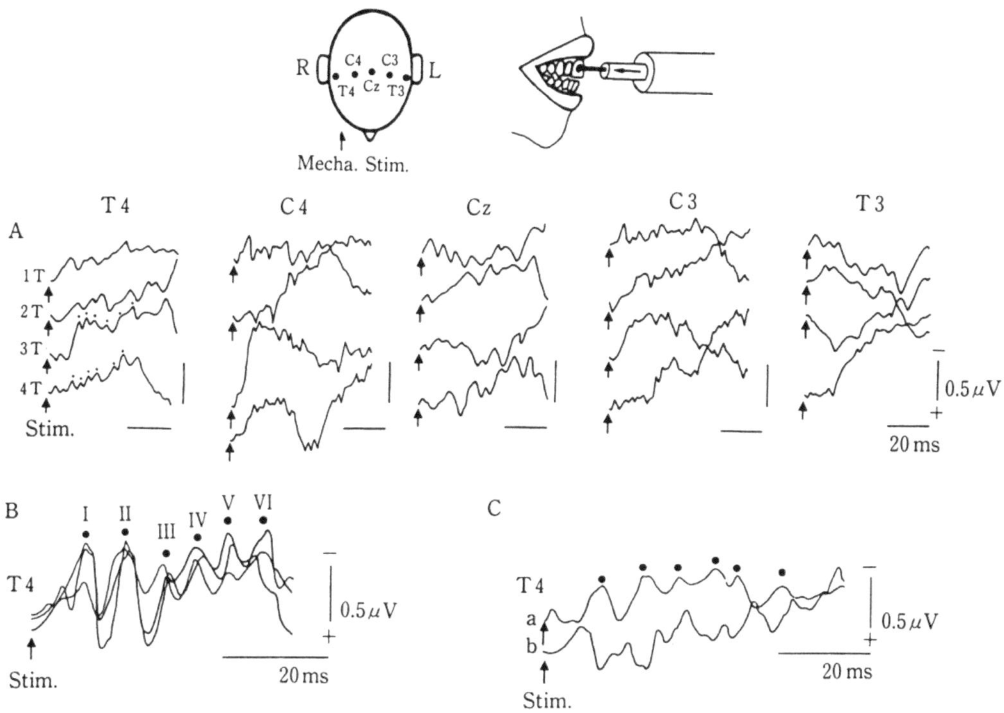

Fig. 8. SEPs and stimulus intensity of right upper first incisor tooth. A: SEPs were recorded from five regions of the human scalp following mechanical stimulation at various intensities: 1T (threshold), 2T, 3T, and 4T. Dots indicate the PM-SEP of T4 with six peaks. T: temporal area. C: central area. Cz: midline-central area. R: right side. L: left side. B: 3 times superimposed PM-SEPs taken at different times for the same subject. I, II, III, IV, V, and VI indicate six waves of the negative component of PM-SEP. C: SEPs before and after induction of local anesthesia of the periodontal ligament. a) PM-SEP before induction of anesthesia. b) Cortical potentials after induction of anesthesia. Each dot indicates six waves of the negative component of PM-SEP. All of these potentials were averaged 100 times.

Tanaka et al. (1991) conducted topographical analysis of periodontal mechanoreceptor-sensory evoked potential induced by mechanical stimulation of a tooth in eight subjects. Sensory evoked potentials (PM-SEPs) were recorded from various regions of the scalp by the mechanical stimulation of a normal tooth (Fig.8). The mechanical stimulation was applied to the right upper first incisor tooth. PM-SEPs were averaged 100 times following the mechanical stimulation of the tooth that produced six waves of SEP at the ipsilateral temporal area (T4) but did not evoke any potential from the other regions. All the six components were abolished after the induction of local anesthesia of the periodontal ligament. They concluded that the six waves of PM-SEP were evoked by the mechanical stimulation of the tooth, suggesting that the sensory cortex receives afferent impulses from the periodontal mechanoreceptors on the ipsilateral side in humans. These findings suggest the possibility that a sensory area on the unilateral hemisphere is responsible for the jaw movements on the ipsilateral side in humans. It is noteworthy that studies using the combination of ERPs and fMRI show great promise in helping researchers to more comprehensively understand the neural basis of behavior, including motor and sensory functions in the maxillofacial regions.

4.3 Overview of CNV

When a human subject is instructed to make a movement in response to the second of two successive stimuli, a slow cortical negative potential appears on the scalp prior to the movement (Walter et al., 1964). A schema of the CNV waveform is shown in Fig. 9.

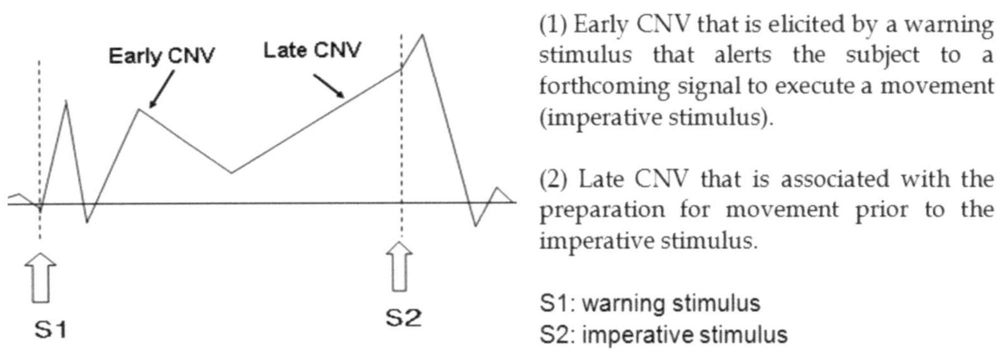

Fig. 9. Schema of CNV waveform.

This potential has been called CNV and is considered to consist of two main components related to the functions of the brain (Rohrbaugh et al., 1976). The first component is an early wave that is elicited by a warning stimulus that alerts the subject to a forthcoming signal to execute a movement (imperative stimulus). The second component is a late wave that is associated with the preparation for movement prior to the imperative stimulus. There are many experimental reports on the CNVs in relation to body movements (Brunia & Vingerhoets, 1981; Rebert & Lowe, 1984; Nakajima et al., 1994; Ulrich et al., 1998).
Previously, CNVs were believed to be one of the MRCPs for the planning or execution of externally paced movements. Recently, however, late CNVs can be detected during some operation in the domain of mental preparation, that is, expectancy and the anticipation for

the imperative stimulus. Oishi and Mochizuki (1998) demonstrated that the amplitude of CNV significantly correlates with blood flow only within the frontal cortex. In addition, subdural recordings of epilepsy patients revealed that BP and CNV are commonly generated from MI and SMA, but that the late component of CNV is also generated from the prefrontal association cortices (Ikeda et al., 1996). Therefore, at present, CNV is considered to reflect activities of the prefrontal cortex associated with cognitive functions (Fuster, 1984; Bares et al., 2007). Hamano et al. (1997) reported the difference between CNVs and BPs recorded from subdural electrodes implanted in patients with intractable epilepsy.

According to their reports, BPs were recorded from the primary motor area (MI), the primary sensory area (SI), and the supplementary sensorimotor area (SSMA). On the other hand, CNVs showed a patchy distribution in the prefrontal area and SSMA for the early component and in the prefrontal area, MI, SI, temporal area, occipital area and SSMA for the late component. These findings suggest that the CNV recorded from the scalp is the summation of multiple cortical potentials that have different origins and different functions. The cortical distribution of late CNV was different from that of BPs. Moreover, clinical neurophysiological studies have proved the diagnostic importance of CNV and MRCP in subcortical generation mechanisms, although both of them commonly share at least some cortical generators, indicating the clinical criteria that late CNV and MRCP are generated from the basal ganglia and cerebellar efferent system, respectively (Ikeda et al., 1994; Ikeda et al.,1996). There is a functional difference between CNV and MRCP in cognitive processes in the beginning of a movement.

4.4 Features of CNV associated with swallowing

There are many research reports on the cortical potentials associated with volitional swallowing. Huckabee et al. (2003) reported that the MRCP associated with volitional swallowing is characterized by a slower slope rising than that obtained during the finger movement. They also explained that this phenomenon is due to a marked absence of late components 500 ms prior to the movement onset, suggesting the close relationship between SMA and brainstem CPG for oral pharyngeal swallowing in neural tracts. Thus, the characteristic of the MRCP associated with volitional swallowing may be explained in terms of the absence of NS'. Satow et al. (2004) also proved by epicortical recording of MRCPs in the patients with epilepsy that the cerebral cortex does not play a significant role in postmovement processing of swallowing.

Dysphagia is characterized by difficulty in swallowing (Bulat & Orlando, 2005). This symptom is common in neurogenic diseases such as stroke, dementia, Parkinson's disease, multiple sclerosis and muscular dystrophy, and often causes aspiration pneumonia. Recent studies have revealed that rehabilitation training induces reorganization of motor areas in the cortex of the patients with stroke (Allred & Jones, 2008; Raboyeau et al., 2008). This reorganization is believed to be due to the plasticity of the human brain. In this rehabilitation technique, the patient holds his/her breath, swallows, and then releases the air by coughing. During rehabilitation, patients are often instructed to initiate an action such as swallowing in response to a cue from a speech therapist (command swallowing). However, the differences in the cognitive functions of the brain between command swallowing and volitional swallowing remain unclarified. Therefore, we investigated the waveforms of the CNVs in the reaction-time swallowing task, to clarify the difference in cortical activity between volitional and command swallowing (Nonaka et al., 2009). Previously, we compared the waveforms of CNV associated with the command swallowing task with those of MRCP associated with the volitional swallowing task in healthy adults to elucidate the effects of human swallowing training on brain activities preceding the onset of swallowing.

In this study, the subjects were instructed to swallow their saliva as quickly as possible in response to a sound signal 4 s after the onset of a self-paced breath holding in the command swallowing task or to swallow their saliva while holding their breath for 4 s in the volitional swallowing task.

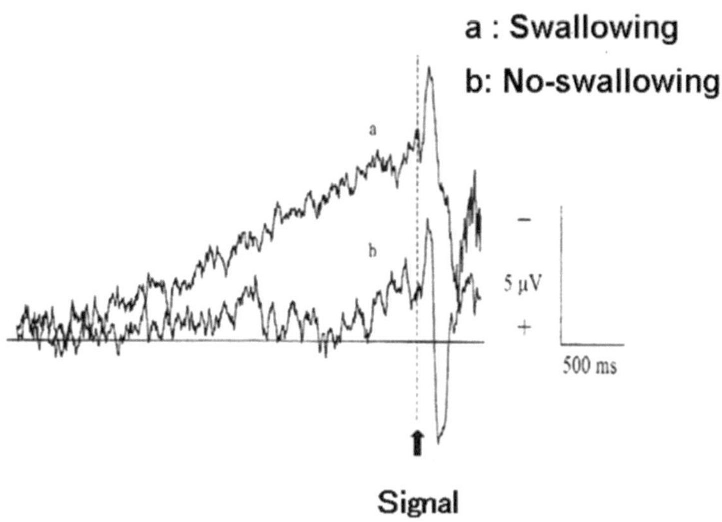

Fig. 10. CNV waveforms obtained during swallowing and no-swallowing task.

Figure 10 shows a comparison between the cortical potentials in the command swallowing task and the no-swallowing (no-motor task) task in the same subject. In the no-swallowing task, a subject was instructed to not swallow his/her saliva in response to the sound signal 4 s after the onset of a self-paced breath holding. The amplitude of CNV was larger in the command swallowing task than in the no-swallowing task. Likewise, the amplitude of CNV tends to increase depending on the intent of swallowing in the subjects. Figure 11 and 12 show a comparison between CNV and MRCP waveforms obtained during both volitional and command swallowing tasks. The amplitudes of CNV recorded at five scalp locations during the command swallowing task were significantly larger than the peak amplitudes of MRCPs during the volitional swallowing task. The findings suggest the possibility that nonsensory/motor regions are activated during the command swallowing task. Considering that the subjects were instructed to not swallow their saliva until the presentation of the signal in this experiment, the generation of CNVs obtained during the command swallowing task in our study may be related to activities of the prefrontal cortex associated with the cognitive functions of attention, memory, and decision. We concluded that CNV is an appropriate index for assessing cognitive functions during the command swallowing.

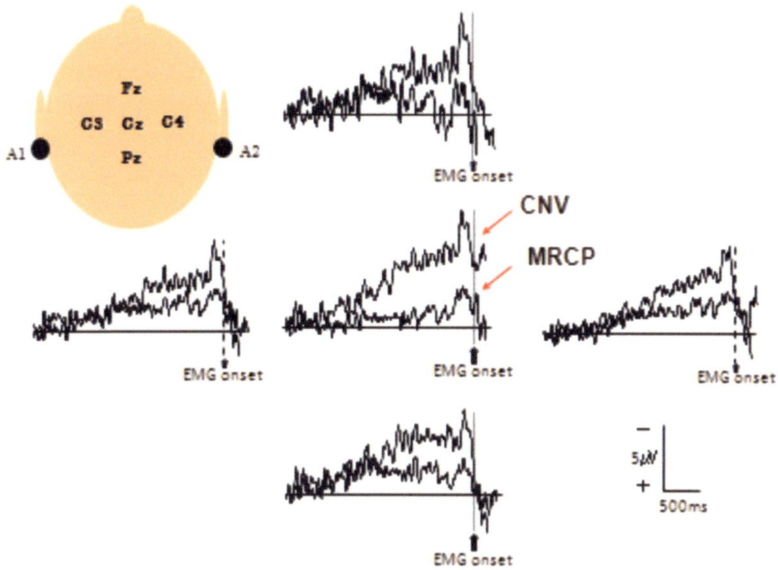

Fig. 11. Comparison between CNV and MRCP waveforms in 10 subjects.
CNV, contingent negative variation; MRCP: Movement-Related Cortical Potentials. (From Nonaka et al., 2009)

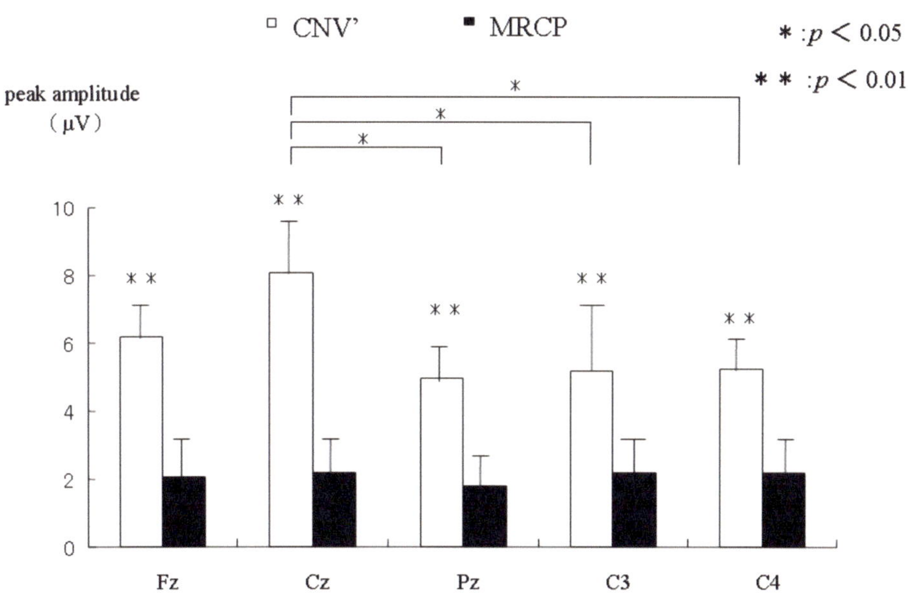

Fig. 12. Mean peak amplitudes of CNV and MRCP at five electrode sites for both swallowing tasks in all subjects. CNVs were significantly larger than MRCPs at five electrode sites and were also significantly smaller at Pz, C3, and C4 than at Cz.
** CNV>MRCP, p<0.01; * CNV smaller than CZ, p<0.05.

5. Wavelet transform analysis for ERPs associated with jaw motor function

Neuroscience is the integrated region of many academic fields, its development contributes to the advance of various science technologies. In particular, the industrial application of neuroscience is expected not only in the medical field but also in many other fields.

A brain–machine interface (BMI) is a direct communication pathway between the brain and an external device. BMIs are developed at assisting, augmenting or repairing human cognitive or sensory-motor functions. For example, BMI provides a new communication pathway for patients with neurological disorders that left them unable to make make voluntary muscle contraction. A potential BMI application is that patients may control a neuro-prosthetic robot directly from their brain so that they can achieve virtual interaction with their environment.

Recently, EEGs have been the most studied potential non-invasive interface, mainly owing to its fine temporal resolution, ease of use, portability and low set-up cost (Akin, 2002; Graimann, 2004; Wei-Yen & Yung-Nien, 2009).

MRCP and CNV are ERPs that reflect human psychological activities, such as the intention and motivation of movement. If MRCP and CNV components can be directly extracted from original brain waves in real time without averaging their components in original brain waves, such a technique will become a new means of information communication for man-machine interfaces. Similarly to the Fourier transform, the wavelet transform is a technique of signal separation.

As a major difference between them, the Fourier transform represents a target signal with an infinite series of sine waves, whereas the wavelet transform represents a target signal with temporally localized waves (wavelets). In other words, the Fourier transform enables the detection of the degree of similarity of a target signal to sine waves, whereas the wavelet transform enables the detection of that of a target signal to wavelets. Compared with the Fourier transform, the wavelet transform has an inferior frequency resolution but a superior temporal resolution. Figure 13 shows a Mexican hat wavelet and a Daubechies wavelet (N=2).

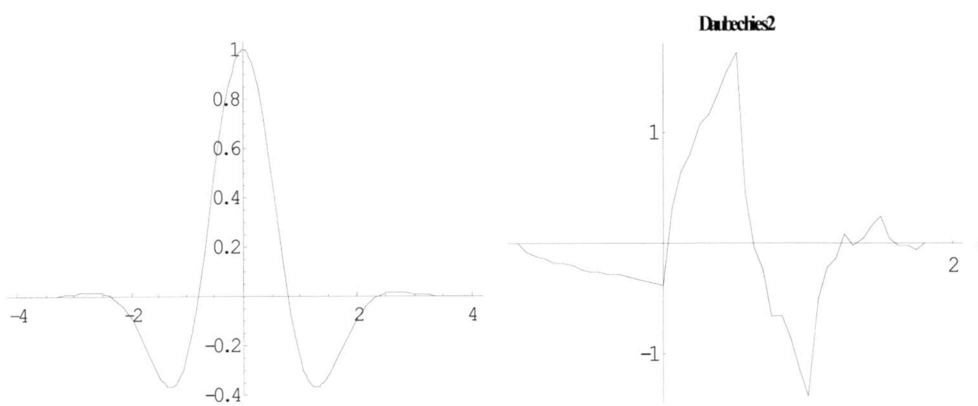

Mexican hat wavelet　　Daubechies wavelet(N=2)

Fig. 13. Examples of wavelet.

In this section, we focus on a case in which the components of brain potentials are extracted using the temporal localization properties and frequency range of the wavelet transform as a means of detecting MRCP and CNV waveforms. In this case, using the wavelet transform, electromyogram components are eliminated from CNV waveforms obtained by measuring the reaction time during a jaw-opening motor task.

Figure 14 (a) shows a waveform obtained simply by averaging brain waves during a jaw-opening movement using S1 as a reference (20 trials). In the figure, CNV is observed in the vertex region (Cz), where the CNV amplitude is maximum.

Although a moderate negative gradient likely to be attributable to CNV is clearly observed between S1 and S2, it is confirmed that noise components caused by the myopotential are mixed in the waveform.

When a discrete wavelet transform is applied to the above waveform obtained by averaging, the waveform can be decomposed into individual wavelets from high- to low-frequency components.

In addition, the original waveform obtained by averaging can be reconstructed by applying the inverse wavelet transform to all the decomposed components. When the amplitudes of particular components are assumed to be zero in this reconstruction, a waveform from which these components are eliminated can be obtained. Using this technique, we reconstructed a signal using particular components alone, compared its waveform with the original waveform obtained by averaging, and eliminated components that are not related to CNV.

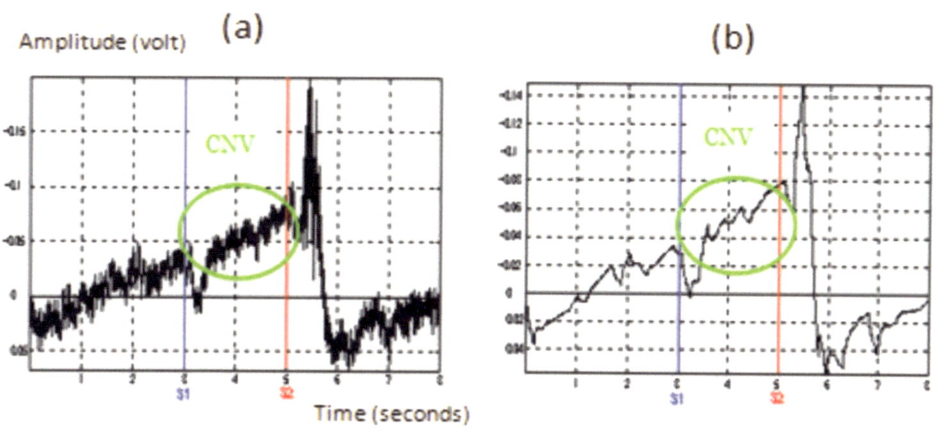

Fig. 14. Wavelet analysis of CNV during jaw-opening movement.
(a) waveform obtained by averaging. (b) waveform obtained after wavelet analysis.

Figure 14 shows a waveform reconstructed after eliminating the first to eighth high-frequency components and using only the ninth and subsequent high-frequency components (sampling frequency = 1.5 kHz). Considering real-time analysis, a fast wavelet transform algorithm developed by Mallat was used for decomposition and reconstruction employing a Daubechies wavelet (N=2). It is confirmed from Fig. 2(b) that noise components were eliminated whereas CNV components were maintained. This finding indicates that CNV is characterized by the ninth and subsequent high-frequency wavelet components. At the same time, we also confirmed a technique of separating artifact components due to, for example, myopotential and eye movements, which disturb the detection of waveforms by machines; such a technique may lead to practical applications of MRCP and CNV to man-machine interfaces.

6. Frequency changes of jaw muscle activity during reaction to a warning signal in the reaction time task

In this chapter, we discuss how MRCPs and CNVs reflect the brain activities corresponding to the onset of oral and facial movements. Actually, they can provide useful information on the control system for these movements. On the other hand, surface electromyography (EMG) is commonly used as a technique for the recording of skeletal muscle activity during a movement. Presently, EMG data are believed to provide information on the muscle contraction only. Recently, however, it has been clarified that the frequency changes of the muscle activity reflect motor preparation in the central nervous system. This changing can be also detected in jaw muscle EMGs.

6.1 Overview of EMG frequency changes preceding rapid movements

Rhythmic slow waves with a periodicity of 20-30 ms in elector spinal muscle EMG appear preceding a rapid voluntary trunk movement in humans (Tanii, 1984; Tanii & Kinugasa, 1986). These waves are is followed often by a silent period. This is similarly observed in the EMG recording in the reaction-time trunk movement task (Tanii at al., 1985). The surface EMG of the elector spinal muscle changes to rhythmic slow waves after a warning signal in this task. The power spectrum of surface EMG frequencies after the warning stimulus shifts to lower in the task, owing to the rhythmic slower waves, in association with motor preparation to perform the movement. The slowing of waves in surface EMG during the preparatory period is believed to reflect the modification of firing rates of individual motor units during the phasic contraction in the movement. On the other hand, motor imagery (MI) is the mental representation of a specific action without any corresponding motor output. Recently, Lebon et al. (2008) demonstrated that the EMG frequency was significantly higher during MI, than under the control condition (during resting). Their findings also suggest that a specific motor program requires recruitment of motor units during motor imagery.

6.2 Frequency changes in jaw muscle EMG during reaction to warning signal

Frequency changes in the masseter muscle EMG were examined in eight healthy subjects during the reaction time in a unilateral jaw-biting paradigm (Nakajima, 1995).

Each subject sat comfortably in an armchair and was presented with a visual warning stimulus (S1) followed 2 s later by a visual imperative stimulus (S2).

He/she was instructed to perform the jaw-biting movement upon the presentation of S2, with a small piece of wood held between the first upper and lower molars on the right side. Subjects were also instructed to make six biting movements, each separated by a 60-s rest period. Bipolar surface EMGs were recorded from the masseter muscle and digastric muscles on the right side as the agonist and antagonist, respectively.

The EMG signals from 1.0 s before S1 to 3.0 s after S1 were digitized. The samples were analyzed by fast Fourier transform (FFT) for each 1-s period. The analysis interval was divided into following three periods:

- The period 0-1 s before presentation of S1 (prestimulus period).
- The period 0-1 s after presentation of S1 (early poststimulus period).
- The period 1-2 s after presentation of S1 (late poststimulus period).

In five subjects, masseter EMG power spectra significantly shifted to lower frequencies in both the early and the late poststimulus period periods than those in the prestimulus period period (Wilcoxon signed rank test, $p<0.05$). In two subjects, the EMG power spectra significantly shifted to lower frequencies in either the early or the late post-stimulus period than those in the pre-stimulus period ($p<0.05$). In one subject, no change was observed ($p>0.05$).

Masseter muscle EMG power spectra shifts to lower frequencies when biting force increases. This shift is well explained in terms of the recruitment of larger motor units at higher bite force. If this is so, our findings suggest that the slowing of waves in the EMG after the first signal is related to the recruitment of larger motor units. Considering the findings of this other previous study, the frequency changes of jaw muscle activity may indicate a state of readiness in the central nervous system for rapid and strong biting movements after the second stimulus.

In conclusion, these findings suggest the possibility of obtaining useful information on higher brain activities from the data of EMG. In the future, the study using the combination of ERP and EMG recordings will show great promise in helping scientists to more comprehensively understand the neural basis of motor functions in the maxillofacial region.

7. Conclusion

We concluded that MRCPs and CNVs are reliable Indicator the study of which may lead to the understanding of the oral and facial motor functions in humans. These cortical potentials have the advantage of temporal resolution for the detection of cortical activities. They are likely to be a very useful tool for elucidating the mechanism underlying the central processing of motor functions, as compared with PET and fMRI. Therefore, in further studies, we should clarify the significance of these cortical potentials in patients with oral motor dysfunctions.

8. Acknowledgment

We would like to thank Dr. Matsumoto Yuji for help in developing the methods of wavelet transform analysis of the ERP associated with jaw movement.

Financial support from a Grant from the Ministry of Education, Culture, Sports, Science and Technology to promote multi-disciplinary research projects is gratefully acknowledged.

This work was supported in part by Sato Fund, Nihon University (2009, 2011) and Grand from Dental Research Center, Nihon University (2010).

9. References

Akin M. (2002). Comparison of wavelet transform and FFT methods in the Analysis of EEG signal. Journal of Medical Systems, Vol. 26, No. 3, (June 2002), pp. 241-247, ISSN 0148-5598

Allred, R. P. & Jones, T. A. (2008). Sensorimotor reorganization by proprioceptive training in musician's dystonia and writer's cramp. Neurology , Vol. 70, No.4, (January 2008), pp. 304-315, ISSN 0028-3878

Andre´, J. (2001). Brain Stem Control of Swallowing: Neuronal Network and Cellular Mechanisms. Physiological Reviews, Vol. 81, No. 2, (April 2001), pp. 929-969, ISSN 0031-9333

Bares, M.; Nestrasil, I. & Rektor, I. (2007). The effect of response type (motor output versus mental counting) on the intracerebral distribution of the slow cortical potentials in an externally cued (CNV) paradigm. Brain Research Bulletin, Vol. 71, No. 4, (January 2007), pp. 428-435, ISSN 0361-9230

Bromm, B. & Chen, A. C. (1995). Brain electrical source analysis of laser evoked potentials in response to painful trigeminal nerve stimulation. Electroencephalography and Clinical Neurophysiology, Vol. 95, No.1, (July 1995), pp. 14-26,ISSN 0013-4694

Brunia, C.H. & Vingerhoets, A. J. (1981). Opposite hemisphere differences in movement related potentials preceding foot and finger flexions. Biological Psychology, Vol. 13, (December 1981), pp. 261-269, ISSN 0301-0511

Bulat, R.S. & Orlando, R.C. (2005). Oropharyngeal Dysphagia. Current Treatment Options in Gastroenterology, Vol. 8, No.4, (August 2005), pp. 269-274, ISSN 1092-8472

Bushnell, M. C.; Duncan, G. H.; Dubner, R.; Jones, R. L. & Maixner, W. (1985). Attentional influences on noxious and innocuous cutaneous heat detection in humans and monkeys. Journal of Neuroscience, Vol. 5, No. 5, (May 1985), pp. 1103-1110, ISSN 0270-6474

Desmedt, J. E.; Tomberg, C.; Noel, P. & Ozaki, I. (1990). Beware of the average reference in brain mapping. Electroencephalography Clinical Neurophysiology, Vol. 41, Suppl . pp. 22–27, ISSN 0013-4694

Dowman, R. (2004). The pain-evoked P2 is not a P3a event-related potential. Brain Topography, Vol. 17, No. 1, (Fall 2004), pp. 3-12, ISSN 0896-0267

Dowman, R.; Darcey, T.; Barkan, H.; Thadani, V. & Roberts, D. (2007). Human intracranially-recorded cortical responses evoked by painful electrical stimulation of the sural nerve. Neuroimage, Vol. 34, No.2, (January 2007), pp. 743-763, ISSN 1053-8119

Dziewas, R.; Soros, P.; Ishii, R.; Chau, W.; Henningsen, H.; Ringelstein, E.B.; Knecht, S. & Pantev, C.(2003). Neuroimaging evidence for cortical involvement in the preparation and in the act of swallowing. Neuroimage, Vol. 20, No. 1, (September 2003), pp.135-144, ISSN 1053-8119

Fuster, J. M. (1984). Behavioural electrophysiology of the prefrontal cortex. Trends Neurosci ence; Vol. 7, No.11, pp. 408-414, ISSN 0166-2236

Graimann, B.; Huggins, J.E.; Levine, S.P. & Pfurtscheller, G. (2004). Toward a direct brain interface based on human subdural recordings and wavelet-packet analysis. IEEE Transactions on Bio-medical Engineering, Vol.51, No.6, (June 2004), pp.954-62, ISSN 0018-9294

Gratton, G.; Bosco, C. M.; Kramer, A. F.; Coles, M.G.; Wickens, C.D. & Donchin, E. (1990). Event-related brain potentials as indices of information extraction and response priming. Electroencephalography Clinical Neurophysiology, Vol. 75, No.5, (May 1990) pp.419-432, ISSN 0013-4694

Hamano, T. ; Lüders, H.O. ; Ikeda, A. ; Collura, T.F. ; Comair, Y.G. & Shibasaki, H. (1997). The cortical generators of the contingent negative variation in humans: a study with subdural electrodes, Electroencephalography Clinical Neurophysiology, Vol. 104, No. 3, (May 1997), pp. 257-268, ISNN 1388-2457

Hamdy, S.; Mikulis, D. J.; Crawley, A.; Xue, S.; Lau, H.; Henry, S. & Diamant, N. E. (1999). Cortical activation during human volitional swallowing: an event-related fMRI study. American Journal of Physiology-Gastrointestinal and Liver Physiology, Vol. 277, No. 1, (July 1999), pp. 219–225, ISSN 0193-1857

Hamdy, S.; Rothwell, J. C.; Aziz, Q. & Thompson, D. G. (2000). Organization and reorganization of human swallowing motor cortex: implications for recovery after stroke. Clinical Science , Vol. 99, No.2, (August 2000), pp.151–157, ISSN 0143-5221

Huckabee, M. L.; Deecke, L.; Cannito, M.P.; Gould, H. J. & Mayr, W. (2003). Cortical control mechanisms in volitional swallowing: the Bereitschaftspotential. Brain Topography, (Fall 2003), Vol.16, No. 1, pp. 3-17,ISNN 0896-0267

Iannetti, G. D.; Truini, A.; Romaniello, A.; Galeotti, F.; Rizzo, C.; Manfredi, M. & Cruccu, G. (1990). Evidence of a specific spinal pathway for the sense of warmth in humans. Journal of Neurophysiology, Vol. 75, No.5, (May 1990), 419-432, ISSN 0013-4694

Ikeda, A.; Luders, H.O.; Burgess, R. C. & Shibasaki, H. (1992). Movement-related potentials recorded from supplementary motor area and primary motor area. Role of supplementary motor area in voluntary movements. Brain, Vol. 115, No. Pt4, (August 1992), pp. 1017-1043, ISSN 0006-8993

Ikeda, A.; Shibasaki, H.; Nagamine, T.; Terada, K.; Kaji, R.; Fukuyama, H. & Kimura, J. (1994). Dissociation between contingent negative variation and Bereitschaftspotential in a patient with cerebellar efferent lesion. Electroencephalogrphy Clinical Neurophysiology, Vol. 90, No. 5, (May 1994), pp. 359-364, ISSN 0013-4694

Ikeda, A.; Luders, H. O.; Collura, T.F.; Burgess, R.C.; Morris, H. H.; Hamano, T. & Shibasaki, H. (1996). Subdural potentials at orbitofrontal and mesial prefrontal areas accompanying anticipation and decision making in humans: a comparison with Bereitschaftspotentials. Electroencephalography Clinical Neurophysiol ogy,Vol. 98, No. 3, (March 1996), pp. 206-212, ISSN 0013-4694

Kakigi , R.; Watanabe, S. & Yamasaki, H. (2000). Pain-related somatosensory evoked potentials. Journal of Clinical Neurophysiology, Vol. 17, No.3, (May 2000), pp.295-308, ISSN 0736-0258

Kern, M.K.; Jaradeh, S.; Arndorfer, R.C. & Shaker, R. (2001). Cerebral cortical representation of reflexive and volitional swallowing in humans. American Journal of Physiology-Gastrointestinal and Liver Physiology, Vol. 280, No. 3, (March 2001), pp. 354-360, ISSN 0193-1857

Kornhuber, H. H., & Deecke, L. (1964). Hirnpotentiala¨nderungen beim Menschen vor und nach Willkurbewegungen, dargestellt mit Magnetband-Speicherung und Ruckwartsanalyse. Pflügers Archiv, Vol. 281, pp. 52. ISSN 0031-6768

Lorenz, J. & Garcia-Larrea, L. (2003). Contribution of attentional and cognitive factors to laser evoked brain potentials. Clinical neurophysiology, Vol. 33, No. 6, (December 2003), 293-301, ISSN 0987-7053

Lebon, F. ; Rouffet, D ; Collet, C. & Guillot, A. (2008). Modulation of EMG power spectrum frequency during motor imagery. Neuroscience Letters, Vol. 435, No.3, (April 2008), 181-185, ISSN 0304-3940

Lund, J P. & Kolta, A. (2006). Generation of the Central masticatory pattern and its modification by sensory feedback. Dysphagia, Vol. 21. No. 3, (July 2006), pp.167-74, ISSN 0179-051X

Michel, C. M.; Murray, M.M.; Lantz, G.; Gonzalez, S.; Spinelli, L. & Gravede, P. R. (2004). EEG source imaging. Clinical Neurophysiology, Vol. 115, No. 10, (October 2004), pp. 2195–2222, ISSN 1388-2457

Miltner, W. H. & Weiss, T. (1998) Brain electrical correlates of pain processing. Zeitschrift für Rheumatologie, Vol. 57, Suppl. 2, pp. 14-18, ISSN 0340-1855

Morimoto, T.; Hamada, T. & Kawamura, Y. (1983). Alteration in directional specificity of interdental dimension discrimination with the degree of mouth opening. Journal of Oral Rehabilitation, Vol. 10, No. 4, (July 1983), pp.335-342, ISSN 0305-182X

Momose, T.; Nishikawa, J.; Watanabe, T.; Sasaki, Y.; Senda, M.; Kubota, K.; Sato, Y.; Funakoshi, M. & Minakuchi, S. (1997). Effect of mastication on regional cerebral blood flow in humans examined by positron-emission tomography with 15O labeled water and magnetic resonance imaging. Archives of Oral Biology, Vol. 42, No.1, (January 1997), pp. 57-61, ISSN 0003-9969

Nakajima, I.; Tanaka, Y.; Uchida, A.; Sakai, T.; Akasaka, M.; Mori, A. & Sumino, R. (1991). Cortical potentials associated with voluntary biting movement in humans. Neuroscience Research, Vol.10, No.4, (May 1991), pp. 285-289, ISSN 0168-0102

Nakajima, I.; Miyauchi, M.; Minowa, K.; Akasaka, M. & Uchida, A. (1994) Contingent negative variations associated with jaw opening in humans. Somatosensory and motor research, Vol.11, No.2, (March 1994), pp. 149-152, ISSN 0899-0220

Nakajima I. (1995). Fast Fourier transform analysis of the masseter muscle EMG during reaction to a warning signal. Electromyography and Clinical Neurophysiology, Vol. 35, No. 5, (August-September 1995), pp. 281-284, ISSN 0301-150X

Nakamura, Y. & Katakura, N. (1995). Generation of masticatory rhythm in the brainstem. Neuroscience Research, Vol. 23. No.1, (August 1995), pp. 1–19, ISSN 0168-0102

Nonaka, T.; Yoshida, M.; Yamaguchi, T.; Uchida, A.; Ohba, H.; Oka, S. & Nakajima I. (2009). Contingent negative variations associated with command swallowing in humans. Clinical Neurophysiology, Vol.120, No.10, (October 2009), pp. 1845-1851, ISSN 1388-2457

Oishi, M. & Mochizuki, Y. (1998). Correlation between the contingent negative variation and regional cerebral blood flow. Clinical Electroencephalograpgy, Vol. 29, No.3, (July 1998), pp. 124-127, ISSN 0009-9155

Oka, S.; Chapman, C.R.; Kim, B.; Nakajima, I.; Shimizu, O. & Oi, Y. (2007). Pupil dilation response to noxious stimulation: effect of varying nitrous oxide concentration. Clinical Neurophysiology, Vol. 118, No.9, (September 2007), pp. 2016-2024, ISSN 1388-2457

Oka, S.; Chapman, C.R.; Kim, B.; Shimizu, O.; Noma N.; Takeichi, O.; Imamura, Y. & Oi, Y. (2010). Predictability of painful stimulation modulates subjective and physiological responses. The Journal of Pain, Vol. 11, No. 3, (March 2010), pp. 239-246, ISSN 1526-5900

Onozuka, M.; Fujita, M. ; Watanabe, K.; Hirano, Y. ; Niwa, M.; Nishiyama, K. & Saito, S. (2002). Mapping brain region activity during chewing: a functional magnetic resonance imaging study. Journal of Dental Research, Vol. 81, No.11, (November 2002), pp.743-746, ISSN 0022-0345

Oono, Y.; Fujii, K.; Motohashi, K. & Umino, M. (2008). Diffuse noxious inhibitory controls triggered by heterotopic CO_2 laser conditioning stimulation decreased the SEP amplitudes induced by electrical tooth stimulation with different intensity at an equally inhibitory rate. Pain, Vol. 136, No.3, (June 2008), pp. 356-365, ISSN 0304-3959

Raboyeau, G.; De Boissezon, X.; Marie, N.; Balduyck, S.; Puel, M.; Bézy, C.; Démonet, J. F. & Cardebat, D. (2008). Translating principles of neural plasticity into research on speech motor control recovery and rehabilitation. Journal of Speech, Language, and Hearing Research, (February 2008), Vol. 51, No. 1, pp. 240-258, ISSN 1092-4388

Rebert, C. S. & Lowe, R. C. (1984). Hemispheric lateralization of event-related potentials in a cued reaction-time task. Biological psychology, Vol. 19, No.3, (December 1984), pp. 189-204, ISSN 0301-0511

Rohrbaugh, J. W.; Syndulko, K, & Lindsley, D.B. (1976). Brain wave components of the contingent negative variation in humans. Science, Vol. 191, No. 4231, (March 1976), pp.1055-1057. ISSN:0036-8075

Sasaki, K.; Gemba, H. & Hashimoto, S. (1981). Premovement slow cortical potentials on self-paced hand movements and thalamocortical and corticocortical responses in the monkey. Experimental Neurology, Vol. 72, No.1, (April 1981), pp. 41-50, ISSN 0014-4886

Satow, T.; Ikeda, A.; Yamamoto, J.; Begum, T.; Thuy, D. H. D.; Matsuhashi, M.; Mima, T.; Nagamine, T. ; Baba, K. ; Mihara, T. ; Inoue, Y. ; Miyamoto, S. ; Hashimoto, N. & Shibasaki, H. (2004). Role of primary sensorimotor cortex and supplementary motor area in volitional swallowing: a movement-related cortical potential study. American journal of physiology. Gastrointestinal and Liver Physiology, Vol. 287, No.2, (August 2004), pp. 459-470. ISSN 0193-1857

Shibasaki, H.; Barret, G. & Halliday, E. (1980). Components of the movement-related cortical potential and their scalp topography. Electroencephalography Clinical Neurophysiology, Vol. 49, No.3-4, (August 1980), pp.213-226, ISSN 0013-4694

Shibasaki, H. (2008). Human brain mapping: Hemodynamic response and electrophysiology. Clinical Neurophysiology, Vol. 119, No. 4, (April 2008), pp. 731-743. ISSN 1388-2457

Tanaka, Y.; Nakajima, I.; Uchida, A.; Akasaka, M.; Mori, A. & Sumino, R. (1991). Somatosensory evoked potentials by mechanical stimulation of tooth in humans. Brain and Nerve, Vol. 43, No.2, (February 1991), pp. 163-168, ISSN 1881-6096 (Abstract in English)

Tanii, K. (1984). Occurrence of a rhythmic slower wave in EMG prior to a rapid voluntary movement. Electroencephalography and clinical neurophysiology, Vol. 57, No. 5, (May 1984), pp. 435 -440, ISSN 0013-4694

Tanii, K.; Sadoyama, T., & Sameshima, M. (1985). Power spectralanalysis of the surface electromyogram before and after a warning signal in a reaction movement. Electroencephalography and clinical neurophysiology, Vol. 60, No.6, (June 1985), pp.532-538, ISSN 0013-4694

Tanii, K. & Kinugasa, T. (1986). Changes in activity of motor units preceding a rapid voluntary movement. Electroencephalography and Clinical Neurophysiology, Vol. 63, No. 2, (February 1986), pp. 188-191. ISSN 0013-4694

Tarkka, I. M. & Treede, R. D. (1993). Equivalent electrical source analysis of pain-related somatosensory evoked potentials elicited by a CO_2 laser. Journal of Clinical Neurophysiology, Vol. 10, No.4, (October 1993), pp. 513-519, ISSN 0736-0258

Toogood, J. A.; Barr, A. M.; Stevens, T. K.; Gati, J.S.; Menon, R.S. & Martin, R. E. (2005). Discrete functional contributions of cerebral cortical foci in voluntary swallowing: a functional magnetic resonance imaging (fMRI) "Go, No-Go" study. Experimental Brain Research, Vol. 161, No.1, (February 2005), pp. 81-90, ISSN 0014-4819

Ulrich, R.; Leuthold, H. & Sommer, W. (1998). Motor programming of response force and movement direction. Psychophysiology, Vol. 35, No.6, (November 1998), pp. 721-728. ISSN 0048-5772

Walter, W.G.; Cooper, R,; Aldridge, V.J.; McCallum, W.C. & Winter, A.L. (1964). Contingent negative variation: An electric sign of sensorimotor association and expectancy in the human brain. Nature, Vol. 203 (July 1964), pp. 380-384, ISSN 0028-0836

Watanabe, Y.; Abe, S.; Ishikawa, T.; Yamada Y. & Yamane, G. Y.(2004). Cortical regulation during the early stage of initiation of voluntary swallowing in humans. Dysphagia, Vol. 19, No.2, (Spring 2004), pp.100-108, ISSN 0179-051X

Wei-Yen, H. & Yung-Nien, S. (2009) EEG-based motor imagery analysis using weighted wavelet transform features. Journal of Neuroscience Methods, Vol.30, No.2, (January 2009), pp. 310–318, ISSN 0165-0270

Yamasaki, H.; Kakigi, R. ; Watanabe, S. & Hoshiyama M. (2000). Effects of distraction on pain-related somatosensory evoked magnetic fields and potentials following painful electrical stimulation. Brain Research. Cognitive Brain Research, Vol. 9, No.2, (March 2000), pp.165-175 ISSN 0926-6410

Yoshida, K.; Kaji, R.; Hamano, T.; Kohara, N.; Kimura, J.; Shibasaki, H. & Iizuka, T. (2000). Cortical potentials associated with voluntary mandibular movements. Journal of Dental Research, Vol. 79, No.7, (July 2000), pp.1514-1518, ISSN 0022-0345